CONTENTS

PEDIATRIC

SECRETS

Fifth Edition

Richard A. Polin, MD
Professor of Pediatrics
Columbia University College of Physicians and Surgeons
Vice Chairman for Clinical and Academic Affairs
Director, Division of Neonatology
Morgan Stanley Children's Hospital of New York, New York

Mark F. Ditmar, MD
Director, AtlantiCare/duPont Pediatric Hospitalist Program
AtlantiCare Regional Medical Center
Atlantic City, New Jersey
Clinical Associate Professor of Pediatrics
Jefferson Medical College
Philadelphia, Pennsylvania

MOSBY

ELSEVIER

1600 John F. Kennedy Blvd.
Ste 1800
Philadelphia, PA 19103-2899

PEDIATRIC SECRETS, FIFTH EDITION   ISBN: 978-0-323-06561-0

NOTICE

Knowledge and best practice in this field are constantly changing. As new research and experience broaden our knowledge, changes in practice, treatment and drug therapy may become necessary or appropriate. Readers are advised to check the most current information provided (i) on procedures featured or (ii) by the manufacturer of each product to be administered, to verify the recommended dose or formula, the method and duration of administration, and contraindications. It is the responsibility of the practitioner, relying on their own experience and knowledge of the patient, to make diagnoses, to determine dosages and the best treatment for each individual patient, and to take all appropriate safety precautions. To the fullest extent of the law, neither the Publisher nor the Editors/Authors assumes any liability for any injury and/or damage to persons or property arising out of or related to any use of the material contained in this book.

Library of Congress Cataloging-in-Publication Data
Pediatric secrets / [edited by] Richard A. Polin, Mark F. Ditmar. – 5th ed.
    p. ; cm. – (Secrets series)
Includes bibliographical references and index.
ISBN 978-0-323-06561-0
    1. Pediatrics–Examinations, questions, etc. 2. Pediatrics. I. Polin, Richard A. (Richard Alan), 1945-
II. Ditmar, Mark F. III. Series: Secrets series.
    [DNLM: 1. Pediatrics–Examination Questions. WS 18.2 P3716 2011]
RJ48.2.P65 2011
618.9200076–dc22

                                                                          2010010434

Acquisitions Editor: James Merritt
Developmental Editor: Andrea Vosburgh
Project Manager: Janaki Srinivasan Kumar

Working together to grow
libraries in developing countries

www.elsevier.com | www.bookaid.org | www.sabre.org

ELSEVIER   BOOK AID International   Sabre Foundation

Printed in Canada
Last digit is the print number: 9   8   7   6   5   4   3   2   1

CONTRIBUTORS

Peter C. Adamson, MD
Professor of Pediatrics and Pharmacology, Department of Pediatrics, University of Pennsylvania School of Medicine; Director, Clinical and Translational Research, The Children's Hospital of Philadelphia, Philadelphia, Pennsylvania

Kwame Anyane-Yeboa, MD
Professor of Clinical Pediatrics, Department of Pediatrics, Columbia University College of Physicians and Surgeons; Attending Pediatrician, Division of Genetics, Department of Pediatrics, Columbia University Medical Center, New York, New York

Richard Aplenc, MD, MSCE
Assistant Professor, Department of Pediatrics, University of Pennsylvania; Assistant Physician, Department of Pediatrics, The Children's Hospital of Philadelphia, Philadelphia, Pennsylvania

Balu H. Athreya, MD
Professor of Pediatrics, Thomas Jefferson University, Philadelphia, Pennsylvania; Division of Rheumatology, Alfred I. DuPont Children's Hospital, Wilmington, Delaware

Bradley A. Becker, MD
Associate Professor, Division of Allergy and Immunology, Department of Pediatrics, Saint Louis University School of Medicine; Co-Director, Asthma Center for Children, Division of Allergy and Immunology, Department of Pediatrics, SSM Cardinal Glennon Children's Medical Center; Division of Allergy and Immunology, Department of Pediatrics and Internal Medicine, Saint Louis University Hospital, St. Louis, Missouri

Joan Bregstein, MD
Assistant Clinical Professor of Pediatrics, Director, Community Outreach, Department of Pediatrics, Division of Pediatric Emergency Medicine, Morgan Stanley Children's Hospital of New York-Presbyterian, New York, New York

Elizabeth Candell Chalom, MD
Assistant Professor, Department of Pediatrics, University of Medicine and Dentistry of New Jersey, Newark, New Jersey; Chief, Pediatric Rheumatology, Department of Pediatrics, Saint Bamabas Medical Center, Livingston, New Jersey

Mark F. Ditmar, MD
Director, AtlantiCare/duPont Pediatric Hospitalist Program, AtlantiCare Regional Medical Center, Atlantic City, New Jersey; Clinical Associate Professor of Pediatrics, Jefferson Medical College, Philadelphia, Pennsylvania

Andrew H. Eichenfield, MD
Chief, Division of Pediatric Rheumatology, Mount Sinai Medical Center, New York, New York; Assistant Clinical Professor of Pediatrics, College of Physicians and Surgeons, Columbia University, New York

Anders Fasth, MD, PhD
Professor, Department of Pediatrics, Institution of Clinical Sciences, University of Gothenburg; Department of Pediatric Immunology, The Queen Silvia Children's Hospital; Director, The Swedish National Cord Blood Bank, Sahlgrenska University Hospital, Gothenburg, Sweden

Mary Pat Gallagher, MD
Assistant Professor of Clinical Pediatrics, Department of Pediatrics, Columbia University College of Physicians and Surgeons; Assistant Attending Physician, Department of Pediatrics, Morgan Stanley Children's Hospital of New York-Presbyterian, New York, New York

Maria C. Garzon, MD
Professor of Clinical Dermatology and Clinical Pediatrics, Columbia University College of Physicians and Surgeons; Director, Department of Pediatric Dermatology, Morgan Stanley Children's Hospital of New York-Presbyterian, New York, New York

Andrew B. Grossman, MD
Clinical Assistant Professor of Pediatrics, Department of Pediatrics, University of Pennsylvania School of Medicine; Attending Physician, Division of Gastroenterology, Hepatology, and Nutrition, The Children's Hospital of Philadelphia, Philadelphia, Pennsylvania

Daniel Esten Hale, MD
Professor of Pediatrics, Department of Pediatrics, University of Texas Health Science Center at San Antonio; Senior Physician, Pediatric Endocrinology and Diabetes, Christus Santa Rosa Children's Hospital; Attending Physician, Children Center at the Texas Diabetes Institute, University Health System, San Antonio, Texas

Constance J. Hayes, MD
Professor of Clinical Pediatrics, Emeritus, Division of Pediatric Cardiology, Department of Pediatrics, Columbia University College of Physicians and Surgeons; Attending Physician, Division of Pediatric Cardiology, Department of Pediatrics, Morgan Stanley Children's Hospital of New York-Presbyterian, New York, New York

Georg A. Holländer, MD
Professor of Molecular Medicine in Paediatrics, Department of Biomedicine, University of Basel; Professor of Molecular Medicine in Paediatrics and Head, Department of Research, The University Children's Hospital of Basel, Basel, Switzerland

Allan J. Hordof, MD
Professor of Clinical Pediatrics, Fellowship Program Director, Division of Pediatric Cardiology, Department of Pediatrics, Columbia University College of Physicians and Surgeons; Senior Attending Physician, Division of Pediatric Cardiology, Department of Pediatrics, Morgan Stanley Children's Hospital of New York-Presbyterian, New York, New York

Kent R. Kelley, MD
Assistant Clinical Professor, University of Chicago Biological Sciences Division, Chief, Pediatric Neurology, Department of Pediatrics, Northshore University Health System, Evanston, Illinois

Chris A. Liacouras, MD
Professor of Pediatric Gastroenterology, University of Pennsylvania School of Medicine; Attending Physician, Division of Gastroenterology, Hepatology, and Nutrition, The Children's Hospital of Philadelphia, Philadelphia, Pennsylvania

Emily G. Lipsitz, MD
Pediatric Hematology-Oncology Fellow, Departments of Hematology and Oncology, The Children's Hospital of Philadelphia, Philadelphia, Pennsylvania

Vivian A. Lombillo, MD, PhD
Attending Physician, Pediatric Dermatology, Pediatric Dermatology Associates, Lake Success, New York

Steven E. McKenzie, MD, PhD
Professor, Departments of Medicine and Pediatrics, Thomas Jefferson University, Philadelphia, Pennsylvania

Kimberly D. Morel, MD
Assistant Professor of Clinical Dermatology and Pediatrics, Department of Dermatology and Pediatrics, Columbia University College of Physicians and Surgeons; Assistant Professor of Clinical Dermatology and Pediatrics, Department of Pediatrics, Morgan Stanley Children's Hospital of New York-Presbyterian, New York, New York

Martin A. Nash, MD
Professor of Clinical Pediatrics, Columbia University College of Physicians and Surgeons; Director of Pediatric Nephrology, Department of Pediatrics, Morgan Stanley Children's Hospital of New York-Presbyterian, New York, New York

Sharon E. Oberfield, MD
Professor of Pediatrics, Columbia University College of Physicians and Surgeons; Director, Pediatric Endocrinology, Morgan Stanley Children's Hospital of New York-Presbyterian, New York, New York

Carlos D. Rosé, MD, CIP
Professor of Pediatrics, Department of Pediatrics, Thomas Jefferson University, Philadelphia, Pennsylvania; Director, Pediatric Rheumatology, Department of Pediatrics, Alfred I. DuPont Children's Hospital, Wilmington, Delaware

Cindy Ganis Roskind, MD
Assistant Clinical Professor of Pediatrics, Division of Pediatric Emergency Medicine, Department of Pediatrics, Columbia University College of Physicians and Surgeons; Division of Pediatric Emergency Medicine, Department of Pediatrics, Morgan Stanley Children's Hospital of New York-Presbyterian, New York, New York

Philip Roth, MD, PhD
Director of Neonatology, Chairman, Department of Pediatrics, Staten Island University Hospital, Staten Island, New York; Associate Professor of Pediatrics, Department of Pediatrics, State University of New York - Downstate Medical Center, Brooklyn, New York

Benjamin D. Roye, MD, MPH
Assistant Professor, Department of Orthopaedic Surgery, Mount Sinai School of Medicine; Attending Physician, Department of Pediatric Orthopaedic Surgery, Morgan Stanley Children's Hospital of New York-Presbyterian, Columbia Medical Center; Attending Physician, Department of Orthopaedic Surgery, Beth Israel Medical Center, New York, New York

Robert L. Seigle, MD
Assistant Professor of Clinical Pediatrics, Division of Pediatric Nephrology, Department of Pediatrics, Columbia University College of Physicians and Surgeons; Assistant Attending Pediatrician, Department of Pediatrics, Morgan Stanley Children's Hospital of New York-Presbyterian, New York, New York

F. Meridith Sonnett, MD
Associate Clinical Professor of Pediatrics, Department of Pediatrics, Columbia University College of Physicians and Surgeons; Chief, Division of Pediatric Emergency Medicine, Morgan Stanley Children's Hospital of New York-Presbyterian, New York, New York

Thomas J. Starc, MD, MPH
Professor of Clinical Pediatrics, Division of Pediatric Cardiology, Department of Pediatrics,
Columbia University College of Physicians and Surgeons; Senior Attending Physician, Division
of Pediatric Cardiology, Department of Pediatrics, Morgan Stanley Children's Hospital of New
York-Presbyterian, New York, New York

Robert W. Wilmott, MD
IMMUNO Professor and Chairperson, Department of Pediatrics, Saint Louis University;
Pediatrician-in-Chief, Department of Pediatrics, Cardinal Glennon Children's Medical Center, St.
Louis, Missouri

PREFACE

It has been more than 20 years (and in the interim one Phillies and two Red Sox World Series championships) since the publication of the initial *Pediatric Secrets*. With this new edition, we strove to continue the principles of past editions by incorporating topics and questions about common (and less common) pediatric issues that are discussed every day in inpatient and outpatient settings. It is a constant dialogue involving pathophysiology, diagnosis, and therapy that leads to greater understanding. We have again tried to highlight major areas in pediatrics that remain controversial and less clearly defined.

We thank the chapter authors for their diligence in revising and updating, particularly in more novel aspects of pediatric medicine. We are very grateful to Andrea Vosburgh of Elsevier for her thoughtful suggestions, attention to detail, and patience with deadlines.

We have watched our own families grow, and in some cases begin families of their own, during the span of these editions. To Helene, Allison, Mitchell, Jessica, and Gregory Polin and to Nina, Erin, Cara, and Grace Ditmar, thank you for providing a lifetime of support and for continuing to leave the light on for us.

Since the publication of our last edition, Dr. Jean Cortner has passed away. Dr. Cortner was physician-in-chief at the Children's Hospital of Philadelphia from 1974 until 1986. He was a mentor, colleague, and friend, as well as a consummate physician with intellectual verve, genuine compassion, and remarkable insight. He is very much missed. We dedicate this 5th edition of *Pediatric Secrets* to his memory.

Richard A. Polin, MD
Mark F. Ditmar, MD

TOP 100 SECRETS

These secrets are 100 of the top board alerts. They summarize the concepts, principles, and most salient details of clinical practice

1. Always consider ovarian torsion in the differential diagnosis of abdominal pain in girls, particularly during the ages of 9 to 14 years, when ovarian cysts as potential lead points are more common because of the maturing reproductive hormonal axis.

2. A pelvic examination is not required before prescribing oral contraceptives for teenagers without risk factors. Appropriate screening for sexually transmitted infections and possible cervical dysplasia can be scheduled, but delaying oral contraception unnecessarily increases the risk for pregnancy.

3. Emergency contraception should be discussed with all sexually active adolescents; 90% of teenage pregnancies are unintended.

4. Nutritional and hormonal interventions may be needed should an active girl or young woman develop the "female athletic triad," which encompasses the distinct but interrelated conditions of disordered eating, amenorrhea, and osteoporosis.

5. Teenagers with attention-deficit/hyperactivity disorder and conduct disorders are at high risk for substance abuse disorders. Substance abuse is often associated with comorbid psychiatric disorders.

6. In preadolescents and younger adolescents, being overweight is more commonly associated with an advanced skeletal age and increased height compared with nonobese peers. Relative short stature in a younger obese patient may indicate endocrine disease.

7. The most common chronic disease of childhood is early dental caries.

8. Calluses over the metacarpophalangeal joints of the index and/or middle fingers (Russell sign) may indicate repetitive trauma from self-induced attempts at vomiting in patients with eating disorders.

9. The three essential features of autism are impaired social interaction, absent or abnormal speech and language development, a narrow range of interests, and stereotyped or repetitive responses to objects.

10. Bilingual children develop speech milestones normally; two-language households should not be presumed as a cause of speech delay.

11. Most amblyopia is unilateral; vision testing solely with both eyes open is inadequate.

12. The "atopic march" is the phenomenon in which about half of infants with atopic dermatitis eventually develop asthma, and two thirds develop allergic rhinitis.

13. Contact dermatitis should be suspected with rashes that are well-demarcated, geometric, and/or linear in nature, and may appear in uncommon or specific areas (e.g., earlobes, weight-bearing surfaces of feet).

14. Patients with atypical Kawasaki disease are usually younger (<1 year old) and most commonly lack cervical adenopathy and extremity changes.

15. Neonates with midline lumbosacral lesions (e.g., sacral pits, hypertrichosis, lipomas) above the gluteal crease should have screening imaging of the spine performed to search for occult spinal dysraphism.

16. Infantile acne necessitates an endocrine workup to rule out precocious puberty.

17. The most common finding on the examination of a child's genitalia after suspected sexual abuse is a normal examination.

18. High-dose epinephrine is no longer recommended in pediatric resuscitation because it has not been shown to be beneficial compared with standard dosing and may actually be harmful in cardiac arrest secondary to asphyxia.

19. The single most important step for treating all chemical exposures (including acts of terrorism) is an initial decontamination strategy of immediate removal of clothing, which can eliminate about 90% of contaminants.

20. In the setting of bites, prophylactic antibiotics have been shown to significantly reduce infections in only two settings: bites to the hands and human bites. Some experts recommend treatment for other "high-risk" injuries, such as cat bites, foot wounds, puncture wounds, and wounds treated more than 12 hours after the injury.

21. Consider the use of prostaglandin E_1 to maintain the patency of the ductus arteriosus in a newborn younger than 1 month who presents in shock with evidence of congestive heart failure and cyanosis because of the possibility of a ductal-dependent cardiac lesion, such as hypoplastic left heart syndrome.

22. The most common cause of overdose deaths in children and adolescents in the United States is acetaminophen, owing to its widespread availability and frequency of use in accidental and suicidal intoxications.

23. Midline neck masses usually involve the thyroid gland or thyroid remnants, such as a thyroglossal duct cyst.

24. Because 20% to 40% of solitary thyroid nodules in adolescents are malignant, an expedited evaluation is needed if a nodule is discovered.

25. An initial bolus of insulin (typically, 0.1 units/kg), previously used as standard treatment for diabetic ketoacidosis, is no longer recommended because it is thought to be unnecessary and may increase the risk for cerebral edema.

26. Unlike patients with type 1 diabetes, most youth with type 2 diabetes have little or no weight loss and absent or mild polyuria or nocturia. Most have glycosuria without ketonuria (although up to 33% can have ketonuria).

27. Acanthosis nigricans is found in 90% of youth diagnosed with type 2 diabetes.

28. More than 40% of infants regurgitate effortlessly more than once a day.

29. Nasogastric lavage is a simple method for differentiating upper gastrointestinal bleeding from lower gastrointestinal bleeding.

30. Potential long-term complications of pediatric inflammatory bowel disease include chronic growth failure, abscesses, fistulas, nephrolithiasis, and toxic megacolon.

31. Bilious emesis in a newborn represents a sign of potential obstruction and is a true gastrointestinal emergency.

32. The most common condition presenting as a food impaction in an adolescent is eosinophilic esophagitis.

33. About 99% of full-term infants pass stool at less than 24 hours after birth. Failure to pass stool within the first 48 hours of life should be considered abnormal until proved otherwise.

34. The most common cause of bloody diarrhea in infants younger than 1 year is allergic (or nonspecific) colitis, usually attributed to cow milk–based formula.

35. About 80% of children will outgrow (that is, develop a tolerance to) certain food allergies, particularly eggs and milk, by age 10 years or earlier. However, only about 20% outgrow a peanut allergy. Food allergies that develop after age 3 years are less likely to be outgrown.

36. In patients with Down syndrome and behavioral problems, do not overlook hearing loss (both sensorineural and conductive); it occurs in up to two thirds of patients with this condition, and it can be a possible contributor to those types of problems.

37. Three or more minor malformations should raise concern about the presence of a major malformation.

38. An infant with nonsyndromic sensorineural hearing loss should be tested for mutations in the connexin 26 gene. Mutations in that gene contribute to at least 50% of autosomal recessive hearing loss and about 10% to 20% of all prelingual hearing loss.

39. Carbon monoxide poisoning is often misdiagnosed because the presenting symptoms can be flu-like.

40. Hospitalization is indicated for significant burns involving the hands, feet, joints, or perineum or if there are circumferential burns.

41. Fecal soiling is almost always associated with severe functional constipation and not Hirschsprung disease.

42. Interpretation of stool tests for *Clostridium difficile* is more problematic in young infants because up to 70% may be colonized with the organism. By the second year of life, this rate declines to about 6%, and above age 2 years to 3%, which is the approximate rate in adults.

43. The classic picture of appendicitis is anorexia followed by pain, then by nausea and vomiting, with subsequent localization of findings to the right lower quadrant. However, there is a large degree of variability, particularly in younger patients.

44. Absence of anemia does not exclude the possibility of iron deficiency because iron depletion is relatively advanced before anemia develops.

45. After iron supplementation for iron deficiency anemia, the reticulocyte count should double in 1 to 2 weeks, and hemoglobin should increase by 1 g/dL in 2 to 4 weeks. The most common reason for persistence of iron deficiency anemia is poor compliance with supplementation.

46. Because 30% of patients with hemophilia have no family history of the disorder and new mutations are the cause, clinical suspicion is important in the presence of excessive and frequent ecchymoses.

47. Up to 20% of adolescents with menorrhagia will have a bleeding disorder, most commonly von Willebrand disease, and screening is recommended.

48. In patients with sickle cell disease, use of transcranial Doppler ultrasound to measure intracranial blood flow and regular transfusions to reduce the hemoglobin S content for those with abnormal values can significantly lower the likelihood of stroke.

49. The determination of immunoglobulin G subclass concentrations is meaningless in children who are younger than 4 years.

50. The most common specific etiology diagnosed in pediatric patients with a systemic febrile illness after international travel is malaria. More than half of the world's population lives in areas where malaria is endemic.

51. A male child with a liver abscess should be considered to have chronic granulomatous disease until it is proved otherwise.

52. Perinatal asphyxia accounts for less than 15% of cases of cerebral palsy.

53. Leukocyte adhesion deficiency should be considered in a newborn with a significantly delayed separation of the umbilical cord (>6 weeks).

54. The most common congenital infection is cytomegalovirus, which in some large screening studies occurs in up to 1.3% of newborns. About 90% to 95% of affected newborns do not have symptoms, but some may later develop hearing loss.

55. Hyperbilirubinemia generally is not an indication for the cessation of breastfeeding but rather for increasing its frequency.

56. Vigorous correction of constipation has been shown to diminish both enuresis and the frequency of urinary tract infections.

57. The two most productive facets of patient evaluation to explain renal disease as a possible cause of symptoms are (1) the measurement of blood pressure and (2) the examination of the first-morning void after the bladder is emptied of urine stored overnight (when a specimen is most likely to be concentrated).

58. The most common cause of persistent seizures is an inadequate serum antiepileptic level.

59. Migraine headaches are usually bilateral in children but unilateral (75%) in adults.

60. Seizures with fever in patients older than 6 years should not be considered febrile seizures.

61. After age and white blood cell count, early response to therapy is the most important prognostic feature for children with acute lymphoblastic leukemia.

62. Leukemias and lymphomas that have a high proliferation and cell turnover rate (e.g., Burkitt lymphoma, T-cell lymphoblastic leukemia) place patients at the highest risk for complications from tumor lysis syndrome.

63. Eighty percent or more of patients who present with acute lymphoblastic leukemia have a normochromic, normocytic anemia with reticulocytopenia.

64. Older children with unexplained unilateral deformities (e.g., pes cavus) of an extremity should have screening magnetic resonance imaging to evaluate for intraspinal disease.

65. Asthma rarely causes clubbing in children. Consider other diseases, particularly cystic fibrosis.

66. Most children with recurrent pneumonia or persistent right middle lobe atelectasis have asthma. But all that wheezes is not asthma.

67. A normal respiratory rate strongly argues against a bacterial pneumonia.

68. Nasal polyps or rectal prolapse in children suggests cystic fibrosis.

69. The three most common causes of anaphylaxis in pediatric hospitals and emergency departments are latex, food, and drugs. Suspected allergies to shellfish, peanuts, and nuts warrant a prescription for an epinephrine pen because of the increased risk for future anaphylaxis.

70. Up to 10% of normal, healthy children may have low-level (1:10) positive antinuclear antibody testing that will remain positive. Without clinical or laboratory features of disease, it is of no significance.

71. The daily spiking fevers of systemic juvenile rheumatoid arthritis can precede the development of arthritis by weeks to months.

72. Abdominal pain (mimicking an acute abdomen) and arthritis can frequently precede the rash in Henoch-Schönlein purpura disease and thus confuse the diagnosis.

73. Premature babies should be immunized in accordance with postnatal chronologic age.

74. Without a booster after age 5 years, pertussis protection against infection is about 80% during the first 3 years after immunization, dropping to 50% after 4 to 7 years, and to near 0% after 11 years.

75. When administering an intramuscular vaccination, aspiration is not necessary because no large blood vessels are located at the recommended sites for injection.

76. About 6% of children are streptococcus carriers and will have positive throat cultures between episodes of pharyngitis.

77. Apgar scores at 1 and 5 minutes do not predict long-term outcome.

78. Sodium bicarbonate should never be administered to newborns without first ensuring adequate ventilation.

79. Coagulase-negative staphylococci are the most common bacterial pathogens responsible for nosocomial infections in the neonatal intensive care unit.

80. In more than 90% of cases, intraventricular hemorrhages in preterm infants occur during the first 3 days of life.

81. Recovery occurs in about 90% of patients with brachial plexus injuries.

82. Isolated primary nocturnal enuresis rarely has identifiable organic pathology.

83. Asymptomatic microscopic hematuria is found in 0.5% to 2% of schoolchildren and is benign in most; evaluation yields no renal or urologic pathology.

84. Significant proteinuria, in addition to hematuria, is much more likely to cause an underlying pathology compared with hematuria alone.

85. Clean-bagged specimens in infants and toddlers are unreliable for culture diagnosis of urinary tract infections because of the high contamination rate.

86. Uncircumcised male infants have a 10-fold greater risk for urinary tract infection compared with circumcised males.

87. During the first year of life, hypotonia is more common than hypertonia in patients who are ultimately diagnosed with cerebral palsy.

88. Monitor patients with cerebral palsy (especially with spastic diparesis) regularly for hip subluxation because earlier identification assists therapy.

89. Headaches that awaken children from sleep, are associated with vomiting without nausea, are made worse by straining or coughing, and have intensity changes with changes in body position are concerning for pathology that is causing increased intracranial pressure.

90. Establishing the maturity level of the skeletal bones in a patient with scoliosis is important because the risk for progression is increased with greater degrees of skeletal immaturity.

91. In adolescents, progressive scoliotic curves are seven times more likely to occur in girls than boys.

92. $Paco_2$ measurements that are normal (40 mm Hg) or rising in asthmatic patients with tachypnea or significant respiratory distress are worrisome for evolving respiratory failure.

93. In half of patients with chlamydial pneumonia, conjunctivitis precedes pneumonia.

94. Hilar adenopathy suggests tuberculosis.

95. In a febrile infant or toddler with a white blood cell count greater than 20,000/mm^3, consider a chest radiograph to look for pneumonia, which can be present in up to 10% without respiratory symptoms.

96. Although the incidence of rheumatic fever is low in the United States, worldwide it is the leading cause of cardiovascular death during the first five decades of life.

97. Because up to 10% of patients can have asymptomatic *Borrelia burgdorferi* infection and both immunoglobulin M and immunoglobulin G antibodies to *B. burgdorferi* can persist for 10 to 20 years, the diagnosis of Lyme disease in older children and adolescents can be tricky in patients with atypical clinical presentations.

98. Compared with viral meningitis, Lyme meningitis is more likely to have a cranial neuropathy (usually facial nerve), papilledema, and a longer duration of symptoms before seeking medical care.

99. About 10% to 20% of patients with Rocky Mountain spotted fever do not develop a rash, so a high index of suspicion is needed for any patient in an endemic area who presents with fever, myalgia, severe headaches, and vomiting.

100. Most pediatric deaths in the United States associated with influenza tend to result from either (1) an exacerbation of an underlying medical condition or invasive procedure, or (2) coinfection from another pathogen, most commonly *Staphylococcus aureus*.

CHAPTER 1

ADOLESCENT MEDICINE

Mark F. Ditmar, MD

CLINICAL ISSUES

1. **What are the major health risks for adolescents?**
   - **Unintentional injury:** The leading cause of death, particularly alcohol-related automobile accidents. Adolescents account for 6% of total drivers but 14% of fatal crash victims.
   - **Violence:** Homicide is the second leading cause of death among 15- to 24-year-olds and the leading cause for black males in this age range. Suicide is the third leading cause of death in adolescents aged 10 to 19 years.
   - **Substance abuse:** In surveys, nearly 10% of 12- to 17-year-old adolescents admit to illicit drug use during the previous 30 days.
   - **Sexually transmitted Infections (STIs):** May involve 1 in 4 teenagers. Up to 30% of all STIs reported annually to the Centers for Disease Control and Prevention (CDC) involve adolescents. Adolescents between 15 and 19 years of age have the highest age-specific rates of chlamydial and gonorrheal infections of any population group.
   - **Teen pregnancy:** 90% are unintended.
   - **Obesity:** 15% of U.S. teenagers are obese (body mass index [BMI] $\geq$95% for age), and 15% are at risk for obesity (BMI between 85% and 95% for age).

2. **Name the major risk factors that are associated with injuries to adolescents.**
   - **Use of alcohol while engaged in activities** (e.g., driving, swimming, boating): 20% of all adolescent deaths are alcohol-related car crashes.
   - **Failure to use safety devices** (e.g., seat belts, motorcycle or bicycle helmets): Seat belt use among adolescents is the lowest of any age group (10% admit to never or rarely using one), and fewer than 10% use bicycle helmets.
   - **Access to firearms:** 50% of deaths among black male teenagers and 20% of deaths among white male teenagers are due to firearms, primarily handguns.
   - **Athletic participation:** Most injuries are reinjuries, which highlights the importance of proper rehabilitation.

3. **Which sport causes the greatest number of catastrophic injuries in teenagers?**
   Catastrophic injuries are those that result in death or permanent severe functional disability. For boys, *football* is the leading cause. For girls, *cheerleading* is number one cause, owing to the gymnastic-type stunts that are performed, which can result in falls from significant heights.

   Mueller FO: Catastrophic head injuries and high school and collegiate sports, *J Athl Train* 36:312–315, 2001.

4. **What diagnoses require mandatory disclosure regardless of confidentiality?**
   In most states . . .
   - Notification of child welfare authorities under state **child-abuse** (physical and sexual) reporting laws
   - Notification of law enforcement officials of **gunshot** and **stab wounds**
   - Warning from a psychotherapist to a reasonably identifiable victim of a patient's **threat of violence**

■ Notification to parents or other authorities if a patient represents a reasonable threat to himself or herself (i.e., **suicidal ideation**)

5. **When can teenagers give their own consent for medical care or procedures?**
   Teenagers who are married, who are parents themselves, who are members of the armed forces, who are living apart from their parents, who are high school graduates, and/or who have evidence of independence (financial or otherwise) may fit the definition of an "emancipated" or "mature" minor. However, the definition varies from state to state.

   Bruce CR, Berg SL, McGuire AL: Please don't call my mom: pediatric consent and confidentiality, *Clin Pediatr* 48:243–246, 2009.

6. **For which services do many states waive the legal requirement for parental consent for patients under age 18?**
   These include care for STIs, contraception services, pregnancy-related care, substance abuse treatment, mental health services, and treatment for rape or sexual assault.

7. **How does the "HEADS FIRST" system assist in adolescent interviewing?**
   This mnemonic, which was originally devised at State University of New York Upstate Medical University, allows for a systematic approach to multiple health issues and risk factors that affect teenagers:
   Home: living arrangements, family relationships, support
   Education: school issues, study habits, achievement, employment, expectations
   Abuse: physical, sexual, emotional, verbal
   Drugs: peer and personal use, alcohol, tobacco, marijuana, cocaine, others
   Safety: injury prevention, safety equipment, seat belts, helmets, hazardous activities
   Friends: peer pressure, interaction, confidants
   Image: self-esteem, body image, weight management
   Recreation: exercise, relaxation, television and media time
   Sexuality: changes, feelings, experiences, orientation, contraception
   Threats: depressed or upset easily, suicidal ideation or attempts, harm to others

   Cavanaugh RM Jr: Managing the transitions of early adolescence, *Adolesc Health Update* 20:1–8, 2008.

EATING DISORDERS

8. **What types of dieting raise concern for the development of an eating disorder?**
   Dieting that is associated with ...
   ■ Decreasing weight goals
   ■ Increasing criticism of body image
   ■ Increasing social isolation
   ■ Amenorrhea or oligomenorrhea

9. **How is the diagnosis of anorexia made?**
   Anorexia nervosa consists of a spectrum of psychological, behavioral, and medical abnormalities. The *1996 Diagnostic and Statistical Manual for Primary Care: Child and Adolescent Version* criteria list five components:
   ■ **Refusal to maintain body weight** or BMI at or above minimal norms for age and height (<85% of expected weight for height or a BMI of <17.5 in an older adolescent)
   ■ **Intense fear of gaining weight** or becoming fat despite being underweight
   ■ **Disturbances of perception** of body shape and size
   ■ **Denial of seriousness** of weight loss or low body weight

■ In postmenarchal girls, **amenorrhea** (i.e., the absence of at least three consecutive menstrual cycles)

National Eating Disorders Association: http://www.nationaleatingdisorders.org.

National Association of Anorexia Nervosa and Associated Disorders: http://www.anad.org.

10. **What are good and bad prognosticators for recovery from anorexia?**
Good: Early age at onset ($<$14 years), high educational achievement, improvement in body image after weight gain, emotionally well-adjusted, supportive family, shorter duration of illness
Bad: Late age at onset, continued overestimation of body size, self-induced vomiting or bulimia, laxative abuse, family dysfunction, male, comorbid mental illness, substance abuse, longer duration of illness

11. **What hormonal abnormalities may be seen in anorexia nervosa?**
Amenorrhea is seen in most cases due to hypothalamic and pituitary dysfunction with very low levels of luteinizing hormone (LH) and follicle-stimulating hormone (FSH). Twenty-five percent of affected girls experience amenorrhea before significant weight loss occurs, which suggests that there is a psychological effect on physiology. Symptoms that are suggestive of **hypothyroidism**—constipation, cold intolerance, dry skin, bradycardia, and hair or nail changes—are common. Thyroid studies, however, have relatively normal results, except for a low triiodothyronine (T_3) and an increased reverse T_3 (rT_3), which is a less active isomer.

The T_3/rT_3 reversal is also seen in conditions that are associated with weight loss, possibly indicating that it is a physiologic means of adapting to a lower energy state. Other abnormalities include a loss of diurnal variation in **cortisol**, diminished plasma catecholamine levels, normal or increased **growth hormone** levels, and flattened glucose tolerance curve.

12. **In addition to underweight and amenorrhea, what other clinical features may be found in patients with anorexia nervosa?**
Symptoms: Cold intolerance, constipation, fatigue, postural dizziness, early satiety, bloating
Signs: Pubertal delay, growth retardation, development of lanugo hair, abnormal skin (dry, hyperkeratotic; sometimes orange due to increased carotene), hypothermia, bradycardia, postural hypotension, acrocyanosis, dependent edema

Morris J, Twaddle S: Anorexia nervosa, *BMJ* 334:894–898, 2007.

13. **What are some indications that a pediatric patient with anorexia nervosa should be admitted to a hospital?**
■ $>$75% of ideal body weight or ongoing weight loss despite intensive management
■ Dehydration
■ Electrolyte abnormalities (e.g., hypokalemia, hyponatremia, hypophosphatemia)
■ Heart rate less than 50 beats per minute daytime, less than 45 beats per minute nighttime
■ Systolic blood pressure less than 80 mm Hg
■ Orthostatic changes in pulse ($>$20 beats per minute) or blood pressure ($>$10 mm Hg)
■ Temperature less than 96°F
■ Cardiac dysrhythmia
■ Acute medical complication of malnutrition (syncope, seizure, congestive heart failure, pancreatitis)
■ Severe coexisting psychiatric disease

American Academy of Pediatrics: Committee on Adolescence: Identifying and tolerating eating disorders, *Pediatrics* 111:204–211, 2003.

14. **What causes sudden cardiac death in patients with anorexia nervosa?**
Chronic emaciation affects the myocardium. Anorectic patients develop depressed cardiovascular function and an altered conduction system. Electrocardiogram (ECG) changes are common. Patients with anorexia have significantly lower heart rates (averaging 20 beats per minute less than peers), lower R values in V6, and longer QRS intervals. These ECG changes often occur without underlying electrolyte abnormalities. The arrhythmogenic potential is heightened if electrolytes (specifically potassium) are distorted by excessive vomiting or laxative abuse. Sudden death is likely as a result of the culmination of chronic myocardial injury in emaciated patients (>35% to 40% below ideal weight) with resultant heart failure and dysrhythmia.

Panagiotopoulos C, McCrindle BW, Hick K, Katzman DK: Electrocardiographic findings in adolescents with eating disorders, *Pediatrics* 105:1100–1105, 2000.

15. **Do males and females with anorexia nervosa have a similar clinical profile?**
It is estimated that less than 5% of anorexia nervosa involves boys. Males are more likely to ...
- Have been obese before the onset of symptoms.
- Be ambivalent regarding the desire to gain or lose weight.
- Have more issues about gender and sexual identity.
- Involve dieting with sports participation.
- Engage in "defensive dieting" (avoiding weight gain after an athletic injury).

Domine F, Berchtold A, Akre C, et al: Disordered eating behaviors: what about boys? *J Adolesc Health* 44:111–117, 2009.

Rosen DS: Eating disorders in adolescent males, *Adolesc Med* 14:677–689, 2003.

KEY POINTS: ANOREXIA NERVOSA

1. Hallmark: Intense fear of gaining weight despite being underweight.
2. BMI < 17.5 in older adolescents strongly suggests anorexia.
3. 95% female, but evidence suggests increasing prevalence among males.
4. Inquire about the possibility of an eating disorder with a direct question: "How do you feel about your weight?"
5. Sedimentation rates: Usually normal in eating disorders; elevation suggests other diagnoses, such as inflammatory bowel disease.
6. Most common causes of death: cardiac dysfunction and suicide.

16. **How is the diagnosis of bulimia nervosa made?**
Bulimia nervosa is a syndrome of voracious, high-caloric overeating and subsequent forced vomiting (by gagging or ipecac) and/or other purging methods (e.g., laxatives, diuretics). This often occurs during periods of frustration or psychological stress. Its incidence is thought to be higher than that of anorexia nervosa, and males are rarely involved. The diagnosis is made using a patient's **history**.

17. **List the medical complications of bulimia nervosa.**
Electrolyte abnormalities: Hypokalemia, hypochloremia, and metabolic alkalosis may occur. The hypokalemia can cause a prolonged QT interval and T-wave abnormalities.
Esophageal: Acid reflux with esophagitis and (rarely) Mallory-Weiss tear may be found.
Cardiac: Ipecac use can result in cardiomyopathy due to a toxic effect of one of its principal components, the alkaloid emetine.

Central nervous system: Neurotransmitters can be affected, thereby causing changes in the patient's perceptions of satiety.

Miscellaneous: Enamel erosion, salivary gland enlargement, cheilosis, and knuckle calluses are signs of recurrent vomiting.

Mehler PS: Bulimia nervosa, *N Engl J Med* 349:875–881, 2003.

18. **How do anorexia nervosa and bulimia nervosa differ?**
See Table 1-1.

TABLE 1-1. COMPARISON OF ANOREXIA NERVOSA AND BULIMIA NERVOSA

Anorexia Nervosa	Bulimia Nervosa
Vomiting or diuretic/laxative abuse uncommon	Vomiting or diuretic/laxative abuse
Severe weight loss	Less weight loss; avoidance of obesity
Slightly younger	Slightly older
More introverted	More extroverted
Hunger denied	Hunger pronounced
Eating behavior may be considered normal	Eating behavior is egodystonic and a source of self-esteem
Sexually inactive	Sexually active
Obsessional fears with paranoid features	Histrionic features
Amenorrhea	Menses irregular or absent
Death from starvation/suicide	Death from hypokalemia/suicide

From Shenker IR, Bunnell DW: Bulimia nervosa. In McAnarmey ER, Kreipe RE, Orr DP, Comerci GD (eds): Textbook of Adolescent Medicine. Philadelphia, W.B. Saunders, 1992, p 545.

19. **What modalities are used to treat eating disorders?**
Nutritional rehabilitation: Patients are often begun on 1200 to 1500 kcal per day, increasing by 500 kcal every 1 to 4 days up to 3500 kcal (for females) and to 4000 kcal (for males). Overnight nasogastric feedings are routinely recommended. Total parenteral nutrition is rarely required.

Medication: Prokinetic agents (e.g., domperidone) are used to minimize postprandial bloating. Antidepressants, including serotonin-specific reuptake inhibitors (e.g., fluoxetine), and atypical neuroleptic mediations (e.g., risperidone) have been used with some limited success.

Psychotherapy: Individual and family therapy may both be useful.

Attia E, Walsh BT: Behavioral management for anorexia nervosa, *N Engl J Med* 360:500–506, 2009.

Yager J, Andersen AE: Anorexia nervosa, *N Engl J Med* 353:1481–1488, 2005.

20. **Name the three features that constitute the "female athletic triad."**
Disordered eating, amenorrhea, and osteoporosis. These three distinct yet interrelated disorders are often seen in active girls and young women. All female athletes are at risk for developing this triad, with 15% to 60% of female athletes demonstrating abnormal weight-control behaviors. Diagnosis is based on history, physical examination, and laboratory evaluation. The basic laboratory workup should include urine human chorionic gonadotropin, thyroid-stimulating hormone, prolactin, FSH, LH, testosterone, dehydroepiandrosterone sulfate (DHEA-S), and progesterone challenge test. Ongoing counseling is often indicated,

as are nutritional and hormonal interventions. Treatment commonly includes calcium supplements and oral contraceptives.

Greydanus DE, Omar H, Pratt HD: The adolescent female athelete: current concepts and conundrums, *Pediatr Clin North Am* 57:697-718, 2010.

American Academy of Pediatrics Committee on Sports Medicine and Fitness: Medical concerns in the female athlete, *Pediatrics* 106:610–613, 2000.

MENSTRUAL DISORDERS

21. **What is the difference between primary and secondary amenorrhea?**
    Primary amenorrhea: No onset of menses by age 16 or within 3 years of onset of secondary sex characteristics or within 1 year of Tanner V breast and pubic hair development
    Secondary amenorrhea: No menses for 3 months after previous establishment of regular menstrual periods or for 6 months if regular cycles have not been established

22. **What causes primary amenorrhea?**
    The key feature in the differential diagnosis is whether the amenorrhea is associated with the development of secondary sex characteristics.
    Amenorrhea *without* secondary sex characteristics:
    ■ Chromosomal or enzymatic defects (e.g., Turner syndrome, chromosomal mosaics, 17α-hydroxylase deficiency)
    ■ Congenital absence of uterus
    ■ Gonadal dysgenesis (with elevated gonadotropins)
    ■ Hypothalamic-pituitary abnormalities (with diminished gonadotropins)
    Amenorrhea *with* secondary sex characteristics:
    ■ Dysfunction of hypothalamic release of gonadotropin-releasing hormone (GnRH) (e.g., stress, excessive exercise, weight loss, chronic illness, polycystic ovary disease, medications, hypothyroidism)
    ■ Abnormalities of pituitary gland (e.g., tumor, empty sella syndrome)
    ■ Ovarian dysfunction (e.g., irradiation, chemotherapy, trauma, viral infection, autoimmune inflammation)
    ■ Abnormalities of genital tract (e.g., cervical agenesis, imperforate hymen, androgen insensitivity with absent uterus)
    ■ Pregnancy

23. **How can estrogen influence be evaluated on vaginal or cervical smears?**
    Vaginal smear: In patients with normal estrogen, 15% to 30% of cells are superficial (small pyknotic nuclei with large cytoplasm), and the remainder are intermediate (larger nuclei with visible nucleolus but still with cytoplasm predominant). If parabasal cells are noted (nuclear-to-cytoplasmic ratio of $\geq$50:50), relative estrogen deficiency should be suspected.
    Cervical smear: Cervical mucus is smeared onto a glass slide and allowed to dry. If a fern pattern appears, estrogen is normal (i.e., because salts crystallize only if estrogen is unopposed by progesterone). No fern pattern occurs during the second half of menses, after ovulation, because of the presence of progesterone. Absence of ferning during pregnancy is also a result of higher progesterone levels.

24. **What is the value of a progesterone challenge test in a patient with amenorrhea?**
    If bleeding ensues within 2 weeks after the administration of oral medroxyprogesterone (5-10 mg daily for 5-10 days) or intramuscular progesterone in oil (5-10 mg daily for 5-10 days), the test is positive. This indicates that the endometrium has been primed by estrogen and that the outflow tract is functioning. No response indicates hypothalamic-pituitary dysfunction or ovarian failure.

25. **A 14-year-old girl has Tanner III features and monthly abdominal pain but no onset of menstrual flow. What is the likely diagnosis?**
An **anatomic abnormality of the vagina** (e.g., imperforate hymen or transverse vaginal septum) or **cervix** (e.g., agenesis).

26. **An obese 16-year-old girl has oligomenorrhea, hirsutism, acne, and an elevated LH/FSH ratio. What condition is likely?**
Polycystic ovary syndrome. This disorder is characterized by the triad of *menstrual irregularities* (amenorrhea or oligomenorrhea), *hirsutism*, and *acne* that begins during puberty. Obesity is common. In these individuals, there is an apparent gonadotropin-dependent, functional ovarian hyperandrogenism with elevated LH (or LH/FSH ratio of >3:1) and insulin resistance. A dysregulation of ovarian and adrenal synthesis of androgens and estrogen is likely. Polycystic ovaries, although commonly found on ultrasound, are not essential for the diagnosis.

Baldwin CY, Witchel SF: Polycystic ovary syndrome, *Pediatr Ann* 35:888–897, 2006.

27. **What is the range of complications of polycystic ovary syndrome?**
■ Infertility
■ Abnormal lipid metabolism
■ Type 2 diabetes
■ Endometrial cancer
■ Cardiovascular disease

Pfeifer SM, Kives S: Polycystic ovary syndrome in the adolescent, *Ob Gyn Clin North Am* 36:129–152, 2009.

28. **What constitutes excessive menstrual bleeding in an adolescent?**
As a rule, most menstrual periods do not last more than 7 days, do not occur more frequently than every 21 to 40 days, and are not associated with more than 80 mL of blood loss. The quantitation can be difficult because pad or tampon numbers correlate poorly with total blood loss. Blood clots or a change in pad numbers appears to have more reliability. Suspicion of excessive loss should prompt an evaluation of hematocrit and/or reticulocyte count.

29. **Differentiate the "rhagia" types of menstrual problems.**
Menorrhagia: Hypermenorrhea or heavy menstrual bleeding with regular cyclic intervals
Metrorrhagia: Irregular bleeding due to varying cycles
Menometrorrhagia: Heavy bleeding that occurs at varying intervals

30. **How common are anovulatory menstrual periods in adolescents?**
Anovulatory cycles (and with them, an increased likelihood of irregular periods) occur in 50% of adolescents for up to 2 years after menarche and in up to 20% after 5 years (the rate in adults). Anovulatory cycles result in unopposed estradiol production, which can cause the following: (1) breakthrough bleeding at varying intervals due to insufficient hormone to support a thickened endothelium, and (2) heavy and prolonged menstrual flow due to lack of progesterone. However, most anovulatory menstrual cycles are normal because the intact negative feedback loop (i.e., rising estradiol lowers FH and LSH, which, in turn, lower estradiol) does not allow for prolonged elevated estrogen with endometrial proliferation.

31. **Describe the evaluation for a patient with dysfunctional uterine bleeding (DUB).**
Dysfunctional uterine bleeding is irregular and/or prolonged vaginal bleeding in the absence of structural pelvic pathology. It remains a diagnosis of exclusion. Depending on the age of the patient and her history of sexual activity, the following studies should be considered:
■ Speculum examination for evidence of trauma or vaginal foreign body
■ Bimanual examination for ovarian mass, uterine fibroid, and signs of pregnancy or pelvic inflammatory disease

- Papanicolaou (Pap) smear for cervical dysplasia
- Pregnancy test
- Serum prolactin
- Thyroid function tests
- Coagulation studies (especially for von Willebrand disease)

Albers JR, Hull SK, Wesley RM: Abnormal uterine bleeding, *Am Fam Physician* 69:1915–1932, 2004.

32. **How can the timing of abnormal uterine bleeding help identify the most likely cause?**
    Abnormal bleeding at the normal time of cyclic shedding:
    - Blood dyscrasia (especially von Willebrand disease)
    - Endometrial pathology (e.g., submuous myoma, intrauterine device)

    Abnormal bleeding at any time during the cycle, but normal cycles:
    - Vaginal foreign body
    - Trauma
    - Endometriosis
    - Infection
    - Uterine polyps
    - Cervical abnormality (e.g., hemangioma)

    Noncyclic bleeding or abnormal cyclic bleeding (<21 days or >45 days, usually associated with anovulatory cycles):
    - Physiologic (especially during early adolescence)
    - Polycystic ovary disease
    - Psychosocial pathology
    - Excessive exercise
    - Endocrine disorders
    - Adrenal and ovarian tumors
    - Ovarian failure

    Adapted from Kozlowski K, Gottlieb A, Graham CJ, Cleveland ER: Adolescent gynecologic conditions presenting in emergency settings, *Adolesc Med* 4:63–76, 1993.

33. **What are the two key clinical features that determine the management of dysfunctional uterine bleeding?**
    Hemoglobin concentration (i.e., anemia) and *signs of* **orthostatic hypotension**. The more severe the clinical feature, the more urgent and aggressive the management must be, particularly in the setting of acute hemorrhage.

34. **How should a very anemic teenager with DUB and positive orthostatic signs be managed?**
    If there are orthostatic changes and the hemoglobin is low (<7 mg/dL) . . .
    - Hospitalize for oral combination medications (e.g., 30 mcg ethinyl estradiol/0.3 mg norgestrel every 6 hours until bleeding slows with a medication taper up to 3 weeks); if bleeding persists after two doses, begin high-dose intravenous conjugated estrogen therapy (e.g., 25 mg IV. May repeat every 4 to 6 hours for up to 4 doses)
    - Begin intravenous fluids and consider transfusion (usually not required)
    - Unresponsive bleeding may require dilation and curettage (also rarely required in adolescents)
    - Coagulation studies (owing to a higher likelihood of underlying coagulopathy; tests for von Willebrand disease should be drawn before therapy because estrogen increases von Willebrand factor concentrations)
    - Begin iron supplementation

    Braverman PK, Breech LL: Menstrual disorders. In Slap GB, editor: *Adolescent Medicine: The Requisites in Pediatrics*, Philadelphia, 2008, Mosby Elsevier, pp 157–160.

KEY POINTS: MENSTRUAL DISORDERS

1. Abnormally heavy bleeding at menarche or unusually long menstrual periods: Consider von Willebrand disease.

2. Irregular menstrual bleeding patterns: Common in early adolescence because regular ovulatory menstrual cycles typically do not develop for 1 to 1½ years after the onset of menarche.

3. Always consider pregnancy in a patient with secondary amenorrhea.

4. Signs of androgen excess (hirsutism and/or acne) in the setting of menstrual irregularities suggest polycystic ovary syndrome.

5. Progressively worsening dysmenorrhea suggests endometriosis as a cause of chronic pelvic pain in adolescents.

6. Ask about dysmenorrhea: It affects >50% of teenage girls and causes considerable school absence.

35. **How common is dysmenorrhea in adolescent females?**
Up to 90% of adolescents are affected by primary dysmenorrhea. The condition remains the single greatest cause of lost school hours in females. However, fewer than 15% of teenage females with dysmenorrhea will seek medical care, so it is important to screen for the problem. Most cases are primary, but about 10% of patients with severe dysmenorrhea symptoms will have uterine or pelvic abnormalities, such as endometriosis.

    Harel Z: Dysmenorrhea in adolescents and young adults: etiology and management, *J Pediatr Adolesc Gynecol* 19:363–371, 2006.

36. **Why is dysmenorrhea more common in *late* rather than *early* adolescence?**
Dysmenorrhea occurs almost entirely with ovulatory cycles. Menses shortly after the onset of menarche is usually anovulatory. With the establishment of more regular ovulatory cycles after 2 to 4 years, primary dysmenorrhea becomes more likely.

37. **In a teenager with dysmenorrhea, what factors suggest an underlying identifiable pathologic problem rather than primary dysmenorrhea?**
Primary dysmenorrhea is painful menses without identifiable pelvic pathology and accounts for most cases in teenagers. However, underlying pathology is more likely if any of the following conditions are present: **menorrhagia; intermenstrual bleeding; pain at times other than menses** (suggesting outflow obstruction); or **abnormal uterine shape** on examination (suggesting uterine malformation).

38. **What two classes of medications are most commonly used for dysmenorrhea?**
Nonsteroidal anti-inflammatory drugs (NSAIDs): Evidence strongly suggests a key role for prostaglandins (especially prostaglandin $F_{2\alpha}$ and prostaglandin $E_{2\alpha}$) in pain because of uterine hyperactivity. NSAIDs can limit local prostaglandin production. Naproxen, ibuprofen, and mefenamic acid may be effective in up to 80% of patients.
Hormonal therapies: Oral contraceptives act by reducing endometrial growth, which limits the total production of endometrial prostaglandin. Ovulation is suppressed, which also minimizes pain. A combined estrogen-progestin pill is preferred. Improvement may not be seen for up to 3 months.

    Braverman PK: Dysmenorrhea and premenstrual syndrome. In Neinstein LS, editor: *Adolescent Health Care*, ed 5, Philadelphia, 2008, Wolters Kluwer, pp 674–686.

39. **What is the most common cause of chronic pelvic pain in adolescents without a history of pelvic inflammatory disease?**
    Endometriosis. This condition results from the implantation of endometrial tissue to areas of the peritoneum outside the uterine cavity. The pain is both noncyclic (may occur with intercourse or defecation) and cyclic (often most severe just before menses, and dysmenorrhea is common). When suspected, initial treatment is with NSAIDs and/or oral contraceptives. Intermenstrual bleeding is common. Definitive diagnosis is by laparoscopy and biopsy. Therapy can be surgical (e.g., excision, coagulation, laser vaporization) and/or medical (e.g., GnRH analogues, combination oral contraceptives, medroxyprogesterone acetate).

    Bulun SE: Endometriosis. *N Engl J Med* 360:268–279, 2009.

    Mounsey AL, Wilgus A, Slawson DC: Diagnosis and management of endometriosis, *Am Fam Physician* 74:594–602, 2006.

40. **What is the peak age for ovarian torsion?**
    In a study of 80 patients, nearly two thirds of cases occurred between the ages of 9 and 14 years, with a mean age of 11 years. This early pubertal peak is thought to be due to the increasing likelihood of the development of ovarian cysts by the maturing reproductive hormonal axis. These cysts then act as lead points for torsion.

    Oltmann S, Fischer R, Barber R, et al: Cannot exclude torsion—a 15-year review, *J Pediatr Surg* 44:1212–1217, 2009.

41. **Why do more ovarian torsions occur on the right than the left?**
    Multiple studies have noted this asymmetry in location, with nearly two thirds of ovarian torsions occurring on the right. A leading theory is that the relative mobility of the cecum allows for more ovarian motion on the right compared with the relatively fixed sigmoid colon on the left. Because torsion manifests almost 100% of the time with pain, this right-sided preference causes ovarian torsion to be commonly confused with appendicitis. Delays in diagnosis are common, which lessens ovarian salvage rates.

    Oltmann S, Fischer R, Barber R, et al: Cannot exclude torsion—a 15-year review, *J Pediatr Surg* 44:1212–1217, 2009.

42. **Is ultrasonography typically diagnostic in the setting of ovarian torsion?**
    The definitive diagnostic feature of torsion that could be detected by ultrasound—visualization of the twisted pedicle—is seen in fewer than 10% of cases. Certain ultrasonographic features can suggest torsion, such as a pelvic mass of 5 cm or larger or diminished or absent arterial or venous (particularly venous) Doppler flow, but they are not diagnostic. In some studies with documented operative torsion, Doppler studies were normal in up to 60%.

    Anders J: Ovarian torsion in the pediatric emergency department: making the diagnosis and the importance of advocacy, *Clin Pediatr Emerg Med* 10:31–37, 2009.

OBESITY

43. **What is the body mass index (BMI)?**
    BMI = (weight [kg]/height [m^2]). As an indicator of body fat, it is recommended by the CDC as the main screening tool for obesity. When plotted on standard charts for age and gender, a BMI from 85% to 95% indicates "at risk for overweight," and a BMI above the 95th percentile indicates "overweight." It is estimated that about 30% to 40% of U.S. adolescents are overweight or at risk for being overweight. BMI growth charts for age and gender are available at http://www.cdc.gov/growthcharts/.

    American Association of Pediatrics: http://www.aap.org/obesity.

    Obesity in America: http://www.obesityinamerica.org.

44. **Why is an obese 10-year-old who is short potentially of more clinical concern than one who is tall?**
Being overweight is more commonly associated with an advanced skeletal age in preadolescents and younger adolescents and thus increased height compared with nonobese peers. Thus, relative short stature in an obese 10-year-old could be a sign of possible endocrine disease.

Schneider MB. Obesity. In Neinstein LS, editor: *Adolescent Health Care*, ed 5, Philadelphia, 2008, Wolters Kluwer, pp 468.

45. **What percentage of obese teenage patients have an identifiable underlying pathologic cause for their obesity?**
5%. 3% have *endocrine* problems (hypothyroidism, Cushing syndrome, hypogonadism), and 2% have *uncommon syndromes* (such as Prader-Willi, Laurence-Moon-Biedl).

Schneider MB: Obesity. In Neinstein LS, editor: *Adolescent Health Care*, ed 5, Philadelphia, 2008, Wolters Kluwer, pp 468.

46. **What are the risk factors for obesity in teenagers?**
   - **Positive family history:** With one obese parent, probability of obesity is 30%; with two obese parents, this increases to 70% to 80%.
   - **Degree of obesity as a child:** More severe obesity is likely to persist.
   - **Socioeconomic status:** 10- to 17-year-olds living below the poverty line are 2½ times more likely to be overweight or obese.
   - **Television viewing:** Increased television viewing appears to correlate with a higher likelihood of obesity.
   - **Race:** Rates for Mexican-Americans are higher than for rates for blacks, which are higher than rates for whites.
   - **Family size:** Obesity decreases as family size increases; it has the greatest prevalence among single children.

Dietz WH, Robinson TN: Overweight children and adolescents, *N Engl J Med* 350:2100–2109, 2005.

47. **Are boys or girls more likely to remain obese teenagers throughout puberty?**
Girls. During puberty, body fat decreases by 40% in boys and increases by 40% in girls. Puberty leads to the normalization of body weight in 70% of obese males but in only 20% of obese females. Girls who have early menarche (age, ≤11 years) are twice as likely to become obese adults as are late maturers (age, ≥14 years). Girls also have significant declines in physical activity during adolescence.

48. **What morbidities can be associated with adolescent obesity?**
   - Hypertension
   - Lipid abnormalities
   - Apnea
   - Orthopedic problems (e.g., slipped epiphyses, Blount disease)
   - Gallstones
   - Steatohepatitis
   - Intracranial hypertension
   - Accelerated pubertal and skeletal development
   - Diabetes mellitus, type 2
   - Polycystic ovary syndrome

Fennoy I: Metabolic and respiratory comorbidities of childhood obesity, *Pediatr Ann* 39:140-146, 2010.

49. **What features constitute the metabolic syndrome?**
   - Central obesity (excessive fat around the abdomen)
   - Lipid abnormalities

- Hypertension
- Insulin resistance and/or glucose intolerance
- Prothrombotic state
- Proinflammatory state (elevated C-reactive protein)
  Well-described in adults with obesity, this constellation of biomarkers and risk factors for adverse cardiovascular outcomes has been increasingly recognized in adolescents. Its presence in adolescence increases the likelihood of cardiovascular disease in adulthood.

Morrison JA, Friedman LA, Gray-McGuire C: Metabolic syndrome in childhood predicts adult cardiovascular disease 25 years later, *Pediatrics* 120:340–345, 2007.

Weiss R, Dziura J, Burgert TS, et al: Obesity and the metabolic syndrome in children and adolescents, *N Engl J Med* 350:2362–2374, 2004.

50. **What features on physical examination are particularly important in the evaluation of the obese patient?**
    - Blood pressure (hypertension)
    - Facial dysmorphic features (evidence of genetic syndrome)
    - Tonsils (hypertrophy; potential for obstructive apnea)
    - Thyroid (goiter, possible hypothyroidism)
    - Acanthosis nigricans (type 2 diabetes)
    - Hirsutism (polycystic ovary syndrome)
    - Striae (Cushing syndrome)
    - Right upper quadrant (RUQ) tenderness (gallbladder disease)
    - Small hands and feet, cryptorchidism (Prader-Willi syndrome)
    - Limited hip range of motion (slipped capital femoral epiphysis)
    - Lower-leg bowing (Blount disease)

Eissa MAH: Overview of pediatric obesity: key points in the evaluation and therapy, *Consultant Pediatr* 2:293–296, 2003.

51. **Do obese children and adolescents become obese adults?**
    In most tracking studies, only 25% to 50% become obese adults. However, in some studies, this rate has ranged as high as 85%. The most important risk factors for persistence of obesity are later age of onset and increased severity of obesity at any age.

Dietz WH, Bellizzi MC: Overweight children and adolescents, *N Engl J Med* 352:2100, 2005.

KEY POINTS: OBESITY

1. Obesity: Most common chronic condition in children.

2. Obesity and short stature—think thyroid abnormalities and evaluate thyroid-stimulating hormone and T_4 levels.

3. Only 5% of obese children have an identifiable underlying pathologic cause.

4. If a child is at risk as a result of family history, the earlier the modifications (e.g., limiting television time), the better.

5. Keep weight reduction or stabilization goals reasonable; if too unrealistic, discouragement and weight cycling are more likely.

52. **What is the long-term outlook for the obese teenager?**
Obesity in adolescence is associated with *medical*, *economic*, and *social* consequences. Obese teenagers, especially females, have lower rates of school completion, lower rates of marriage, lower household incomes, and higher rates of poverty. Even if weight corrections occur later, the early obesity is associated with increased atherosclerotic heart disease in men and women, with colorectal cancer and gout in men, and with arthritis in women.

Schwimmer JB, Burwinkle TM, Varni JW: Health-related quality of life of severely obese children and adolescents, *JAMA* 289:1813–1819, 2003.

53. **How effective are intervention and treatment for obesity in adolescents?**
Weight-reduction regimens involving behavior modification and dietary therapy are modestly effective with regard to short-term results, but they are notoriously ineffective for the achievement of long-term weight loss.

Appetite suppressants are uncommonly used in adolescents owing to problems of side effects and limited data on efficacy. Gastric bypass and banding (bariatric surgery) can be considered for those with a BMI higher than 40, particularly if associated with complicating problems such as diabetes mellitus or sleep apnea.

Wilfley DE, Stein RI, Saelens BE, et al: Efficacy of maintenance treatment approaches for childhood overweight: a randomized controlled trial. *JAMA* 298:1661–1673, 2007.

Dietz WH: What constitutes successful weight management in adolescents? *Ann Intern Med* 145:81–90, 2006.

SEXUAL DEVELOPMENT

54. **What is Tanner staging for boys?**
In 1969 and 1970, Dr. James Tanner categorized the progression of stages of puberty, dividing pubertal development in boys into pubic and genital development (Table 1-2).

TABLE 1-2. TANNER STAGING FOR BOYS	
Stage	**Description**
Pubic Hair	
I	None
II	Countable; straight; increased pigmentation and length; primarily at base of penis
III	Darker; begins to curl; increased quantity
IV	Increased quantity; coarser texture; covers most of pubic area
V	Adult distribution; spread to medial thighs and lower abdomen
Genital Development	
I	Prepubertal
II	Testicular enlargement (>4 mL volume); slight rugation of scrotum
III	Further testicular enlargement; penile lengthening begins
IV	Testicular enlargement continues; increased rugation of scrotum; increased penile breadth
V	Adult

55. **What is the normal progression of sexual development and growth for boys during puberty?**
Nearly all boys begin puberty with testicular enlargement. This is followed in about 6 months by pubic hair and then about 6 to 12 months later by phallic enlargement. For boys, puberty lasts an average of 3.5 years and begins an average of 2 years later than it does in girls (Fig. 1-1).

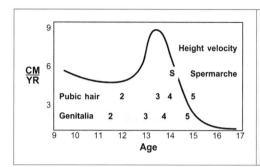

Figure 1-1. Summary of pubertal development in boys. (From Rosen DS: Physiologic growth and development during adolescence. Pediatr Rev 25:194–200, 2004.)

56. **What are the ranges of normal in the stages of pubertal development in girls?**
Tanner divided pubertal development in girls according to pubic hair and breast development (Table 1-3).

TABLE 1-3. TANNER STAGES FOR GIRLS	
Stage	Description
Pubic Hair	
I	None
II	Countable; straight; increased pigmentation and length; primarily on medial border of labia
III	Darker; begins to curl; increased quantity on mons pubis
IV	Increased quantity; coarser texture; labia and mons well covered
V	Adult distribution with feminine triangle and spread to medial thighs
Breast Development	
I	Prepubertal
II	Breast bud present; increased areolar size
III	Further enlargement of breast; no secondary contour
IV	Areolar area forms secondary mound on breast contour
V	Mature; areolar area is part of breast contour; nipple projects

57. **What is the normal progression of sexual development and growth for girls during puberty?**
About 85% of girls begin puberty with the initiation of breast enlargement, whereas 15% have axillary hair as the first sign. Menarche usually occurs about 18 to 24 months after the onset of breast development. For girls, the duration of puberty is about 4.5 years, which is longer than that of boys (Fig. 1-2).

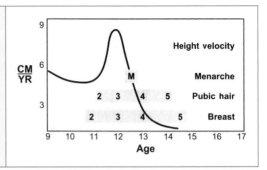

Figure 1-2. Summary of pubertal development in girls. (From Rosen DS: Physiologic growth and development during adolescence. Pediatr Rev 25:198, 2004.)

58. **Has the age of menarche declined in the United States during the past 80 years?**
Survey data of women from aged 20 to 80 years do indicate a decline over this time period of about 15 months for black girls, 12 months for Mexican-American girls, and 10 months for white girls. A variety of factors may be contributing, including environmental (dietary changes and increasing obesity), socioeconomic, and genetic.

   McDowell MA, Brody DJ, Hughes JP: Has age at menarche changed? Results from the National Health and Nutrition Examination Survey (NHANES), *J Adolesc Health* 40:227–231, 2007.

59. **When do boys develop the ability to reproduce?**
The average age of **spermarche** (as demonstrated by the presence of spermatozoa in the first morning urine) is 13.3 years. Unlike what occurs in girls (in whom menarche follows the peak height velocity), in boys, spermarche occurs before the growth spurt.

60. **When is delayed sexual development a concern?**
Boys who are 14 years of age without testicular enlargement (>4 mL) or pubic hair and girls who are 13 years without signs of breast development are considered to have delayed puberty. By definition, this is about 2.5% of healthy teens in the United States (2.5 standard deviations below the mean). In girls with immature breast development, lack of menarche by age 15 years or within 5 years of onset of puberty is also considered abnormal. A girl with normal breast and pubic hair development but no menarche by age 16 years more properly has primary amenorrhea.

61. **Why should the sense of smell be tested in a teenager with delayed puberty?**
Kallmann syndrome is characterized by a defect in GnRH with resultant gonadotropin deficiency and hypogonadism. Maldevelopment of the olfactory lobes occurs, with resultant anosmia or hyposmia. Less commonly, cleft palate, congenital deafness, and color blindness can occur. These patients require hormonal therapy to achieve puberty and fertility.

62. **What is the most common cause of delayed puberty?**
Constitutional delay of growth and maturity, the cause in 70% to 90% of cases, is a form of hypogonadotropic hypogonadism, in which there is delayed secretion of GnRH and activation of the gonadal axis. There is often a family history of late-onset puberty indicating a strong genetic component. Children often are small for their age (5%) but have grown steadily. Bone age is delayed.

63. **What features suggest constitutional delay of puberty?**
- Family history of delayed puberty
- Often short (3rd to 25th percentile) compared with peers

- Growth velocity slowed (4 to 7 cm/year) compared with same-age, same-sex peers (8 to 11 cm/year)
- Bone age delayed (from 1.5 to 4 years) compared with chronologic age
- Normal prepubertal anatomy, sense of smell, prepubertal LH, FSH levels

64. **Which laboratory tests should you consider in a boy or girl with delayed puberty?**

If history or physical examination does not suggest an underlying cause (e.g., anorexia nervosa, chronic disease), tests should include **LH, FSH, testosterone** (male), and **bone age**. These tests help categorize the condition as *hypergonadotropic* with increased GnRH, LSH, and LH (implying possible gonadal defects, androgen insensitivity, or enzyme defects) or *hypogonadotropic* with decreased GnRH and low to normal FSH and LH (implying constitutional delay or primary hypothalamic-pituitary problems). Most cases involve decreased GnRH.

Further testing is predicated on the results of these initial tests. For example, a 14.5-year-old male with a bone age of 11.5 years and a total testosterone of 23 ng/dL (normal prepubertal level is <10 ng/dL) will probably begin to show outward evidence of puberty within the subsequent few months. Therefore, no further studies are warranted. On the other hand, if this boy has a bone age of 12.5 years, a testosterone level of less than 10 ng/dL, and no elevation of FH and LSH, specific testing of the hypothalamic-pituitary axis is indicated.

65. **What is the most common cause of primary gonadal failure in boys?**

Klinefelter syndrome. The frequency of this condition is 1 in every 500 to 1000 males. It is characterized in adolescence by gynecomastia and small, firm testes with seminiferous tubule dysgenesis, and it is found in more than 80% of XXY males (i.e., males with 47 chromosomes). Levels of FSH and LH are elevated in these patients.

66. **Can puberty be safely accelerated?**

In some teenagers—more commonly boys—the constitutional delay in puberty has significant psychological effects. Studies have shown that, in *boys*, puberty can be accelerated without any compromise in expected adult height. In boys older than 14 years with plasma testosterone levels of less than 10 ng/dL, 50 to 200 mg of intramuscular testosterone enanthate can be given every 2 to 4 weeks for 4 to 6 months. Treatment for *girls* who are constitutionally delayed is less well studied. Conjugated estrogen (0.3 mg [e.g., Premarin]) or micronized estradiol (0.5 mg) orally daily or transdermal estradiol, 12.5-25 mcg daily for 4 to 6 months has been used in girls older than 13 years without breast buds.

Kaplowitz PB: Delayed puberty, *Pediatr Rev* 31:189-195, 2010.

KEY POINTS: SEXUAL DEVELOPMENT

1. If no signs of puberty by age 13 in girls and age 14 in boys, evaluate for an underlying pathologic medical cause.

2. Most cases of late puberty are constitutional (genetic) delay.

3. Nearly all boys begin puberty with testicular enlargement; 85% of girls begin puberty with breast enlargement.

4. Gynecomastia occurs in up to 50% to 75% of boys during Tanner genital stages II and III.

5. Mean time between the onset of breast development and menarche is slightly more than 2 years.

67. **How do you evaluate a breast lump noted by a teenage girl on self-examination?**

Although the incidence of cancerous lesions is extremely low in adolescents, it is not zero, and breast lumps do require careful evaluation. *Fibrocystic changes* (i.e., the proliferation of stromal and epithelial elements, ductal dilation, cyst formation) are common in later adolescence and are characterized by variations in size and tenderness with menstrual periods. The most common tumor (70% to 95%) is a fibroadenoma, which is a firm, discrete, rubbery, smooth mass that is usually found laterally. Other causes of masses include lipomas, hematomas, abscesses, simple cysts, and rarely, adenocarcinoma (especially if a bloody nipple discharge is present).

The size, location, and other characteristics of a mass should be documented and reevaluated over the next one to three menstrual periods. A persistent or slowly growing mass should be evaluated with *fine-needle aspiration*. *Ultrasound* can be helpful for distinguishing cystic from solid masses. *Mammography* is a very poor tool for identifying distinct pathologic lesions in teenagers because the breast density of adolescents makes interpretation difficult.

Huppert JS, Zidenberg N: Breast disorders in females. In Slap GB, editor: *Adolescent Medicine: The Requisites in Pediatrics*, Philadelphia, 2008, Mosby Elsevier, pp 146–151.

68. **Should breast self-examination be taught and emphasized for all teenage girls?**

Because the incidence of malignancy is very low in this age group, no data support benefits for breast self-examination, and indeed it may cause unnecessary anxiety and testing. Exceptions would be all adolescents with a history of malignancy, those who have had radiation therapy to the chest more than 10 years ago, and adolescents 18 to 21 years old whose mothers carry the *BRCA1* or *BRCA2* gene.

Huppert JS, Zidenberg N: Breast disorders in females. In Slap GB, editor: *Adolescent Medicine: The Requisites in Pediatrics*, Philadelphia, 2008, Mosby Elsevier, p 150.

SEXUALLY TRANSMITTED INFECTIONS

69. **How does the prevalence of sexually transmitted infections (STIs) in adolescents compare with that of adults?**

Among sexually active people, adolescents have a **higher likelihood** than adults of being infected with an STI. About 25% of adolescents contract at least one STI by the time of high school graduation. Reasons for the increased susceptibility include the following:

- Cervical ectropion: *Neisseria gonorrhoeae* and *Chlamydia trachomatis* more readily infect columnar epithelium, and the adolescent ectocervix has more of this type of epithelium than does that of an adult.
- Cervical metaplasia in the transformation zone (from columnar to squamous epithelium) is more susceptible to human papillomavirus (HPV) infection.
- There is less frequent use of barrier methods of contraception among this population.

70. **What is the best way to screen for STIs?**

The gold standard for STIs, particularly in any case of possible sexual abuse, is **culture**. However, nonculture techniques, particularly involving nucleic acid amplification tests (NAATs), such as polymerase chain reaction or transcription-mediated amplification, are widely used and widely studied, primarily for chlamydial and gonococcal infections.

Advantages of NAATs include more rapid results and less invasiveness. Disadvantages include higher costs and lack of antibiotic sensitivity testing.

71. **What should be the screening practice for STIs in male adolescents?**
National recommendations for heterosexual males who are sexually active are less explicit because of uncertainties related to cost-effectiveness and public health benefits. Screening for *N. gonorrhoeae* and *C. trachomatis* should be considered for high-risk males (multiple partners, inconsistent condom use). Universal screening for human immunodeficiency virus (HIV) is recommended. For males who have had sex with males, CDC recommendations include annual HIV and syphilis serology. Annual or more frequent screening should be based on specific sexual practices.

Holland-Hall C: Sexually transmitted infections in teens, *Contemp Pediatr* 25:56–65, 2008.

Centers for Disease Control and Prevention: Revised recommendations for HIV testing of adults, adolescents and pregnant women in health-care settings, *Mortal Morb Wkly Rep* 5:1, 2008.

72. **What is the most common STI in sexually active teenage males?**
Urethritis, both gonococcal and nongonococcal. Nongonococcal urethritis, particularly due to *C. trachomatis*, is more common and is often asymptomatic. Other less common causes of nongonococcal urethritis include *Ureaplasma urealyticum*, *Trichomonas vaginalis*, herpes simplex, HPV, and yeast.

73. **What should be the screening practice for STIs in female adolescents?**
For all sexually active females younger than 25 years, the U.S. Preventive Services Task Force recommends screening *annually* for *C. trachomatis* and *N. gonorrhoeae*. Other experts recommend screening annually for *T. vaginalis* infections as well. Females at higher risk, such as those with previous infections, irregular condom use, or multiple partners, may require screening more frequently. Universal screening for HIV is recommended. Screening for syphilis and hepatitis B is on a case-by-case basis. Screening for herpes is not recommended.

Holland-Hall C: Sexually transmitted infections in teens, *Contemp Pediatr* 25:56–65, 2008.

Centers for Disease Control and Prevention: Revised recommendations for HIV testing of adults, adolescents and pregnant women in health-care settings, *Mortal Morb Wkly Rep* 55:1, 2008.

74. **Are pelvic examinations with specula always required to obtain specimens for possible STIs in teenagers?**
Trends in screening for STIs in teenage girls are shifting from endocervical sampling to urine-based and vaginal swab collection because:
- Urine testing for chlamydia and gonorrhea using nucleic acid amplification techniques approaches the sensitivity and specificity of specimens obtained using a speculum.
- Vaginal specimens obtained without the use of a speculum have a high screening validity for trichomonas, bacterial vaginosis, and yeast infections.
- Self-collection by teenagers of vaginal specimens have yielded comparable results compared with physician-obtained cervical specimens when nucleic acid amplification testing was used.

Fang J, Husman C, DeSilva L, et al: Evaluation of self-collected vaginal swab, first void urine, and endocervical swab specimens for the detection of *Chlamydia trachomatis* and *Neisseria gonorrhoeae* in adolescent females, *J Pediatr Adolesc Gynecol* 21:355–360, 2008.

75. **Which STI is most closely linked to cervical cancer?**
Human papillomavirus. HPV affects 20% to 40% of sexually active adolescent females. More than 100 HPV types have been identified, of which about 40% are known to infect the genital tract. They differ in their likelihood of leading to cancer. High-risk HPV includes types

16 and 18. Because of this association, the quadrivalent vaccine Gardasil and the bivalent vaccine Cervarix have been recommended by the Advisory Committee on Immunization Practices for adolescent females beginning at the 11 to 12-year visit.

76. **What are the presentations of HPV infections?**
Presentations of HPV are typically **subclinical** but can include **anogenital condyloma acuminatum** and **cervical infection,** which may lead to cervical dysplasia. HPV is also a cause of nonsexually transmitted disease, including **deep plantar warts, palmar warts,** and **common warts.** When compared with older adults, studies have demonstrated that the natural history of cervical HPV infection in teenage girls is for spontaneous clearing of both the low-risk types (90%) and the high-risk types (75%) over a 6- to 8-month period.

77. **When are Pap smears indicated in teenagers?**
The American Cancer Society recommends a Pap screen within 3 years after the initiation of sexual activity or by age 21 years, whichever comes first, with follow-up frequency dependent on cytology and HPV DNA testing. This reflects the high rates of regression of both HPV infection and abnormal cytology (particularly low-grade squamous intraepithelial lesions) in adolescents.

Greydanus DE, Omar H, Patel DR: Cervical cancer screening in adolescents, *Pediatr Rev* 30:23–25, 2009.

78. **Is the presence of an ectropion noted on pelvic examination a concern?**
An **ectropion** is the outward rolling of a margin. A cervical ectropion is the extension of the erythematous columnar epithelium from the os onto the duller, pink cervix. It is a relatively common finding in adolescents. However, large ectropions extending to the vaginal wall or an abnormal cervical shape can be associated with diethylstilbestrol exposure *in utero* or chronic cervicitis.

79. **Describe the appearance of condylomata acuminata.**
Condyloma acuminata (anogenital warts) are soft, fleshy, wet, polypoid or pedunculated papules that appear in the genital and perianal area (Fig. 1-3). They may coalesce and take on a cauliflower-like appearance. Visualization of anogenital warts can be enhanced by wetting the area with 3% to 5% acetic acid (vinegar), which whitens the lesions.

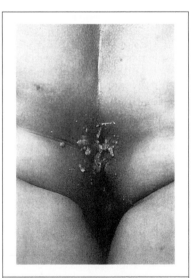

Figure 1-3. Perianal condylomata acuminata. (From Gates RH: Infectious Disease Secrets, 2nd ed. Philadelphia, Hanley & Belfus, 2003, p 221.)

80. **What is the natural history of genital warts?**
Left untreated, 40% of genital warts may spontaneously resolve, but the timing is unpredictable (months to years). The lesions are not oncogenic and will not progress to malignancy. Treatment, often done for cosmetic purposes or symptoms of itching or burning, consists of topical products (Podofilox 0.5% solution or Imiquimod 5% cream), cryotherapy, or surgical removal. Recurrence rates can be as high as one third.

81. **What are pearly penile papules?**
This is a common condition in teenage males and is often misdiagnosed as condylomas. Multiple smooth, round, skin-colored papules develop most commonly at the corona of the glans penis and histologically are angiofibromas. These are benign and have no association with papillomavirus.

Kluger N, Dereure O: Penile papules. *N Engl J Med* 360:1336, 2009.

82. **What is the typical presentation of chlamydial genital infections in both female and male teenagers?**
Most are **asymptomatic,** which can persist for several months. In females with symptoms, the disease should be suspected if vaginal discharge and bleeding are noted, especially after intercourse; this may be due to endocervical friability. In males, the most typical symptoms are dysuria and a penile discharge.

Peipert JF: Genital chlamydial infections, *N Engl J Med* 349:2424–2430, 2003.

83. **A sexually active 17-year-old girl with adnexal and RUQ tenderness probably has what condition?**
Fitz-Hugh-Curtis syndrome. This is an infectious perihepatitis that is caused by gonococci or, less commonly, by chlamydiae. It should be suspected in any patient with pelvic inflammatory disease (PID) who has RUQ tenderness. It may be mistaken for acute hepatitis or cholecystitis. The pathophysiology is thought to be the direct spread from a pelvic infection along the paracolic gutters to the liver, where inflammation develops and capsular adhesions form (the so-called violin-string adhesions seen on surgical exploration). If RUQ pain persists despite treatment for PID, ultrasonography should be done to rule out a perihepatic abscess.

84. **A teenage girl develops migratory polyarthritis, fever, and scattered petechial lesions several days before menses. What condition should be suspected?**
Gonococcal-arthritis-dermatitis syndrome (GADS). After a migratory polyarthritis or polyarthralgia, the arthritis settles in one or two large joints. The patient then develops painful tenosynovitis over the tendon sheaths in addition to a characteristic crop of embolic skin lesions over the trunk and extremities. Diagnosis is confirmed by culturing gonococci from blood, synovial fluid, and/or rectal or genitourinary sites.

85. **What is the typical appearance of *N. gonorrhoeae* on Gram stain?**
Intracellular gram-negative diplococci (Fig. 1-4).

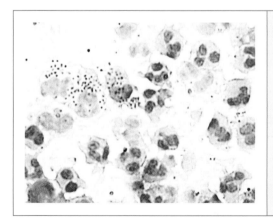

Figure 1-4. Gram stain of *Neisseria gonorrhoeae*. (From Gates RH: Infectious Disease Secrets, 2nd ed. Philadelphia, Hanley & Belfus, 2003, p 207.)

KEY POINTS: SEXUALLY TRANSMITTED INFECTIONS

1. Regardless of the pathogen, most STIs in adolescents are asymptomatic.

2. Nucleic acid amplification tests for chlamydia and gonorrhea are particularly useful when screening for urethritis in males and cervicitis in females.

3. STI screening in girls is shifting from endocervical sampling to urine-based and vaginal swab collection.

4. The most common STI in adolescent males is urethritis due to *Chlamydia trachomatis*.

5. Despite higher rates of STIs being found among adolescents than any other age group, clinicians frequently do not inquire about sexual activity, risk factors, or means of reducing risks.

86. **What is the minimal criteria for the diagnosis of Pelvic inflammatory disease (PID)?**
Any one of the following must be present:
- Uterine tenderness
- Cervical motion tenderness
- Adnexal tenderness

87. **What additional criteria support the diagnosis of PID?**
- Oral temperature higher than 38.3°C (101°F)
- Abnormal cervical or vaginal discharge (with leukocytes > epithelial cells)
- Elevated erythrocyte sedimentation rate (usually >15 mm/hour)
- Elevated C-reactive protein
- Cervical infection with *N. gonorrhoeae* or *C. trachomatis*

Because no single clinical aspect or laboratory test is definitive for PID, a constellation of findings is used to support the diagnosis.

Centers for Disease Control and Prevention: Sexually transmitted diseases treatment guidelines, *Mortal Morb Wkly Rep* 55:48, 2002.

88. **How is the diagnosis of PID definitively made?**
- **Endometrial biopsy** with histopathologic evidence of endometritis (rarely done in teenagers due to low likelihood of endometrial cancer)
- **Transvaginal** or **abdominal ultrasonography** revealing tubo-ovarian abscess or fallopian tube abnormalities (e.g., thickened, fluid-filled fallopian tubes with or without free pelvic fluid)
- **Laparoscopy** revealing abnormalities consistent with PID

American Academy of Pediatrics: Pelvic inflammatory disease. In Pickering LK, editor: *2009 Red Book*, ed 28, Elk Grove Village, IL, 2009, American Academy of Pediatrics, pp 501–502.

89. **What are the sequelae of PID?**
Twenty-five percent of patients with a history of PID will have one or more major sequelae of the disease, including the following:
- Tubo-ovarian abscess
- Recurrent infection
- Chronic abdominal pain: May include exacerbated dysmenorrhea and dyspareunia related to pelvic adhesions in about 20% of patients with PID
- Ectopic pregnancy: Risk is increased threefold to sevenfold
- Infertility: Up to 11% after one episode of PID, 30% after two episodes, and 55% after three or more episodes

Bortot AT, Risser WL, Cromwell, PF: Coping with pelvic inflammatory disease in the adolescent, *Contemp Pediatr* 21:33–48, 2004.

90. **Which adolescents with PID should be hospitalized for intravenous antibiotics?**
    Those with any of the following conditions:
    - Surgical emergency (e.g., appendicitis or ectopic pregnancy [or if such a diagnosis cannot be excluded])
    - Severe illness (e.g., overt peritonitis, vomiting)
    - Tubo-ovarian abscess
    - Pregnancy
    - High suspicion for unreliable compliance or timely follow-up within 72 hours
    - Failure of outpatient therapy

    American Academy of Pediatrics: Pelvic inflammatory disease. In Pickering LK, editor: *2009 Red Book*, ed 28, Elk Grove Village, IL, 2009, American Academy of Pediatrics, p 502.

KEY POINTS: PELVIC INFLAMMATORY DISEASE

1. The highest rate of PID occurs in adolescents.

2. No single clinical aspect or laboratory test is definitive for PID.

3. Key clinical finding: adnexal, cervical motion, or lower abdominal tenderness.

4. Cultures are often negative in PID because the disease is in the upper genital tract, but specimens; however, specimens are obtained from the lower tract.

5. Ectopic pregnancy can mimic PID.

6. Hospitalization: Indicated for patients with PID with surgical emergencies, severe illness, immunodeficiency, pregnancy, unreliable compliance, or failure of outpatient therapy.

91. **How do symptoms of infectious endocervicitis vary in relation to menses?**
    Gonorrhea is much more likely to present *during menstruation*. Of patients with gonorrhea, 85% develop symptoms during the first 7 days of menses, compared with only 33% of patients with chlamydial infections.

92. **How are the genital ulcer syndromes differentiated?**
    Genital ulcers may be seen in herpes simplex, syphilis, chancroid, lymphogranuloma venereum, and granuloma inguinale (donovanosis). Herpes and syphilis are the most common, and granuloma inguinale is very rare. Although there is overlap, clinical distinction is summarized in Table 1-4.

93. **What are risk factors for the acquisition of genital ulcer disease?**
    - Male
    - Lack of circumcision
    - High-risk sexual behaviors (men having sex with men have sixfold increased risk)
    - Infection with HIV

    Braverman PK: Genital ulcer disease: herpes simplex virus, syphilis, and chancroid. In Slap GB, editor: *Adolescent Medicine: The Requisites in Pediatrics*, Philadelphia, 2008, Mosby Elsevier, p 211.

TABLE 1-4. DIFFERENTIATION OF GENITAL ULCER SYNDROMES

	Herpes Simplex	Syphilis (Primary, Secondary)	Chancroid	Lymphogranuloma Venereum
Agent	Herpes simplex virus	*Treponema pallidum*	*Haemophilus ducreyi*	*Chlamydia trachomatis*
Primary lesions	Vesicle	Papule	Papule-pustule	Papule-vesicle
Size (mm)	1-2	5-15	2-20	2-10
Number	Multiple, clusters (coalesce ±)	Single	Multiple (coalesce ±)	Single
Depth	Superficial	Superficial or deep	Deep	Superficial or deep
Base	Erythematous, nonpurulent	Sharp, indurated, nonpurulent	Ragged border, purulent, friable	Varies
Pain	Yes	No	Yes	No
Lymphadenopathy	Tender, bilateral	Nontender, bilateral	Tender, unilateral, may suppurate, unilocular fluctuance	Tender, unilateral, may suppurate, multilocular fluctuance

From Shafer MA: Sexually transmitted disease syndromes. In McAnarmey ER, Kreipe RE, Orr DP, Comerci GD (eds): Textbook of Adolescent Medicine. Philadelphia, W.B. Saunders, 1992, p 708.

94. **How do recurrent episodes of genital herpes simplex infections compare with the primary episode?**
    - Usually less severe, with faster resolution
    - Less likely to have prodromal symptoms (buttock, leg, or hip pain or tingling)
    - Less likely to have neurologic complications (e.g., aseptic meningitis)
    - More likely to have asymptomatic infections
    - Duration of viral shedding is shorter (4 versus 11 days)

    Kimberlin DW, Rouse DJ: Genital herpes, *N Engl J Med* 350:1970–1977, 2004.

95. **How are the three most common causes of postpubertal vaginitis clinically distinguished?**
    Candidal vaginitis: Vulvar itching and erythema, vaginal discharge (thick, white, curdlike)
    Trichomonal vaginitis: Vulvar itching and erythema, vaginal discharge (gray, yellow-green, frothy; rarely malodorous)
    Bacterial vaginosis: Minimal erythema, vaginal discharge (malodorous; thin white discharge clings to vaginal walls)

96. **How does the vaginal pH help indicate the cause of a vaginal discharge?**
    Ordinarily, the vaginal pH of a pubertal girl is less than 4.5 (compared with 7.0 in prepubertal girls). If the pH is greater than 4.5, infection with trichomonal or bacterial vaginosis should be suspected.

97. **How does evaluation of the vaginal discharge help to identify the etiology?**
    See Table 1-5.

TABLE 1-5. EVALUATION OF VAGINAL DISCHARGE			
	Candidal Vaginitis	**Trichomonal Vaginitis**	**Bacterial Vaginosis**
pH	≤4.5	>4.5	>4.5
KOH prep	Mycelia pseudohyphae	Normal	Fishy odor (positive "whiff" test)
NaCl prep	Few WBCs	Many WBCs; motile trichomonads	Few WBCs

KOH = potassium hydroxide, NaCl = sodium chloride (salt), WBCs = white blood cells.

98. **How is trichomoniasis diagnosed?**
    Wet mount microscopy and **culture.** Rapid antigen tests are also becoming available for the protozoan *T. vaginalis.* For a wet mount, a sample of vaginal fluid is rolled onto a glass slide, and normal saline is added; look for the lashing flagella and jerky motility of the trichomonads (Fig. 1-5). Although inexpensive and offering immediate results, wet mount studies are positive in only about two thirds of culture-positive trichomonal infections.

    Gallion HR, Dupree LJ, Scott TA, et al: Diagnosis of *Trichomonas vaginalis* in female children and adolescents evaluated for possible sexual abuse: a comparison of the InPouch *Trichomonas vaginalis* culture method and wet mount microscopy. *J Pediatr Adolesc Gynecol* 32:300–305, 2009.

99. **What are "clue cells"?**
    Clue cells are vaginal squamous epithelial cells to which many bacteria are attached. This gives the cell a stippled appearance when viewed in a normal saline preparation (Fig. 1-6). Clue cells are characteristic—but not diagnostic—of bacterial vaginosis.

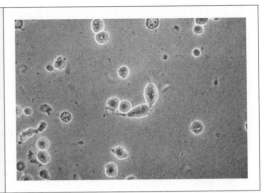

Figure 1-5. Wet mount of vaginal secretions with leukocytes and flagellated trichomonads. (From Mandell GL, Bennett JE, Dolin R [eds]: Principles and Practice of Infectious Diseases, 6th ed. Philadelphia, Churchill Livingstone, 2004, p. 1361.)

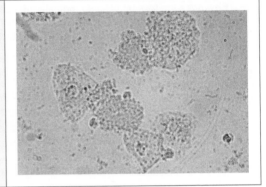

Figure 1-6. "Clue cells" are squamous cells with folded cytoplasm and numerous bacteria (typically *Gardnerella vaginalis*) attached to their surface. (From Mandell GL, Bennett JE, Dolin R [eds]: Principles and Practice of Infectious Diseases, 6th ed. Philadelphia, Churchill Livingstone, 2004, p. 1366.)

100. What is the etiology of bacterial vaginosis?

Formerly called nonspecific, *Gardnerella*, or *Haemophilus* vaginitis, bacterial vaginosis is the replacement of normal vaginal lactobacilli with a variety of bacteria, including *Gardnerella vaginalis*, genital mycoplasmas, and an overgrowth of anaerobic species. *G. vaginalis* can be found in small numbers in up to 30% of nonsexually active adolescents, so vaginal cultures are of limited value.

101. How common is bacterial vaginosis in prepubertal girls?

Very uncommon. A clinical diagnosis of bacterial vaginosis in this patient population should prompt evaluation for the possibility of sexual abuse.

102. What are the criteria for the diagnosis of bacterial vaginosis?

Clinical diagnosis requires three of the four following criteria (Amsel criteria):
- Homogeneous thin white or gray homogeneous vaginal discharge
- Discharge pH greater than 4.5
- On wet mount, more than 20% of cells are clue cells
- Positive "whiff" test: addition of 10% KOH to discharge results in fishy odor

Hwang LY, Shafer M-A: Vaginitis and vaginosis. In Neinstein LS, editor: *Adolescent Health Care*, ed 5, Philadelphia, 2008, Wolters Kluwer, pp 728–729.

103. **Is there an effective treatment for bacterial vaginosis?**
Optimal management remains unclear. Acceptable treatment options include oral metronidazole (Flagyl), 0.75% metronidazole gel, or 2% clindamycin cream. Treatment failure is about 15%. Relapse rates as high as 30% may occur within 3 months.

SUBSTANCE ABUSE

104. **What are the stages of alcohol and drug abuse by teenagers?**
Stage 1: **Potential for abuse** (decreased impulse control, peer pressure, ready availability)
Stage 2: **Experimentation** (learning the euphoria; few consequences, little behavior change)
Stage 3: **Regular use** (seeking the euphoria; increased frequency; use alone; buying or stealing drugs)
Stage 4: **Regular use** (preoccupation with the "high"; daily use, loss of control, risk taking, estrangement from "sober" friends)
Stage 5: **Burnout** (use of drugs to feel normal; multiple addictions, physical and mental deterioration, self-destructive behavior)

Barangan CJ, Alderman EM: Management of substance abuse, *Pediatr Rev* 23:123–130, 2002.

105. **What are the categories of abused drugs?**
- **Sedative-hypnotics:** Alcohol, barbiturates, benzodiazepines, γ-hydroxybutyrate, flunitrazepam (Rohypnol), other sedatives
- **Stimulants:** Caffeine, cocaine, amphetamines, decongestants
- **Tobacco**
- **Cannabinoids:** Marijuana, hashish
- **Opioids:** Heroin, opium, pharmaceutical opioid painkillers, methadone, oxycodone (OxyContin)
- **Hallucinogens:** Lysergic acid diethylamide (LSD), phencyclidine, mescaline, psilocybin, hallucinogenic mushrooms, ecstasy
- **Inhalants:** Aliphatic, halogenated, and aromatic hydrocarbons; nitrous oxide; ketones; esters
- **Steroids**

Liepman MR, Calles JL, Kizilbash L, et al: Genetic and nongenetic factors influencing substance abuse by adolescents, *Adolesc Med* 13:375–401, 2002.

106. **What is the CRAFFT screen?**
This is a six-item screening test for adolescent substance abuse. Two or more "yes" answers indicate more than 90% sensitivity and more than 80% specificity for significant substance abuse. A number of screening instruments are available for interviewing adolescents, and the search for alcohol or drug use should be part of routine medical care.
- **C**ar: Have you driven a car (or ridden with a driver) under the influence of drugs or alcohol?
- **R**elax: Do you use drugs or alcohol to relax, feel better, or fit in?
- **A**lone: Do you use drugs or alcohol while you are alone?
- **F**orget: Do you sometimes forget what you did while using drugs or alcohol?
- **F**amily/Friends: Do they ever tell you to cut down on drug or alcohol use?
- **T**rouble: Have you gotten into trouble when using drugs or alcohol?

American Academy of Pediatrics, Committee on Substance Abuse: policy statement—alcohol use by youth and adolescents: a pediatric concern, *Pediatrics* 125: 1078-1087, 2010.

107. **What are characteristic physical signs of illicit drug use?**
See Table 1-6.

TABLE 1-6. PHYSICAL SIGNS OF ILLICIT DRUG USE

Physical Sign	Drug of Abuse
Hypothermia	Phencyclidine, ketamine
Hyperthermia	Mescaline, LSD
Increased heart rate	Amphetamine, cocaine, marijuana, MDMA (ecstasy), LSD
Increased blood pressure	Amphetamine, cocaine, phencyclidine, MDMA, LSD
Decreased gag reflex	Heroin, morphine, oxycodone, other opiates, benzodiazepines
Conjunctival redness	Marijuana
Pinpoint pupils	Heroin, morphine, oxycodone, other opiates
Sluggish pupillary response	Barbiturates
Irritation/ulceration of nasal mucosa	Intranasal cocaine, heroin, inhalants
Oral sores/burns, perioral pyodermas	Inhalants
Cutaneous scars ("tracks")	Intravenous use
Gynecomastia, small testes	Marijuana
Subcutaneous fat necrosis	Intravenous and intradermal use
Tattoos in antecubital fossa	Intravenous use
Skin abscesses and cellulitis	Intravenous and intradermal use

Kaul P, Coupey SM: Clinical evaluation of substance abuse, Pediatr Rev 23:85–94, 2002.

108. **Should an adolescent be screened for drug abuse without his or her consent?**
This is an area of contention. The official position of the American Academy of Pediatrics is that testing should not be done without consent in a competent older adolescent, even if a parent wishes otherwise. Others have argued that a teenager's right to privacy and confidentiality does not supersede potential risks for serious damage from drug abuse, particularly if there is strong clinical suspicion or parental concern. The legal ramifications are evolving and vary from state to state. In 1995, the U.S. Supreme Court ruled that random drug testing of high-school athletes was legal.

109. **A teenager who is being screened for drug abuse submits a suspicious urine specimen for testing. How can you tell if it is urine?**
- pH should be between 4.6 and 8.0.
- Temperature should range between 90.5°F and 98.6°F (32.5°C to 37°C).
- Urine submitted at body temperature will exceed 90.5°F (32.5°C) for 15 to 20 minutes. If the temperature is below this level during the first 4 minutes, the specimen should be considered suspect.
- Urine creatinine concentration should exceed 0.2 mg/mL.
- Urine specific gravity should be not less than 1.003.

110. **How long do illicit drugs remain detectable in urine specimens?**
There is variability depending on a patient's hydration status and method of intake, but, as a rule, metabolites can be detected after ingestion, as shown in Table 1-7. Most urine screens are very sensitive and may detect drugs up to 99% of the time in concentrations

established as analytic cut-off points. However, the screens can be much less specific, sometimes with false-positive rates of up to 35%. Therefore, second tests using the analytic methodology most specific for the suspected drug should be used.

TABLE 1-7. DETECTION OF ILLICIT DRUG METABOLITES	
Alcohol	7-12 hours
Amphetamines	48 hours
Barbiturates (short acting)	24 hours
Benzodiazepines (short acting)	3 days
Cocaine	2-4 days
Marijuana	3 days for light smoker; >30 days for heavy smoker
Morphine	48-72 hours
Oxycodone	2-4 days
Phencyclidine	8 days

Moeller KE, Lee KC, Kissack JC: Urine drug screening: practical guide for clinicians, Mayo Clin Proc 83:66–76, 2008.

111. **What is the genetic predisposition of alcoholism?**
A male child of an alcoholic father is four times more likely to become alcoholic than a child with a nonalcoholic father. If a monozygotic twin is alcoholic, the likelihood of the other twin becoming alcoholic is 55%; for dizygotic twins, the likelihood is 25%.

112. **Which type of substance abuse is more common in younger adolescents than older adolescents?**
Inhalants. In some surveys, up to 20% of 8th graders report recent use of inhalants (or "huffing"), compared with about 15% of 12th graders. Household products are typically abused, including aliphatic hydrocarbons (e.g., gasoline, butane in cigarette lighters), aromatic hydrocarbons (e.g., benzene and toluene in glues and acrylic paints), alkyl halides (e.g., methylene chloride and trichloroethylene in paint thinners and spot removers), and ketones (e.g., acetone in nail polish remover). Inhalant abusers appear to have a greater risk for long-term substance abuse compared with users of other psychoactive drugs. Inhalants have short durations of action and usually cannot be detected by toxic screen. However, they can cause cerebral atrophy and death (by asphyxiation or cardiac arrhythmia).

113. **What is the leading cause of fatality related to inhalant abuse?**
Sudden sniffing death syndrome. The volatile hydrocarbons sensitize the myocardium to the effect of epinephrine and also affect depolarization of the myocardial cell membranes. Abnormal propagation of impulses can occur, sometimes associated with adrenaline surge (as when hallucinating or running from an authority figure), and a fatal arrhythmia results. In adolescents who die from this entity, about 1 in 5 are using inhalants for the first time.

Williams JF, Storck M: Inhalant abuse, *Pediatrics* 119:1009–1017, 2007.

114. **What are the toxicities of chronic marijuana use?**
Pulmonary: Decreased pulmonary function. Compared with cigarette smoke, marijuana smoke contains more carcinogens and respiratory irritants and produces higher carboxyhemoglobin levels and greater tar deposition. Long-term studies will determine whether there is a link between chronic marijuana smoke exposure and lung cancer.

Endocrine: Associated with decreased sperm count and motility; may interfere with hypothalamic-pituitary function and increase the likelihood of anovulation; antagonizes insulin, which may affect diabetic management.

Behavioral: Short-term memory impairment, interference with learning, possible "amotivational syndrome."

115. **What performance-enhancing drugs are used by teenagers?**
In a study of 10,000 adolescents between the ages of 12 and 18 years, 12% of males and 8% of females used products to improve appearance or strength, including protein shakes, anabolic steroids, creatine, androstenedione, and human growth hormone. Thirty percent of adolescents using these products do not participate in sports but take these products in an effort to improve their appearance.

Castillo EM, Comstock RD: Prevalence of use of performance-enhancing substances among United States adolescents, *Pediatr Clin N Am* 54:663–675, 2007.

Field AE, Austin SB, Camargo CA, et al: Exposure to the mass media, body shape concerns, and use of supplements to improve weight and shape among male and female adolescents, *Pediatrics* 116:e214, 2005.

116. **List the potential side effects of anabolic steroids**
See Table 1-8.

TABLE 1-8. POTENTIAL SIDE EFFECTS OF ANABOLIC STEROIDS

Endocrine	In males—testicular atrophy, oligospermia, gynecomastia
	In females—amenorrhea, breast atrophy, clitoromegaly
Musculoskeletal	Premature epiphyseal closure
Dermatologic	Acne, hirsutism, striae, male pattern baldness
Hepatic	Impaired excretory function with cholestatic jaundice, elevated liver function test results, peliosis hepatitis (a form of hepatitis in which hepatic lobules have microscopic pools of blood), benign and malignant tumors
Cardiovascular	Hypertension, decreased high-density lipoprotein, thrombosis
Psychological	Aggressive behavior, mood swings, depression

Smith DV, McCambridge TM: Performance-enhancing substances in teens, Contemp Pediatr 26:41, 2009.

117. **What are the risks of smokeless tobacco?**
As a result of the decreased gingival blood flow caused by nicotine, chronic ischemia and necrosis can occur. Chronic use results in **gingival recession** and **inflammation, periodontal disease,** and **oral leukoplakia** (a premalignant change). The risk for oral and pharyngeal cancer is increased. Although more commonly used by males, smokeless tobacco used by pregnant females may be associated with low-birthweight infants and premature birth. Smokeless tobacco, like cigarettes, is addictive.

118. **When does cigarette smoking begin?**
In the United States, about three fourths of daily adult smokers started smoking when they were between the ages of 13 and 17 years. Worldwide, the average age is lower. Cigarette smoking remains the major preventable cause of premature death in the world. Of the estimated 1.25 billion smokers in the world, 800 million live in developing countries. In the United States, rates for teenagers younger than 18 years have been declining since the late 1990s.

119. **What are the three main reasons that cigarette smoking begins?**
   - Peer pressure (the strongest influence)
   - Curiosity or wanting to experiment
   - Family members smoke

   Lenney W, Enderby B: "Blowing in the wind": a review of teenage smoking, *Arch Dis Child* 93:72–75, 2008.

120. **What are the 5 "As" of smoking cessation counseling?**
   - Ask about tobacco use
   - Advise to quit
   - Assess willingness to attempt quitting
   - Assist in attempt to quit (e.g., pharmacotherapy such as nicotine gum or patch)
   - Arrange follow-up

   Klein JD, Camenga DR: Tobacco prevention and cessation in pediatric patients, *Pediatr Rev* 25:17–26, 2004.

121. **How effective are school-based youth smoking cessation programs?**
   In general, success rates are low (5% to 17%) when looking at cessation 6 to 7 months after the intervention. This is true for a variety of programs: structured educational courses, nicotine replacement therapy, and computer-based education. Clearly, this is an area in which new approaches and strategies are needed.

   Wiehe SE, Garrison MM, Christakis DA, et al: A systemic review of school-based smoking prevention trials with long-term follow-up, *J Adolesc Health* 36:162–169, 2005.

122. **Are tattoos a tip-off to high-risk behaviors?**
   Yes. Permanent tattoos are obtained by 10% to 16% of adolescents between the ages of 12 and 18 years in the United States. They are strongly associated with high-risk behaviors, including substance abuse, early initiation of sexual intercourse, interpersonal violence, and school failure.

   Roberts TA, Ryan SA: Tattooing and high-risk behavior in adolescents, *Pediatrics* 110:1058–1063, 2002.

TEENAGE MALE DISORDERS

123. **How common is gynecomastia in teenage boys?**
   As many as 50% to 75% of boys between the ages of 12 and 14½ years have some breast development. In about 25%, it lasts for more than 1 year and, in 7%, for more than 2 years. It occurs most commonly during Tanner genital stages II and III, and it usually consists of subareolar enlargement (breast bud). It may be unilateral or bilateral. The breast bud may be tender, which indicates the recent rapid growth of tissue. Obese boys often have breast enlargement due to the deposition of adipose tissue, and differentiation from gynecomastia (true breast budding) is sometimes difficult.

   Cakan N, Kamat D: Gynecomastia: evaluation and treatment recommendations for primary care providers, *Clin Pediatr* 46:487–490, 2007.

124. **Why does gynecomastia occur so commonly?**
   Early during puberty, the production of estrogen (a stimulator of ductal proliferation) increases relatively faster than does that of testosterone (an inhibitor of breast development). This slight imbalance causes the breast enlargement. In obese teenagers, the enzyme aromatase (found in higher concentrations in adipose tissue) converts testosterone to estrogen.

125. **What drugs are associated with gynecomastia?**
The drugs that cause this effect can be easier to recall using the CHEST acronym:
- **C**alcium-channel blockers: Verapamil, nifedipine
- **H**ormonal medications: Anabolic steroids, oral contraceptives
- **E**xperimental/illicit drugs: Marijuana, heroin, amphetamines, methadone
- p**S**ychoactive drugs: Phenothiazines, tricyclic antidepressants, diazepam
- **T**estosterone antagonists: Spironolactone, ranitidine, cimetidine, ketoconazole

126. **Which boys with gynecomastia warrant further evaluation?**
- Prepubertal boys
- Pubertal-age boys with little or no virilization and small testes
- Boys with hepatomegaly or abdominal mass palpated
- Boys with central nervous system complaints

   Evaluations may include testing for hypothalamic or pituitary disease, feminizing tumors of the adrenal or testes, and genetic abnormalities (e.g., Klinefelter syndrome). Although breast cancer is nearly reportable if it occurs in boys and is extremely rare in men (0.2%), in patients with Klinefelter syndrome, the rate increases to 3% to 6%.

127. **What treatment options are available for developmental gynecomastia?**
Treatment usually depends on the amount of breast tissue present and the degree of psychological problems that this causes. There are three primary options:
- **Reassurance:** Explanation of the process and expected resolution usually suffices for most adolescents. They should be told that most cases resolve within 1 year of onset.
- **Pharmacotherapy:** These agents may include antiestrogens (clomiphene citrate, tamoxifen), aromatase inhibitors (testolactone), nonaromatizable androgens (dihydrotestosterone), and weak androgens (danazol).
- **Surgery:** This should be done by a plastic surgeon who has experience in breast reduction.

   Nordt CA, DiVasta AD: Gynecomastia in adolescents, *Curr Opin Pediatr* 20:375–382, 2009.

128. **What are the clinical manifestations of testicular torsion?**
Testicular torsion in adolescents usually presents with acute-onset hemiscrotal pain that radiates to the groin and lower abdomen. Nausea and vomiting are common, but fever is rare. The testis is acutely tender and swollen, and it may be high riding. The cremasteric reflex (the testicle retracts after light stroking of the ipsilateral thigh) is absent. Many patients report previous episodes of severe acute scrotal pain.

129. **How is testicular torsion diagnosed?**
Radionuclide imaging of the scrotum with techneticum-99m pertechnetate and/or color Doppler ultrasound demonstrates low or absent blood flow and can be helpful in equivocal cases. However, testis salvage depends on the timely restoration of blood flow, and obtaining such studies should not delay a highly suspect case from surgical exploration. The spermatic cord sometimes can be untwisted manually; this will give temporary relief, but surgical exploration is still required for fixation to prevent recurrence. Both testes may be secured because the underlying suspension defect is often bilateral.

   Gatti JM, Murphy JP: Acute testicular disorders, *Pediatr Rev* 29:235–240, 2008.

130. **How is testicular torsion clinically differentiated from other causes of the acute painful scrotum?**
- **Epididymitis:** Usually slower in onset; pain is initially localized to epididymis, but as inflammation spreads, whole testis may become painful; not usually associated with vomiting; pain does not usually radiate to the groin; usually associated with dysuria, pyuria, and discharge; often caused by *C. trachomatis* and *N. gonorrhoeae*; history of STIs is suggestive; unusual in prepubertal boys and in nonsexually active teenagers

- **Orchitis:** Usually slower in onset; often systemic symptoms (nausea, vomiting, fever, chills) as a result of diffuse viral infection; in patients with mumps, occurs about 4 to 6 days after parotitis; bilateral involvement more common
- **Torsion of appendix testis:** Sudden onset of pain; localized, isolate tender nodule at upper pole (occasionally with bluish discoloration, the so-called blue-dot sign); nausea and vomiting uncommon; more common in prepubertal boys
- **Incarcerated hernia:** Acute onset; pain not localized to hemiscrotum; usually palpable inguinal mass; testes not painful; symptoms and signs of bowel obstruction (vomiting, abdominal distention, guarding, rebound tenderness)

Yin S, Trainor JL: Diagnosis and management of testicular torsion, torsion of the appendix testis, and epididymitis, *Clin Pediatr Emerg Med* 10:38–44, 2009.

131. **How does the Prehn sign help distinguish between epididymitis and testicular torsion?**
Classically, relief of pain with elevation of the testis (*positive Prehn sign*) is associated with epididymitis, whereas persistent or increased pain (*negative Prehn sign*) is more indicative of testicular torsion. However, there is considerable overlap, and this relatively nonspecific sign should be interpreted in the context of other signs and symptoms.

132. **If complete testicular torsion has occurred, how long is it before irreversible changes develop?**
Irreversible changes develop in **4 to 6 hours.** However, it is clinically impossible to distinguish partial from complete torsion, and thus duration of symptoms should not be used as a gauge for determining viability. Duration of symptoms does correlate with abnormal testicles on follow-up examination, which underscores the need for prompt diagnosis. Two thirds of patients with testicles salvaged between 12 and 24 hours after the onset of symptoms have palpable evidence of testicular atrophy during later evaluation, compared with only 10% when the diagnosis is made in less than 6 hours.

133. **What is the most frequent solid cancer in older adolescent males?**
Testicular cancer. The most common type is a seminoma, which, if detected when confined to the testicle (stage I), has a cure rate of up to 97% with orchiectomy and radiation. Although its overall effectiveness is debated, most authorities recommend that all adolescent males be taught testicular self-examination so that irregularities or changes in size can be noted early.

134. **What is the significance of a varicocele in a teenager?**
A *varicocele* is an enlargement of either the pampiniform or cremasteric venous plexus of the spermatic cord, which results in a boggy enlargement ("bag of worms") of the upper scrotum. These are rare before puberty. About 15% of boys between the ages of 10 and 15 years have a varicocele, and in 2%, the varicoceles are very large. Most are asymptomatic. Longitudinal studies of adolescents show that large varicoceles may interfere with normal testicular growth and result in decreased spermatogenesis. Surgical correction can prevent the progressive damage.

Hayes JH: Inguinal and scrotal disorders, *Surg Clin North Am* 86:371–381, 2006.

135. **Which varicoceles warrant surgical intervention?**
- More than 20% volume difference between testes, implying a hypotrophic testes
- Large varicocele
- Bilateral varicoceles (higher potential for infertility)
- Testicular pain
- Poor patient compliance with follow-up

Raj GV, Wiener JS: Varicoceles in adolescents: when to observe, when to intervene, *Contemp Pediatr* 21:39–56, 2004.

136. **On which side do varicoceles more commonly occur?**
The **left** side. The left spermatic vein drains into the left renal vein at a right angle, and the right spermatic vein drains into the inferior vena cava at an obtuse angle. These hemodynamics favor higher left-sided pressures, which predispose patients to left-sided varicoceles. Unilateral left-sided varicoceles are the most common types, occurring in 90% of patients; the remainder are bilateral. A unilateral right-sided lesion is rare, and many experts consider its finding a reason to search for other causes of venous obstruction, such as a renal or retroperitoneal tumor, using ultrasound, computed tomography, or magnetic resonance imaging.

137. **An adolescent who boasts of his overpowering "hircismus" is likely in need of what?**
Both a dictionary and a shower. *Hircismus* is offensive axillary odor.

TEENAGE PREGNANCY

138. **How common is teenage pregnancy in the United States?**
Teenage pregnancy rates declined by 34% from 1991 to 2005, but increased by 3% in 2006. The rates remain among the highest for a developed country. About 1 in 14 young women less than 20 years become pregnant each year (about 800,000 pregnancies). Fifteen thousand pregnancies occur in teenagers between the ages of 10 and 14 years. The likelihood that an adolescent will become pregnant before age 20 years is about 1 in 4. Eighty percent to 90% of these pregnancies are unintended. About 50% progress to delivery, 35% are terminated by abortion, and 15% end by miscarriage.

139. **What factors make it more likely that a teenager will become pregnant?**
   - **Early initiation of sexual intercourse:** Risk factors for early initiation include low socioeconomic status, low future-achievement orientation, and academic difficulties.
   - **Influence from peers and sisters:** If surrounded by sexually active friends and siblings, a teenager is more likely to be permissive with regard to sexual behavior and pregnancy itself. Many teens do not view pregnancy as a negative experience.
   - **History of physical or sexual abuse**
   - **Family history of adolescent pregnancy**
   - **Lack of family support and structure**
   - **Barriers to contraception:** Inaccurate information, lack of accessibility, improper use
   - **History of pregnancy**
   - **History of negative pregnancy tests**
   - **Race:** Blacks and Hispanics have higher rates of pregnancy than whites, although rates significantly vary by race according to socioeconomic status.

   Cox JE: Teenage pregnancy. In Neinstein LS, editor: *Adolescent Health Care*, ed 5, Philadelphia, 2008, Wolters Kluwer, pp 565–569.

140. **If a teenager has been pregnant once, how likely is she to become pregnant again during her teenage years?**
Repeat adolescent pregnancy is common. Up to 25% of teenagers will become pregnant again by age 20 years. Factors associated with a likely second teen pregnancy include age younger than 16 years at first conception, boyfriend older than 20 years, school dropout, below expected grade level at the time of first pregnancy, welfare dependency after the first pregnancy, complications during the first pregnancy, and departure from the hospital without birth control.

141. **What are the risks for infants of teenage mothers?**
Teenage mothers have a disproportionately increased risk for having babies who have a low birthweight, are premature, or are small for gestational age. In addition, infant mortality is

two to three times greater for the infants of teenage mothers. These infants also have higher likelihoods of abuse and cognitive, behavioral, and emotional problems. Studies conflict with regard to whether these risks are due to inherent biologic difficulties with pregnancy at a young age or to sociodemographic factors associated with teenage pregnancy (e.g., poverty, inadequate prenatal care).

Paranjothy S, Broughton H, Adappa R, et al: Teenage pregnancy: who suffers? *Arch Dis Child* 94: 239–245, 2009.

142. **How soon after conception will a urine pregnancy test become positive?**
Human chorionic gonadotropin (hCG) is a glycoprotein (with α and β subunits) that is produced by trophoblastic tissue. Urine levels of 25 mIU/mL are detectable by the most sensitive methods (i.e., radioimmunoassay or enzyme immunoassay to the β subunit) by about 7 days after fertilization. Although many home pregnancy tests can detect these low levels, some are less sensitive and detect levels of hCG that are about 1500 mIU/mL. This occurs, on average, about 3 weeks after fertilization (or 1 week after the missed menstrual period).

143. **In what setting should ectopic pregnancy be suspected?**
Amenorrhea with **unilateral abdominal** or **pelvic pain** and **irregular vaginal bleeding** is ectopic pregnancy until proved otherwise. A teenager with a ruptured ectopic pregnancy can present with features of shock (hypotension, tachycardia) and rebound tenderness. Sequential hCG levels can help with differentiating an ectopic from an intrauterine pregnancy. Ordinarily, the doubling time of hCG levels is about 48 hours; in ectopic pregnancy, there is usually a significant lag. Other causes of lag include missed abortion and spontaneous abortion. Abdominal or transvaginal ultrasound is also useful for diagnosis. Laparoscopy may be necessary if the diagnosis remains unclear.

Barnhart KT: Ectopic pregnancy, *N Engl J Med* 361:379–387, 2009.

144. **How likely are teenagers to use contraception at the time of first intercourse?**
About one third of teenagers use no contraception at the time of first intercourse. The approximate time between onset of intercourse and seeking medical services for adolescent females is nearly 1 year. This in large part explains why 20% of all adolescent pregnancies occur during the first month after initiating sexual activity and why 50% occur within the first 6 months. If abstinence is not an option for a teenager, discussion of contraception should be initiated by the clinician early during adolescence to prevent unintended pregnancy.

Rimsza ME: Counseling the adolescent about contraception, *Pediatr Rev* 24:162–170, 2003.

145. **Is a pelvic examination mandatory before starting a patient on oral contraceptive pills?**
No. Numerous professional organizations, including the American College of Obstetricians and Gynecologists, have advised that a pelvic examination is not required for safe use of oral contraception. A large percentage of teenagers will delay seeking contraceptive care if they believe a pelvic examination is required. Annual screening should subsequently be done for STIs. The estimated risk for death from contraceptive use in a nonsmoking teenager (0.3/100,000) is substantially less than the risk for death during childbirth in the same age group (11.1/100,000).

Rimsza ME: Counseling the adolescent about contraception, *Pediatr Rev* 24:162–170, 2003.

146. **What oral treatment is most commonly used for emergency postcoital contraception (e.g., in a rape case)?**
Plan B is a U.S. Food and Drug Administration (FDA)-approved progestin-only method with 1 tablet (0.75 mg of levonorgestrel) taken as soon as possible after intercourse and repeated in 12 hours. A single dose of 1.5 mg Plan B One Step appears to be as effective. Progestin-only emergency contraception appears to act by inhibiting or delaying ovulation, disrupting follicular development, thickening cervical mucus to impede sperm penetration, and affecting the

maturation of the corpus luteum. Plan B can reduce the risk for pregnancy by at least 75% when given within 72 hours of unprotected intercourse. Some studies have shown effectiveness when taken up to 120 hours later.

Gupta N, Corrado S, Goldstein M: Hormonal contraception for the adolescent, *Pediatr Rev* 29:386–396, 2009.

TEENAGE SUICIDE

147. How commonly do adolescents attempt suicide in the United States?
About 3500 teenagers die from suicide each year, but data about the frequency of attempts are hampered by underreporting. For each death by suicide, there are an estimated 8 to 200 attempts that fail, placing the number of attempts between 32,000 and 800,000. From 1950 to 2004, the suicide rate for adolescents in the 15- to 19-year-old group increased by 200%, compared with a 17% increase for the general population.

148. Who are more likely to attempt suicide, males or females?
Up to nine times as many females as males attempt suicide. However, males (particularly white males) are much more likely to succeed, due in large part to the choice of more lethal methods (especially firearms). Females more commonly try ingestions or wrist slashing. In younger patients (10 to 14 years), suffocation (such as hanging) is the most common method used.

149. Which adolescents are at increased risk for suicide?
Those with any of the following characteristics:
- History of previous attempts, especially those involving very lethal methods and those within the past 2 years
- Signs of current major depressive disorder
- Substance abuse (likelihood of suicide is increased up to ninefold)
- Easy access to firearms (most common location for teenage suicide involving firearms is in the home)
- Family history of psychiatric problems, including suicide and depression
- Personal history of "acting out" behavior (e.g., delinquency, truancy, sexual promiscuity)
- Living out of the home (in a correctional facility or group home)
- Gay or bisexual adolescents (likelihood of suicide is increased fourfold)
- History of physical or sexual abuse

Pfeffer CR: Suicidal behavior in children and adolescents: causes and management. In Martin A, Volkmar FR, editors: *Lewis' Child and Adolescent Psychiatry*, ed 4, Philadelphia, 2007, Wolters Kluwer, pp 529–538.

150. Which adolescents who have attempted suicide should be hospitalized?
Although many programs admit all patients, even if they are medically stable, those adolescents with failed attempts who should strongly be considered for inpatient evaluation include those with the following:
- Recurrent attempts
- Evidence of psychosis or persisting pervasive wish to die
- Method other than ingestion (e.g., jumping, use of firearm, attempted asphyxiation by hanging or carbon monoxide inhalation)
- Attempt at remote location (with less likelihood of discovery)
- Inadequate home, social, and supervisory situation

American Academy of Child and Adolescent Psychiatry: Practice Parameter for the Assessment and Treatment of Children and Adolescents with Suicidal Behavior, *J Am Acad Child Adolesc Psychiatry* 40: 245–515, 2001.

CHAPTER 2

BEHAVIOR AND DEVELOPMENT

Mark F. Ditmar, MD

ATTENTION–DEFICIT/HYPERACTIVITY DISORDER

1. **What characterizes attention-deficit/hyperactivity disorder (ADHD)?**
   ADHD is a chronic neurodevelopmental and behavioral disorder, considered to have neurobiologic origins, that is diagnosed on the basis of the number, severity, and duration of three clusters of behavioral problems: *inattention*, *hyperactivity*, and *impulsivity*. It is the most commonly diagnosed behavior disorder in children. According to the *Diagnostic and Statistical Manual of Mental Disorders IV Text Revision* (DSM-IV-TR), symptoms of inattention, hyperactivity, and impulsivity must have lasted for more than 6 months and be inconsistent with the child's developmental level. These symptoms have to involve more than one setting and result in significant functional impairment at home, school, or in social settings. Some symptoms must have begun before the age of 7 years.

   Pliszka S: American Academy of Child and Adolescent Psychiatry Work Group on Quality Issues. Practice parameter fro the assessment and treatment of children and adolescents with attention-deficit/hyperactivity disorder, *J Am Acad Child Adolesc Psychiatry* 46:894–921, 2007.

   National Resource Center on ADHD: http://www.help4adhd.org.

   Attention Deficit Disorder Association: http://www.add.org.

2. **How common is ADHD?**
   Community prevalence studies indicate that 4% to 12% of school-aged children are affected by ADHD.

3. **Are boys or girls more likely to be diagnosed with ADHD?**
   Males are three to four times more frequently diagnosed with ADHD. Their symptoms tend to be more disruptive, particularly with hyperactivity, whereas girls present more commonly with problems of attention.

4. **Is there a genetic predisposition to ADHD?**
   ADHD has a **high rate of heritability.** In studies of identical twins raised apart, if one twin has ADHD, the other has up to a 75% likelihood of being diagnosed with ADHD. In nonidentical twin studies, the concordance rate is as high as 33%. Studies of siblings of patients with ADHD indicate a 20% to 30% likelihood. About 25% of children with ADHD have at least one parent with symptoms or diagnosis of ADHD.

5. **What conditions can mimic ADHD?**
   Medical: Lead toxicity, iron deficiency, thyroid dysfunction, visual or hearing impairment, sleep disorders, mass lesions (e.g., hydrocephalus), seizures, complex migraines, fetal alcohol syndrome, fragile X syndrome, Williams syndrome, neurofibromatosis, tuberous sclerosis, medication side effects (e.g., cold preparations, steroids), and substance abuse.

Developmental or learning disorders: Mental retardation (MR), autistic spectrum disorders (e.g., pervasive developmental disorder, Asperger syndrome), and specific learning disabilities. Central auditory processing difficulties have also been investigated, although it is still unclear as to whether such difficulties are a different disorder or whether they represent the cognitive deficits seen with ADHD.

Behavioral or emotional disorders: Affective disorders (e.g., dysthymia, bipolar disorder), anxiety disorders, stress reactions (e.g., posttraumatic stress disorder, adjustment disorder), other disruptive behavior disorders (e.g., oppositional defiant disorder), and personality disorders.

Psychosocial factors: Family dysfunction, parenting dysfunction, and abuse.

6. **What are the comorbid disorders commonly seen with ADHD?**
   - Anxiety
   - Bipolar disorder
   - Conduct disorder
   - Depression
   - Language problems
   - Learning disorders
   - Mental retardation
   - Oppositional defiant disorder
   - Sleep problems
   - Tic disorders

7. **Is there a definitive diagnostic test for ADHD?**
   No. Diagnosis requires evidence of characteristic symptoms occurring in high frequency over an extended period of time. This information, which is ideally obtained from at least two settings or sources (e.g., school and home), can be garnered from observation, narrative histories, and the use of various standardized rating scales. A practitioner's ADHD toolkit, with scales for diagnosis, is available from the National Initiative for Children's Healthcare Quality at http://www.nichq.org/resources/toolkit.

   Carter S, Syed-Sabir H: How to use: a rating score to diagnose attention deficit hyperactivity disorder, *Arch Dis Child Educ Pract Ed* 93:159–162, 2008.

8. **How should ADHD be treated?**
   A multimodal approach is recommended, which may include psychotropic medication, behavioral therapies, family education and counseling, and educational interventions.

   Jellinek M: ADHD treatments: going beyond the meds, *Contemp Pediatr* 25:39–48, 2008.

   Pliszka S: American Academy of Child and Adolescent Psychiatry Work Group on Quality Issues. Practice parameter for the assessment and treatment of children and adolescents with attention-deficit/hyperactivity disorder, *J Am Acad Child Adolesc Psychiatry* 46:894–921, 2007.

9. **What are the best medications for treating ADHD?**
   Stimulant medications (methylphenidate and dextroamphetamine). Randomized, controlled trials support their benefits, usually by demonstrating the improvement of core ADHD symptoms in 70% to 80% of children. Of the 20% to 30% of nonresponders to one medication, about half will respond to the other stimulant. Other medications used include atomoxetine (a nonstimulant approved in 2003), α-adrenergic agonists (e.g., clonidine), tricyclic antidepressants, and atypical antidepressants (e.g., bupropion). There is concern about the possible overuse of stimulants in children of all ages.

   Rappley MD: Attention-deficit/hyperactivity disorder, *N Engl J Med* 352:165–173, 2005.

10. **Is a positive response to stimulant medication diagnostic of ADHD?**
A positive response is not diagnostic because (1) children without symptoms of ADHD given stimulants demonstrate positive responses in sustained and focused attention, and (2) observer bias (i.e., parent or teacher) can be considerable. Thus, many experts recommend a placebo-controlled trial when stimulant medication is used.

Nahlilk J: Issues in diagnosis of attention-deficit/hyperactivity disorder in adolescents, *Clin Pediatr* 43:1–10, 2004.

11. **Is an electrocardiogram (ECG) required before beginning patients on stimulant medication for ADHD?**
This is controversial. There were concerns expressed through the U.S. Food and Drug Administration (FDA) regarding a potential increased risk for sudden death for ADHD patients on stimulant medication. However, studies did not demonstrate an increased risk compared with the background rate of sudden death. The Council on Cardiovascular Disease in the Young (part of the American Heart Association) listed the indication for an ECG in this setting as class II, indicating uncertainty as to its need or lack of need. Many pediatric cardiologists do not recommend the study because, in a population with a very low risk, the ECG as a screening test has low predictive values, both positive and negative. However, if there are risk factors by patient history (e.g., syncope during exercise), family history (e.g., first-degree relative with early sudden death), or examination (e.g., abnormal murmur or absent femoral pulses), a cardiac evaluation is indicated.

Vetter VL, Elia J, Erickson C, et al: Cardiovascular monitoring of children and adolescents with heart disease receiving stimulant drugs, *Circulation* 117:2407–2423, 2008.

Perrin JM, Friedman RA: Cardiovascular monitoring and stimulant drugs for attention-deficit/hyperactivity disorder, *Pediatrics* 122:451–453, 2008.

12. **How young is "too young" to diagnose ADHD and prescribe stimulant medications?**
The diagnosis is considered difficult to make in children younger than 4 to 6 years because the validity and reliability of the diagnosis of ADHD in these age groups have not been demonstrated. Although dextroamphetamine is approved by the FDA for this age group, methylphenidate carries a warning against its use in children younger than 6 years. Concerns exist regarding the unproven treatment of children at such a young age and the potential deleterious effect of psychotropic drugs on brain development. A National Institute of Mental Health study in children 3 to 5.5 years treated with methylphenidate found improvement in ADHD symptoms, but 30% had moderate to severe adverse events. There has been a dramatic increase in the "off-label" use of stimulant medication since 1990 for children 2 to 4 years old. The evaluation and most ideal treatment of these younger children remain a challenge.

Lerner M, Wigal T: Long-term safety of stimulant medications used to treat children with ADHD, *Pediatr Ann* 37:37–45, 2008.

Wigal T, Greenhill L, Chuang S, et al: Safety and tolerability of methylphenidate in preschool children with ADHD, *J Am Acad Child Adolesc Psychiatry* 45:1284–1293, 2006.

13. **What are the risks for adolescents with ADHD?**
Increased high-risk behaviors, including higher rates of sexually transmitted infections and pregnancies, and **increased school problems,** including higher rates of grade failure, dropping out, and expulsion. Untreated ADHD has also been found to be a significant risk factor for future substance abuse.

Wolraich ML, Wibbelsman CJ, Brown TE, et al: Attention-deficit/hyperactivity disorder among adolescents: a review of the diagnosis, treatment, and clinical implications, *Pediatrics* 115:1734–1746, 2005.

KEY POINTS: THE "I"SSENTIALS OF ADHD

Inattention
Increased activity
Impulsiveness
Impairment in multiple settings
Inappropriate (for developmental stage)
Incessant (persists for >6 months)

14. **Does sugar or food additives make children hyperactive?**
    Although it would be gratifying if complex behavioral problems could be attributable solely or in large measure to dietary causes, the results have been mixed. In a double-blind, controlled trial involving excessive dietary intakes of sucrose or aspartame, no adverse behavioral or cognitive changes were noted. However, another study in which children were given a drink containing artificial colors, sodium benzoate, or neither, those taking the beverage with food additives had significantly increased adverse effects.

    McCann D, Barrett A, Cooper A, et al: Food additives and hyperactive behaviour in 3-year-old and 8/9-year-old children in the community: a randomised, double-blinded, placebo-controlled trial, *Lancet* 370:1560–1567, 2007.

    Wolraich ML, Wilson DB, White JW: The effect of sugar on behavior or cognition in children: a meta-analysis, *JAMA* 274:1617–1621, 1995.

15. **Are alternative or complementary therapies beneficial for ADHD?**
    Many are tried by frustrated parents (often unbeknownst to the primary care provider), such as megadose vitamin therapy, herbals, antifungal therapy, and others. However, randomized controlled trials are few and, when done, typically demonstrate no benefit.

    Weber W, Vander Stoep A, McCarty RL, et al: *Hypericum perforatum* (St John's Wort) for attention-deficit/hyperactivity disorder in children and adolescents, *JAMA* 299:2633–2641, 2008.

    Sadiq AJ: Attention-deficit/hyperactivity disorder and integrative approaches, *Pediatr Ann* 36:508–515, 2007.

16. **Do children with ADHD become teenagers and adults with ADHD?**
    Ongoing observations of children initially diagnosed with ADHD note that 70% to 80% will continue to have symptoms present during adolescence and up to 60% will show symptoms as adults. Of the features of ADHD, hyperactivity is the symptom most likely to be outgrown. Inattention, distractibility, and failure to finish things are more likely to persist. Adolescents and adults also have continued problems with anxiety and depression as well as with tobacco and substance abuse. Motor vehicle infractions, employment difficulties, and intimate relationships have also been described as problematic for adults. Children and adolescents with symptoms of conduct disorder as well as ADHD are at the highest risk for severe problems as adults.

    Wolraich ML, Wibbelsman CJ, Brown TE, et al: Attention-deficit/hyperactivity disorder among adolescents: a review of the diagnosis, treatment, and clinical implications, *Pediatrics* 115:1734–1746, 2005.

    Children and Adults with Attention Deficit/Hyperactivity Disorder: http://www.chadd.org.

AUTISM

17. **What are the autism spectrum disorders?**
    Also called *pervasive developmental disorders*, these are five complex neuropsychiatric syndromes (as listed in DSM-IV-TR) that are characterized by problems with social interaction, verbal and nonverbal communication, and repetitive behaviors with varying

degrees of severity. The syndromes include the following: (1) autistic disorder (autism); (2) Asperger syndrome; (3) Rett syndrome; (4) childhood disintegrative disorder (with developmental deterioration after 24 months of age); and (5) pervasive developmental disorder, not otherwise specified (PDD-NOS).

American Psychiatric Association: *Diagnosis and Statistical Manual of Mental Disorders: DSM-IV-TR*, Washington, DC, 2000, American Psychiatric Association.

Autism Society of America: http://www.autism-society.org.

Autism Speaks: http://www.autism.org.

Autism Research Institute: http://www.autismwebsite.com.

18. **What are the three essential features of autism?**
    1. Impaired social interaction (extreme aloneness, failure to make eye contact)
    2. Absent or abnormal speech and language development
    3. Narrow range of interest and stereotyped or repetitive responses to objects

KEY POINTS: THREE ESSENTIAL FEATURES OF AUTISM

1. Impaired social interaction

2. Absent or abnormal speech and language development

3. Narrow range of interest and stereotyped or repetitive responses to objects

19. **Which behaviors of children should arouse suspicion of possible autism?**
    - Avoidance of eye contact during infancy ("gaze aversion")
    - Relating to only part of a person's body (e.g., the lap) rather than to the whole person
    - Failure to acquire speech or speech acquisition in an unusual manner (e.g., echolalia [repeating another person's speech])
    - Failure to respond to name when called
    - Spending long periods of time in repetitive activities and fascination with movement (e.g., spinning records, dripping water)
    - Failure to look in the same direction when directed by an adult ("gaze monitoring")
    - Absence of pointing to show or request something ("protodeclarative pointing")
    - Excessively lining up toys or other objects
    - Limited pretend or symbolic play

    Johnson CP, Myers SM: Identification and evaluation of children with autism spectrum disorders, *Pediatrics* 120:1183–1215, 2007.

20. **When should screening be done for autism?**
    The American Academy of Pediatrics (AAP) recommends that all children receive autism-specific screening at 18 and 24 months and whenever there is a concern for autism. Younger siblings of patients with autism have a 10- to 20-fold increased risk. Problems with preverbal gestural language and deficits in social skills are present in most children by 18 months of age. Early recognition of autism can lead to earlier intervention, which can improve outcomes markedly. The 23-question M-CHAT (modified version of the Checklist for Autism in Toddlers) is probably the most commonly used screening questionnaire. Positive results warrant referral for more detailed testing.

    Pinto-Martin JA, Young LM, Mandell DS, et al: Screening strategies for autism spectrum disorders in pediatric primary care, *J Dev Behav Pediatr* 29:345–350, 2008.

    Pander J, Verbalis A, et al: Screening for autism in older and younger toddlers with the Modified Checklist for Autism in Toddlers, *Autism* 12:513, 2008.

21. **What studies should be considered in the evaluation of a child with suspected autism?**
    - Hearing screening
    - Metabolic screening: Urine for organic acids, serum for lactate, amino acids, ammonia, and very long-chain fatty acids (if developmental regression, MR, dysmorphic features, hypotonia, vomiting or dehydration, feeding intolerance, early-onset seizures, episodic vomiting)
    - Chromosomal analysis, other genetic testing (if dysmorphic features or MR; more than two dozen genetic syndromes are associated with autism)
    - DNA fragile X analysis (if MR or phenotype of long, thin face and prominent ears)
    - Electroencephalogram (especially if history of seizures, staring spells, or regression of milestones)
    - Neuroimaging with magnetic resonance imaging (especially if abnormal head shape or circumference, focal neurologic abnormalities, or seizures)
    - Lead level (if history of pica)

    Pickler L, Elias E: Genetic evaluation of the child with an autism spectrum disorder, *Pediatr Ann* 38:26–29, 2009.

22. **Is the prevalence of autism increasing?**
    It is clear that more children are being diagnosed with autistic spectrum disorders. A 2007 Centers for Disease Control and Prevention (CDC) report estimates an overall national prevalence rate of 6.6 per 1000 in 8-year-old children or about 1 in 150 compared with 0.4 per 1000, 40 years ago. There is disagreement regarding whether this represents a true increase or changes in diagnostic and classification practices, such as greater awareness of the condition, broader definitions of autism (including PDD-NOS), better diagnostic definitions or diagnostic substitution (developmental language disorders of the 1980s now being classified as autistic variants).

    Peacock G, Yeargin-Allsopp M: Autism spectrum disorders: prevalence and vaccines, *Pediatr Ann* 38:22–25, 2009.

23. **Do vaccines cause autism?**
    Many claims have been made regarding possible environment triggers for autism, especially vaccines, particularly measles-mumps-rubella (MMR), and vaccine components, particularly thimerosal (a mercury-containing compound used as a preservative in some vaccines). The Institute of Medicine has found no link between the use of thimerosal or MMR as a cause of autism. The debate still lingers with additional claims that underlying medical conditions, such as mitochondrial deficits, may have encephalopathic features triggered by vaccines.

    Gust DA, Darling N, Kennedy A, Schwartz B: Parents with doubts about vaccines: which vaccines and why, *Pediatrics* 122:718–725, 2008.

    Offit PA: Vaccines and autism revisited—the Hannah Poling Case, *N Engl J Med* 358:2089–2091, 2008.

    Offitt PA: *Autism's False Prophets*, New York, 2008, Columbia University Press.

    Institute of Medicine: *Immunization Safety Review: Vaccines and Autism*, Washington, DC, 2004, National Academies Press.

24. **What distinguishes Asperger syndrome and PDD-NOS from autism?**
    There is debate about whether clear boundaries divide these pervasive developmental disorders as defined by DSM-IV-TR criteria. In general, *Asperger syndrome* is characterized by better early language development (both expressive and receptive) without significant delay, better self-help skills, and better cognitive development, but with impairments in social interaction with behaviors (e.g., stereotypical) and restricted interests as seen in autism. Although formal language skills are adequate, conversational and

pragmatic language abilities are impaired. Although Asperger syndrome is commonly referred to as "higher-functioning autism," some experts feel these categories are also distinct. *PDD-NOS*, which is diagnosed more frequently than the other two categories combined, refers to those children with problems of social interaction, communication, and restricted interests who do not fit the specific diagnostic criteria. This category tends to be a diagnostic catch-all for patients who do not fit the specific criteria of other conditions.

Walker DR, Thompson A, Zwaigenbaum, L, et al: Specifying PDD-NOS: a comparison of PDD-NOS, Asperger syndrome and autism, *J Am Acad Child Adolesc Psychiatry* 43:172–180, 2004.

25. **Does early intervention and/or therapy improve the outcome in children with autism?**
In general, earlier diagnosis and involvement of therapies for children with autism does appear to improve outcomes such as a decreased need for special education in later years and an increase in the chance for independence as an adult. Certain subsets of children with autism, such as those with no coexisting cognitive deficits, will fare better. Additionally, earlier recognition and intervention may assist families in understanding and coping with potentially challenging medical comorbidities and social and behavioral issues.

Zwaigenbaum L, Bryson S, Lord C, et al: Clinical assessment and management of toddlers with suspected autism spectrum disorder: insights from studies of high-risk infants, *Pediatrics* 123:1383–1391, 2009.

26. **What is Rett syndrome?**
A rare condition in females (1 in 15,000 to 22,000; likely lethal *in utero* in males) characterized by normal head circumference at birth and normal early development followed, at 5 to 48 months, by deceleration of head growth, onset of stereotypical hand movements (handwringing, handwashing), decline in coordinated gait and trunk movements, and progression of marked impairment of expressive and receptive language. Mutations or large deletions involving the methyl-CpG-binding protein 2 (MeCP2) occur in most cases.

BEHAVIOR PROBLEMS

27. **What are the most common types of behavior problems in children?**
   - **Problems of daily routine** (e.g., food refusal, sleep abnormalities, toilet difficulties)
   - **Aggressive-resistant behavior** (e.g., temper tantrums, aggressiveness with peers)
   - **Overdependent-withdrawing behavior** (e.g., separation upset, fears, shyness)
   - **Hyperactivity**
   - **Undesirable habits** (e.g., thumb-sucking, head banging, nail biting, playing with genitals)
   - **School problems**

Chamberlin RW: Prevention of behavioral problems in young children, *Pediatr Clin North Am* 29:239–247, 1982.

28. **How much do babies normally cry each day?**
In Brazelton's oft-quoted 1962 study of 80 infants, it was found that, at 2 weeks of age, the average crying time was nearly 2 hours per day. This increased to nearly 3 hours per day at 6 weeks and then declined to about 1 hour per day at 12 weeks.

Brazelton TB: Crying in infancy, *Pediatrics* 29:579–588, 1962.

29. **What is infantile colic?**
Colic is excessive crying or fussiness, which occurs in 5% to 20% of infants depending on the criteria used. For study purposes, it is defined as paroxysms of crying in an

otherwise healthy infant for more than 3 hours per day on more than 3 days per week for more than 3 weeks. The typical clinical picture is that of an otherwise healthy and well-fed baby (usually between the ages of 2 weeks and 3 months) who cries intensely and inconsolably for several hours at a time, usually during the late afternoon or evening. Often the infant appears to be in pain and has a slightly distended abdomen, with the legs drawn up; occasional temporary relief occurs if gas is passed.

The symptoms nearly always resolve by the time the infant is 3 to 4 months old, but the problem can have repercussions, including early discontinuation of breastfeeding, multiple formula changes, heightened maternal anxiety and distress, diminished maternal-infant interaction, and increased risk for child abuse.

30. **What causes colic?**
No precise cause has been identified, and the etiology is likely multifactorial. Theories have involved gastrointestinal dysfunction (e.g., intolerance or allergy to cow milk or soy protein, gastroesophageal reflux, lactose intolerance, immaturity of the gastrointestinal tract), neurologic problems (immaturity of the central nervous system, neurotransmitter imbalance), hormonal processes (e.g., increased serotonin), difficult infant temperament, and interaction problems between the infant and the caregiver (e.g., misinterpreted infant cues, transfer of parental anxiety).

31. **Are there any treatments that are useful for colic?**
As is the case for most self-resolving conditions without a known cause, **counseling** is the most effective treatment. However, multiple interventions with minimal effectiveness are often tried, and these often involve the gastrointestinal tract: elimination of cow milk from the breastfeeding mother's diet, formula changes (to soy or to protein hydrolysates), or a trial of herbal tea or simethicone to decrease intestinal gas. Medications such as antispasmodics are not recommended because of the risk for side effects. Other sensory modifiers (e.g., car rides, massage, swaddling) are also attempted to provide some course of action until the expected 3- to 4-month resolution.

Cohen-Silver J, Ratnapalan S: Management of infantile colic: a review, *Clin Pediatr* 48:14–17, 2009.

32. **What evaluations should be done for the excessively crying infant?**
The infant with acute excessive crying, interpreted by caretakers as differing in quality and persisting beyond a reasonable time (generally 1 to 2 hours) without adequate explanation, can be a taxing problem for pediatricians and emergency room physicians. The differential diagnosis is broad, but infantile colic remains most common diagnosis (but a diagnosis of exclusion). History and physical examination make the diagnosis in most infants. However, other tests to consider include stool for occult blood (possible intussusception), fluorescein testing of both eyes (possible corneal abrasion), urinalysis and urine culture (possible urinary tract infection), pulse oximetry (hypoxia from cardiac causes may manifest as increased irritability), and electrolytes and blood glucose (possible endocrine or metabolic disturbance).

Freedman SB, Al-Harthy N, Thull-Freedman J: The crying infant: diagnostic testing and frequency of serious underlying disease, *Pediatrics* 123:841–848, 2009.

Ditmar MF: Crying. In Schwartz MW, editor: *The 5-Minute Pediatric Consult*, ed 5, Philadelphia, 2008, Wolters Kluwer, pp 232–233.

33. **How should children be punished?**
The goal of punishment should be to teach children that a specific behavior was wrong and to discourage the behavior in the future. To meet this goal, punishment should be consistent and relatively brief. It should be carried out in a calm manner as soon as possible after the infraction. Time-out from ongoing activity and removal of privileges are two punishment

techniques that can be used. The use of corporal punishment is controversial. Although spanking and other physical forms of punishment are widely practiced, most developmental authorities argue against their use because they do not foster the internalization of rules of behavior and may legitimize violence.

Larsen MA, Tentis E: The art and science of disciplining children, *Pediatr Clin North Am* 50:817–840, 2003.

34. **How valid is the proverb "spare the rod and spoil the child" as a defense for corporal punishment?**
The actual biblical proverb (Proverbs 13:24) reads, "He who spares the rod hates his son, but he who loves him is careful to discipline him." Although the proverb has often been used as a justification for spanking, in actuality it does not refer to specific discipline strategies but rather to the need for love and discipline. In addition, the rod may refer to the shepherd's staff, which was used to guide—rather than hit—sheep.

Carey TA: Spare the rod and spoil the child: is this a sensible justification for the use of punishment in child rearing? *Child Abuse Negl* 18:1005–1010, 1994.

35. **Is physical injury a concern in children with head banging?**
Head banging, which is a common problem that occurs in 5% to 15% of normal children, rarely results in physical injury. When injury does occur, it is usually in children with autism or other developmental disabilities. Normal children often show signs of bliss as they bang away, and the activity usually resolves by the time the child is 4 years old. (It may resume spontaneously during pediatric board examinations.)

36. **What is the difference between a "blue" breath-holding spell and a "white" breath-holding spell?**
Both are syncopal attacks with involuntary cessation of breathing that occur in up to 4% of children between the ages of 6 months and 4 years.
"Blue" or cyanotic spell: More common. Vigorous crying provoked by physical or emotional upset leads to apnea at end of expiration. This is followed by cyanosis, opisthotonus, rigidity, and loss of tone. Brief convulsive jerking may occur. The episode lasts from 10 to 60 seconds. A short period of sleepiness may ensue.
"White" or pallid spell: More commonly precipitated by an unexpected event that frightens the child. Crying is limited or absent. Breath holding and loss of consciousness occur simultaneously. On testing, children prone to these spells demonstrate increased responsiveness to vagal maneuvers. This parasympathetic hypersensitivity may cause cardiac slowing, diminished cardiac output, and diminished arterial pressure, which result in a pale appearance.

37. **When should a diagnosis of seizure disorder be considered rather than a breath-holding spell?**
- Precipitating event is minor or nonexistent
- History of no or minimal crying or breath holding
- Episode lasts >1 minute
- Period of postepisode sleepiness lasts >10 minutes
- Convulsive component of episode is prominent and occurs before cyanosis
- Occurs in child <6 months or >4 years old
- Associated with incontinence

38. **Does treatment with iron decrease the frequency of breath-holding spells?**
In the 1960s, it was observed that children with breath-holding spells had lower hemoglobin levels than controls. Treatment with iron has decreased the frequency of breath-holding spells in some children, most notably those with iron deficiency anemia. Interestingly, some of

the children whose breath-holding spells respond to iron are not anemic, and the mechanism by which iron decreases breath-holding spells is not known.

Boon R: Does iron have a place in the management of breath-holding spells? *Arch Dis Child* 87:77–78, 2002.

39. **When does prolonged thumb-sucking warrant intervention?**
If frequent thumb-sucking persists in a child who is older than 4 to 5 years or in whom permanent teeth have begun to erupt, treatment is usually indicated. Persistent thumb-sucking after the eruption of permanent teeth can lead to malocclusion.

40. **What treatments are used for thumb-sucking?**
Treatment commonly has two components: (1) physical modifications such as an application of a substance with an unpleasant taste at frequent intervals (such products are commercially available) and/or use of a thumb splint or glove for nighttime sucking, and (2) behavior modification with positive reinforcement (small rewards) given when a child is observed not sucking his or her thumb. Occlusive dental appliances are generally not needed.

41. **When should "toilet training" be started?**
When a child has language readiness (use of two-word phrases and two-step commands), understands the cause and effect of toileting, seems to desire independence without worsening oppositional behaviors, and has sufficient motor skills and body awareness, training can be begun. The physical prerequisite of the neurologic maturation of bladder and bowel control usually occurs between 18 and 30 months of age. The child's emotional readiness is often influenced by his or her temperament, parental attitudes, and parent-child interactions. The "potty chair" is typically introduced when the child is between 2 and 3 years old. In the United States, about one fourth of children achieve daytime continence by 2 years and 98% by 3 years. There are distinct racial disparities regarding parental beliefs. Black parents believe training should be initiated around 18 months compared with 25 months for white parents.

Horn IB, Brenner R, Rao M, et al: Beliefs about the appropriate age for initiating toilet training: are there racial and socioeconomic differences? *J Pediatr* 149:165–168, 2006.

42. **Are girls or boys toilet trained earlier?**
On average, **girls** are toilet trained earlier than boys. With regard to most other developmental milestones during the first years of life, however, there do not appear to be significant sex differences (i.e., in walking or running, sleep patterns, or verbal ability). Girls do show more rapid bone development.

43. **When is masturbation in a child considered pathologic?**
Masturbation (the rhythmic self-manipulation of the genital area) is considered a normal part of sexual development. However, if masturbation occurs to the exclusion of other activities (compulsive masturbation), if it occurs in public places when the child is older than 6 years, or if the child engages in activities that mimic adult sexual behavior, evaluation for sexual abuse, central nervous system abnormalities, or psychological pathology would be appropriate.

CRANIAL DISORDERS

44. **How many fontanels are present at birth?**
Although there are six fontanels present at birth (two anterior lateral, two posterior lateral, one anterior, and one posterior), only two (the anterior and posterior fontanels) are usually palpable on physical examination (Fig. 2-1).

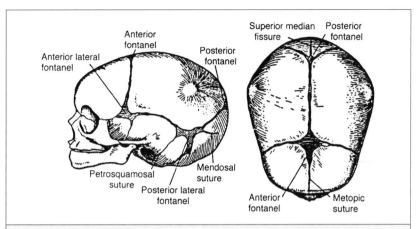

Figure 2-1. The cranium at birth, showing major sutures and fontanels. No attempt is made to show molding or overlapping of bones, which sometimes occurs at birth. (From Silverman FN, Kuhn JP [eds]: Caffey's Pediatric X-ray Diagnosis, 9th ed. St. Louis, Mosby, 1993, p 5.)

45. **When does the anterior fontanel close?**
    Usually when the infant is **between 10 and 14 months** old. However, it may not be palpable as early as 3 months, or it may remain open until 18 months.

46. **Which conditions are most commonly associated with premature or delayed closure of the fontanel?**
    Premature closure: Microcephaly, high calcium-to-vitamin D ratio in pregnancy, craniosynostosis, hyperthyroidism, or variation of normal
    Delayed closure: Achondroplasia, Down syndrome, increased intracranial pressure, familial macrocephaly, rickets, or variation of normal

47. **When is an anterior fontanel too big?**
    The size of the fontanel can be calculated using the formula: (length + width)/2, where length equals anterior-posterior dimension and width equals transverse dimension. However, there is wide variability in the normal size range of the anterior fontanel. Mean fontanel size on day 1 of life is 2.1 cm, with an upper limit of normal of 3.6 cm in white infants and 4.7 cm in black infants. These upper limits may be helpful for identifying disorders in which a large fontanel may be a feature (e.g., hypothyroidism, hypophosphatasia, skeletal dysplasias, increased intracranial pressure). Of note is that the posterior fontanel is normally about the size of a fingertip or smaller in 97% of full-term newborns.

    Kiesler J, Ricer R: The anterior fontanel, *Am Fam Physician* 67:2547–2552, 2003.

48. **What are the types of primary craniosynostosis?**
    Craniosynostosis is the premature fusion of various cranial suture lines that results in the ridging of the sutures, asymmetrical growth, and deformity of the skull. Suture lines (with resultant disorders listed in parentheses) include sagittal (scaphocephaly or dolichocephaly), coronal (brachycephaly), unilateral coronal or lambdoidal (plagiocephaly), and metopic (trigonocephaly). Multiple fused sutures can result in a high and pointed skull (oxycephaly or acrocephaly) (Fig. 2-2).

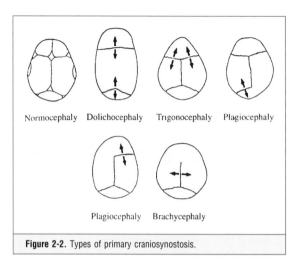

Figure 2-2. Types of primary craniosynostosis.

49. **What is the most common type of primary craniosynostosis?**
Sagittal (60%); coronal synostosis accounts for 20% of cases.

50. **What causes craniosynostosis?**
Most cases of isolated craniosynostosis have no known etiology. *Primary* craniosynostosis may be observed as part of craniofacial syndromes, including Apert, Crouzon, and Carpenter syndromes. *Secondary* causes can include abnormalities of calcium and phosphorus metabolism (e.g., hypophosphatasia, rickets), hematologic disorders (e.g., thalassemia), mucopolysaccharidoses, and hyperthyroidism. Inadequate brain growth (e.g., microcephaly) can lead to craniosynostosis.

Williams H: Lumps, bumps and funny shaped heads, *Arch Dis Child Educ Pract Ed* 93:120–128, 2008.

51. **What is positional or deformational plagiocephaly?**
Since the implementation of the "back-to-sleep" program by the AAP in 1992 to reduce the risk for sudden infant death syndrome (SIDS), about 1 in 60 infants has developed occipital flattening (posterior or lambdoidal plagiocephaly) due to transient calvarial deformation from prolonged supine sleeping positions. The condition can be prevented by varying the infant's head position during sleep and feeding and by observing prone positioning ("tummy time") for at least 5 minutes daily during the first 6 weeks of life. Therapy for severe cases consists of repositioning, physiotherapy, helmet treatment, and rarely surgery.

Xia JJ, Kennedy KA, et al: Nonsurgical treatment of deformational plagiocephaly, *Arch Pediatr Adolesc Med* 162:719–727, 2008.

Saeed NR, Wall SA, Dhariwal DK: Management of positional plagiocephaly, *Arch Dis Child* 93:82–84, 2008.

American Academy of Pediatrics Committee on Practice and Ambulatory Medicine: Prevention and management of positional skull deformities in infants, *Pediatrics* 112:119–202, 2003.

52. **How is positional plagiocephaly differentiated from plagiocephaly caused by craniosynostosis?**
Synostotic lambdoidal plagiocephaly is much more rare. It is usually associated with ridging of the involved suture lines, and it causes a different pattern of frontal bossing and ear displacement when the infant's head is viewed from above (Fig. 2-3).

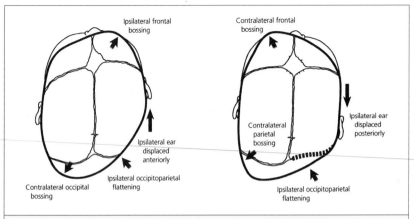

Figure 2-3. Factors distinguishing (*left*) positional plagiocephaly from (*right*) lambdoidal craniosynostosis. (From Kabbani H, Raghuveer TS: Craniosynostosis. Am Fam Physician 69:2866, 2004.)

53. **What conditions are associated with skull softening?**
   - Cleidocranial dysostosis
   - Craniotabes
   - Lacunar skull (associated with spina bifida and major central nervous system anomalies)
   - Osteogenesis imperfecta
   - Multiple wormian bones (associated with hypothyroidism, hypophosphatasia, and chronic hydrocephalus)
   - Rickets

54. **What is the significance of craniotabes?**
   In this condition, abnormally soft, thin skull bones buckle under pressure and recoil like a ping-pong ball. It is best elicited on the parietal or frontal bones and is often associated with rickets in infancy. It may also be seen in hypervitaminosis A, syphilis, and hydrocephalus. Craniotabes may be a normal finding during the first 3 months of life.

55. **What evaluations should be done in a child with microcephaly?**
   The extent of evaluation depends on various factors: prenatal versus postnatal acquisition, presence of minor or major anomalies, developmental problems, and neurologic abnormalities. The diagnosis can be as straightforward as a simple familial variant (autosomal dominant) in a child with normal intelligence, or it can range to a variety of conditions associated with abnormal brain growth (e.g., intrauterine infections, heritable syndromes, chromosomal abnormalities). Evaluation may include the following:
   - Parental head-size measurements
   - Ophthalmologic evaluation (abnormal optic nerve or retinal findings may be found in various syndromes)
   - Karyotype
   - Neuroimaging (cranial magnetic resonance imaging or computed tomography to evaluate for structural abnormalities or intracranial calcifications)
   - Metabolic screening
   - Cultures and serology if suspected intrauterine infection

56. **What are the three main general causes of macrocephaly?**
   - **Increased intracranial pressure:** Caused by dilated ventricles (e.g., progressive hydrocephalus of various causes), subdural fluid collections, intracranial tumors, or benign increased intracranial pressure (i.e., pseudotumor cerebri) from various causes

- **Thickened skull:** Caused by cranioskeletal dysplasias (e.g., osteopetrosis) and various anemias
- **Megalencephaly** (enlarged brain): May be familial or syndromic (e.g., Sotos syndrome) or caused by storage diseases, leukodystrophies, or neurocutaneous disorders (e.g., neurofibromatosis)

DENTAL DEVELOPMENT AND DISORDERS

57. **When do primary and permanent teeth erupt?**
Mandibular teeth usually erupt first. The central incisors appear by the age of 5 to 7 months, with about 1 new tooth per month thereafter until 23 to 30 months, at which time the second molars (and thus all 20 primary or deciduous teeth) are in place. Of the 32 permanent teeth, the central incisors erupt first between 5 and 7 years, and the third molars are in place by 17-22 years.

American Academy of Pediatric Dentistry: http://www.aapd.org.

American Society of Dentistry for Children: http://www.ucsf.edu/ads/asdc.html.

58. **What is the significance of natal teeth?**
Occasionally, teeth are present at birth (natal teeth) or erupt within 30 days after birth (neonatal teeth). When x-rays are taken, 95% of natal teeth are primary incisors, and 5% are supernumerary teeth or extra teeth. Very sharp teeth that can cause tongue lacerations and very loose teeth that can be aspirated should be removed. Females are affected more commonly than males, and the prevalence is 1 in 2000 to 3500. Most cases are familial and without consequence, but natal teeth can be associated with genetic syndromes, including the Ellis-van Creveld and Hallermann-Streiff syndromes.

59. **How common is the congenital absence of teeth?**
The congenital absence of primary teeth is very rare, but up to 25% of individuals may have an absence of one or more third molars, and up to 5% may have an absence of another secondary or permanent tooth (most commonly the maxillary lateral incisors and mandibular second premolar).

60. **What are mesiodentes?**
These are **peg-shaped supernumerary teeth** that occur in up to 5% of individuals, and they are most commonly situated in the maxillary midline. They should be considered for removal because they interfere with the eruption of permanent incisors.

61. **What is a ranula?**
A large **mucocele,** usually bluish, painless, soft, and unilateral, that occurs under the tongue. Most of these self-resolve. If a patient has a large one, surgical marsupialization can be done. If the ranula is recurrent, excision may be needed.

62. **Where are Epstein pearls located?**
These white, superficial, mobile nodules are usually midline and often paired on the hard palate in many newborns. They are keratin-containing cysts that are asymptomatic, do not increase in size, and usually exfoliate spontaneously within a few weeks.

63. **What is the most common chronic disease of childhood?**
Early childhood dental caries affects more than half of 7-year-olds, which is about triple the rate of obesity and five times the rate of asthma. By 17 years old, only 15% to 20% of individuals are free from dental caries, and the average child has 8 decayed, missing, or filled tooth surfaces. Prevention of dental caries involves decreasing the frequency of tooth exposure to carbohydrates (frequency is more important than total amount), using fluoride, brushing the teeth, and using sealants.

Section on Pediatric Dentistry and Oral Health, American Academy of Pediatrics: Preventive oral health intervention for pediatricians, *Pediatrics* 122:1387–1394, 2008.

64. **What are milk-bottle caries?**

Frequent contact of cariogenic liquids (e.g., milk, formula, breast milk, juice) with teeth, as occurs in infants who fall asleep with a bottle or who are breastfed frequently at night after the age of 1 year ("nursing caries"), has been associated with a significant increase in the development of caries (Fig. 2-4). The AAP recommends that infants not be put to sleep with a bottle (unless it is filled with water), that nocturnal ad lib breast feeding be limited as dental development progresses, and that cup feedings be introduced when the child is 1 year old.

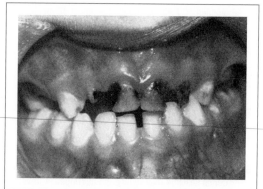

Figure 2-4. Classic nursing bottle decay involving the maxillary anterior teeth. Mandibular incisors are protected by the tongue during feeding and are usually caries free. (From Gessner IH, Victorica BE: Pediatric Cardiology: A Problem-Oriented Approach. Philadelphia, W.B. Saunders, 1993, p 232.)

65. **Which children are at higher risk for caries?**

Family history (parents, siblings) of caries, visible white spots or plaques on teeth, suboptimal exposure to fluoridated water, nighttime milk or juice feedings from bottles, frequent intake of sugar-laden food between meals. The American Academy of Pediatric Dentistry has a rapid screening tool to assess the risk for caries. The higher the risk, the earlier a dental visit should take place.

American Academy of Pediatric Dentistry: *Policy on use of a caries-risk assessment tool (CAT) for infants, children and adolescents.* Available at: http://www.aapd.org/media/Policies_Guidelines/P_CariesRiskAssess.pdf. Accessed on October 1, 2009.

Silk H: Making oral health a priority in your preventive pediatric visits, *Clin Pediatr* 49:103-109, 2010.

66. **How does fluoride minimize the development of dental caries?**

■ Topical fluoride from toothbrushing is thought to increase the remineralization of enamel.

■ Bacterial fermentation of sugar into acid plays a major role in the development of caries, and fluoride inhibits this process.

■ As teeth are developing, fluoride incorporates into the hydroxyapatite crystal of enamel, thereby making it less soluble and less susceptible to erosion.

67. **What is fluorosis?**

Exposure to excessive levels of fluoride during tooth development, primarily in a patient younger than 8 years, can damage enamel, causing changes that range from mild (lacy white markings) to severe (pitting, mottling, striations).

68. **How long should fluoride supplementation be continued?**

Fluoride supplementation should continue until a child is 14 to 16 years old, when the third molar crowns are completely calcified.

KEY POINTS: DENTAL PROBLEMS

1. Prolonged pacifier use beyond the age of 18 months can result in oral and dental distortions.

2. Dental caries is the most common chronic disease of childhood.

3. Appropriate use of fluoride and dental sealants could prevent caries in most children.

4. Use of formula or breastfeeding at bedtime after dental eruption leads to higher incidences of caries.

5. Excessive fluoride is associated initially with a white, speckled, or lacy appearance of the enamel.

---

69. **How effective are dental sealants for preventing cavities?**
Dental sealants may reduce the development of caries by up to 80% compared with rates in untreated teeth. Although fluoride acts primarily by protecting smooth surfaces, dental sealants (commonly bisphenol A and glycidyl methacrylate) act by protecting the pits and fissures of the surface, especially in posterior teeth. Reapplication may be needed every 2 years. As a preventive dental procedure, it is relatively underused.

70. **How common is gingivitis in children?**
Gingivitis is **extremely common,** affecting nearly 50% of children. The disorder is usually painless and is manifested by the bluish-red discoloration of gums, which are swollen and bleed easily. The cause is bacteria in plaque deposits between teeth; the cure is improved dental hygiene and daily flossing.

71. **What is the largest health-related expense before adulthood for normally developing children?**
Dental braces. More than 50% of children have dental malocclusions that could be improved with treatment, but only 10% to 20% have severe malocclusions that require treatment. For others, the costs and benefits of braces need to be weighed individually. Besides the financial expense, the costs of braces include physical discomfort and some increases in the risk for tooth decay and periodontal disease.

72. **What causes halitosis is children?**
Halitosis (bad breath) is usually the result of oral factors, including microbial activity on the dorsal tongue and between the teeth. Conditions associated with postnasal drip, including chronic sinusitis, upper and lower respiratory tract infections, and various systemic diseases, are also causes.

Amir E, Shimonov R, Rosenberg M: Halitosis in children, *J Pediatr* 134:338–343, 1999.

73. **Pacifiers: friend or foe?**
Pros: Appear to reduce the risk for SIDS (for this reason, use in infancy is now encouraged by the AAP after breastfeeding is well established); role as soother
Cons: May (or may not) promote early discontinuation of breastfeeding; may modestly increase the risk for otitis media; if improperly cleaned, may serve as bacterial reservoir; with two-piece design, potential for aspiration; potential for compulsive use (pacifier addiction); persistent use (years) can interfere with normal teeth positioning.

O'Connor NR, Tanabe KO, et al: Pacifiers and breastfeeding: a systematic review, *Arch Pediatr Adolesc Med* 163:378–382, 2009.

Schwartz RH, Guthrie KL: Infant pacifiers: an overview, *Clin Pediatr* 47:327–331, 2008.

DEVELOPMENTAL ASSESSMENT

74. **What are primitive reflexes?**
Primitive reflexes are *automatisms* that are usually triggered by an external stimulus. They are thought to emanate from primitive regions of the central nervous system: the spine, the inner ear labyrinths, and the brainstem. Examples are rooting, which is triggered by touching the corner of the mouth, and the asymmetrical tonic neck reflex (ATNR), which is triggered by rotating the head. Some reflexes (e.g., rooting, sucking, and grasp) have survival value. Others, such as the ATNR or the tonic labyrinthine reflex, have no obvious purpose. Placing and stepping reflexes usually disappear by 2 months. Moro and grasp reflexes and the ATNR usually disappear by 5 months.

75. **What three primitive reflexes, if persistent beyond 4 to 6 months, can interfere with the development of the ability to roll, sit, and use both hands together?**
Moro reflex: Sudden neck extension results in extension, abduction, and then adduction of the upper extremities with flexion of fingers, wrists, and elbows.
ATNR: In a calm supine infant, turning of the head laterally results in relative extension of the arm and leg on the side of the turn and flexion of both on the side away from the turn (the "fencer" position).
Tonic labyrinthine reflex: In an infant who is being held suspended in the prone position, flexion of the neck results in shoulder protraction and hip flexion, whereas neck extension causes shoulder retraction and hip extension.

> Zafeiriou DI: Primitive reflexes and postural reactions in the neurodevelopmental examination, *Pediatr Neurol* 31:1–8, 2004.

76. **At what age do children develop handedness?**
Usually by **18 to 24 months.** Hand preference is usually fixed by the time a child is 5 years old. Handedness before 1 year may be indicative of a problem with the nonpreferred side (e.g., hemiparesis, brachial plexus injury).

77. **What percentage of children are left-handed?**
Various studies put the prevalence at **between 7% and 10%.** However, in former premature infants without cerebral palsy, the rate increases to 20% to 25%. Although antecedent brain injury has been hypothesized to account for this increase in prevalence of left-handedness, studies of unilateral intraventricular hemorrhage and handedness have not demonstrated a relationship. Of note is that animals such as mice, dogs, and cats show paw preferences, but, in these groups, 50% prefer the left paw and 50% prefer the right paw.

> Marlow N, Roberts BL, Cooke RW: Laterality and prematurity, *Arch Dis Child* 64:1713–1716, 1989.

78. **What are the major developmental landmarks for motor skills during the first 2 years of life?**
See Table 2-1.

79. **What are the most common causes of gross motor delay?**
Normal variation is the most common, followed by **mental retardation. Cerebral palsy** is a distant third, and all other conditions combined (e.g., spinal muscular atrophy, myopathies) run a distant fourth. The most common pathologic cause of gross motor delay is MR, although most children with this condition have normal gross motor milestones.

TABLE 2-1. MAJOR DEVELOPMENTAL LANDMARKS FOR MOTOR SKILLS	
Developmental Landmark	Age Range (mo)
Major Gross Motor	
Steadiness of head when placed in supported position	1-4
Sits without support for >30 seconds	5-8
Cruises or walks holding on to things	7-13
Stands alone	9-16
Walks alone	9-17
Walks up stairs with help	12-23
Major Fine Motor	
Grasp	2-4
Reach	3-5
Transfers objects from hand to hand	5-7
Fine pincer grasp with index finger and thumb apposition	9-14
Spontaneous scribbling	12-24

80. **Do infant walkers promote physical strength or development of the lower extremities?**

No. On the contrary, published data confirm that infants in walkers actually manifest mild but statistically significant gross motor delays. Infants with walkers were found to sit and crawl later than those without walkers. However, most walk unaided within a normal time frame. Safety hazards can include head trauma, fractures, burns, finger entrapments, and dental injuries. Most of the serious injuries involve falls down stairs.

Pin TP, Eldridge B, Galea MP: A review of the effects of sleep position, play position and equipment use on motor development in infants, *Dev Med Child Neuro* 49:858–867, 2007.

81. **Do twins develop at a rate that is comparable to infants of single birth?**

Twins exhibit **significant verbal and motor delay** during the first year of life. The difficulty lies not in the lack of potential but in the relative lack of individual stimulation. In general, children who are more closely spaced in a family have slower acquisition of verbal skills. Twins with significant language delay or with excessive use of "twin language" (language understood only by the twins themselves) may be candidates for interventional therapy.

82. **Do premature infants develop at the same rate as term infants?**

For the most part, premature infants do develop at the same rate as term infants. In ongoing developmental assessments, they eventually "catch up" to their chronologic peers, not by accelerated development, but rather through the arithmetic of time. As they age, their degree of prematurity (in months) becomes less of a percentage of their chronologic age. Early in life, the extent of prematurity is key and must be taken into account during assessments. Such "correction factors" are generally unnecessary after the age of 2 to 3 years, depending on the degree of prematurity.

83. **When can an infant smell?**

The sense of smell is present **at birth.** Newborn infants show preferential head turning toward gauze pads soaked with their mother's milk as opposed to the milk of another woman.

In one study, infants exposed to familiar odors prior to heelstick procedures had lower pain responses.

Goubet N, Strasbaugh K, Chesney J: Familiarity breeds content? Soothing effect of a familiar odor on full-term newborns, *J Dev Behav Pediatr* 28:189–194, 2007.

84. **What are the best measures of cognitive development?**
Ideally, cognitive development should be assessed in a fashion that is free of motor requirements. **Receptive language** is the best measure of cognitive function. Even an eye blink or a voluntary eye gaze can be used to assess cognition independently of motor disability. Adaptive skills such as tool use (e.g., spoon, crayon) are also useful, although they may be delayed because of purely motoric reasons. Gross motor milestones such as walking raise concerns about MR if they are delayed, but normal gross motor milestones cannot be used to infer normal cognitive development.

85. **What do the stages of play tell us about a child's development?**
A well-taken history of a child's play is a valuable adjunct to more traditional milestones such as language and adaptive skills (Table 2-2).

TABLE 2-2. PLAY ACTIVITY AND CHILD DEVELOPMENT		
Age Range (mo)	Play Activity	Underlying Skills
3	Midline hand play	Sensorimotor; self-discovery
4-5	Bats at objects	Ability to affect environment
6-7	Directed reaching; transfers	
7-9	Banging and mouthing objects	
12	Casting ("I throw it down, and you pick it up for me"); explores objects by visual inspection and handling rather than orally	Object permanence; social reciprocity; use of pointing, joint attention (eye gaze), and simple language to effect response in caregiver
16-18+	Stacking and dumping; exploring; lids; light switches; simple mechanical toys (jack-in-the-box; shape ball)	Means-ends behavior: experimenting with causality
24	Imitative play ("helping" with the dishes; doll play with a physical doll)	Language and socialization; development of "inner language"
36	Make-believe play (e.g., doll play with a pillow to represent the doll)	Distinguish between "real" and "not real"
48	Simple board games, rule-based playground games (e.g., "tag")	Concrete operations (Piaget)

Data from http://www.parentcenter.com.

86. **What can one learn about a child's developmental level with regard to the use of a crayon?**
A lot. At less than 9 months, the infant will use the crayon as a teething object. Between 10 and 14 months, the infant will make marks on a piece of paper, almost as a by-product of holding the crayon and "banging" it against the paper. By 14 to 16 months, the infant will make marks spontaneously, and, by 18 to 20 months, he or she will make marks with vigorous scribbling. By 20 to 22 months, an infant will begin copying specific geometric patterns as presented by the examiner (Table 2-3). The ability to execute these figures requires visual-perceptual, fine motor, and cognitive abilities. Delay in the ability to complete these tasks suggests difficulty with one or more of these underlying streams of development.

TABLE 2-3. CRAYON USE AND DEVELOPMENT LEVEL

Age	Task
20-22 mo	Alternates from scribble to stroke on imitation of examiner
27-30 mo	Alternates from horizontal to vertical on imitation of examiner
36 mo	Copies circle from illustration
3 yr	Copies cross
4 yr	Copies square
5 yr	Copies triangle
6 yr	Copies "Union Jack"

87. **What is the value of the Goodenough-Harris drawing test?**
This "draw a person" test is a screening tool used to evaluate a child's cognition and intellect, visual perception, and visual-motor integration. The child is asked to draw a person, and a point is given for each body part drawn with pairs (e.g., legs) that is considered as one part. An average child that is 4 years and 9 months will draw a person with three parts; most children by the age of 5 years and 3 months will draw a person with six parts.

LANGUAGE DEVELOPMENT AND DISORDERS

88. **What are average times for the development of expressive, receptive, and visual language milestones?**
See Table 2-4.

TABLE 2-4. DEVELOPMENT OF EXPRESSIVE, RECEPTIVE, AND VISUAL LANGUAGE

Age (mo)	Expressive	Receptive	Visual
0-3	Coo	Alerts to voice	Recognizes parents; visual tracking
4-6	Monosyllabic babbling, laugh, "raspberry"	Turns to voice and sounds	Responds to facial expressions
7-9	Polysyllabic babbling; mama/dada, nonspecific	Recognizes own name; inhibits to command "No"	Imitates games (patty cake; peek-a-boo)

(continued)

TABLE 2-4. DEVELOPMENT OF EXPRESSIVE, RECEPTIVE, AND VISUAL LANGUAGE *(continued)*

Age (mo)	Expressive	Receptive	Visual
10-12	Mama/dada specific; first word other than mama/dada or names of other family members or pets	Follows at least 1 one-step command without a gestural cue (e.g., "Come here," "Give me")	Points to desired objects
16-18	Uses words to indicate wants	Follows many one-step commands; points to body parts on command	
22-24	Two-word phrases	Follows two-step commands	
30	Telegraphic speech	Follows prepositional commands	
36	Simple sentences		

89. **What are signs of significantly delayed receptive and expressive speech delay warranting evaluation?**
See Table 2-5.

TABLE 2-5. SIGNS OF SPEECH–LANGUAGE PROBLEMS ABSOLUTELY NEEDING FURTHER EVALUATION

At Age (mo)	Receptive	Expressive
15	Does not look/point at 5-10 objects/people named by parent	Not using three words
18	Does not follow simple commands ("roll the ball")	No use of single words (including mama, dada)
24	Does not point to pictures or body parts when they are named	Single-word vocabulary of ≤10 words
30	Does not verbally respond or nod/shake head to questions	Not using unique two-word phrases, including noun-verb combinations; unintelligible speech
36	Does not understand prepositions or action words; does not follow two-step directions	Vocabulary <200 words; does not ask for things by name; echolalia to questions; regression of language after acquiring two-word phrases

Data from Harlor ADB Jr, Bower C, et al: Clinical report—hearing assessment in infants and children: recommendations beyond neonatal screening. Pediatrics 124:1252–1263, 2009; and Schum RL: Language screening in the pediatric office setting. Pediatr Clin N Am 54:432, 2007.

American Speech-Language-Hearing Association: http://www.asha.org.

90. **Do deaf infants babble?**
Yes. Babbling begins at about the same time in both deaf and hearing infants, but deaf infants stop babbling without the normal progression to meaningful communicative speech.

Locke JL: Babbling and early speech: continuity and individual differences, *First Language* 9:191–205, 1989.

Laurent Clerc National Deaf Education Center: http://clerccenter.gallaudet.edu.

91. **At what age does a child's speech become intelligible?**
Intelligibility increases by about 25% per year. A 1-year-old child has about 25% intelligibility, a 2-year-old has 50%, a 3-year-old has 75%, and a 4-year-old has 100%. Significantly delayed intelligibility should prompt a hearing and language evaluation.

92. **What are the most common causes of so-called delayed speech?**
The most common causes of speech or language delay include the following: developmental language disorders (i.e., normal cognition, impaired intelligibility, and delayed emergence of phrases, sentences, and grammatical markers), MR, hearing loss, and autistic spectrum disorder.

Feldman HM: Evaluation and management of language and speech disorders in preschool children, *Pediatr Rev* 26:131–142, 2005.

93. **What causes flat tympanograms?**
Tympanometry is an objective measurement of the compliance of the tympanic membrane and the middle ear compartment that involves varying the air pressure in the external ear canal from about -200 to $+400$ mm H_2O while measuring the reflected energy of a simultaneous acoustic tone. A normal tracing looks like an inverted "V," with the peak occurring at an air pressure of 0 mm H_2O; this indicates a functionally normal external canal, an intact tympanic membrane, and a lack of excess of middle ear fluid. Flat tympanograms occur with perforation of the tympanic membrane, occlusion of the tympanometry probe against the wall of the canal, obstruction of the canal by a foreign body or impaction by cerumen, or large middle ear effusion. Flat tympanograms due to middle ear effusion are usually associated with a 20- to 30-dB conductive hearing loss, although in occasional instances, the loss may be as great as 50 dB.

94. **A toddler with a bifid uvula and hypernasal speech most likely has what condition?**
Velopharyngeal insufficiency with a possible submucosal cleft palate. The velum (soft palate) moves posteriorly during swallowing and speech, thereby separating the oropharynx from the nasopharynx. Velopharyngeal insufficiency exists when this separation is incomplete, which may occur after cleft palate repair or adenoidectomy (usually transient). In severe cases, nasopharyngeal regurgitation of food may occur. In milder cases, the only manifestation may be hypernasal speech as a result of the nasal emission of air during phonation. If a bifid uvula is present, one should palpate the palate carefully for the presence of a submucous cleft.

KEY POINTS: LANGUAGE DEVELOPMENT

1. Very red flags: No meaningful words by 18 months or no meaningful phrases by 2 years.

2. Intelligibility should increase yearly by 25%, from 25% at 1 year of age up to 100% at 4 years of age.

3. Stuttering is common in younger children, but beyond the age of 5 to 6 years, it warrants speech evaluation.

4. Autism, mental retardation, and cerebral palsy can present with speech delay.

5. Evaluation of hearing is mandatory in any setting of significant speech delay.

95. **When is stuttering abnormal?**

Stuttering is a common characteristic of the speech of preschool children. However, most children do not persist with stuttering beyond 5 or 6 years of age. Preschoolers at increased risk for persistence of stuttering include those with a positive family history of stuttering and those with anxiety-provoking stress related to talking. A child older than 5 or 6 years who stutters should be referred to a speech-language pathologist for assessment and treatment.

National Center for Stuttering: http://www.stuttering.com.

96. **What advice should be given to parents of a child who stutters?**

■ Do not give the child directives about how to deal with his or her speech (e.g., "Slow down" or "Take a breath").

■ Provide a relaxed, easy speech model in your own manner of speaking to the child.

■ Reduce the need and expectations for the child to speak to strangers, adults, or authority figures or to compete with others (such as siblings) to be heard.

■ Listen attentively to the child with patience and without showing concern.

■ Seek professional guidance if speech is not noticeably more fluent in 2 to 3 months.

97. **Which infants with "tongue tie" should have surgical correction?**

"Tongue tie," complete or partial ankyloglossia, is the restriction of mobility of the tongue due to a short or thickened lingual frenulum (Fig. 2-5). Complete ankyloglossia, with the tongue unable to protrude past the alveolar ridge or to move laterally, is uncommon but, when present, requires frenuloplasty. Partial ankyloglossia with

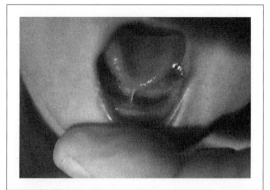

Figure 2-5. Newborn with ankyloglossia. (From Clark DA: Atlas of Neonatology. Philadelphia, W.B. Saunders, 2000, p 146.)

variability in lingual range of motion occurs in up to 5% of newborns. There is a wide range of opinion regarding the need for "clipping." Partial ankyloglossia can interfere with breastfeeding when there is limited lingual extension or inability to touch the hard palate with the mouth wide open. Although in recent history, it has been infrequently performed, in-office lingual frenotomy is an option (procedure is viewable at http://www.youtube.com/watch?v=XN-vVYd1m-o). Ankyloglossia is less commonly associated with speech problems.

Martin MS, Schwartz RH: Tackling ankyloglossia in the office, *Contemp Pediatr* 25:59–64, 2008.

Krol DM, Keels MA: Oral conditions, *Pediatr Rev* 28:17–18, 2007.

Lalakea ML, Messner AH: Ankyloglssia: does it matter? *Pediatr Clin N Am* 50:381–397, 2003.

MENTAL RETARDATION

98. **How is mental retardation defined?**

There are efforts to add adaptive behaviors to the definition as well as the traditional subaverage level of intellectual function. The American Association on Mental Retardation (AMMR) defines MR as "significantly sub-average general intellectual functioning [IQ of

70 to 75] accompanied by significant limitations in adaptive functioning in at least two of the following skill areas: communication, self-care, social skills, self-direction, academic skills, work, leisure, health, and/or safety. These limitations manifest themselves before 18 years of age." DSM-IV-TR criteria rely more heavily on IQ scores.

99. **Should the term *mental retardation* be changed?**
There is controversy that the term is stigmatizing and pejorative. Alternatives proposed include *intellectual disability* or *cognitive-adaptive disorder*. The AAMR reflects those concerns by its name change to the American Association on Intellectual and Developmental Disabilities (AAIDD). However, because of numerous statutes and programs that use the term *mental retardation* and thus carry legal ramifications, the change will likely be a gradual process.

Schalock RL, Luckasson RA, Shogren KA, et al: The renaming of mental retardation: understanding the change to the term intellectual disability, *Intellect Dev Disabil* 45:116–124, 2007.

100. **How is intelligence classified with IQ scores?**
Most IQ tests are constructed to yield a mean IQ of 100 and a standard deviation of 15 points (Table 2-6).

TABLE 2-6. CONSTRUCTION OF INTELLIGENCE QUOTIENT SCORES

Intelligence Quotient	Standard Deviation	Category
>130	>+2	Very superior
116-130	+1 to +2	High average to superior
115-85	Mean ± 1	Average
84-70	−1 to −2	Low average to borderline MR
69-55	−2 to −3	Mild MR
54-40	−3 to −4	Moderate MR
39-25	−4 to −5	Severe MR
<25	<−5	Profound MR

MR, mental retardation.

101. **What features can indicate cognitive problems in infants and young children?**
In younger infants and toddlers, fine motor skill development and especially language development are the usual best correlates of cognitive achievement. As the child ages, the various milestones can be evaluated. Significant sequential delay should warrant referral for formal developmental testing to evaluate the possibility of MR (Table 2-7).

First LR, Palfrey JS: The infant or young child with developmental delay, *N Engl J Med* 330:478–483, 1994.

102. **Worldwide, what is the most common preventable cause of MR?**
Iodine deficiency leads to maternal and fetal hypothyroxinemia during gestation, which causes brain developmental injury. Severe endemic iodine deficiency can cause cretinism (characterized by deaf-mutism, severe intellectual deficiency, and often hypothyroidism) and may occur in 2% to 10% of isolated world communities. Moderate iodine deficiency, which is even more common, leads to milder degrees of cognitive impairment.

Zimmermann MB, Jooste PL, Pandav CS: Iodine-deficiency disorders, *Lancet* 372:1251–1262, 2008.

Cao XY, Jiang XM, Dou ZH, et al: Timing of vulnerability of the brain to iodine deficiency in endemic cretinism, *N Engl J Med* 331:1739–1744, 1994.

TABLE 2-7. SIGNS OF SEQUENTIAL DELAY IN COGNITIVE ACHIEVEMENT	
2-3 mo	Not alerting to mother with special interest
6-7 mo	Not searching for dropped object
8-9 mo	No interest in peek-a-boo
12 mo	Does not search for hidden object
15-18 m	No interest in cause-and-effect games
2 yr	Does not categorize similarities (e.g., animals versus vehicles)
3 yr	Does not know own full name
4 yr	Cannot pick shorter or longer of two lines
4½ yr	Cannot count sequentially
5 yr	Does not know colors or any letters
5½ yr	Does not know own birthday or address

PSYCHIATRIC DISORDERS

103. **What is the prevalence of childhood psychiatric disorders?**
Overall, 15% to 20% of children 4 to 20 years old in community samples are diagnosed with a specific psychiatric disorder. The most common disorders are as follows:
■ Attention deficit hyperactivity disorder (4% to 10%)
■ Separation anxiety (3% to 5%)
■ Oppositional disorder (5% to 10%)
■ Overanxious disorder (2% to 5%)
■ Conduct disorder (1% to 5%)
■ Depression (2% to 6%)

   National Institute of Mental Health: http://www.nimh.nih.gov.

   American Academy of Child and Adolescent Psychiatry: http://www.aacap.org.

104. **If a parent has an affective disorder, what is the likelihood that an offspring will have similar problems?**
Approximately 20% to 25% of these children will develop a major affective disorder, and as many as 40% to 45% will have a psychiatric problem.

105. **How does mania differ in children and adolescents?**
Mania occurs in about 0.5% to 1% of adolescents and occurs less frequently in prepubertal children. *Younger children* may present with extreme irritability, emotional lability, and aggression. Dysphoria, hypomania, and agitation may be intermixed. Hyperactivity, distractibility, and pressured speech often occur in all age groups. Symptoms in *adolescents* more closely resemble those seen in adults. They include elated mood, flight of ideas, sleeplessness, bizarre behavior, delusions of grandeur, paranoia, and euphoria.

106. **What ritualistic behaviors are common in children with obsessive-compulsive disorder?**
The most common rituals involve **excessive cleaning, repeating gross motor rituals** (e.g., going up and down stairs), and **repetitive checking behaviors** (e.g., checking that doors are locked or that homework is correct). Obsessions most commonly deal with fear of

contamination. Symptoms tend to wax and wane in severity, and the specific obsessions or compulsions change over time. Most children attempt to disguise their rituals. Anxiety and distress that interfere with school or family life can occur when children fail in their efforts to resist the thoughts or activities. Cognitive behavioral therapy and selective serotonin-reuptake inhibitor (SSRI) medications (e.g., sertraline), particularly in combination, can be beneficial.

Gilbert AR, Maalouf FT: Pediatric obsessive-compulsive disorder: management in primary care, *Curr Opin Pediatr* 20:544–550, 2008.

107. **What distinguishes a conduct disorder from an oppositional defiant disorder?**
Both are disruptive behavior disorders of childhood and early adolescence. **Conduct disorder** is the more serious disorder in that it is diagnosed when the child's behaviors violate the rights of others (e.g., assault) or are in conflict with major societal norms (e.g., stealing, truancy, setting fires). Children with conduct disorder are at risk for developing the antisocial personality disorder seen in adults. **Oppositional defiant disorder** is characterized by recurrent negative and defiant behaviors toward authority figures.

108. **What are common symptoms of depression in children and adolescents?**
- Sadness
- School problems
- Tearfulness
- Somatic complaints
- Irritability
- Suicidal ideation
- Negative self-imagery
- Changes in appetite
- Lack of concentration
- Unintended weight changes
- Decreased interest in usual activities
- Sleep problems, including hypersomnia
- Fatigue
- Delusions

109. **How is depression in children diagnosed?**
The DSM-IV-TR criteria require the presence of five or more symptoms from the categories of sleep, interest, guilt, concentration, appetite, psychomotor, and suicide during the same 2-week period. A variety of ratings scales (e.g., the Hamilton Depression Rating Scale, the Childhood Depression Inventory, the Child Behavioral Checklist, the Beck Depression Inventory) are available to assist with evaluation.

110. **What are treatments for major depressive disorder in children and adolescents?**
Psychotherapy: Various types of therapy may be used, including cognitive-behavioral therapy, interpersonal therapy, and family therapy.
Psychopharmacology: SSRIs have been recommended by the American Academy of Child and Adolescent Psychiatry as the treatment of choice for children who warrant pharmacotherapy. There have been controversial warnings by regulatory agencies in Britain and the United States that antidepressant medications may be associated with an increased risk for suicide.
Electroconvulsive therapy: This treatment is reserved for psychotic or life-threatening depression that is unresponsive to other treatments.

U.S. Preventive Services Task Force: Screening and treatment for major depressive disorder in children and adolescents: U.S. Preventive Services Task Force recommendation statement, *Pediatrics* 123:1223–1228, 2009.

Zuckerbrot RA, Cheung A, Jensen PS, et al: Guidelines for adolescent depression in primary care—GLAD PC—part 1, *Pediatrics* 120:e1299–e1312, 2007.

111. **Are any laboratory tests indicated in the evaluation of possible depression in children?**
Depending on the history and the physical examination, laboratory and radiographic studies may be indicated if an organic cause of symptoms is suspected. Thyroid function studies, a complete blood count to evaluate for anemia, pregnancy testing in postpubertal girls, and toxicology testing (if drug abuse is suspected) should be considered.

Jackson B, Lurie S: Adolescent depression: challenges and opportunities, *Adv Pediatr* 53:111–163, 2006.

112. **How likely is it that a depressed teenager will be a depressed adult?**
Despite being a treatable condition, depression is chronic and recurrent, and up to 60% of teenagers will have recurrence as an adult.

Weissman MM, Wolk S, Goldstein RB, et al: Depressed adolescents grow up, *JAMA* 281: 1707–1713, 1999.

113. **What are types of anxiety disorders in children?**
Separation anxiety disorder: Developmentally inappropriate, unrealistic, persistent fears of separation from caregivers that interfere with daily activities
Panic disorder: Recurrent, discrete periods of intense fear or discomfort; rare in prepubertal children; may occur with or without agoraphobia (fear or distress in or about places that may limit egress, such as a restaurant)
Social anxiety disorder: Extreme anxiety about social interactions with peers and adults; may manifest as generalized or specific (e.g., public speaking)

114. **Which is preferable for children with anxiety disorders, cognitive behavioral therapy (CBT) or medication?**
Actually, a **combination of both.** In a study of 488 children using CBT alone, medication (sertraline) alone, combination therapy, or placebo, the combination therapy resulted in 80% very much or much improved as measured by ratings scales compared with either therapy alone or placebo.

Walkup JT, Albano AM, Piacentini J, et al: Cognitive behavioral therapy, sertraline, or a combination in childhood anxiety, *N Engl J Med* 359:2753–2766, 2008.

115. **What characterizes bipolar disorder?**
This is a *mood disorder* with fluctuations of *mania* followed by *depression* and interludes of relatively normal behavior. In children, there are often out-of-control mood swings with dramatic behavior changes including marked irritability and rage.
- **Manic episode:** Inflated self-esteem, decreased need for sleep, flight of ideas or racing thoughts, distractibility, increase in goal-directed activity, excessive involvement in dangerous activities that have a high potential for dangerous consequences
- **Major depressive episode:** Depressed mood, markedly diminished interest or pleasure in activities, significant changes in weight and appetite, insomnia or hypersomnia, fatigue or loss of energy, diminished ability to concentrate, indecisiveness, recurrent thoughts of death or suicide

Cummings CM, Fristad MA: Pediatric bipolar disorder: recognition in primary care, *Curr Opin Pediatr* 20:560–565, 2008.

116. **How does pediatric bipolar disorder differ from adult bipolar disorder?**
    ■ More irritability than euphoria
    ■ More complex cycling and mixing of mood states
    ■ High levels of comorbidity, especially ADHD

    Wozniak J, Biederman J: Bipolar disorder in children. In Parker S, Zuckerman B, Augustyn M, editors: *Developmental and Behavioral Pediatrics*, ed 2, Philadelphia, 2005, Lippincott Williams & Wilkins, pp 132–135.

PSYCHOSOCIAL FAMILY ISSUES

117. **How likely is it that children in the United States will experience the separation or divorce of their parents?**
    More than 50% of first marriages end in divorce. In the United States, about 1.5 million children experience parental divorce each year. It is estimated that nearly 75% of black children and 40% of white children born to married parents will experience their parents' divorce before they are 18 years old. An addition to this stressor is that 50% of individuals who divorce will remarry within 5 years, thus creating another major family transition for a child.

118. **How do children of different ages vary in their response to parental divorce?**
    Preschool age (2½ to 5 years): Most likely to show regression in developmental milestones (e.g., toilet training); irritability; sleep disturbances; preoccupation with fear of abandonment; demanding with remaining parent
    Early school age (6 to 8 years): Most likely to demonstrate open grieving; preoccupied with fear of rejection and of being replaced; half may have a decrease in school performance
    Later school age (9 to 12 years): More likely to demonstrate profound anger at one or both parents; more likely to distinguish one parent as the culprit causing the divorce; deterioration in school performance and peer relationships; sense of loneliness and powerlessness
    Adolescence: Significant potential for acute depression and even suicidal ideation; acting-out behavior (substance abuse, truancy, sexual activity); self-doubts about own potential for marital success

    Hetherington EM: Divorce and the adjustment of children, *Pediatr Rev* 26:163–169, 2005.

    Kelly JB: Children's adjustment in conflicted marriage and divorce: a decade review of research, *J Am Acad Child Adolesc Psychiatry* 39:963–973, 2000.

119. **What factors are central to a good outcome after a divorce?**
    ■ Ability of parents to set aside or resolve conflicts without involving children
    ■ Emotional and physical availability of custodial parent to the child
    ■ Parenting skills of custodial parent
    ■ Extent to which child does not feel rejected by noncustodial parent
    ■ Child's temperament
    ■ Presence of supportive family network
    ■ Absence of continuing anger or depression in the child

    Cohen GJ: Helping children deal with divorce and separation, *Pediatrics* 110:1019–1023, 2002.

120. **What is the "vulnerable child syndrome"?**
    The *vulnerable child syndrome* is characterized by excessive parental concern about the health and development of their child. It usually occurs after a medical illness in which the parents are understandably upset or worried about the child's health (e.g., prematurity,

congenital heart disease). However, this concern persists despite the child's recovery. Problems of the syndrome can include pathologic separation difficulties for parent and child, sleep problems, overprotectiveness, and overindulgence. Children are at risk for behavioral, school, and peer-relationship problems.

Pearson SR, Boyce WT: The vulnerable child syndrome, *Pediatr Rev* 25:345–348, 2004.

121. **How does the cognitive understanding of death evolve?**
Toddler (<2 years): Death as separation, abandonment, or change; may become irritable or withdrawn
Preschool (2 to 6 years): Prelogical thought with magical and egocentric beliefs that the child may be responsible for the death; death as temporary and reversible
School age (6 to 10 years): Concrete logical thinking; death as permanent and universal but due to a specific illness or injury rather than as a biologic process; death is something that occurs to others; may develop a morbid interest in death
Adolescence (>10 years): Abstract logical thinking; more complete comprehension of death; death as a possibility for self

Linebarger JS, Sahler OJZ, Egan KA: Coping with death, *Pediatr Rev* 30:350–355, 2009.

122. **Should adopted children be informed of their adoption?**
Yes. It should not occur as a one-time event, but rather increasing amounts of information can be given over time. Most preschool children will not understand the process or meaning of adoption, and for them, disclosure should be guided by what the child wants to know. School-age children should be aware of their adoption and feel comfortable discussing it with their parents.

Borchers D, for the American Academy of Pediatrics Committee on Early Childhood, Adoption, and Dependent Care: Families and adoption: The pediatrician's role in supporting communication, *Pediatrics* 112:1437–1441, 2003.

123. **How common is domestic violence?**
Statistics indicate that 10% to 40% of families are afflicted by domestic violence. The potential impact on children in these families is enormous, including behavioral problems, developmental delay, and abuse. The AAP has recommended that all pediatricians incorporate screening for domestic violence as part of anticipatory guidance.

Parkinson GW, Adams RC, Emerling FG: Maternal domestic violence screening in an office-based pediatric practice, *Pediatrics* 108:e43–e51, 2001.

124. **Does participation in day care during infancy and the toddler years have negative effects on cognitive development?**
This question has been examined in a large multisite study funded by the National Institute of Child Health and Human Development. At 24 and 36 months of age, there has been no demonstrable relationship between the number of hours in day care and any of the measures of cognitive or language development. However, child care of higher quality was associated with better language and cognitive outcomes. The frequency of language stimulation in the child care setting seemed to be the most important variable.

125. **Who are "latchkey" children?**
The term refers to the millions of children younger than 18 years who are in unsupervised care after school because they are members of families in which one or two parents work. Because of the enormous variability of circumstances, the consequences may be positive (e.g., increased maturity, self-reliance) or negative (e.g., isolation, feelings of neglect). Increased after-school programs may minimize negative consequences.

126. **What are the effects of heavy television watching in young children?**
It is not hard to overestimate the television exposure of children. Thirty percent of preschoolers have a television in their bedroom. Young children in some studies spend up to one third of their waking hours watching television. Although the AAP discourages television viewing in the first 2 years of life, most children begin watching television at 5 months of age. Studies have documented the effects of heavy television viewing in the following areas: increased aggressive behavior (if exposed to more violent programming), increase in general level of arousal, increased risk for attentional problems, increased obesity, and decreased school performance. The long-term implications of this excessive early exposure to television are unclear, but negative effects on development, cognition, and attention have been demonstrated.

Christakis DA: The effects of infant media usage: what do we know and what should we learn? *Acta Paediatr* 98:8–16, 2009.

Schmidt ME, Rich M: Media and child health: pediatric care and anticipatory guidance for the information age, *Pediatr Rev* 27:289–297, 2006.

SCHOOL PROBLEMS

127. **How is "learning disability" defined?**
Currently, as defined by federal legislation, *learning disability* (LD) "means a disorder in one or more of the basic psychological processes involved in understanding or in using language, spoken or written, which may manifest itself in an imperfect ability to listen, think, speak, read, write, spell, or to do mathematical calculations." Such difficulties are not due to visual, hearing, or motor handicaps; emotional problems; MR; or environmental, social, cultural, or economic issues. This implies a discrepancy between academic achievement and that expected for age, schooling, and intelligence.

Dworkin PH: School failure. In Parker S, Zuckerman B, Augustyn M, editors: *Developmental and Behavioral Pediatrics*, ed 2, Philadelphia, 2005, Lippincott Williams & Wilkins, pp 280–284.

128. **What distinguishes dyslexia, dyscalculia, and dysgraphia?**
Dyslexia is a reading LD. It is the most common LD, affecting 3% to 15% of school-aged children. About 80% of children identified as learning disabled have dyslexia (or a specific reading difficulty) as their primary diagnosis. Characterized by problems decoding single words (i.e., reading single words in isolation), dyslexia is usually the result of deficits in phonological processing.
Dyscalculia, or specific mathematics disability, affects 1% to 6% of children. Mathematics disabilities involve difficulties in computation, math concepts, and/or the application of those concepts to everyday situations.
Dysgraphia, or disorder of written expression, affects up to 10% of children. Difficulties with writing have several possible etiologies, including problems with fine motor control, linguistic abilities, visual-spatial skills, motor planning, proprioception, attention, memory, and sequencing.

Feder KP, Majnemer A: Handwriting development, competency, and intervention, *Dev Med Child Neurol* 49:312–317, 2007.

Shaywitz SE, Shaywitz BA: Dyslexia. *Pediatr Rev* 24:147–152, 2003.

129. **What are clues that a school-aged child may have dyslexia?**
Problems in speaking: Mispronunciation of multisyllable words; hesitant, choppy speech; imprecise language
Problems in reading: Trouble reading and sounding out unfamiliar words; reading aloud is hesitant and choppy; handwriting is very messy; extremely poor speller; great difficulties in learning a foreign language; often a family history of reading or spelling difficulties

Shaywitz SE, Gruen JR, Shaywitz BA: Management of dyslexia, its rationale, and underlying neurobiology, *Pediatr Clin North Am* 54:609–623, 2007.

130. **In addition to learning disabilities, what factors may contribute to academic underachievement?**
   - Hearing or visual problems
   - MR
   - Developmental language disorders
   - ADHD
   - Emotional and psychiatric disorders
   - Disorganized home environment
   - Lack of social support
   - Sleep problems
   - Chronic medical conditions
   - Medications (e.g., anticonvulsants, antihistamines)

131. **How are the two types of school avoidance behaviors distinguished?**
   - **Anxiety-related avoidance:** Excessive fears (about peers, potential for teasing, grades); often an overprotective parent; typically excellent students with no classroom behavioral issues; girls affected more often than boys; symptoms are often physiologic manifestations of anxiety (e.g., headache, abdominal pain)
   - **Secondary-gain avoidance:** No anxiety about school; absence often follows lingering illness; "rewarded" at home for absence (e.g., sympathy, television); often are poor students; boys affected more often than girls; symptoms are fabricated or exaggerated (e.g., sore throat, extremity pain)

   Schmitt BD: School avoidance. In Parker S, Zuckerman B, Augustyn M, editors: *Developmental and Behavioral Pediatrics*, ed 2, Philadelphia, 2005, Lippincott Williams & Wilkins, pp 275–279.

132. **How much of a problem are bullies?**
   Bullying is defined as "intentional, unprovoked abuse of power by one or more children to inflict pain or cause distress to another child on repeated occasions." It is a universal problem in schools worldwide. The victims frequently experience a range of psychological, psychosomatic, and behavioral problems that include anxiety, insecurity, low self-esteem, sleeping difficulties, bedwetting, sadness, and frequent bouts of headache and abdominal pain. In this age of new media technology, electronic bullying (or cyberbullying) is a rapidly growing problem.

   Kowalksi RM, Limber SP: Childhood bullying among middle school students, *J Adolesc Health* 41: S22–S30, 2007.

   Lyznicki JM, McCaffree MA, Robinowitz CB: Childhood bullying: implications for physicians, *Am Fam Physician* 70:1723–1728, 2004.

SLEEP PROBLEMS

133. **What is the average daily sleep requirement by age?**
   - Newborns: 16 to 20 hours
   - 6 months: 13 to 14 hours
   - Toddlers (1 to 3 years): 12 hours
   - Preschoolers (3 to 6 years): 11 to 12 hours
   - Middle childhood (6 to 12 years): 10 to 11 hours
   - Adolescents (>12 years): 9 hours

   Chamness JA: Taking a pediatric sleep history, *Pediatr Ann* 37:503, 2008.

134. **Why is the supine sleeping position recommended for infants?**
   In countries that have advocated the supine sleeping position as a preventive measure for SIDS, there have been dramatic decreases in the incidence of the syndrome. Hypotheses on

why the prone position is more dangerous for infants have included the potential for airway obstruction and the possibility of rebreathing carbon dioxide, particularly when soft bedding is used.

135. **When do infants begin to sleep through the night?**
By the time they are about 3 months old, about 70% of infants (slightly more for bottle-fed babies and slightly less for breastfed babies) will not cry or awaken their parents between midnight and 6 AM. By 6 months, 90% of infants fit into this category, but between 6 and 9 months, the percentage of infants with night awakenings increases.

136. **What advice to parents may minimize the problem of night waking?**
- After a parent-child bedtime routine, place the infant in the sleep setting while he or she is still awake (i.e., do not rock an infant to sleep).
- The parent should not be present as the child falls asleep.
- Gradually eliminate night feedings (infants by 6 months receive sufficient daytime nutrition to allow this).
- Transitional objects (e.g., blanket, teddy bear) may minimize separation issues.
- Create a consistent sleep schedule and a bedtime routine.
- Avoid giving a child items in late afternoon or evening that contain caffeine (e.g., chocolate, soda).

Meltzer LJ, Mindell JA: Nonpharmacologic treatments for pediatric sleeplessness, *Pediatr Clin North Am* 51:135–151, 2004.

137. **How common are sleep problems in elementary school-aged children?**
About 40% of children between 7 and 12 years old experience sleep-onset delay, 10% experience night awakening, and 10% have significant daytime sleepiness. Some studies have shown that the extent of sleep is also inversely related to teacher-reported psychiatric symptoms.

Chamness JA: Taking a pediatric sleep history, *Pediatr Ann* 37:503, 2008.

138. **What are parasomnias?**
Parasomnias are undesirable physical phenomena that occur during sleep. Examples include night terrors, nightmares, sleepwalking, sleeptalking, nocturnal enuresis, sleep bruxism, somniloquy, and body rocking. Between the ages of 3 and 13 years, nearly 80% of all children will have had at least one parasomnia.

139. **At what age do sleepwalking and sleeptalking occur?**
Sleepwalking occurs most commonly between the ages of 5 and 10 years. As many as 15% of children between the ages of 5 and 12 years may have somnambulated once, and as many as 10% of 3- to 10-year-old children may sleepwalk regularly. The sleepwalking child is clumsy, restless, and walking without purpose, and the episode is not remembered. Injury is common during this outing. **Sleeptalking** is monosyllabic and often incomprehensible. Both conditions usually end before the age of 15 years. Severe cases may benefit from diazepam or imipramine therapy.

140. **What is the difference between nightmares and night terrors?**
Nightmares are frightening dreams that occur during rapid eye movement (REM) sleep (usually during the last half of the night) and that may be readily recalled on awakening. The child is aroused without difficulty and is usually easily consolable, but returning to sleep after a nightmare may be problematic.

Night terrors are brief episodes that occur during non-REM stage IV sleep. They usually last 30 seconds to 5 minutes, during which a child sits up, screams, and appears aroused, often staring and sweating profusely. The child cannot be consoled, rapidly goes back to sleep, and does not recall the episode in the morning. The onset of night terrors in an older child or persistent multiple attacks may indicate more serious psychopathology.

141. **What recommendation should be given to a parent whose child is having night terrors?**
An explanation of the phenomenon to the parent, with emphasis on the fact that the child is still asleep during the episode and should not be awakened, is all that is needed. If stress or sleep deprivation coincides with the night terrors, these factors should be addressed. If this is not successful, other approaches may be considered.
- When night terrors occur at the same time each night, the parent may awaken the child 15 minutes before the anticipated event over a 7-day period and keep him or her awake for at least 5 minutes. This often disrupts the sleep cycle and results in resolution of the problem.
- Rarely, for severe night terrors, a short course of diazepam will suppress REM sleep, reset the sleep cycles, and result in cessation of the problem.

VISUAL DEVELOPMENT AND DISORDERS

142. **How well does a newborn see?**
Because of the short diameter of the eye as well as retinal immaturity, a newborn's visual acuity is roughly 20/200 to 20/400. The human face is the most preferred object of fixation during early infancy. The light sense is one of the most primitive of all visual functions and is present by the 7th fetal month.

143. **Do babies make tears?**
Alacrima, or the absence of tear secretion, is not uncommon during the newborn period, although some infants may produce reflexive tearing at birth. In most others, tearing is delayed and typically not seen until the infant is 2 to 4 months old. Persistent lack of tearing is seen in Riley-Day syndrome (familial dysautonomia). This is a rare genetic syndrome seen in the Ashkenazi Jewish population, affecting 1 in 10,000 newborns. Other symptoms include diaphoresis, skin blotching or marbling, hyporeflexia, and indifference to pain.

144. **At what age does an infant's eye color assume its permanent color?**
A neonate's eyes will never be lighter than they are at birth. The pigmentation of the iris in all races increases over the first 6 to 12 months. The eye color is usually defined by 6 months and always by 1 year.

145. **A 2-week-old infant with intermittent eye discharge and clear conjunctiva has what likely diagnosis?**
Nasolacrimal duct obstruction, seen in roughly 5% of newborns, is typically due to an intermittent blockage at the lower end of the duct. Massaging the area and watchful waiting are generally all that is needed. Almost all cases (95%) resolve by 6 months, and a few resolve thereafter. Ophthalmologic referral during the first 6 months is usually unnecessary, unless there are multiple episodes of acute dacryocystitis or a large congenital mucocele. Most ophthalmologists advise referral between 6 and 13 months because during this period, simple probing of the duct is curative in 95% of patients. After 13 months, the cure rate by probing alone falls to 75%, and silicone intubation of the duct is often necessary.

146. **What are the valves of Rosenmüller and Hasner?**
These are narrowings of the nasolacrimal drainage system where blockage can commonly occur in infancy, particularly at the Hasner valve due to persistence of an embryonic membrane (Fig. 2-6).

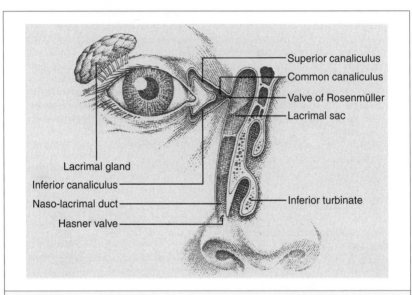

Figure 2-6. The nasolacrimal drainage system. (From Ogawa GSH, Gonnering RS: Congenital nasolacrimal duct obstruction. J Pediatr 119:13, 1991.)

147. **What is normal visual acuity for children?**
- **Birth to 6 months:** Gradually improves from 20/400 to 20/80
- **6 months to 3 years:** Improves from 20/80 to 20/50
- **2 to 5 years:** Improves to 20/40 or better, with a less than two-line difference between left and right eyes on visual charts
- **>5 years:** 20/30 or better, with a less than two-line difference between eyes on visual charts
It should be noted that almost 20% of children require eyeglasses for correction of refractive errors before adulthood.

148. **When do binocular fixation and depth perception develop in children?**
Binocularity of vision depends primarily on the adequate coordination of the extraocular muscles and is normally established by 3 to 6 months of age. At about 6 to 8 months, early evidence of depth perception is seen, but it is still poorly developed. Depth perception becomes very accurate at 6 or 7 years and continues to improve through the early teenage years.

149. **How does refractive capacity vary with age?**
The newborn infant is typically slightly hyperopic (farsighted). The mild hyperopia actually increases slowly for about the first 8 years. It then decreases gradually until adolescence, when vision is emmetropic (no refractive error). After 20 years, there is a tendency for myopia (nearsightedness).

150. **How are the degrees of blindness classified?**
The World Health Organization defines blindness as follows:
- **Visual impairment:** Snellen visual acuity of $\leq 20/60$ (best eye corrected)
- **Social blindness:** Snellen visual acuity of $\leq 20/200$ or a visual field of ≤ 20
- **Virtual blindness:** Snellen visual acuity of $< 20/1200$ or a visual field of ≤ 10
- **Total blindness:** No light perception

American Foundation for the Blind: http://www.afb.org.

Prevent Blindness America: http://www.preventblindness.org.

151. **What is strabismus?**
Strabismus is the misalignment of the eyes with either an in-turning (esotropia), out-turning (exotropia), or up-turning (hypertropia) of one eye.

152. **A 2-month-old baby is noted to have eyes that appear to turn outward rather than looking forward. Is this strabismus?**
Yes, but intervention is not needed unless the symptom persists beyond 2 to 3 months of age. Strabismus is defined as any deviation from perfect ocular alignment. However, most newborns (up to 70%) will be found to have an exodeviated alignment (i.e., looking somewhat out) rather than an orthotropic (i.e., straight) alignment. Most infants will become orthotropic by the time they are 4 months old.
Infants do not focus well because the macula and fovea are poorly developed at birth. Therefore, it is not uncommon for infants to occasionally have an inward crossing of the eyes or for their eyes to be turned slightly outward to 10 or 15 degrees. Persistent in-turning of the eyes for more than a few seconds or outward deviation of more than 10 to 15 degrees requires ophthalmologic referral.

153. **Name the types of childhood strabismus**
- **Strabismus of visual deprivation** occurs when normal vision in one or both eyes is disrupted by any cause. The most serious varieties occur with tumors (e.g., retinoblastoma). In children with ocular tumors, strabismus may be the presenting sign.
- **Infantile** or **congenital esotropia** occurs within the first few months of life, usually as an isolated condition and often with large-angle strabismus. Corrective surgery is usually required.
- **Accommodative esotropia** commonly occurs between the ages of 3 months and 5 years in very farsighted (hyperopic) children. These children use extra lens accommodation because of their visual problems, which leads to persistent convergence. Eyeglasses to correct the hyperopia often correct the esotropia.
- **Intermittent exotropia** appears between the ages of 2 and 8 years as misalignment that is often brought on by fatigue, visual inattention, or bright sunlight. There is a strong hereditary component. Surgery is often necessary after the correction of refractive errors and the elimination of any pathology that might have caused visual deprivation.
- **Incomitant strabismus** is caused by limited eye movement due to restriction (e.g., periocular scarring) or muscle paresis, most commonly from neurologic (e.g., cranial nerve palsies) or muscle pathology. The size of the deviation changes depending on the gaze because of the restrictions of eye movement.

Wright KW. *Pediatric Ophthalmology for Primary Care*, ed 3, Elk Grove Village, IL, 2008, American Academy of Pediatrics, pp 49–70.

154. **What separates pseudostrabismus from true strabismus?**
Often a cause of unnecessary ophthalmologic referrals, **pseudostrabismus** is the appearance of ocular misalignment (usually esotropia) that occurs in children with a broad and flat nasal bridge and prominent epicanthal folds. The iris appears to be shifted to the midline, with differing

amounts of white sclera on each side (Fig. 2-7). This is a common condition that may occur in up to 30% of newborns. No treatment is required. It may be distinguished from true esotropia (or strabismus) by the observation of full extraocular movements, by symmetrical reflections of a flashlight on the cornea from a distance of about 12 inches (although this test as a measure of strabismus is more accurate in infants ≥6 months old), and by normal visualization of red reflexes by direct ophthalmoscopy.

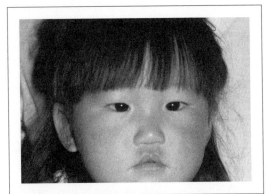

Figure 2-7. Pseudoesotropia. Note that the wide nasal bridge and prominent epicanthal folds create the illusion of an esotropia. The corneal light reflexes are centered in each eye; therefore, the eyes are straight. (From Gault JA: Ophthalmology Pearls. Philadelphia, Hanley & Belfus, 2003, p 45.)

Ticho BH: Strabismus, *Pediatr Clin North Am* 50:173–188, 2003.

155. **What is amblyopia?**
     Amblyopia refers to decreased visual acuity in one eye that is not correctable by glasses and is a result of decreased visual stimulation of that eye. The visual cortex adheres to the concept of "use it or lose it." Amblyopia is the most common cause of vision loss in children younger than 6 years, and it occurs in 1% to 2% of this age group and in 2% to 2.5% of the general population.

156. **What are the causes of amblyopia?**
     ■ **Strabismus:** Input from one eye is suppressed to avoid double vision.
     ■ **Anisometropic amblyopia:** Significant refraction differences cause the suppression of images from the weaker eye.
     ■ **Deprivation:** Images received are unclear (e.g., from congenital cataracts or ptosis).
     ■ **Occlusion amblyopia:** This is typically iatrogenic. Prolonged covering of the preferred eye as a treatment for amblyopia can cause changes in visual acuity in the preferred eye.

     Mittelman D: Amblyopia, *Pediatr Clin N Am* 50:189–196, 2003.

157. **Which treatments are effective for amblyopia?**
     The first step involves providing a clear retinal image with use of eyeglasses or contact lenses for refractive errors and with removal of any obstructing opacities such as cataracts. Occlusion of the good eye allows stimulation of the visual cortex correlating to the amblyopic eye. Traditionally, prolonged patching has been the therapeutic mainstay. By causing papillary dilation and paralysis of accommodation, 1% atropine drops in the better eye cause blurring, particularly for patients who are hyperopic, and reliance on the amblyopic eye. Recent studies have shown that both atropine and patching are effective treatments for patients from 3 to 12 years and that shorter durations of patching are as effective as longer periods.

     Pediatric Eye Disease Investigator Group: Patching vs atropine to treat amblyopia in children aged 7 to 12 years, *Arch Ophthalmol* 126:1634–1642, 2008.

158. **What is the red reflex test?**
     An essential component of any eye examination in an infant or child, the red reflex test is an evaluation of reflected light off the ocular fundus. A direct ophthalmoscope, set to a lens

power of "0," is projected onto both eyes from a distance of 18 inches. A red image, symmetrical from both eyes, should be visible. Abnormal color (particularly white), incomplete coloring (dark spots present), or asymmetrical coloring warrant ophthalmologic consultation because these can represent cataracts, glaucoma, retinoblastoma, strabismus, or high refractive errors.

American Academy of Pediatrics, Section on Ophthalmology: Red reflex examination in neonates, infants, and children, *Pediatrics* 112:1401–1404, 2008.

159. **Why are early diagnosis and treatment critical for patients with congenital cataracts?**
Delay in treatment can lead to irreversible vision loss as a result of deprivation amblyopia. Cataracts undiagnosed for as little as 4 to 8 weeks after birth can result in permanent deficits. In general, the younger the child, the more urgent the need for evaluation if cataracts are suspected.

160. **What is ectopia lentis?**
Ectopia lentis refers to the displacement or dislocation of the lens. It may be due to trauma, but it has also been associated with systemic diseases such as Marfan syndrome, homocystinuria, and congenital syphilis.

161. **What diseases may present with a white pupil?**
Leukocoria, or white pupil, may be a result of any mass behind the pupillary space. This includes infants with cataracts, retinoblastoma, or retinopathy of prematurity who develop retinal detachment.

162. **How common are unequally sized pupils?**
Up to 20% of the normal population can have physiologic **anisocoria** (inequality of pupil size) of up to 0.5 mm. The percentage of difference remains the same in bright or dim lighting.

163. **Is heterochromia normal?**
Yes, if it is an *isolated* finding. Heterochromia irides, or difference in iris colors, can be a familial autosomal dominant trait. It is also seen in some syndromes (e.g., Waardenburg, Horner). However, changes in color can occur from trauma, hemorrhage, inflammation (uveitis, iridocyclitis), malignancy (retinoblastoma, neuroblastoma), or glaucoma, or after intraocular surgery.

KEY POINTS: VISION

1. Red reflex testing should be done routinely for all infants.

2. Suspected cataracts require urgent evaluation, particularly in newborns and younger infants.

3. Uncorrected visual acuity errors in children <8 years old can cause irreversible, lifelong problems.

4. Amblyopia accompanies strabismus in 30% to 60% of cases.

5. Pseudoesotropia, a normal variant, mimics strabismus as a result of widened epicanthal folds. Unlike strabismus, corneal light reflections are equal.

6. Nasolacrimal duct obstruction is common in infants and resolves spontaneously in >95% of cases by 6 months of age.

164. **How is color blindness inherited?**

Color blindness typically involves the variable loss of the ability to distinguish colors, especially red, green, and blue. The defects can be partial (anomaly) or complete (anopia). Defects in appreciating red or green color are transmitted in an X-linked recessive manner and affect up to 1% and 6%, respectively, of the male population. Blue color blindness is an autosomal dominant phenomenon and occurs in 0.1% of the population.

ACKNOWLEDGMENT

The editors gratefully acknowledge contributions by Drs. Nathan J. Blum, Mark Clayton, and James Coplan that were retained from the first three editions of *Pediatric Secrets*.

CARDIOLOGY

Thomas J. Starc, MD, MPH, Constance J. Hayes, MD,
and Allan J. Hordof, MD

CHAPTER 3

CLINICAL ISSUES

1. **Is cardiac pathology the most common cause of chest pain in children?**
   On the contrary, a cardiac cause is uncommon. More common identifiable causes include *musculoskeletal* pain (e.g., strained intercostal muscles, costochondritis, precordial catch syndrome), *pulmonary* disease (e.g., asthma, cough illness, pneumonia), and *gastrointestinal* disease (e.g., esophagitis, gastroenteritis). Other possibilities include *psychogenic* and the always present *idiopathic* diseases (which may represent the largest category).

   Gokhale J, Selbst SM: Chest pain and chest wall deformity, *Pediatric Clin N Am* 56:49–65, 2009.

2. **A child with sharp, stabbing, very localized chest pain, which occurs at rest and resolves completely without associated symptoms after 1 minute, likely has what condition?**
   Precordial catch syndrome. Also called *Texidor twinge* after the original 1955 describer, this may be an underappreciated phenomenon in children with very characteristic features that often prompts extensive, and unproductive, diagnostic workups. It manifests as a sudden-onset chest pain in children, very localized (patient points to area with one or two fingers), which occurs most commonly over the left sternal border, right anterior chest, or flanks with variation of site from episode to episode. The pain occurs typically at rest without provocation, is exacerbated by deep breaths (so the patient breathes very shallowly), and usually lasts 30 seconds to 3 minutes. Unlike cardiac, pulmonary, gastrointestinal, or chest wall causes, there is a paucity of associated symptoms (e.g., no palpitations, pallor, flushing, fever, tenderness, or near-syncope). Physical examination, when done during the episode, is normal. The cause is unknown. Pain may originate from the parietal pleura or chest wall (e.g., rib or cartilage), but is not cardiac or pericardial in origin. Ancillary testing, when done, is normal. Management is expectant with reassurance.

   Gumbiner CH: Precordial catch syndrome, *South Med J* 96:38–41, 2003.

3. **Is mitral valve prolapse (MVP) always pathologic?**
   Some studies show that up to 13% of normal children have some degree of posterior leaflet prolapse on echocardiography. There is a spectrum of anatomic abnormalities, the most minor of which are a variation of normal. Children with clinical features of mitral valve insufficiency constitute the pathologic category. Whenever auscultation reveals the classic findings of MVP, referral to a pediatric cardiologist is recommended. This allows for evaluation of the child for possible accompanying cardiac abnormalities (e.g., mitral insufficiency, secundum atrial septal defects) and confirmation of the diagnosis.

4. **What connective tissue diseases may be associated with MVP?**
   Marfan syndrome, Ehlers-Danlos syndrome, pseudoxanthoma elasticum, osteogenesis imperfecta, and Hurler syndrome.

5. **During physical examination, what patient maneuvers can increase the likelihood of detecting MVP on auscultation?**
   In patients with MVP, the leaflets of the mitral valve apparatus billow into the left atrium. Maneuvers that decrease left ventricular size and volume (and thus increase the relative size of the leaflets) increase the likelihood of hearing the click or murmur. These include the straining phase of a Valsalva maneuver, inspiration, and change from a supine to a sitting position or from a squatting to a standing position. The left lateral decubitus position may also be facilitative.

6. **Can a patient with heart disease simultaneously be polycythemic and iron deficient?**
   Yes. Patients with cyanotic heart disease may develop both clinical entities. Initially, as a response to cyanosis, the hematocrit rises. In patients with iron deficiency, the hematocrit may remain elevated, and the mean corpuscular volume will be lower than normal. Detailed studies of iron stores often reveal a concurrent deficiency. Children with a history of poor nutrition and blood loss (e.g., previous surgery) are especially at risk for developing iron deficiency.

7. **What syndrome should come to mind for the patient with pulmonary stenosis and hypercholesterolemia?**
   Alagille syndrome is associated with peripheral pulmonary stenosis and liver disease. These children have chronic cholestasis secondary to decreased intrahepatic interlobular bile ducts. Hypercholesterolemia is thought to be secondary to the liver disease. Other findings are peculiar facies, butterfly-like vertebral arch defects, and growth defects.

8. **What are the common types of vascular rings and slings?**
   Vascular rings occur when the trachea and/or the esophagus is encircled by aberrant vascular structures. Vascular slings are compressions (typically anterior) that are caused by nonencircling aberrant vessels (Table 3-1).

TABLE 3-1. VASCULAR RINGS AND SLINGS

	Frequency (%)	Symptoms	Treatment
"Complete" Rings			
Double aortic arch	50	Respiratory difficulty, worsened by feeding or exertion (onset <3 mo)	Surgical division of a smaller arch (usually the left)
Right aortic arch with left ligamentum arteriosum	45	Mild respiratory difficulty (onset later in infancy); swallowing dysfunction	Surgical division of ligamentum arteriosum
"Incomplete" Rings			
Anomalous innominate artery	<5	Stridor and/or cough in infancy	Conservative management or surgical suturing of artery to the sternum

(continued)

TABLE 3-1. VASCULAR RINGS AND SLINGS *(continued)*			
	Frequency (%)	Symptoms	Treatment
Aberrant right subclavian artery	<5	Occasional swallowing dysfunction	Usually no treatment necessary
Vascular sling or anomalous left pulmonary artery	Rare	Wheezing and cyanotic episodes during first weeks of life	Surgical division of anomalous left pulmonary artery (from right pulmonary artery) and anastomosis to the main pulmonary artery

Adapted from Park MK: Pediatric Cardiology for Practitioners, 5th ed. St. Louis, 2008, p 578.

9. **What evaluations are commonly done if a vascular ring is suspected?**
   - **Chest radiograph:** For detection of possible right-sided aortic arch
   - **Barium esophagram:** Historically considered the gold standard for diagnosis; confirms external indentation of esophagus in up to 95% of cases (Fig. 3-1)
   - **Magnetic resonance imaging (MRI):** Noninvasive and now used as the primary diagnostic modality
   - **Arteriogram:** Precise delineation of vascular anatomy; rarely needed because of MRI
   - **Echocardiogram:** Not helpful for identifying the ring itself, but important when evaluating for possible congenital heart disease, which can occur in patients with vascular rings

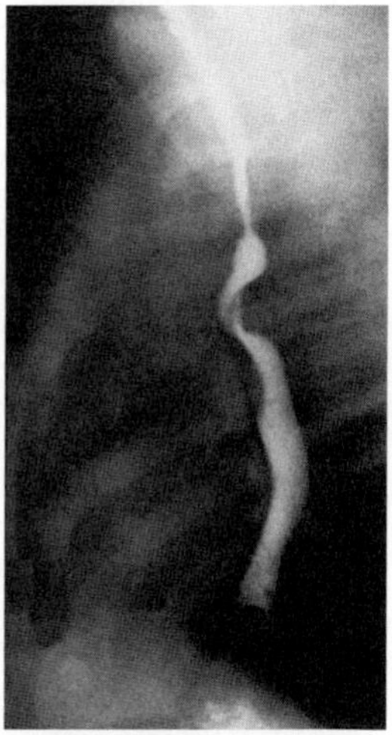

Figure 3-1. Barium swallow in a toddler with posterior compression of the esophagus and trachea from a vascular ring. (From Zitelli BJ, Davis HW: Atlas of Pediatric Physical Diagnosis, 4th ed. St. Louis, Mosby, 2002, p 540.)

10. **Describe four categories of cardiomyopathy in children.**
    - **Dilated cardiomyopathy** is the most common. Etiology is usually unknown. Anatomically, the heart is normal, but both ventricles are dilated. Older children present symptoms of congestive heart failure (CHF). Infants show symptoms of poor weight gain, feeding difficulty, and respiratory distress. In all pediatric age groups, a more acute presenting symptom can be shock.
    - **Hypertrophic cardiomyopathy with left ventricular (LV) outflow obstruction** is also known as idiopathic hypertrophic subaortic stenosis and asymmetrical septal hypertrophy. Of patients with this condition, most have some degree of LV outflow tract obstruction as a

result of abnormal hypertrophy of the subaortic region of the intraventricular septum. Most of these defects are inherited in an autosomal dominant fashion.

- **Hypertrophic cardiomyopathy without LV outflow obstruction** is also usually of unknown etiology. It may be associated with systemic metabolic disease, particularly storage disease. Cardiomegaly is a constant feature.
- **Restrictive cardiomyopathy** is associated with abnormal diastolic function of the ventricles. The ventricles may be of normal size, or they may be hypertrophied with normal systolic function. The atria are typically enlarged. The etiology is usually unknown but may be storage disease.

Maron BJ: Hypertrophic cardiomyopathy in childhood, *Pediatr Clin North Am* 51:1305–1346, 2004.

Shaddy RE: Cardiomyopathies in adolescents: dilated, hypertrophic, and restrictive, *Adolesc Med* 12:35–45, 2001.

11. **Should a child with a cardiomyopathy be referred for genetic evaluation?**
   Yes. Hypertrophic cardiomyopathy is commonly familial with the 14q1 chromosome a major locus. Dilated cardiomyopathy and restrictive cardiomyopathy are less often associated with a genetic abnormality.

   Morita H, Rehm HL, Menesses A, et al: Shared genetic causes of cardiac hypertrophy in children and adults, *N Engl J Med* 358:1899–1908, 2008.

12. **What mineral is added to hyperalimentation fluids to prevent a potential cardiomyopathy?**
   Selenium is routinely added to hyperalimentation fluids to prevent selenium deficiency, which can be a cause of both skeletal weakness and cardiomyopathy. This "acquired" heart disease has been described in patients on long-term hyperalimentation (before modern hyperalimentation); patients with AIDS, chronic diarrhea, and wasting disease; and children living in the Keshan province of China, where the soil is naturally low in selenium. It is typically reversible with the addition of selenium to the diet or intravenous fluids.

13. **What are the cardiac causes of sudden cardiac death in children and adolescents?**
   Sudden death occurs because of ventricular fibrillation in the setting of myocardial or coronary abnormalities or primary rhythm disorders. The main structural causes are hypertrophic cardiomyopathy (particularly with extreme LV hypertrophy), anomalies of the coronary artery, Marfan syndrome, and arrhythmogenic right ventricular (RV) dysplasia. Coronary artery anomalies (congenital or acquired) may be a consideration. Prolonged QT syndrome and Wolff-Parkinson-White (WPW) syndrome have also been implicated. Children with CHD (e.g., aortic stenosis, Ebstein anomaly) are at higher risk for sudden death.

   Rowland T: Sudden unexpected death in young athletes: reconsidering "hypertrophic cardiomyopathy." *Pediatrics* 123:1217–1222, 2009.

   Shirley KW, Adrim RA: Sudden cardiac death in young athletes, *Clin Pediatr Emerg Med* 6:194–199, 2005.

14. **What is the likely diagnosis in a 10-year-old little leaguer who develops sudden cardiac arrest after being struck in the chest by a batted baseball?**
   Commotio cordis. This is a life-threatening dysrhythmia or arrhythmia that occurs as a result of a blunt, nonpenetrating direct blow to the chest. The precordial force is often only low or moderate and typically not associated with structural injury. Ventricular fibrillation is thought to occur when impact is applied during the vulnerable phase of repolarization, which occurs 30 to 15 milliseconds before the peak of the T wave. Prompt cardiopulmonary resuscitation followed by defibrillation improves the chance of survival.

   Maron BJ, Estes NAM III: Commotio cordis, *N Engl J Med* 362:917–927, 2010.

15. **What historical features may identify the patient who is at risk for sudden death?**
   - Sudden death may be associated with previous symptoms of exertional chest discomfort, dizziness or prolonged dyspnea with exercise, syncope, and palpitations.
   - Family history of premature cardiovascular disease (<50 years), hypertrophic or dilated cardiomyopathy, Marfan syndrome, long QT syndrome, other clinically significant dysrhythmias or sudden death may be associated with these patients. For example, although 40% of cases of hypertrophic cardiomyopathy are sporadic, 60% are inherited in an autosomal dominant fashion.
   - History of seizure-like activity.

   Papapakis M, Whyte G, Sharma S: Preparticipation screening for cardiovascular abnormalities in young competitive athletes, *BMJ* 337:806–812, 2008.

16. **How can the preparticipation sports physical examination identify patients at risk for sudden death?**
   - Marfanoid features: Tall and thin habitus, hyperextensible joints, pectus excavatum, click and murmur suggestive of MVP
   - Pathologic murmurs (any systolic murmur grade 3/6 or greater, any diastolic murmur)
   - Weak or delayed femoral pulses
   - Dysrhythmia: Rapid or irregular heartbeat

   Singh A, Silberbach M: Cardiovascular preparticipation sports screening, *Pediatr Rev* 27:418–423, 2006.

17. **Should an electrocardiogram (ECG) be included in the preparticipation screening of athletes?**
   This remains a hotly debated topic. The potential value is that an ECG could identify at-risk athletes with hypertrophic cardiomyopathy, arrhythmogenic RV cardiomyopathy, and long QT syndrome. The European Society of Cardiology recommends ECG screening, but the American Heart Association believes it has not been sufficiently studied to prove its effectiveness.

   Chaitman BR: An electrocardiogram should not be included in routine preparticipation screening of young athletes, *Circulation* 116:2610–2615, 2007.

   Myerburg RJ, Vetter VL: Electrocardiograms should be included in preparticipation screening of athletes, *Circulation* 116:2610–2615, 2007.

18. **In which patients is syncope more likely to be of a cardiac nature?**
   - Sudden onset without any prodromal period of dizziness or imminent awareness
   - Syncope during exercise or exertion
   - History of palpitations or abnormal heartbeat before event
   - Syncope leading to a fall which results in an injury
   - Family history of sudden death

19. **What arrhythmias may be associated with syncope?**
   See Table 3-2.

20. **What is the most common cause of syncope in children?**
   In otherwise healthy children, **neurally mediated syncope** is most common. This entity goes by a number of terms, including vasovagal syncope, neurocardiogenic syncope, and autonomic syncope. Individuals who experience an orthostatic challenge may paradoxically respond with a decreased heart rate and increased peripheral vasodilation, which results in hypotensive syncope. Treatment for recurrent episodes may involve mineralocorticoids, salt and extra fluids, and β-blockers.

   Sapin SO: Autonomic syncope in pediatrics: a practice-oriented approach to classification, pathophysiology, diagnosis, and management, *Clin Pediatr* 43:17–23, 2004.

TABLE 3-2. SYNCOPE

Diagnosis	History and Physical Examination	Electrocardiographic Findings
WPW	Family history of WPW, known hypertrophic cardiomyopathy, or Ebstein anomaly	Short PR interval, presence of delta waves
Prolonged QT syndrome	Family history of prolonged QT, sudden death, and/or deafness	QTc = >0.44 sec
Atrioventricular block	Myocarditis, Lyme disease, acute rheumatic fever, maternal history of lupus	First-, second-, or third-degree heart block
Arrhythmogenic right ventricular dysplasia	Syncope, palpitations, positive family history	PVCs, V tachycardia, left bundle branch block
Ventricular tachycardia	Most ventricular tachycardia occurs in abnormal hearts; requires extensive evaluation	V tachycardia

WPW = Wolff-Parkinson-White syndrome; PVCs = premature ventricular contractions; QTc = corrected QT interval.
From Feinberg AN, Lane-Davies A: Syncope in the adolescent. Adolesc Med 13:553–567, 2002.

KEY POINTS: SYNCOPE MORE LIKELY TO BE OF A CARDIAC NATURE

1. Occurring during exercise

2. Sudden onset without prodromal symptoms or awareness

3. Complete loss of tone or awareness leading to injury

4. Palpitations or abnormal heartbeat noted before event

5. Abnormal heart rate (fast or slow) after event

6. Family history of sudden death

21. **What are the most common clinical signs of coarctation of the aorta (Fig. 3-2) in older children?**
    - Differential blood pressure: arms > legs (100%)
    - Systolic murmur or bruit in the back (96%)
    - Systolic hypertension in the upper extremities (96%)
    - Diminished or absent femoral or lower-extremity pulses (92%)

    Ing FF, Starc TJ, Griffiths SP, Gersony WM: Early diagnosis of coarctation of the aorta in children: a continuing dilemma, *Pediatrics* 98:378–382, 1996.

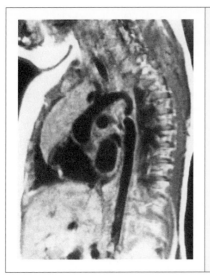

Figure 3-2. Magnetic resonance imaging of coarctation of the aorta. (From Clark DA: Atlas of Neonatology. Philadelphia, W.B. Saunders, 2000, p 119.)

22. **What is the difference between isotonic and isometric exercise?**
    Isotonic exercise is dynamic exercise (e.g., running), whereas *isometric* exercise is static (e.g., lifting weights). Static exercise causes pressure overload on the heart, so dynamic exercise is usually preferred for patients with congenital heart disease.

CONGENITAL HEART DISEASE

23. **What are the common etiologies for CHD?**
    Only a small percentage of cases have identifiable causes:
    - Primary genetic factors (e.g., chromosomal abnormalities, single gene abnormalities): 10%
    - Environmental factors (e.g., chemicals; drugs such as isotretinoin or Accutane; viruses such as rubella; maternal disease): 3% to 5%
    - Genetic-environmental interactions (i.e., multifactorial): 85%

24. **What prenatal maternal factors may be associated with cardiac disease in the neonate?**
    See Table 3-3.

25. **In a cyanotic newborn, how can you distinguish pulmonary disease from cyanotic CHD?**
    With the **hyperoxia test**. The infant is placed on 100% oxygen, and an arterial blood gas level is obtained. A Pao_2 of greater than 100 mm Hg is usually achieved in infants with primary lung disease, whereas a Pao_2 of less than 100 mm Hg is characteristic of heart disease. Typically, children with cyanotic heart disease also have a low or normal Pco_2, whereas children with lung disease have an elevated Pco_2. Unfortunately, the hyperoxia test does not usually distinguish children with cyanotic heart disease from those with persistent pulmonary hypertension.

26. **Which congenital heart lesions commonly appear with cyanosis during the newborn period?**
    Independent pulmonary and systemic circulations (severe cyanosis)
    - Transposition of great arteries with an intact ventricular septum

TABLE 3-3. PRENATAL MATERNAL FACTORS ASSOCIATED WITH CARDIAC DISEASE IN NEONATES

Prenatal Historical Factor	Associated Cardiac Defect
Diabetes mellitus	Left ventricular outflow obstruction (asymmetric septal hypertrophy, aortic stenosis), D-transposition of great arteries, ventricular septal defect
Lupus erythematosus	Heart block, pericarditis, endomyocardial fibrosis
Rubella	Patent ductus arteriosus, pulmonic stenosis (peripheral)
Alcohol use	Pulmonic stenosis, ventricular septal defect
Aspirin use	Persistent pulmonary hypertension syndrome
Lithium	Ebstein anomaly
Diphenylhydantoin	Aortic stenosis, pulmonary stenosis
Coxsackie B infection	Myocarditis

From Gewitz MH: Cardiac disease in the newborn infant. In Polin RA, Yoder MC, Burg FD (eds): Workbook in Practical Neonatology, 3rd ed. Philadelphia, W.B. Saunders, 2001, p 269.

Inadequate pulmonary blood flow (severe cyanosis)
- Tricuspid valve atresia
- Pulmonary valve atresia with intact ventricular septum
- Tetralogy of Fallot
- Severe Ebstein anomaly of the tricuspid valve

Admixture lesions (moderate cyanosis)
- Total anomalous pulmonary venous return
- Hypoplastic left heart syndrome
- Truncus arteriosus

Victoria BE: Cyanotic newborns. In Gessner IH, Victoria BE, editors: *Pediatric Cardiology: A Problem Oriented Approach*. Philadelphia, 1993, W.B. Saunders, p 101.

KEY POINTS: CARDIAC CAUSES OF CYANOSIS IN THE NEWBORN

1. Transposition of the great arteries

2. Tetralogy of Fallot

3. Truncus arteriosus

4. Pulmonary atresia

5. Total anomalous pulmonary venous return

6. Tricuspid atresia

7. Hypoplastic left heart

27. **In the patient with suspected heart disease, what bony abnormalities seen on a chest radiograph increase the likelihood of CHD?**
   - **Hemivertebrae, rib anomalies:** Associated with tetralogy of Fallot, truncus arteriosus, and VACTERL syndrome (vertebral abnormalities, anal atresia, cardiac abnormalities, tracheoesophageal fistula and/or esophageal atresia, renal agenesis and dysplasia, and limb defects)
   - **11 ribs:** Seen in patients with Down syndrome
   - **Skeletal chest deformities** (scoliosis, pectus excavatum, narrow anterior-posterior diameter): Associated with Marfan syndrome and mitral valve prolapse
   - **Bilateral rib notching:** Coarctation of the aorta (usually seen in older children)

28. **How do pulmonary vascular markings on a chest radiograph help in the differential diagnosis of a cyanotic newborn with suspected cardiac disease?**
   The chest radiograph may help to differentiate the types of congenital heart defects. The increase or decrease in pulmonary vascular markings is indicative of pulmonary blood flow:
   Decreased pulmonary markings (diminished pulmonary blood flow)
   - Pulmonary atresia or severe stenosis
   - Tetralogy of Fallot
   - Tricuspid atresia
   - Ebstein anomaly
   Increased pulmonary markings (increased pulmonary blood flow)
   - Transposition of great arteries
   - Total anomalous pulmonary venous return
   - Truncus arteriosus

29. **What ECG findings are considered characteristic for various congenital heart malformations?**
   - **Left axis deviation:** Endocardial cushion defects (both complete atrioventricular [AV] canal and ostium primum atrial septal defects), tricuspid atresia
   - **WPW syndrome:** Ebstein anomaly, L-transposition of the great arteries (L-TGA)
   - **Complete heart block:** L-TGA, polysplenia syndrome

30. **What chest radiograph findings (Fig. 3-3) are considered characteristic for various CHDs?**
   - **Boot-shaped heart:** Tetralogy of Fallot
   - **Egg-shaped heart:** Transposition of great arteries
   - **Snowman silhouette:** Total anomalous pulmonary venous return (supracardiac)
   - **Rib notching:** Coarctation of the aorta (older children)

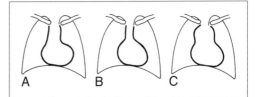

Figure 3-3. Abnormal cardiac silhouettes. *A*, Boot-shaped heart seen in cyanotic tetralogy of Fallot or tricuspid atresia. *B*, Egg-shaped heart seen in transposition of the great arteries. *C*, Snowman silhouette seen in total anomalous pulmonary artery venous return (supracardiac type). (From Park MK: Pediatric Cardiology for Practitioners, 4th ed. St. Louis, Mosby, 2002, p 54.)

31. **What are the common ductal-dependent cardiac lesions?**
   Ductal-dependent pulmonary blood flow
   - Critical pulmonary valve stenosis
   - Pulmonary atresia

- Tetralogy of Fallot with severe pulmonary stenosis
- Tricuspid atresia with pulmonary stenosis or pulmonary atresia
  Ductal-dependent systemic blood flow
- Coarctation of the aorta
- Hypoplastic left heart syndrome
- Interrupted aortic arch

32. **What types of CHDs are associated with the right aortic arch?**
    - Tetralogy of Fallot with pulmonary atresia (50%)
    - Truncus arteriosus (35%)
    - Classic tetralogy of Fallot (25%)
    - Double-outlet right ventricle (25%)
    - Single ventricle (12.5%)

    Crowley JJ, Oh KS, Newman B, et al: Telltale signs of congenital heart disease, *Radiol Clin N Am* 31:573–582, 1993.

33. **Which genetic syndromes are most commonly associated with CHD?**
    See Table 3-4.

TABLE 3-4. GENETIC SYNDROMES ASSOCIATED WITH CONGENITAL HEART DISEASE		
Syndrome	Percentage of Patients with CHD	Predominant Heart Defects
Down	50	ECD, VSD, TOF
Turner	20	COA
Noonan	65	PS, ASD, ASH
Marfan	60	MVP, AoAn, AR
Trisomy 18	90	VSD, PDA
Trisomy 13	80	VSD, PDA
DiGeorge	80	IAA-B, TA
Williams	75	SVAS, peripheral PS

AoAn = aortic aneurysm; AR = aortic regurgitation; ASD = atrial sepal defect; ASH = asymmetrical septal hypertrophy; CHD = congenital heart disease; COA = coarctation of the aorta; ECD = endocardial cushion defect; IAA-B = interrupted aortic arch type B; MVP = mitral valve prolapse; PDA = patent ductus arteriosus; PS = pulmonary stenosis; SVAS = supravalvular aortic stenosis; TA = truncus arteriosus; TOF = tetralogy of Fallot; VSD = ventricular septal defect. From Frias JL: Genetic issues of congenital heart defects. In Gessner IH, Victoria BE (eds): Pediatric Cardiology: A Problem Oriented Approach. Philadelphia, W.B. Saunders, 1993, p 238.

34. **Which infants with CHD should be evaluated for other anomalies?**
    In the evaluation of the newborn with heart disease, several known associations between CHD and other anomalies should be considered, especially for the patient with more complex disease. Syndromes such as CHARGE (coloboma, heart disease, choanal atresia, retarded growth and development or central nervous system anomalies, genital hypoplasia, ear anomalies and/or deafness) or VACTERL may first be identified by the presence of heart disease. An association between conotruncal defects (tetralogy of Fallot, truncus arteriosus, and interrupted aortic arch) and deletions on chromosome 22 is often seen. Some of these

patients may have DiGeorge syndrome or velocardiofacial syndrome, but others may have only minimal palatal dysfunction. For this reason, patients with conotruncal cardiac defects should undergo screening for deletions on chromosome 22; if these are found, these patients should be referred to a geneticist for special testing and evaluation.

35. **Describe the clinical manifestations of a large patent ductus arteriosus (PDA).**
   - Tachypnea and tachycardia
   - Bounding pulses
   - Hyperdynamic precordium
   - Wide pulse pressure
   - Continuous murmur (older child)
   - Systolic murmur (premature infant)
   - Labile oxygenation (premature infant)
   - Apnea (premature infant)

36. **How commonly do PDAs occur in premature infants?**
   They are evident in 40% to 60% of infants with a birthweight of 501 to 1500 g.

37. **Is a "to-and-fro" murmur a good description for the heart murmur of a PDA?**
   No. The heart murmur of a typical patent ductus arteriosus is usually continuous or at least "spills from systole into diastole." The direction of blood flow is from the aorta to the pulmonary artery in systole and continues from the aorta to the pulmonary artery during diastole. A to-and-fro murmur describes blood flow in a complex valvular lesion such as the combination of aortic stenosis with aortic insufficiency or pulmonary stenosis with pulmonary insufficiency. The blood flow in these examples goes "antegrade" during systole and "retrograde" during diastole. This back and forth flow is aptly described as to-and-fro.

38. **How can you explain a Pao$_2$ of more than 400 mm Hg in a blood sample from an umbilical catheter in a newborn with transposition of the great arteries?**
   A very elevated Pao$_2$ can be observed if the umbilical vein catheter has passed from the inferior vena cava to the right atrium and into the left atrium. The Po$_2$ in the left atrium represents the pulmonary venous oxygenation and not the arterial oxygen level. In cyanotic heart disease, the alveolar and pulmonary vein Po$_2$ are usually normal. It is the arterial oxygenation that is severely diminished in children with cyanotic heart disease.

39. **How do an ostium primum and an ostium secundum defect differ?**
   Atrial septal defects are categorized by their location. An **ostium secundum** is an isolated defect that involves a persistently enlarged opening at the fossa ovalis, which is in the center of the septum. An **ostium primum** defect is located more inferiorly and is part of an AV canal defect, often in association with tricuspid or mitral valve abnormalities.

40. **How do the presenting symptoms of ventricular septal defect (VSD) and atrial septal defect (ASD) differ?**
   VSD: In an infant with a large VSD, signs of CHF generally appear at 4 to 8 weeks of age, when the pulmonary vascular resistance drops and pulmonary blood flow increases. CHF is due to a large left-to-right shunt and increased pulmonary blood flow and may be associated with failure to thrive or recurrent respiratory infections. The child with a small VSD may have a systolic murmur during the first few weeks of life. These infants do not develop CHF, and spontaneous closure often occurs.

ASD: Most children with an isolated ASD are not clinically diagnosed until they are 3 to 5 years old. Most are asymptomatic at the time of diagnosis. Rarely, infants with an ASD demonstrate signs of CHF during the first year of life.

41. **What is the primary concern of the pediatric cardiologist if a child with a large VSD is lost to follow-up and comes back after 2 years of age?**
Although even large VSDs may close spontaneously in many children, the child with a large VSD can develop irreversible pulmonary vascular disease as a sequela of the long-term increased pulmonary blood flow and pulmonary hypertension (Eisenmenger syndrome). This complication is usually preventable if the VSD is closed before 18 to 24 months of age.

42. **What clinical features are suggestive of pulmonary hypertension?**
The condition should be suspected in any child with excessive shortness of breath, who fatigues easily (perhaps with feedings in infants) and who has no evidence of pulmonary or cardiac disease (or decompensation if previous disease was identified). Physical examination may reveal an RV lift and a loud pulmonary component of the second heart sound. Eventually, signs of right heart failure with peripheral edema, ascites, and hepatomegaly may develop. The condition as noted previously can be seen in CHD (particularly left-sided lesions) but may also be seen in a variety of conditions: idiopathic, familial, connective tissue disease, respiratory disease (e.g., chronic obstructive pulmonary disease, interstitial lung disease, alveolar hypoventilation disorders) and chronic thrombotic or embolic disease.

> Rothstein R, Paris Y, Quizon A: Pulmonary hypertension, *Pediatr Rev* 30:39–46, 2009.

> Haworth SG: The management of pulmonary hypertension in children, *Arch Dis Child* 93:620–625, 2008.

43. **What is the anomaly in Ebstein anomaly?**
The septal and posterior leaflets of the tricuspid valve are thickened and displaced inferiorly into the right ventricle. In its most severe form, the tricuspid valve is severely incompetent, profound right atrial enlargement results, and signs of congestive heart failure predominate.

44. **What are the four structural abnormalities of tetralogy of Fallot?**
   - Pulmonary stenosis with RV outflow tract obstruction
   - VSD
   - Aorta overriding the VSD
   - RV hypertrophy

45. **What occurs during a "Tet spell"?**
Tet spells are cyanotic and hypoxic episodes that occur in patients with tetralogy of Fallot. The pathophysiology is thought to be related to a change in the balance of systemic-to-pulmonary vascular resistance. Spells may be initiated by events that cause a decrease in systemic vascular resistance (e.g., fever, crying, hypotension) or by events that cause an increase in pulmonary outflow tract obstruction. Both types of events lead to more right-to-left shunting and increased cyanosis. Hypoxia and cyanosis can result in metabolic acidosis and systemic vasodilation, which cause a further increase in cyanosis. Anemia may be a predisposing factor. Although most episodes are self-limited, a prolonged Tet spell can lead to stroke or death; therefore, a spell is an indication for surgery.

46. **Name two conditions in which the murmur has disappeared or diminished in intensity and yet the patient is actually worse.**
In **tetralogy of Fallot**, the systolic heart murmur represents blood flow across the narrow RV outflow tract. With worsening RV outflow tract obstruction or during a cyanotic spell, less

blood crosses the valve, and the heart murmur consequently diminishes and may actually disappear completely.

In a child with a **VSD with Eisenmenger syndrome**, the left-to-right shunt across the VSD diminishes because of the increase in pulmonary vascular resistance. The heart murmur lessens and may disappear. A "honeymoon period" with no shunting is then followed by the progression of increased right-to-left shunting and cyanosis. The pulmonary component of the second heart sound begins to increase in intensity, and visible cyanosis and clubbing of the nail beds are often seen.

47. **After what age does a presumed peripheral pulmonic branch stenosis murmur deserve more detailed study?**
    The murmur of peripheral pulmonic branch stenosis—a low-intensity systolic ejection murmur heard frequently in newborns—is the result of the relative hypoplasia of the pulmonary arteries as well as the acute angle of the branching of pulmonary arteries in the early newborn period. A murmur which persists **beyond 6 months of age** should be investigated.

48. **What should parents be told about the risk for recurrence of common heart defects?**
    The risk for CHD in pregnancies after the birth of one affected child is about 1% to 4%. With two affected first-degree relatives, the risk is about 10%. With three affected children, the family may be considered at even higher risk.

    Congenital Heart Information Network: http://www.tchin.org.

CONGESTIVE HEART FAILURE

49. **Identify the clinical signs and symptoms associated with CHF in children.**
    These may be grouped into three categories:
    - **Signs or symptoms of impaired myocardial performance:** Cardiomegaly, tachycardia, gallop rhythm, cold extremities or mottling, growth failure, sweating with feeding, pallor
    - **Signs or symptoms of pulmonary congestion:** Tachypnea, wheezing, rales, cyanosis, dyspnea, cough
    - **Signs or symptoms of systemic venous congestion:** Hepatomegaly, neck vein distention, peripheral edema (seen in the older patient)

50. **How is heart size assessed in older children?**
    Cardiothoracic (CT) ratio: This is derived by comparing the largest transverse diameter of the heart to the widest internal diameter of the chest: CT ratio = (A + B)/C, as shown in Fig. 3-4. A CT ratio of greater than 0.5 indicates cardiomegaly.

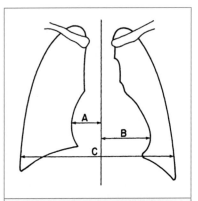

Figure 3-4. The cardiothoracic ratio is obtained by dividing the largest horizontal diameter of the heart (A + B) by the longest internal diameter of the chest (C). (From Park MK: Pediatric Cardiology for Practitioners, 4th ed. St. Louis, Mosby, 2002, p 51.)

51. **In infancy, how does the likely cause of CHF vary by age?**
    See Table 3-5.

TABLE 3-5. CAUSES OF CONGESTIVE HEART FAILURE

Age of Onset	Cause
At birth	HLHS with restrictive foramen ovale
	Volume overload lesions:
	Severe tricuspid or pulmonary insufficiency (i.e., severe Ebstein, tetralogy of Fallot with absent pulmonary valve)
	Large systemic arteriovenous fistula
	Arrhythmia
0-7 days	TGA
	PDA in small premature infants
	HLHS
	TAPVR, particularly those with pulmonary venous obstruction
	Systemic arteriovenous fistula
	Critical AS or PS
1-6 wk	COA isolated or with associated anomalies
	Critical AS
	Large left-to-right shunt lesions (VSD, PDA, AVC)
	All other lesions previously listed
6 wk-4 mo	Large VSD
	Large PDA
	Others such as anomalous left coronary artery from the PA

AS = aortic stenosis; COA = coarctation of the aorta; ECD = endocardial cushion defect;
HLHS = hypoplastic left heart syndrome; PA = pulmonary artery; PDA = patent ductus arteriosus;
PS = pulmonary stenosis; TAPVR = total anomalous pulmonary venous return; TGA = transposition of
the great arteries; VSD = ventricular septal defect.
Adapted from Park, Myung K: Pediatric Cardiology for Practitioners, 5th ed. St. Louis, Mosby,
2008, p 462.

KEY POINTS: COMMON CARDIAC CAUSES OF CONGESTIVE HEART FAILURE IN A 6-WEEK-OLD INFANT

1. Ventricular septal defect

2. AV canal

3. Patent ductus arteriosus

4. Coarctation of the aorta

52. **What are the typical ages for the presentation of CHF with CHD?**
    As a general rule, large-volume overload lesions present soon after birth, ductal-dependent lesions present in the first week when the ductus closes, and lesions with significant

left-to-right shunting present over the first 1 to 2 months as the normal pulmonary vascular resistance falls (with increased systemic-to-pulmonary shunting).

53. **If a patient develops CHF and cardiomegaly during the newborn period, but no heart murmur is heard, what is the differential diagnosis?**
    - Myocarditis
    - Cardiomyopathy as a result of asphyxia, hypoglycemia, or hypocalcemia
    - Glycogen storage disease (Pompe disease)
    - Cardiac dysrhythmia: paroxysmal supraventricular tachycardia, congenital heart block, atrial flutter
    - Arteriovenous malformations (e.g., liver, vein of Galen)
    - Sepsis

54. **If a patient develops CHF and cardiomegaly after the newborn period, but no murmur is heard, what is the differential diagnosis?**
    Myocardial diseases
    - Myocarditis (viral or idiopathic)
    - Glycogen storage disease (Pompe disease)
    - Endocardial fibroelastosis
    Coronary artery diseases resulting in myocardial insufficiency
    - Anomalous origin of left coronary artery from pulmonary artery
    - Kawasaki syndrome (acute vasculitis of infancy and early childhood)
    - Calcification of the coronary arteries
    CHD with severe heart failure
    - Coarctation of the aorta in infants
    - Ebstein anomaly (may have gallop rhythm)

ELECTROCARDIOGRAMS AND DYSRHYTHMIAS

55. **How does the ECG of a term infant differ from that of the older child?**
    - **Birth:** At birth, the ECG reflects RV dominance. The QRS complex consists of a tall R wave in the right precordial leads (V_1 and V_2) and an S wave in the left precordial leads (V_5 and V_6). The axis is also rightward (90 to 150 degrees).
    - **Toddler age (2 to 4 years):** There is an axis shift from the right to the normal quadrant, and the R wave diminishes over the right precordial leads. The S wave disappears from the left precordium.
    - **School age:** At this age, the wave has a nearly adult tracing, with a small R and a dominant S in the right precordial leads and an axis in the normal quadrant.

56. **What are the characteristic features of the ECG of a premature infant?**
    In the premature infant, there is less RV dominance. The R wave may be small in the right precordial leads, and there may be no significant S wave over the left precordium. The electrical axis is often in the normal quadrant (0 to 90 degrees).

57. **Describe the ECG abnormalities associated with potassium and calcium imbalances.**
    See Fig. 3-5.

58. **What is the difference between a QT interval and a corrected QT interval (QTc)?**
    The QT interval represents the time required for ventricular depolarization and repolarization. It begins at the onset of the QRS complex and continues through the end of the T wave. This interval varies with the heart rate. The QTc adjusts for heart rate differences. As a rule, a

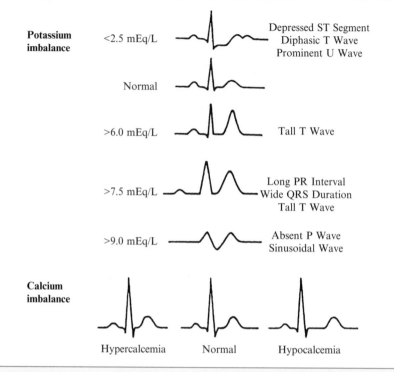

Figure 3-5. Electrocardiogram abnormalities associated with potassium and calcium imbalances. (From Park MK, Guntheroth WG: How to Read Pediatric ECGs, 3rd ed. St. Louis, Mosby, 1992, pp 106–107.)

prolonged QTc interval is diagnosed when the QTc exceeds 0.44 second using the following formula, known as the *Bazett formula*:

$$QTc = QT \text{ (in seconds)}/\sqrt{RR} \text{ (in seconds)}$$

Al-Khatib SM, LaPointe NM, Kramer JM, Califf RM: What clinicians should know about the QT interval, *JAMA* 289:2120–2127, 2003.

59. **What causes a prolonged QT interval?**
Congenital long QT syndrome
- Hereditary form: ion channelopathies (genetic defects in specific potassium and sodium channel genes), Jervell-Lange-Nielsen syndrome (associated with deafness), Romano-Ward syndrome
- Sporadic type

Acquired long QT syndrome
- Drug-induced (especially antidysrhythmics, tricyclic antidepressants, phenothiazines)
- Metabolic and electrolyte abnormalities (hypocalcemia, hypokalemia, very-low-energy diets)
- Central nervous system and autonomic nervous system disorders (especially after head trauma or stroke)
- Cardiac disease (myocarditis, coronary artery disease)

Morita H, Wu J, Zipes DP: The QT syndromes: long and short, *Lancet* 372:750–763, 2008.

Roden DM: Long-QT syndrome, *N Engl J Med* 358:169–176, 2008.

KEY POINTS: ELECTROCARDIOGRAMS ✓

1. As compared with adults, newborns and infants normally have right ventricular dominance.

2. Premature atrial beats in children are usually benign.

3. QT intervals must be corrected for heart rates.

4. A QTc should not exceed 0.44 second, except in infants <6 months old, in whom up to 0.49 second may be normal.

60. **What ECG features are found in the long QT syndromes?**
    These are disorders of repolarization with prolongation of the QT interval, corrected for heart rate (QTc). In addition to a prolonged QTc, other ECG findings are relative bradycardia, T-wave abnormalities, and episodic ventricular tachyarrhythmias, particularly torsades de pointes (Fig. 3-6).

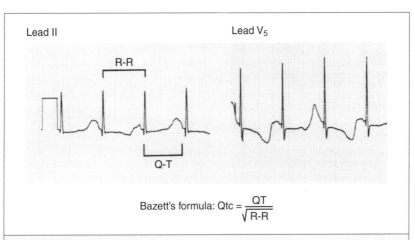

Lead II   Lead V₅

R-R

Q-T

Bazett's formula: $Qtc = \dfrac{QT}{\sqrt{R\text{-}R}}$

Figure 3-6. Long QT syndrome, leads II and V5. Note long QT interval and T-wave alternans (alternating upright and downgoing T waves). (From Towbin JA: Molecular genetic basis of sudden cardiac death. Pediatr Clin N Am 51:1230, 2004, Fig. 1.)

61. **What characterizes torsades de pointes?**
    From the French for "to turn on a point," this is a ventricular tachycardia of varying forms characterized by abrupt changes in amplitude and polarity (Fig. 3-7). It is a pathologic tachyarrhythmia seen in patients with prolonged QT syndromes and the use of certain drugs (e.g., cisapride, thioridazine). Treatment, per the Pediatric Advanced Life Support algorithm, is the infusion of magnesium.

62. **When should amiodarone not be used as the first-line therapy in patients with ventricular tachycardia?**
    In patients with torsades de pointes (polymorphic ventricular tachycardia with a long QT interval) or with ventricular tachycardia and a long QT interval, amiodarone should not be used. Amiodarone is a class III antiarrhythmic agent and will lengthen the QT interval, predisposing the patient to further arrhythmias.

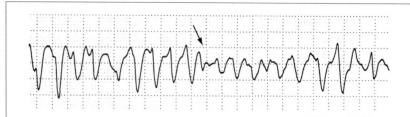

Figure 3-7. Torsades de pointes polymorphic ventricular tachycardia. Note the phase change (*arrow*) with change is QRS polarity. (From Samson RA, Atkins RA: Tachyarrhythmias and defibrillation. Pediatr Clin N Am 55:891, 2008, Fig. 4.)

63. **What are the ECG findings in patients with complete heart block?**
    The atrial and ventricular activities are entirely independent. P waves are regular, and QRS complexes are also regular, with a rate slower than the P rate (Fig. 3-8).

Figure 3-8. Complete heart block. Tracing demonstrates atrial activity (*arrows*) independent of slower ventricular rhythm. (From Zitelli BJ, Davis HW: Atlas of Pediatric Physical Diagnosis, 4th ed. St. Louis, Mosby, 2002, p 144.)

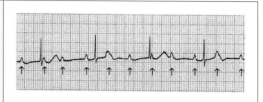

64. **How abnormal are premature atrial contractions?**
    Premature atrial beats are usually benign, with the exception of patients with an electrical or anatomic substrate for supraventricular tachycardia (SVT) or atrial flutter.

65. **How does SVT in children differ from physiologic sinus tachycardia?**
    SVT typically has the following features:
    ■ Sudden onset and termination rather than a gradual change in rate
    ■ Persistent ventricular rate of >180 beats/minute
    ■ Fixed or almost fixed RR interval on ECG
    ■ Abnormal P-wave shape or axis or absent P waves
    ■ Little change in heart rate with activity, crying, or breath holding

66. **When are isolated premature ventricular contractions (PVCs) usually benign in the otherwise healthy school-aged child?**
    ■ Structurally normal heart
    ■ ECG intervals, especially QTc, are normal
    ■ No evidence of myocarditis, cardiomegaly, or ventricular tumor
    ■ No history of drug use
    ■ Electrolytes and glucose are normal
    ■ They decrease with exercise

67. **Name the two most common mechanisms of SVT.**
    ■ Wolff-Parkinson-White (WPW) syndrome (due to an accessory bypass tract)
    ■ AV nodal reentry

68. **What are the clinical settings in which SVT may occur?**
    - Structurally normal heart: Accessory bypass tract or AV nodal reentry
    - Congenital heart disease (pre- or postoperatively): Ebstein anomaly, L-TGA with VSD and pulmonic stenosis; after Mustard, Senning, Fontan procedures
    - Hypertrophic cardiomyopathy
    - Dilated cardiomyopathy
    - Drug-induced: Sympathomimetics (e.g., cold medications, theophylline, beta agonists)
    - Infections: Myocarditis
    - Hyperthyroidism

69. **What are some of the causes of a wide QRS complex?**
    - Premature ventricular contraction
    - Ventricular tachycardia
    - Premature atrial contraction with aberrant conduction
    - SVT with aberrant conduction
    - Bundle branch blocks
    - Pre-excitation syndromes (WPW syndrome)
    - Electrolyte abnormalities
    - Myocarditis
    - Cardiomyopathy
    - Electronic ventricular pacemaker

70. **What vagal maneuvers are used to treat paroxysmal SVT in children?**
    Infants
    - Placement of plastic bag filled with crushed ice over forehead and nose
    - Gagging with tongue blade

    Older children and adolescents
    - Above methods
    - Unilateral carotid massage
    - Valsalva maneuver (abdominal straining while holding breath)
    - Doing a headstand

    In general, the Valsalva maneuver and carotid massage are not as effective for children younger than 4 years. Ocular pressure is not recommended because it has been associated with retinal injury. Vagal stimulation slows conduction in the AV node and prolongs refractoriness of the AV node, thereby interrupting the reentrant circuit.

71. **In addition to vagal maneuvers, what treatments are used acutely for managing SVT?**
    If a patient's clinical condition has deteriorated, synchronized direct-current **cardioversion** is indicated. In patients who are stable and for whom vagal maneuvers have failed, **adenosine** has replaced digoxin and verapamil as the first drug of choice. An initial bolus of 100 mg/kg will exert an effect in 10 to 20 seconds by slowing conduction through the AV node. If this is ineffective, the dose can be increased in increments of 50 to 100 mcg/kg every 1 to 2 minutes to a maximum single dose of 300 mcg /kg. The usual starting dose in adults is 6 mg and then 12 mg if the tachycardia persists.

72. **Why should an electrographic tracing (preferably with multiple leads) be carried out while administering intravenous adenosine?**
    Adenosine is used to convert reentrant SVT to sinus rhythm. During the conversion, observation of the termination of the arrhythmia on ECG can often reveal the mechanism of the tachycardia. In addition, if the tachycardia does not terminate other information can be obtained including the following:
    - The tachycardia is atrial in origin; one can observe varying degrees of AV block with the atrial tachycardia persisting (e.g., atrial flutter).

- The tachycardia is junctional or ventricular with 1:1 ventriculoatrial (VA) conduction; adenosine may induce VA block with VA dissociation.
- The tachycardia terminated and was immediately restarted by a premature atrial beat.

73. **When should the dose of adenosine be modified for suspected cardiac arrhythmia?**
Adenosine should not be routinely used in post–cardiac transplantation patients. Previous experience with adenosine in these patients has produced asystole with no underlying escape rhythm. Because the heart in these patients does not have normal sympathetic and parasympathetic innervation following transplantation, the response to catecholamines is typically blunted, and the heart rate is typically slower than normal. Additionally, many cardiac transplant recipients are taking dipyridamole (Persantine), which potentiates the effects of adenosine, thereby prolonging the duration of AV block. In patients with working pacing wires, it may be possible to use a lower dose of adenosine.

Due to the abnormal flow patterns in patients with the Fontan procedure, these patients frequently require higher doses of adenosine for the treatment of cardiac arrhythmias.

74. **Which children are candidates for transcatheter ablation techniques for SVT?**
Ablation therapy is used most commonly in children with dysrhythmias that are refractory to medical management and in those with life-threatening symptoms or possible lifelong medication requirements. Ablation is now commonly performed in children who are symptomatic from WPW or AV nodal reentrant tachycardia. Recommendations for transcatheter ablation are changing as evidence from increased experience with the safety and efficacy of the procedure is gathered. Recommendations vary with the age of the patient, the severity of the dysrhythmia, the type of lesion, the difficulty with medical control of the dysrhythmia, and the skill of the operator.

75. **What is the lethal arrhythmia of WPW syndrome?**
The lethal arrhythmia in patients with WPW is atrial fibrillation with a rapid ventricular response that degenerates into ventricular fibrillation. The rate of the ventricular response in these patients is dependent on the effective refractory period of the accessory pathway and not the AV node. This can result in ventricular rates of 250 to 300 beats per minute. Following ablation of the accessory pathway, these patients are no longer at risk for atrial fibrillation.

76. **How is WPW syndrome diagnosed on the baseline ECG?**
An accessory pathway bypasses the AV node, thereby resulting in early ventricular depolarization (pre-excitation). It is the most common cause of SVT in children. In infants and younger children with rapid heart rates, the delta wave may not be as evident. Additional clues that may be suggestive of WPW include the following:
- PR interval of <100 msec
- QRS duration of >80 msec
- No Q wave in left chest leads
- Left axis deviation

Perry JC, Giuffre RM, Garson A Jr: Clues to the electrocardiographic diagnosis of subtle Wolff-Parkinson-White syndrome in children, *J Pediatr* 117:871–875, 1990.

INFECTIOUS AND INFLAMMATORY DISORDERS

77. **How many blood cultures should be obtained in patients suspected of bacterial endocarditis?**
At least three separate blood cultures should be obtained. The use of multiple sites may decrease the likelihood of mistaking a contaminant for the true etiologic agent.

78. **Why might properly collected blood cultures be negative in the setting of clinically suspected bacterial endocarditis?**
    - Prior antibiotic use
    - The bacterial endocarditis may be right-sided
    - Nonbacterial infection: Fungal (e.g., *Aspergillus, Candida*) or unusual organisms (e.g., *Rickettsia, Chlamydia*)
    - Unusual bacterial infection: Slow-growing organisms or anaerobes
    - Lesions may be mural or nonvalvular (i.e., less likely to be hematogenously seeded)
    - Nonbacterial thrombotic endocarditis (sterile platelet-fibrin thrombus formations following endocardial injury)
    - Incorrect diagnosis

    Starke JR: Infectious endocarditis. In Feigin RD, Cherry JD, Demmler GJ, Kaplan S, editors: *Textbook of Pediatric Infectious Diseases*, ed 5, Philadelphia, 2004, W.B. Saunders, p 362.

79. **When is antibiotic prophylaxis for a dental procedure recommended?**
    In 2007, the American Heart Association made significant changes in antibiotic recommendations for cardiac patients. Only those with the highest risk for adverse outcomes from endocarditis are advised to receive dental prophylaxis. Prophylaxis with dental procedures is recommended for the following:
    - Prosthetic cardiac valve
    - Previous endocarditis
    - CHD*: Unrepaired cyanotic CHD, including palliative shunts and conduits; repaired CHD with prosthetic material or device, whether placed by surgery or by catheter intervention, during the first 6 months after the procedure[†]; repaired CHD with residual defects at the site of a prosthetic patch or prosthetic device (which inhibit endothelialization)
    - Cardiac transplantation recipients who develop cardiac valvulopathy

    Wilson W, Taubert KA, Gewitz M, et al: Prevention of infective endocarditis: guidelines from the American Heart Association, *Circulation* 116:1736–1754, 2007.

80. **How reliable is the echocardiogram for diagnosing bacterial endocarditis (BE)?**
    Echocardiography can sometimes identify an intracardiac mass that is attached either to the wall of the myocardium or to part of the valve. Although the yield of echocardiography for diagnosing BE is low, the likelihood of a positive finding is increased under certain conditions (e.g., indwelling catheters, prematurity, immunosuppression, evidence of peripheral embolization). BE is a clinical and laboratory diagnosis (physical examination and blood cultures, respectively) and not solely an "echocardiographic" diagnosis. A negative study does not rule out BE.

    Baddour LM, Wilson WR, Bayer AS, et al: Infective endocarditis: diagnosis, antimicrobial therapy and management of complications, *Circulation* 111:3167–3184, 2005.

81. **How do Osler nodes and Janeway lesions differ?**
    Both are noted in individuals with bacterial endocarditis. Pain is a key discriminator. Osler nodes are painful, tender nodules that are found primarily on the pads of the fingers and toes. Janeway lesions are painless, nontender, hemorrhagic nodular lesions seen on the palms and soles, especially on thenar and hypothenar eminences. Both lesions are rare in children with endocarditis.

    Farrior JB, Silverman ME: A consideration of the differences between a Janeway's lesion and an Osler's node in infectious endocarditis, *Chest* 20:239–243, 1976.

---

*Except for the conditions listed previously, antibiotic prophylaxis is no longer recommended for any other form of CHD.

[†]Prophylaxis is recommended because endothelialization of prosthetic material occurs within 6 months after the procedure.

82. **When should myocarditis be suspected?**
   The presenting symptoms of myocarditis can be variable, ranging from subclinical to rapidly progressive CHF. It should be considered in any patient who experiences unexplained heart failure. Clinical signs include tachycardia out of proportion to fever, tachypnea, a quiet precordium, muffled heart tones, gallop rhythm without murmur, and hepatomegaly.

   Cooper LT Jr: Myocarditis. *N Engl J Med* 360:1526–1538, 2009.

83. **What conditions are associated with the development of myocarditis?**
   Infections
   - Bacterial: Diphtheria
   - Viral: Coxsackie B (most common), coxsackie A, human immunodeficiency virus, echoviruses, rubella
   - Mycoplasmal
   - Rickettsial: Typhus
   - Fungal: Actinomycosis, coccidioidomycosis, histoplasmosis
   - Protozoal: Trypanosomiasis (Chagas disease), toxoplasmosis
   Inflammatory
   - Kawasaki disease
   - Systemic lupus erythematosus
   - Rheumatoid arthritis
   - Eosinophilic myocarditis
   Chemical and physical agents
   - Radiation injury
   - Drugs: Doxorubicin
   - Toxins: Lead
   - Animal bites: Scorpion, snake

84. **When should steroids be given to a child with myocarditis?**
   The use of steroids in patients with myocarditis is controversial. Some authorities feel that the use of steroids may inhibit interferon synthesis and increase viral replication. If the inflammatory process is secondary to rheumatic fever, however, steroids may be indicated.

85. **A child visiting from South America presents symptoms including unilateral eye swelling and new-onset acute CHF. What is a likely diagnosis?**
   Acute myocarditis as a result of **Chagas disease** (American trypanosomiasis) is likely. Seen in 25% to 50% of patients in endemic areas with early Chagas disease, Romaña sign is unilateral, painless, violaceous, palpebral edema often accompanied by conjunctivitis. The swelling occurs near the bite site of the parasitic vector: the reduviid or Triatominae bug. Chagas disease, a protozoan infection, is a common cause of acute and chronic myocarditis in Central and South America.

86. **What are the common clinical signs and symptoms of pericarditis?**
   - **Symptoms:** Chest pain, fever, cough, palpitations, irritability, abdominal pain
   - **Signs:** Friction rub, pallor, pulsus paradoxus, muffled heart sounds, neck vein distention, hepatomegaly

87. **What is the position of comfort in the patient with pericarditis?**
   The typical patient with pericarditis prefers to sit up and lean forward.

88. **What is Kawasaki disease?**
A multisystem disease characterized by a vasculitis of small and medium-sized blood vessels. If untreated, this can lead to coronary artery aneurysms and myocardial infarction. In the developed world, Kawasaki disease is the most common cause of acquired heart disease.

   Kawasaki Disease Foundation: http://www.kdfoundation.org.

89. **What are the principal diagnostic criteria for Kawasaki disease?**
The mnemonic **My HEART** may be helpful:
   - **M**ucosal changes, especially oral and upper respiratory; dry and chapped lips; "strawberry tongue"
   - **H**and and extremity changes, including reddened palms and soles and edema; desquamation from fingertips and toes is a later finding (second week of illness)
   - **E**ye changes, primarily a bilateral conjunctival infection without discharge
   - **A**denopathy that is usually cervical, often unilateral, and ≥1.5 cm in diameter
   - **R**ash that is usually a truncal exanthem without vesicles, bullae, or petechiae
   - **T**emperature elevation, often to 40°C (104°F) or above, lasting for >5 days

90. **How many diagnostic criteria are required for Kawasaki disease?**
The presence of fever and at least four of the other five features are needed for the classic diagnosis. However, a significant number of cases of *atypical* Kawasaki disease (20% to 60% of total) have been reported. These feature less than five of the criteria and occur particularly in children younger than 1 year; the symptoms are subsequently accompanied by the typical coronary artery changes. A high index of suspicion is important because Kawasaki disease has replaced acute rheumatic fever as the leading cause of identifiable acquired heart disease in children in the United States.

   Chang FY, Hwang B, Chen SJ, et al: Characteristics of Kawasaki disease in infants younger than six months of age, *Pediatr Infect Dis J* 25:241–244, 2006.

   Rowley AH: Incomplete (atypical) Kawasaki disease, *Pediatr Infect Dis J* 21:563–565, 2002.

91. **What conditions should be considered in the differential diagnosis of Kawasaki disease?**
   - Viral infections (including adenovirus, enterovirus, Epstein-Barr virus, measles)
   - Scarlet fever
   - Staphylococcal scalded skin syndrome
   - Toxic shock syndrome
   - Bacterial cervical lymphadenitis
   - Drug hypersensitivity
   - Stevens-Johnson syndrome
   - Juvenile idiopathic arthritis
   - Leptospirosis
   - Mercury hypersensitivity reaction (acrodynia)

   Fimbres AM, Shulman ST: Kawasaki disease, *Pediatr Rev* 29:308–311, 2008.

92. **What laboratory tests are often abnormal in the first 7 to 10 days of the illness?**
   - **Complete blood count:** 50% of patients have an elevated white blood cell count (>15,000) with neutrophilia; a progressive normochromic, normocytic anemia; platelet count increases (with peak in the second or third week of the season)
   - **Urinalysis:** pyuria without bacteriuria (culture usually negative)
   - **Acute phase reactants:** C-reactive protein, erythrocyte sedimentation rate significantly elevated in 80%

- **Blood chemistry:** Mild increase in hepatic transaminases, low serum sodium, protein and/or albumin
- **Cerebrospinal fluid:** Pleocytosis (usually lymphocytic) with normal protein and glucose

Harnden A, Takahashi M, Burgner D: Kawasaki disease, *BMJ* 338:1133–1138, 2009.

93. **What is the typical age of children with Kawasaki disease?**
80% of cases occur between the ages of 6 months and 5 years. However, cases can occur in infants and teenagers. Both of these groups appear to be at increased risk for developing coronary artery sequelae. The diagnosis is often delayed, particularly in infants, because signs and symptoms of the illness may be atypical or subtle.

Genizi J, Miron D, Spiegel R, et al: Kawasaki disease in very young infants: high prevalence of atypical presentation and coronary arteritis, *Clin Pediatr* 42:263–267, 2003.

94. **What should be the clinical suspicion for a visiting 11-month-old Pakistani girl with fever for 5 days and marked erythema and induration around her bacille Calmette-Guérin (BCG) scar?**
In the Japanese literature (where the incidence of Kawasaki disease is much greater), the local inflammatory reactivation of a BCG inoculation site has been shown to be a specific (though not sensitive) early sign of Kawasaki disease. It is not recognized in the United States as an official criterion toward the diagnosis, but its presence should heighten suspicion of Kawasaki disease. Of course, with any localized induration in the setting of fever, one must also be certain that no soft-tissue infection is present.

Sinha R, Balakumar T: BCG reactivation: a useful diagnostic tool even for incomplete Kawasaki disease, *Arch Dis Child* 90:891, 2005.

KEY POINTS: DIAGNOSTIC FEATURES OF KAWASAKI DISEASE

1. Erythema of oral cavity and dry, chapped lips

2. Conjunctivitis: Bilateral and without discharge

3. Edema and erythema and/or desquamation of hands and feet

4. Cervical lymphadenopathy

5. Polymorphous exanthem on trunk, flexor regions, and perineum

6. Fever, often up to 40°C (104°F), lasting ≥5 days

7. No other identifiable diagnostic entity to explain signs and symptoms

8. Atypical Kawasaki disease (fever but fewer than four of the other criteria) is common in children <1 year of age.

95. **Why should all children with Kawasaki disease receive intravenous immunoglobulin (IVIG) therapy?**
IVIG has been demonstrated to decrease the incidence of coronary artery abnormalities in children with Kawasaki disease. Additionally, fever and laboratory indices of inflammation resolve more quickly after treatment. The most common dosing is a single infusion over 8 to 12 hours of 2 g/kg. In children who remain febrile 36 hours after the first infusion, a second dose of 2 g/kg is recommended.

When administered 5 to 10 days after the start of fever, IVIG improves outcome, with coronary artery dilation developing in less than 5% of patients and giant coronary aneurysms developing in less than 1% of patients. At present, there is no reliable means of predicting which children with Kawasaki disease will develop coronary artery abnormalities. Therefore, all children with Kawasaki disease should receive parental immunoglobulin.

96. Is aspirin therapy of benefit for children with Kawasaki disease?
By itself, high-dose aspirin (80 to 100 mg/kg per day divided into doses taken every 6 hours) is effective for decreasing the degree of fever and discomfort in patients during the acute stages of illness. It is unclear whether high-dose aspirin has an additive effect for decreasing the incidence of coronary artery abnormalities when used in conjunction with γ-globulin. Aspirin may be beneficial when administered in low doses after the resolution of fever owing to its effects on platelet aggregation and prevention of the thrombotic complications seen in children with Kawasaki disease. Therefore, when fever has been absent for 48 hours, the patient is switched to aspirin in low doses (3 to 5 mg/kg/day) which is continued for about 6 to 8 weeks. If a follow-up echocardiogram at that time reveals no coronary abnormalities, therapy is usually discontinued. If abnormalities are present, therapy is continued indefinitely.

97. What is the likelihood of a patient developing coronary artery pathology with and without treatment for Kawasaki disease?
In 30% to 50% of patients, a mild diffuse dilation of coronary arteries begins 10 days after the start of fever. If untreated, 20% to 25% of these will progress to true aneurysms (Fig. 3-9). In about 1% of cases, giant aneurysms (>8 mm diameter) develop, which may heal with stenosis and lead to distal myocardial ischemia. With IVIG therapy, the incidence of aneurysms is reduced to less than 5%.

Harnden A, Takahashi M, Burgner D: Kawasaki disease, *BMJ* 338:1133–1138, 2009.

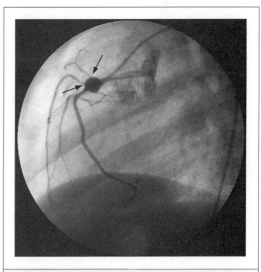

Figure 3-9. Lateral view of coronary angiogram showing right coronary artery with saccular aneurysm. (From Vetter VL [ed]: Pediatric Cardiology: The Requisites in Pediatrics. Philadelphia, Mosby, 2006, p 135.)

98. What factors are most strongly associated with the development of coronary artery disease in patients with Kawasaki disease?
- Duration of fever of >14 days
- Recurrence of fever after an afebrile period of 48 hours
- Cardiomegaly
- Male gender
- Age of <1 year or >8 years

PHARMACOLOGY

99. **How valuable are digoxin levels?**
Digoxin levels are only useful as a guide to digoxin therapy. Digoxin levels may not be as helpful in infants and younger children because of the presence of endogenous digoxin-like immunoreactive substances, which cross-react with immunoassay antibodies to digoxin. Digoxin levels may be helpful, however, in older children and adolescents (especially in the presence of dysrhythmias).

100. **How long before oral digoxin begins to work?**
Oral digoxin reaches peak plasma levels 1 to 2 hours after administration, but a peak hemodynamic effect is not evident until 6 hours after administration (versus 2 to 3 hours for intravenous digoxin).

101. **A child with WPW syndrome and SVT is given digoxin, and the attending cardiologist is dismayed. Why?**
Digoxin can enhance conduction through a bypass tract while slowing down conduction through the AV node. Ventricular fibrillation has been reported in patients with WPW treated with digoxin. This effect is believed to be due to enhanced conduction down the bypass tract. For this reason, propranolol has replaced digoxin as the drug of choice for the treatment of children with SVT and WPW. Of note, verapamil can both shorten the effective refractory period of the accessory pathway and raise the risk for sudden death in WPW patients should they develop atrial fibrillation.

102. **When should indomethacin be administered to newborns with a PDA?**
Indomethacin is effective for closing a PDA within the first 10 days of life. The drug is indicated for preterm infants with a hemodynamically significant PDA, which is defined as one in which there is deteriorating respiratory status (e.g., tachypnea, apnea, CO_2 retention, increased ventilatory support, failure to wean ventilatory support, poor cardiac output, or evidence of congestive heart failure).

Schneider DJ, Moore JW: Patent ductus arteriosus. *Circulation* 114:1873–1882, 2006.

103. **What are the side effects of indomethacin in the neonate?**
- Mild but usually transient decreased renal function
- Hyponatremia
- Hypoglycemia
- Platelet dysfunction producing a prolonged bleeding time
- Occult blood loss from the gastrointestinal tract

104. **What are the contraindications for indomethacin therapy?**
Indomethacin is contraindicated if the creatinine level is more than 1.8 mg/dL, the platelet count is less than 60,000/mm^3, and there is evidence of a bleeding diathesis.

105. **What are the indications for prostaglandin E_1 (PGE_1) in the neonate?**
PGE_1 is indicated in cardiac lesions that depend on a PDA to maintain adequate pulmonary or systemic blood flow or to promote adequate mixing.
- Inadequate pulmonary blood flow (e.g., pulmonary atresia with intact ventricular septum, tricuspid atresia with intact ventricular septum, critical pulmonary stenosis)
- Inadequate systemic blood flow (e.g., critical coarctation of the aorta, interrupted aortic arch, hypoplastic left heart syndrome)
- Inadequate mixing (e.g., transposition of the great vessels)

106. **What are the major side effects of PGE_1?**
Apnea, fever, cutaneous flushing, seizures, hypotension, and bradycardia or tachycardia.

107. **How do α, β, and dopaminergic receptors differ?**
α: In vascular smooth muscle, these cause vasoconstriction.
β_1: In myocardial smooth muscle, these increase inotropic (contractile) force, chronotropic (cardiac rate) effect, and AV conduction (dromotropic).
β_2: In vascular smooth muscle, these cause vasodilation.
Dopaminergic: In renal and mesenteric vascular smooth muscle, these cause vasodilation.

108. **How do relative receptor effects differ by drug type?**
See Table 3-6.

TABLE 3-6. RELATIVE RECEPTOR EFFECTS BY DRUG TYPE				
Drug	α	β_1	β_2	Dopaminergic
Epinephrine	+++	+++	+++	0
Norepinephrine	+++	+++	+ to +	0
Isoproterenol	0	+++	+++	0
Dopamine*	0 to +++	++ to +++	++	+++
	(dose related)	(dose related)	(dose related)	
Dobutamine	0 to +	+++	+	0

*For dopamine, at low doses (2-5 µg/kg/min), dopaminergic effects predominate. At high doses (5-20 µg/kg/min), increased α and β effects are seen. At very high doses (>20 µg/kg/min), a markedly increased α effect with decreased renal and mesenteric blood flow occurs. For dobutamine, β_1 inotropic effects are more pronounced than are chronotropic effects.
Effect of medication: 0 = none; + = small; ++ = moderate; +++ = large.

109. **How are emergency infusions for cardiovascular support prepared?**
See Table 3-7.

TABLE 3-7. EMERGENCY INFUSIONS FOR CARDIOVASCULAR SUPPORT		
Catecholamine	Mixture	Dose
Isoproterenol, epinephrine, norepinephrine	0.6 mg × body wt (in kg), added to diluent to make 100 mL	1 mL/hr delivers 0.1 mcg/kg/min
Dopamine, dobutamine	6 mg × body wt (in kg), added to diluent to make 100 mL	1 mL/hr delivers 1 mcg/kg/min

PHYSICAL EXAMINATION

110. **What causes the first heart sound?**
The first heart sound is caused by the closure of the mitral and tricuspid valves.

111. **What causes the second heart sound?**
The second heart sound is caused by the closure of the aortic and pulmonary valves.

112. **In what settings can an abnormal second heart sound be auscultated?**
Widely split S$_2$
- Prolonged RV ejection time
- RV volume overload: Atrial septal defect, partial anomalous pulmonary venous return
- RV conduction delay: Right bundle branch block

Single S$_2$
- Presence of only one semilunar valve: Aortic or pulmonary atresia, truncus arteriosus
- P$_2$ not audible: Tetralogy of Fallot, transposition of great arteries
- A$_2$ delayed: Severe aortic stenosis
- May be normal in a newborn

Paradoxically split S$_2$ (A$_2$ follows P$_2$)
- Severe aortic stenosis
- Left bundle branch block

Loud P$_2$
- Pulmonary hypertension

113. **When can S$_3$ and S$_4$ be considered normal findings during a pediatric cardiac examination?**
An S$_3$ occurs early in diastole. It may be benign, but it can be abnormal in children with dilated ventricles and decreased compliance (e.g., in patients with CHF). An S$_4$ occurs late in diastole. It is usually abnormal in children.

114. **What is the difference between pulsus alternans and pulsus paradoxus?**
- **Pulsus alternans** is a pulse pattern in which there is alternating (beat-to-beat) variability of pulse strength due to decreased ventricular performance. This is sometimes seen in patients with severe CHF.
- **Pulsus paradoxus** indicates an exaggeration of the normal reduction of systolic blood pressure during inspiration. Associated conditions include cardiac tamponade (e.g., effusion, constrictive pericarditis), severe respiratory illness (e.g., asthma, pneumonia), and myocardial disease that affects wall compliance (e.g., endocardial fibroelastosis, amyloidosis).

115. **How is pulsus paradoxus measured?**
To measure a pulsus paradoxus, determine the systolic pressure by noting the first audible Korotkoff sound. Then retake the blood pressure by raising the manometer pressure to at least 25 mm Hg higher than the systolic pressure, and allow it to fall very slowly. Stop as soon as the first sound is heard. Note that the sound disappears during inspiration. Lower the pressure slowly, and note when all pulsed beats are heard. The difference between these two pressures is the pulsus paradoxus. Normally, in children, there is an 8- to 10-mm Hg fluctuation in systolic pressure with different phases of respiration.

116. **Is palpation for femoral pulses a reliable screening tool for coarctation of the aorta in infants and older children?**
The detection of decreased lower extremity pulses seen in coarctation can be subtle and unreliable. In some infants, a patent ductus arteriosus may provide blood flow to the lower extremities, thus bypassing a severe coarctation. Upper and lower pulses may be equal as long as the ductus remains open. As the ductus closes, signs of coarctation of the aorta may appear with respiratory distress and cardiac failure. Decreased or absent pulses may then be noted. In older children, simultaneous palpation of upper and lower extremity pulses is important. If collaterals have developed, a delay in pulse rather than diminished volume may be noted. In a study of older patients (>1 year old) with documented coarctation, only 20% had absent lower extremity pulses, and distinguishing differences between upper extremity and lower extremity

pulses was unreliable. Thus, some authors recommend that screening for coarctation of the aorta be done by measuring blood pressure in both arms and one leg.

Ing FF, Starc TJ, Griffiths SP, Gersony WM: Early diagnosis of coarctation of the aorta in children: a continuing dilemma, *Pediatrics* 98:378–382, 1996.

117. **What is the differential diagnosis for a systolic murmur in each auscultatory area?**
See Fig. 3-10.

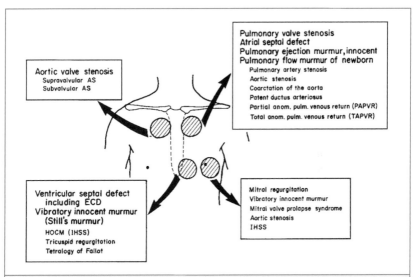

Figure 3-10. Systolic murmurs audible at various locations. Many may radiate to other areas. Less common conditions are shown in smaller type. (From Park MK: Pediatric Cardiology for Practitioners, 4th ed. St. Louis, Mosby, 2002, p 32.)

118. **What are the most common innocent murmurs?**
See Table 3-8.

TABLE 3-8. MOST COMMON INNOCENT MURMURS		
Type (Timing)	Description of Murmur	Common Age Group
Classic vibratory murmur; Still murmur (systolic)	Maximal at MLSB or between LLSB and apex Grade 2-3/6 Low-frequency vibratory, "twanging string," or musical	3-6 years old; occasionally in infancy
Pulmonary ejection murmur (systolic)	Maximal at ULSB Early to midsystolic Grade 1-2/6 in intensity	8-14 years old

(continued)

TABLE 3-8. MOST COMMON INNOCENT MURMURS *(continued)*		
Type (Timing)	Description of Murmur	Common Age Group
Pulmonary flow murmur of newborn (systolic)	Maximal at ULSB Transmits well to left and right chest, axillae, and back Grade 1-2/6 intensity	Premature and full-term newborns; usually disappears by 3-6 months of age
Venous hum (continuous)	Maximal at right (or left) supraclavicular and infraclavicular areas Grade 1-2/6 intensity Inaudible in supine position Intensity changes with rotation of head and compression of jugular vein	3-6 years old
Carotid bruit (systolic)	Right supraclavicular area and over carotids Grade 2-3/6 intensity Occasional thrill over a carotid artery	Any age

LLSB = lower-left sternal border; MLSB = mid-left sternal border; ULSB = upper-left sternal border.

119. **What is the effect of sitting up on the typical innocent murmur?**
Sitting up usually brings out or increases the intensity of the murmur of a venous hum. In contrast, the typical vibratory innocent murmur along the lower left sternal border in the supine child will diminish in intensity and sometimes disappear while sitting upright.

120. **What features are suggestive of a pathologic murmur?**
- Diastolic murmurs
- Late systolic murmurs
- Pansystolic murmurs
- Murmurs associated with a thrill
- Associated cardiac abnormalities (e.g., asymmetrical pulses, clicks, abnormal splitting)
- Continuous murmurs

McCrindle BW, Shaffer KM, Kan JS, et al: Cardinal clinical signs in the differentiation of heart murmurs in children, *Arch Pediatr Adolesc Med* 150:169–174, 1996.

Rosenthal A: How to distinguish between innocent and pathologic murmurs in childhood, *Pediatr Clin North Am* 31:1229–1240, 1984.

121. **If a murmur is detected, what other factors suggest that the murmur is pathologic?**
- Evidence of growth retardation (most commonly seen in murmurs with large left-to-right shunts)
- Associated dysmorphic features (e.g., valvular disease in Hurler syndrome, Noonan syndrome)

■ Exertional cyanosis, pallor, or dyspnea, especially if associated with minor exertion such as climbing a few stairs (may be a sign of early CHF)
■ Short feeding times and volumes in infants (may be a sign of early CHF)
■ Syncopal or presyncopal episodes (may be seen in hypertrophic cardiomyopathy)
■ History of intravenous drug abuse (risk factor for endocarditis)
■ Maternal history of diabetes mellitus (associated with asymmetrical septal hypertrophy, VSD, D-transposition), alcohol use (associated with pulmonic stenosis and VSD), or other medications
■ Family history of congenital heart disease

KEY POINTS: PATHOLOGIC MURMURS

1. Diastolic

2. Pansystolic

3. Late systolic

4. Continuous

5. Thrill present on examination

6. Additional cardiac abnormalities (e.g., clicks, abnormal splitting, asymmetric pulses)

SURGERY

122. **What are shunt operations?**
Shunts between a systemic artery and the pulmonary artery are used to improve oxygen saturation in patients with cyanotic CHD and diminished pulmonary blood flow. Venoarterial shunts that connect a systemic vein and the pulmonary artery are also used for similar purposes.

123. **Name the major shunt operations (Fig. 3-11) for CHD.**
■ The **Blalock-Taussig** shunt consists of an anastomosis between a subclavian artery and the ipsilateral pulmonary artery. The subclavian artery can be divided and the distal end anastomosed to the pulmonary artery (classic BT shunt), or a prosthetic graft (Gore-Tex) can be interposed between the two arteries (modified BT shunt). It allows for pulmonary blood flow in children with severe pulmonary stenosis or atresia.

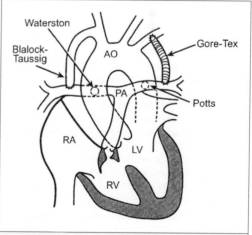

Figure 3-11. Major shunt operations. (From Park MK: Pediatric Cardiology for Practitioners, 4th ed. St. Louis, Mosby, 2002, p 194.)

- The **Waterston** shunt is an anastomosis between the ascending aorta and the right pulmonary artery. This procedure is rarely performed today.
- The **Potts** shunt is an anastomosis between the descending aorta and the left pulmonary artery. This procedure is rarely performed today.

124. **For which congenital heart disorder is the arterial switch operation done?**
Transposition of the great arteries. This procedure restores the aorta and the pulmonary artery to their correct anatomic positions, and it involves the reimplantation of the coronary arteries.

125. **What is the purpose of the Fontan procedure?**
The Fontan procedure (or operation) is designed to reroute systemic venous blood from the superior and inferior vena cava directly to the pulmonary arteries, thus bypassing the ventricle. It is most commonly used for any cardiac lesion with only a single functional ventricle. A common current approach is to anastomose the superior vena cava to the right pulmonary artery and also redirect flow from the inferior vena cava toward the lower superior vena cava through either a baffle or an extracardiac conduit. This deoxygenated blood flows passively to the lungs and returns to the ventricle to be pumped to the systemic circulation.

Tsai W, Klein BL: The postoperative cardiac patient. *Clin Pediatr Emerg Med* 6:216–221, 2005.

126. **What are the most common rhythm disturbances after the Fontan procedure?**
Because of the extensive atrial surgery in the Fontan procedure, there are two major cardiac rhythm issues.
- **Loss of sinus rhythm** with either a nonsinus atrial rhythm or junctional rhythm. Atrial pacing may be required in these patients to either increase heart rate or restore AV synchrony.
- **Intra-atrial reentrant tachycardia** was more common following the old-style Fontan procedure because of the incisional scars and size of the atrium. Although less common with the newer surgical techniques, it remains a major clinical problem in these patients and is often drug resistant and requires either catheter or surgical ablation.

127. **What are the indications for repair of a VSD?**
- **VSD:** Infants with a large VSD that is refractory to medical therapy (thereby causing failure to thrive and/or repeated respiratory tract infections) should be referred for surgery. Pulmonary hypertension is another indication for surgery. In older children with normal pulmonary artery pressure but with significantly increased pulmonary blood flow or left ventricular dilation, surgical closure is sometimes advised.
- **ASD:** Asymptomatic children should be scheduled for repair between 3 and 5 years of age.

128. **What are the indications for closure of an atrial septal defect?**
Asymptomatic children with a secundum atrial septal defect associated with RV dilation and increased pulmonary blood flow typically undergo elective closure between 3 and 5 years of age. Children with a typical secundum atrial septal defect can usually be closed with catheterization techniques. A primum or sinus venous atrial septal defect is closed with surgery. In addition, a very large secundum defect or associated lesions are typically closed at surgery. The rare infant with a symptomatic atrial septal defect should undergo surgery at the time of diagnosis.

129. **Is there any surgical therapy for hypoplastic left heart syndrome?**
In patients with this condition, severe underdevelopment of the left ventricle, mitral valve, aortic valve, and ascending aortic arch occurs. Newborns develop signs of severe CHF and cyanosis. Two surgical options are available: the **Norwood procedure** and **heart transplantation.**

130. **Of all patients wait-listed for solid organ transplantation in the United States, which group has the highest waiting list mortality regardless of age?**
Children listed for heart transplantation. Of 3098 children younger than 18 years (median age, 2 years) listed for a heart transplantation between 1999 and 2006, 17% died, 63% received transplants, 8% recovered, and 12% remain listed.

Almond CSD, Thiagarajan RR, Piercey GE, et al: Waiting list mortality among children listed for heart transplantation in the United States, *Circulation* 119:717–727, 2009.

131. **What is the typical timing for the three operations for children with hypoplastic left heart syndrome?**
- Newborn: Norwood procedure: reconstruction of the new aorta, atrial septectomy, and pulmonary shunt
- 4 to 8 months: Glenn shunt (hemi-Fontan)—superior caval to pulmonary artery connection
- 2 to 4 years: Fontan procedure—inferior vena cava to pulmonary artery connection

Barron DJ, Kilby MD, Davies MD, et al: Hypoplastic left heart syndrome, *Lancet* 374:551–564, 2009.

132. **What is the long-term prognosis for heart transplantation during infancy and childhood?**
Survival statistics have improved dramatically during the past 10 years with the use of newer and safer immunosuppressive agents such as cyclosporine and FK506. However, children who receive transplanted hearts are at increased risk for cardiac rejection, infection, accelerated coronary artery disease, and lymphoproliferative syndromes. Recent estimated 5-year survival rates vary between 65% and 80%.

Conway J, Dipchand AI: Heart transplantation in children, *Pediatr Clin North Am* 57:353–373, 2010.

ACKNOWLEDGMENT

The editors gratefully acknowledge the contributions by Dr. Bernard J. Clark III that were retained from the first three editions of *Pediatric Secrets*.

CHAPTER 4

DERMATOLOGY

*Kimberly D. Morel, MD, Vivian A. Lombillo, MD, PhD,
and Maria C. Garzon, MD**

ACNE

1. **When is acne most likely to develop?**
   The development of micro comedones is typically the earliest sign of acne. Studies have shown that comedones occur in three fourths of premenarchal girls at an average age of 10 years and in about half of 10- to 11-year-old boys. They may herald (or predate) the onset of puberty.

2. **What are the four key factors in acne pathogenesis?**
   1. Abnormal follicular keratinization leading to follicular plugging
   2. Increased sebum production
   3. Proliferation of *Propionibacterium acnes*
   4. Inflammation

3. **How do a "blackhead" and a "whitehead" differ histopathologically?**
   Both lesions are produced by obstruction and distention of the sebaceous follicle with sebum and cellular debris. When the follicular contents tent the overlying skin but are not exposed to the atmosphere, a **whitehead** occurs. If the contents project out of the follicular opening, oxidation of the exposed mass of debris produces a color change and a **blackhead.**

4. **What is the difference between neonatal acne and infantile acne?**
   Neonatal acne occurs in up to 20% of newborns and typically presents during the first 4 weeks after birth. Erythematous papulopustules develop on the face, especially the cheeks. It has been attributed to the transient elevation of androgenic hormones (both maternally derived and endogenous) that are present in a newborn infant. The lesions typically resolve within 1 to 3 months as androgen levels fall. *Neonatal cephalic pustulosis* is a term that has been proposed to replace neonatal acne. Because lesions have been shown to contain *Malassezia* species, neonatal "acne" may actually represent an inflammatory reaction to this yeast flora and not true acne.

   Infantile acne affects a smaller number of infants on a delayed basis (3 to 6 months) and is characterized by greater degrees of inflammatory papules and pustules. Open and closed comedones and sometimes nodules are also present. This type is similar to acne vulgaris and may persist for years. The cause is unknown. Most patients with this condition have no evidence of precocious puberty or increased hormonal levels, although severe acne in this age group warrants evaluation for hyperandrogenism. Systemic therapy is sometimes required.

---

*Off-label use of medications are discussed in this chapter. This chapter is not designed to provide specific treatment guidelines. The authors have no conflicts of interest relevant to the material discussed.

KEY POINTS: MORPHOLOGIC DESCRIPTIONS OF PRIMARY CUTANEOUS LESIONS

1. **Macule:** A circumscribed, flat area, recognizable by color variation from surrounding skin, ≤ 1 cm

2. **Patch:** A large macule, >1 cm

3. **Papule:** A circumscribed elevation, ≤ 1 cm

4. **Plaque:** A large superficial papule, >1 cm

5. **Nodule:** A circumscribed solid elevation, ≤ 1 cm

6. **Vesicle** (small blister): A clear, fluid-filled elevation, ≤ 1 cm

7. **Bullae** (large blister): A fluid-filled elevation, >1 cm

8. **Pustule:** A circumscribed elevation of skin filled with pus

5. **Which disorders resemble neonatal and infantile acne?**
   - **Miliaria rubra** or **pustulosa,** often in areas of occlusion and skin folds
   - **Milia,** white papules without surrounding erythema
   - **Sebaceous hyperplasia,** typically on the nose and yellowish papules
   - **Seborrheic dermatitis,** erythematous scaly patches rather than pustules

6. **Is an infant with acne more likely to be a teenager with acne?**
   The presence or severity of acne in an infant who is younger than 3 months is not thought to correlate with an increased likelihood of adolescent acne. However, delayed acne between 3 and 6 months of age (especially if persistent and severe) does have a higher correlation with the likelihood of more severe adolescent acne. Family history of severe acne also increases the likelihood of future problems.

   Herane MI, Ando I: Acne in infancy and acne genetics, *Dermatology* 206:24–28, 2003.

7. **How are the types and severity of acne categorized?**
   No universal classification exists, but acne is typically categorized as noninflammatory (comedones, open and closed) or inflammatory. Inflammatory acne is then classified by the predominant lesion: papules, pustules, nodes, and/or cysts. *Mild* acne generally involves comedonal acne with a few papules or pustules, *moderate* acne adds more extensive papules or papules with a few nodules, and *severe* acne encompasses all types of inflammatory lesions.

8. **What factors exacerbate acne?**
   - Vigorous scrubbing or picking of lesions
   - Use of comedogenic make-up or other facial products
   - Medications: Anabolic steroids and corticosteroids, lithium, barbiturates, and some oral contraceptives
   - Sweating and tight-fitting clothes or sports equipment
   - Hormone dysregulation, such as polycystic ovarian syndrome

KEY POINTS: MAIN FACTORS IN ACNE PATHOGENESIS

1. Abnormal follicular keratinization

2. Androgen-dependent sebum production

3. Proliferation of *Propionibacterium acnes*

4. Inflammation

9. **What are the most severe forms of acne?**

Acne fulminans is a rare but severe disorder that has also been called *acute febrile ulcerative acne*. It occurs in teenage boys as extensive, inflammatory, ulcerating lesions on the trunk and chest that are usually associated with fever, malaise, arthralgia, and leukocytosis. The etiology remains unclear, but immune complexes are thought to be involved. Treatment is systemic and includes the following: antibiotics, glucocorticoids, and retinoids.

Acne conglobata is a severe form of acne that presents with comedones, papules, pustules, nodules, and abscesses. It is associated with significant scarring. It often arises in early adulthood, more typically in females. Systemic retinoid therapy is the treatment of choice.

James WD: Acne, *N Engl J Med* 352:1463–1472, 2005.

10. **What are the therapeutic approaches to acne?**

Acne therapies, including comedolytics, antibacterial agents, and hormonal modulators, target various factors involved in the pathogenesis of acne.

■ **Topical agents,** including erythromycin, clindamycin, erythromycin-benzoyl peroxide, clindamycin-benzoyl peroxide, benzoyl peroxide, and azelaic acid reduce the population of *Propionibacterium acnes.*

■ **Systemic antibiotics** (e.g., tetracycline and its derivatives) are most frequently used for moderate to severe papulopustular acne.

■ **Topical retinoids** are comedolytic and prevent the formation of new keratin plugs.

■ **Systemic retinoid** isotretinoin (Accutane) is used in cases of severe acne vulgaris. The exact mechanism of action of isotretinoin is not known but appears to be related to the inhibition of sebaceous gland activity.

■ **Hormonal modulation** is most commonly accomplished with oral contraceptive pills, although antiandrogenic agents (e.g., spironolactone) have been used in teenage girls with premenstrual flares, hirsutism, and male-pattern alopecia.

■ **Intralesional corticosteroids:** Sometimes used in severe nodular acne.

For most patients with acne, *combination therapy* (such as a topical retinoid with either a topical or oral antibiotic and benzoyl peroxide) is recommended for patients with both comedonal and inflammatory acne.

Tom WL, Friedlander SF: Acne through the ages: case-based observations through childhood and adolescence, *Clin Pediatr* 47:639–651, 2008.

Zaenglein AL, Thiboutot DM: Expert committee recommendations for acne management, *Pediatrics* 118:1188–1199, 2006.

11. **When is the use of oral isotretinoin indicated in teenagers with acne?**

Isotretinoin, which is 13-*cis*-retinoic acid (Accutane), is most appropriately used for nodulocystic acne, acne conglobata, or scarring acne that has been unresponsive to standard modes of treatment (e.g., oral and topical antibiotics, topical retinoids). Its most dangerous side effect is teratogenicity, and rigorous monitoring and definitive contraceptive counseling are mandatory. The U.S. Food and Drug Administration (FDA) and the manufacturers of isotretinoin created a registry, called iPLEDGE, in an effort to reduce the risk for fetal exposure to isotretinoin. This program monitors patients on isotretinoin with monthly laboratory tests and verification of contraception and knowledge of risks.

Merritt B, Burkhart CN, Morrell DS: Use of isotretinoin for acne vulgaris, *Pediatr Ann* 38:311–320, 2009.

http://www.fda.gov/ohrms/dockets/ac/07/briefing/2007-4311b1-00-index.htm.

12. **What serious side effects may be associated with systemic minocycline therapy for acne?**
Tetracyclines, including the derivative minocycline, are widely prescribed oral antibiotics for acne and have been used safely over long periods of time. They are contraindicated for patients younger than 8 years because of the potential for permanent dental staining. Rare reactions—particularly to minocycline—have included skin discoloration, pneumonitis, autoimmune hepatitis, drug-induced lupus, serum-sickness-like reactions, and severe hypersensitivity reactions.

Brown RJ, Rother KI, Artman H, et al: Minocycline-induced drug hypersensitivity syndrome followed by multiple autoimmune sequelae, *Arch Dermatol* 142:862–868, 2009.

Sturkenboom MC, Meier CR, Jick H, Stricker BH: Minocycline and lupuslike syndrome in acne patients, *Arch Intern Med* 159:493–497, 1999.

13. **What guidelines can help to maximize the compliance of teenagers with therapy for acne?**
- Reassure the teenager that acne is both common and treatable.
- Explain that acne cannot be scrubbed away.
- Do not overload teens with data. A few "take-home" messages are optimal.
- Allow teenagers to ask questions.
- Remember to treat the teenager's back and chest if they are involved, not just the face.
- Give the teenager choices whenever possible
- Be aware of the cost of the medications.
- Do not take noncompliance personally.

Strasburger VC: Acne: what every pediatrician should know about treatment, *Pediatr Clin North Am* 44:1519–1520, 1997.

CLINICAL ISSUES

14. **What are accessory tragi?**
Accessory tragi are fleshy papules that are typically anterior to the normal tragus, or less commonly on the cheek or jawline. They contain variable amounts of cartilage. In most cases, accessory tragi are isolated cutaneous findings. Extensive defects may be associated with hearing loss. Newborns with accessory tragi should have their hearing tested. Less commonly, they are associated with other first branchial arch abnormalities, such as cleft lip and palate, or rare syndromes, such as Treacher Collins, VACTERL, or oculoauriculovertebral syndrome. Accessory tragi are treated by surgically excising the papule and its cartilaginous stalk.

15. **What conditions cause ringlike rashes on the skin?**
Not all rings are ringworm. Annular (ringlike) skin lesions can be seen in a wide variety of skin diseases in children. Common causes of these lesions include the following:
- Tinea corporis
- Dermatitis (atopic, nummular, or contact)

- Granuloma annulare (often composed of small papules without overlying scale)
- Erythema migrans
- Systemic lupus erythematosus

For online photo atlas, see: http://dermatlas.com/derm.

KEY POINTS: DIFFERENTIAL DIAGNOSES OF RING-LIKE SKIN RASHES

1. Tinea corporis

2. Dermatitis (atopic, nummular, or contact)

3. Psoriasis

4. Granuloma annulare (often composed of small papules without overlying scale)

5. Erythema migrans

6. Systemic lupus erythematosus

16. **What is the appearance and natural history of molluscum contagiosum?**
    Molluscum contagiosum is a common skin infection caused by a poxvirus. Lesions are small pinkish-tan, dome-shaped papules that often have a dimpled or umbilicated center. They are usually asymptomatic, but they may be associated with an eczematous dermatitis and itch. Superinfection may complicate the course, require antibiotic therapy, and increase the likelihood of scarring after resolution. In healthy children, the course is self-limited but may last for 2 years. In some cases, persistent and widespread molluscum may require screening for congenital or acquired immunodeficiencies.

17. **What is the best way to eradicate molluscum contagiosum?**
    If watchful waiting is not desired, therapeutic options are primarily destructive methods. Curettage (with core removal), cryotherapy, and peeling agents (salicylic and lactic acid preparations, topical retinoids applied sparingly) can be used. An increasingly popular method is the use of cantharidin, a blistering agent, which is applied in the physician's office to individual lesions. Immunomodulating (e.g., imiquimod, cimetidine) and antiviral therapies remain unproved in children.

    Coloe J, Burkhart CN, Morrell DS: Molluscum contagiosum: what's new and true? *Pediatr Ann* 38:321–325, 2009.

    Lio P: Warts, molluscum and things that go bump on the skin: a practical guide, *Arch Dis Child Educ Pract Ed* 92:ep119–ep124, 2007.

18. **What are the common causes of acute urticaria in children?**
    In children, the most common causes of acute urticaria include the five **I**s:
    - **I**nfection (viral and bacterial are the most frequent, but fungal pathogens may also cause urticaria)
    - **I**nfestation (parasites)
    - **I**ngestion (medication and foods)
    - **I**njections or infusions (immunizations, blood products, and antibiotics)
    - **I**nhalation (allergens such as pollens and molds)

    Weston W, Orchard D: Vascular reactions. In Schachner LA, Hansen RC, editors: *Pediatric Dermatology*, ed 3, St. Louis, 2003, Mosby, pp 801–831.

KEY POINTS: COMMON CAUSES OF URTICARIA—THE FIVE Is

1. Infection (viral and bacterial are the most frequent, but fungal pathogens may also cause urticaria)

2. Infestation (parasites)

3. Ingestion (medications and foods)

4. Injections or infusions (immunizations, blood products, and antibiotics)

5. Inhalation (allergens such as pollens and molds)

19. **Describe the characteristic clinical picture of erythema nodosum.**
A prodrome of fever, chills, malaise, and arthralgia may precede the typical skin findings. Crops of red to blue tender nodules appear over the anterior shins. Lesions may be seen on the knees, ankles, thighs, and, occasionally, the lower extensor forearms and face. They may evolve through a spectrum of colors that resemble a bruise. Often the changes are misdiagnosed as cellulitis or are secondary to a traumatic event. This condition is associated with a variety of infectious (e.g., group A β-hemolytic streptococcus, tuberculosis) and noninfectious (e.g., ulcerative colitis, leukemia) causes.

20. **What, technically, are warts?**
Benign epidermal tumors caused by multiple types of human papillomaviruses.

21. **How are plantar warts distinguished clinically from calluses?**
Plantar warts are painful warts on the soles of the feet. They are flat or slightly raised areas of firm hyperkeratosis with a collarette of normal skin (Fig. 4-1). Unlike calluses, with which they can be confused, plantar warts cause obliteration of the normal skin lines (dermatoglyphics).

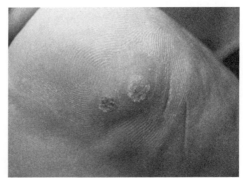

Figure 4-1. Plantar warts. Note disruption of skin lines. Characteristic black dots in the warts are thrombosed capillaries. (From Cohen BA: Pediatric Dermatology, 2nd ed. London, Mosby, 1999, p 115.)

22. **How can common warts be treated?**
The mode of therapy depends on the type and number of warts, the location on the body, and the age of the patient. No matter what treatment is used, warts can always recur; there are no absolute cures. The major goal is to remove warts without residual scarring. Of course, another option is no treatment at all because many warts self-resolve, but they may take years to do so (about 65% disappear within 2 years). Therapies include liquid nitrogen (topical), topical tretinoin cream, cantharidin (if not facial), salicylic acid

preparations, balneotherapy (hot-water therapy), duct tape application, curettage, and electrodesiccation.

Other treatment modalities, including pulsed dye laser, topical imiquimod, and contact immunotherapy, have been used to treat recalcitrant warts in children. In some case reports, oral cimetidine has been effective, perhaps owing to its immunomodulatory activity. Candida antigen injection as an immunotherapy has also recently been shown to be efficacious.

Herman BE, Corneli HM: A practical approach to warts in the emergency department, *Pediatr Emerg Care* 24:246–251, 2008.

Maronn M, Salm C, Lyon V, Galbraith S: One year experience with candida antigen immunotherapy for warts and molluscum, *Pediatric Dermatol* 25:189–192, 2008.

23. **What are the most common causes of lumps and bumps in the skin of children?**

Although most parents fear malignancy, nodules or tumors in the skin are rarely malignant. A study of 775 excised and histologically diagnosed superficial lumps in children revealed the following:

Epidermal inclusion cysts: 59%
Congenital malformations (pilomatrixoma, lymphangioma, hemangioendothelioma, branchial cleft cyst): 17%
Benign neoplasms (neural tumors, lipoma, adnexal tumors): 7%
Benign lesions of undetermined etiology (xanthomas, xanthogranulomas, fibromatosis, fibroma): 6%
Self-limited processes (granuloma annulare, urticaria pigmentosa, persistent insect bite reaction): 6%
Malignant tumors: 1.4%
Miscellaneous: 4%

American Academy of Dermatology: http://www.aad.org.

Wyatt AJ, Hansen RC: Pediatric skin tumors, *Pediatr Clin North Am* 47:937–963, 2000.

Knight PJ, Reiner CB: Superficial lumps in children: what, when, and why? *Pediatrics* 72:147–153, 1983.

24. **Why is a pyogenic granuloma neither pyogenic nor a granuloma?**

A *pyogenic granuloma*, which is also called a *lobular capillary hemangioma*, is a common acquired lesion that develops typically at the site of obvious or trivial trauma on any part of the body. Local capillary proliferation occurs, often rapidly, and bleeding may develop (Fig. 4-2). Curettage and electrodesiccation of the base are curative. The lesion is neither an infectious pyoderma nor a granuloma on biopsy.

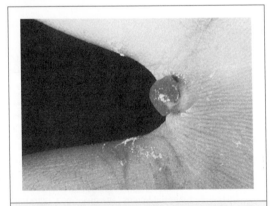

Figure 4-2. Pyogenic granuloma in the web space between fingers. (From Cohen BA: Pediatric Dermatology, 2nd ed. London, Mosby, 1999, p 127.)

25. **An 8-year-old has a hard, nontender, freely mobile nodule of the neck with a slightly bluish hue of the skin. What is the most likely diagnosis?**
    Pilomatrixoma (pilomatricoma). Also called the *benign calcifying epithelioma of Malherbe*, this is a benign tumor that often arises in children and adolescents on the face and neck. It is usually not confused with a malignant condition, but excision is often recommended because these nodules may increase in size or become infected.

26. **What condition is classically diagnosed by the Darier sign?**
    Mastocytoma. This is a benign lesion composed of mast cells that arises at birth or during early infancy. It appears as a pink-tan plaque or nodule, often with a peau d'orange surface. *Darier sign* refers to the eliciting of erythema and an urticarial wheal by stroking or rubbing the lesion. The skin changes are caused by the release of histamine from the mechanically traumatized mast cells.

    Briley LD, Phillips CM: Cutaneous mastocystosis, *Clin Pediatr* 47:757–761, 2008.

27. **What disorder can present as "freckles" associated with hives?**
    Urticaria pigmentosa (mastocytosis). Presenting at birth or during early infancy, multiple mastocytomas appear as brown macules, papules, or plaques (vesicle formation can also occur) and are often mistaken for freckles or melanocytic nevi. Lesions are usually only cutaneous but infrequently may affect other organ systems (e.g., lungs, kidney, gastrointestinal tract, central nervous system). The Darier sign is a key feature of diagnosis.

28. **What is impetigo?**
    Impetigo is a superficial skin infection that is caused by *Staphylococcus aureus* or *Streptococcus pyogenes* (group A streptococcus). Historically, streptococcus was the most prevalent agent. However, during the past few decades, *S. aureus* has become the predominant organism, although mixed infections may also occur. Bullous impetigo is usually caused by *S. aureus*. Community-associated methicillin-resistant *S. aureus* (CA-MRSA) is dramatically increasing in prevalence as a cause of skin and soft tissue infections.

    Gorwitz RJ: A review of community-associated methicillin-resistant *Staphylococcus aureus* skin and soft tissue infections, *Pediatr Infect Dis J* 27:1–7, 2008.

29. **Is topical or systemic therapy better for impetigo?**
    Treatment usually requires an antibiotic that is active against both streptococci and staphylococci. Topical antibiotics (e.g., mupirocin) can be used in localized disease. Systemic antibiotics are usually indicated for extensive involvement; outbreaks among household contacts, schools, or athletic teams; or if topical therapy has failed. Cephalosporins (e.g., cephalexin, cefadroxil), amoxicillin-clavulanate, and dicloxacillin are most effective for non-MRSA infections. If the prevalence of MRSA in the community is more than 10%, other antibiotics should be used. Most MRSA strains remain sensitive to trimethoprim-sulfamethoxazole and clindamycin, but trimethoprim-sulfamethoxazole is ineffective against *S. pyogenes*. Obtaining a culture when possible at the onset of treatment can help guide therapy in the event of unresponsive lesions.

    Silverberg N, Block S: Uncomplicated skin and skin structure infections in children: diagnosis and current treatment options in the United States, *Clin Pediatr* 47:211–219, 2008.

30. **What dermatologic sign starts from a scratch?**
    Dermographism (dermatographism) occurs when the skin is stroked firmly with a pointed object. The result is a red line that is followed by an erythematous flare, which is eventually followed by a wheal. This "triple response of Lewis" usually occurs within 1 to 3 minutes.

Dermographism (or skin writing) is an exaggerated triple response of Lewis and is seen in patients with urticaria. The tendency to be dermographic can appear at any age and may last for months to years. The cause is often unknown. White dermographism is seen in patients with an atopic diathesis, in whom the red line is replaced by a white line without a subsequent flare and wheal.

31. **Do geographic tongues vary in the northern and southern hemispheres?**
Despite the Hubble telescope, more research awaits. *Geographic tongue* refers to the benign condition in which denudations of the filiform papillae on the lingual surface occur, giving the tongue the appearance of a relief map (Fig. 4-3). The patterns change over hours and days, and the histopathology resembles that of psoriasis. The patient is usually asymptomatic. No treatment is effective or necessary because self-resolution is the rule. Etiology in either hemisphere is unknown.

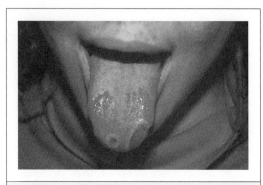

Figure 4-3. Geographic tongue. (From Sahn EE: Dermatology Pearls. Philadelphia, Hanley & Belfus, 1999, p 162.)

32. **What diseases are associated with a strawberry tongue?**
Scarlet fever caused by group A β-hemolytic streptococcus and **Kawasaki disease** are the most common disorders associated with a strawberry tongue. The strawberry-like surface characteristics are caused by prominent lingual papillae. A white strawberry tongue is caused by fibrinous exudate overlying the tongue. Red strawberry tongues lack the fibrinous exudate.

33. **A 2-year-old boy with eczema, fine and sparse hair, primary teeth that are peg shaped, and problems with overheating with exercise has what likely diagnosis?**
Hypohidrotic ectodermal dysplasia. This is most commonly an X-linked recessive disease affecting the skin, hair, teeth, and sweat glands. Genetic mutations affecting a transmembrane protein (ectodysplasin A) involved in ectodermal structures are the likely cause.

ECZEMATOUS DISORDERS

34. **What is the difference between eczema and atopic dermatitis?**
The term *eczema* derives from the Greek word *exzein,* which means to erupt: *ex* (out) plus *zein* (to boil). To most physicians, eczema is synonymous with atopic dermatitis, a chronic skin disease manifested by intermittent skin eruption. **Eczema** is primarily a morphologic term used to describe an erythematous, scaling, inflammatory eruption with itching, edema, papules, vesicles, and crusts. There are other eczematous eruptions (nummular eczema, allergic contact dermatitis), but "garden variety" eczema is certainly the most common.

Atopic dermatitis is a broader allergic tendency with multiple dermal manifestations that are mostly secondary to pruritus. Atopic dermatitis has been called an "itch that rashes, not a rash that itches." Its manifestations are dry skin, chronic and recurrent dermatitis, low threshold to pruritus, hyperlinear palms, eyelid pleats (Dennie-Morgan folds), pityriasis alba, and keratosis pilaris, among others.

Bieber T: Atopic dermatitis, *N Engl J Med* 358:1483–1494, 2008.

National Eczema Association: http://www.nationaleczema.org.

35. **What is the usual distribution of rash in atopic dermatitis?**
    - **Infant:** Cheeks, trunk, and extensor surfaces of extremities, knees, and elbows
    - **Child:** Neck, feet, and antecubital and popliteal fossae
    - **Older child:** Neck, hands, feet, and antecubital and popliteal fossae

KEY POINTS: MAIN FEATURES OF ATOPIC DERMATITIS

1. Extensor surface involvement in infancy

2. Flexural surface involvement in older children

3. Lichenification with chronic scratching

4. Dennie-Morgan folds under eyes

5. Part of atopic triad: atopic dermatitis, asthma, and allergic rhinitis

36. **Describe the five key battle plans to treat atopic dermatitis.**
    1. **Reduce pruritus.** Topical corticosteroids and bland emollients help reduce pruritus. Oral antihistamines may also be used for their sedative effect at night and may reduce pruritus.
    2. **Hydrate the skin.** Emollients (petrolatum and fragrance-free ointments and creams) prevent the evaporation of moisture through occlusion and are best applied immediately after bathing, when the skin is maximally hydrated, to "lock in" moisture. A "soak-and-smear" protocol is advisable in refractory cases.
    3. **Reduce inflammation.** Topical steroids are invaluable as anti-inflammatory agents and can hasten the clearing of eruptions that are erythematous (inflamed). Medium-strength corticosteroids can be used on areas other than the face and occluded regions (diaper area); low-strength steroids (e.g., 1% hydrocortisone) may be used in these thin-skinned areas for limited periods of time. Newer immunomodulators, such as topical tacrolimus and pimecrolimus, are approved for the intermittent treatment of moderate to severe atopic dermatitis in children 2 years and older. However, their long-term side effects have not been fully evaluated.
    4. **Control infection.** Superinfection with *S. aureus* is extremely common. First-generation cephalosporins such as cephalexin are the usual antibiotics of choice for infected atopic dermatitis. Dilute bleach baths are sometimes recommended two to three times per week to reduce staphylococcal colonization.
    5. **Avoid irritants.** Gentle fragrance-free soaps and shampoos should be used; wool and tight synthetic garments should be avoided; tight nonsynthetic garments may help minimize the itchy feeling; consider furniture, carpeting, pets, and dust mites as possible irritants and/or trigger factors.

Krakowski AC, Eichenfield LF, Dohil MA: Management of atopic dermatitis in the pediatric population. *Pediatrics* 122:812–824, 2008.

Palmer CM, Lyon VB: Stepwise approach to topical therapy for atopic dermatitis, *Clin Pediatr* 47:423–434, 2008.

Gutman AB, Kligman AM, Sciacca J, James WD. Soak and smear: a standard technique revisited, *Arch Dermatol* 141:1556–1559, 2005.

37. **Do soaps or clothes make any difference in atopic dermatitis?**
Yes. Soap-free cleansers designed for sensitive skin are better than drying or fragrance soaps. "Bubble baths" should be avoided. Woolen fibers can also irritate the skin and trigger the itch-scratch cycle. Soft fibers are the least irritating (e.g., cotton jerseys).

38. **What is the most common side effect of topical pimecrolimus and tacrolimus?**
These topical immunomodulating creams are used for intermittent therapy. The most common side effect is burning or stinging, which can occur in up to 10% of patients, especially with initial use. This side effect tends to improve with continued use. Use on open skin sores should be avoided. The long-term side effects of chronic use are still under investigation. Patients should be instructed about the importance of sun protection while using topical immunosuppressive medications.

   Eichenfield LF, Hanifin JM, Luger TA, et al: Consensus conference on pediatric atopic dermatitis, *J Am Acad Dermatol* 49:1088–1095, 2003.

39. **Why shouldn't fluorinated (halogenated) steroids be used on the face?**
There are several reasons:
- Facial skin is thinner, and therefore percutaneous absorption is higher.
- Telangiectasias or spider veins can occur.
- Cutaneous atrophy can occur.
- Perioral dermatitis or poststeroid rosacea can occur with rebound symptoms that are worse than the original rash.

40. **Is there a genetic basis for atopic dermatitis?**
It is likely that both genetic and environmental factors play a role. Susceptibility to atopic dermatitis is found in patients with mutations in filaggrin, an epithelial protein that cross-links keratin. Many children with atopic dermatitis have a family history of atopy. If one parent has an atopic diathesis, 60% of offspring will be atopic; if two parents do, 80% of children are affected. Monozygotic twins are often concordant for atopic disease.

   Palmer CN, Irvine AD, Terron-Kwiatkowski A, et al: Common loss-of-function variants of the epidermal barrier protein filaggrin are a major predisposing factor for atopic dermatitis, *Nat Genet* 38:441–446, 2006.

41. **Are there consistent immunologic alterations in children with atopic dermatitis?**
Humoral changes include elevated immunoglobulin E levels and a higher-than-normal number of positive skin tests (type I cutaneous reactions) to common environmental allergens. Cell-mediated abnormalities have been found only during acute flares of the dermatitis; these include mild to moderate depression of cell-mediated immunity, a 30% to 50% decrease in lymphocyte-forming E-rosettes, decreased phagocytosis of yeast cells by neutrophils, and chemotactic defects of polymorphonuclear and mononuclear cells.

42. **What skin infections are more likely in patients with atopic dermatitis?**
- **Secondary bacterial infections:** Up to 90% of patients are colonized with *S. aureus*; a flare of eczema can result in colonization progressing to infection.
- **Eczema herpeticum:** Also known as *herpes simplex virus–associated Kaposi varicelliform eruption*, this refers to skin infected with either type 1 or type 2 herpes simplex virus; grouped patterns of vesicles or erosions are typical; severe involvement requires hospitalization and use of systemic antiviral therapy.
- **Molluscum contagiosum:** Molluscum contagiosum infections tend to be more widespread in children with eczema.
- **Eczema vaccinatum:** This diffuse skin disease could potentially result from contact with the smallpox vaccine.

   Treadwell PA: Eczema and infection, *Pediatr Infect Dis J* 27:551–552, 2008.

43. **How commonly do food allergies contribute to eczema?**
About 35% to 40% of children with moderate to severe atopic dermatitis have food allergies. Although usually not successful as a sole treatment, elimination diets can contribute to improvements in the condition. In a patient with problematic eczema, testing for food allergy and confirmation by elimination diets and food challenges may be beneficial.

Forbes LR, Rushani RW, Spergel JM: Food allergies and atopic dermatitis: differentiating myth from reality, *Pediatr Ann* 38:84–90, 2009.

Rancé F: Food allergy in children suffering from atopic eczema, *Pediatr Allergy Immunol* 19:279–284, 2008.

44. **What other skin conditions mimic atopic dermatitis?**
- Seborrheic dermatitis
- Scabies
- Psoriasis
- Tinea capitis
- Lichen simplex chronicus
- Acrodermatitis enteropathica
- Contact dermatitis
- Langerhans cell histiocytosis
- Xerotic eczema (dry skin)
- Immunodeficiency disorders (e.g., Wiskott-Aldrich syndrome, hyperimmunoglobulin E syndrome, severe combined immunodeficiency)
- Nummular eczema
- Metabolic disorders (e.g., phenylketonuria, essential fatty acid deficiency, biotinidase deficiency)

45. **What is the "atopic march"?**
About half of infants with atopic dermatitis will develop asthma, and two thirds will develop allergic rhinitis. Thus, the one condition in infancy marches toward others. Studies are under way to interrupt this progression.

Spergel JM, Paller AS: Atopic dermatitis and the atopic march, *J Allergy Clin Immunol* 112:S118–S127, 2003.

46. **What features help to differentiate seborrheic from atopic dermatitis during infancy?**
See Table 4-1.

TABLE 4-1. SEBORRHEIC DERMATITIS VERSUS ATOPIC DERMATITIS

	Seborrheic Dermatitis	Atopic Dermatitis
Color	Salmon	Pink or red (if inflamed)
Scale	Yellowish, greasy	White, not greasy
Age	Infants <6 mo or adolescents	May begin at 2-12 mo and continue through childhood
Itching	Not present	May be severe
Distribution	Face, postauricular scalp, axillae, and groin	Cheeks, trunk, and extensors of extremities
Associated features	None	Dennie-Morgan folds, allergic shiners, hyperlinear palms
Lichenification	None	May be prominent
Response to topical steroids	Rapid	Slower

47. **How should parents cope with cradle cap?**

    Seborrheic dermatitis of the scalp—also known as "cradle cap"—during infancy presents as a yellow, greasing, scaling adherent rash on the scalp that may extend to the forehead, eyes, ears, eyebrows, nose, and the back of the head. It appears during the first few months of life and generally resolves in several weeks to a few months. Treatment includes the application of mineral oil followed by shampooing with a mild antidandruff shampoo containing selenium sulfide. Parents should be cautioned to take extra care when washing the scalp because these shampoos may irritate the infant's eyes. A mild-potency topical steroid such as hydrocortisone (1% to 2.5%) may be needed for inflamed lesions. Families should be advised not to scrub or pick off the scale because the underlying skin is often tender and inflamed.

    Naldi L, Rebora A: Seborrheic dermatitis, *N Engl J Med* 360:387–396, 2009.

    Fleischer AB Jr: Diagnosis and management of common dermatoses in children: atopic, seborrheic, and contact dermatitis, *Clin Pediatr* 47:332–346, 2008.

48. **What condition causes bumps on the cheeks, upper arms, and thighs?**

    Keratosis pilaris. Associated both with atopic dermatitis and ichthyosis vulgaris, this condition runs in families and is asymptomatic. It is characterized by spiny follicular papules, giving involved areas a "chicken skin" or "gooseflesh" feel. Usual treatment is with bland emollients or emollients that contain a mild peeling agent, such as lactic acid or α-hydroxy acid preparation.

49. **What are the causes of irritant contact diaper rash?**

    A variety of local factors are involved. Diapers contribute to the chafing of the skin and the prevention of moisture evaporation, thus increasing epidermal hydration and permeability to irritants. Proteolytic enzymes in urine and stool and ammonia in urine irritate chafed skin. Seasoned pediatricians will advise that alcohol-based diaper wipes also "feed the flames" of diaper rash.

    Adam R: Skin care of the diaper area, *Pediatr Dermatol* 25:427–433, 2008.

50. **What features of diaper rash suggest more sinister diseases?**

    - Marked tenderness, rapid onset (staphylococcal scaled skin syndrome)
    - Deep ulcerations, vesicles (herpes simplex)
    - Beefy red, erosive, extensive lesions (particularly intertriginous) that are poorly responsive to topical steroids and antifungals (Langerhans cell histiocytosis, acrodermatitis enteropathica, immunodeficiency states)
    - Extensive and severe lesions with pungent odor (abuse or neglect with infrequent changing)

    Boiko S: Making rash decisions in the diaper area, *Pediatr Ann* 29:50–56, 2000.

51. **Are cloth diapers better than disposables?**

    There is no clear answer here, although there are parties who swear by one or the other. Studies, however, have shown both a decreased incidence of diaper rash with disposable diapers and a documented decrease in skin moisture and incidence of rash with superabsorbent diapers as a result of decreased leakage and less alkaline pH. The adjective "better" implies a value judgment, and other factors such as cost, environmental impact, and convenience must be considered. More than 97% of the diapers used in the United States are of the disposable variety.

52. **Are topical steroid and antifungal preparations useful for treating children with diaper dermatitis?**

    Most diaper dermatitis is diagnosed as either irritant contact dermatitis or candidal dermatitis. Irritant diaper dermatitis responds well to very-low-potency topical corticosteroids (as a result of their anti-inflammatory properties) and a topical barrier such as zinc oxide ointment.

Candidiasis of the diaper area responds well to topical antifungal preparations; rarely, an oral anticandidal medication is also necessary. In both types of diaper dermatitis, frequent diaper changes, exposure to air, and avoidance of excessive moisture are helpful. Combination preparations containing both antifungal and corticosteroid medications are not recommended to treat diaper dermatitis because the strength of the steroid component in these products is usually too high for use in the diaper area.

Kazaks EL, Lane AT: Diaper dermatitis, *Pediatr Clin North Am* 47:909–920, 2000.

53. **Which dietary deficiencies may be associated with an eczematous dermatitis?**
Zinc, biotin, essential fatty acids, and protein (kwashiorkor).

54. **What are the two main types of contact dermatitis?**
Irritant and allergic. *Irritant* contact dermatitis arises when agents such as harsh soaps, bleaches, or acids have direct toxic effects when they come into contact with the skin. *Allergic* contact dermatitis is a T-cell–mediated inflammatory immune reaction that requires sensitization to a specific antigen.

55. **When should contact dermatitis be clinically suspected?**
Although it can be confused with atopic dermatitis, contact dermatitis should give localized features of pruritic, eczematous plaques at the site of exposure. The rash can be well-demarcated and geometric and/or linear in nature, and it may appear in uncommon or specific areas (e.g., earlobes, weight-bearing surfaces of feet). Bear in mind that unrecognized contact dermatitis can contribute to clinical worsening in patients with preexisting atopic dermatitis. It should be considered a possibility in patients with recalcitrant atopic dermatitis.

56. **What types of agents can cause allergic contact dermatitis in children?**
Allergic contact dermatitis can occur in all age groups, but it is often underrecognized in children. Sensitizers include plant resins (poison ivy, sumac, or oak); nickel in jewelry, metal snaps, and belts; topical neomycin ointment; preservatives (formaldehyde releasers); and fabric dyes and materials used in shoes, including adhesives, rubber accelerators, and leather tanning agents.

Lee PW, Elsaie ML, Jacob SE: Allergic contact dermatitis in children: common allergens and treatment. A review, *Curr Opin Pediatr* 21:491–498, 2009.

57. **When does the rash in poison ivy appear relative to exposure?**
Poison ivy, or rhus dermatitis, is a typical delayed hypersensitivity reaction. The time between exposure and cutaneous lesions is usually 2 to 4 days. However, the eruption may appear as late as 1 week or more after contact in individuals who have not been previously sensitized (this explains why lesions continue to erupt after the initial "outbreak" of rash).

58. **Are the vesicles in poison ivy contagious?**
No. The contents of blisters do not contain the allergen. Washing the skin removes all surface oleoresin and prevents further contamination.

59. **What is the "id" reaction?**
Your superego will be stroked if you identify the *id* reaction in a confusing dermatologic case. This reaction is the generalization of a local inflammatory dermatitis (e.g., contact dermatitis, tinea capitis following treatment) to sites that have not been directly involved with the offending agent. The exact mechanism remains unclear, but it may be immune complex mediated.

60. **How does the vehicle used in a dermatologic preparation affect therapy?**
In general, **acute lesions** (moist, oozing) are best treated with aqueous, drying preparations. **Chronic, dry lesions** fare better when a lubricating, moisturizing vehicle is used. As a rule,

any vehicle that enhances hydration of the skin enhances the percutaneous absorption of topical medications (most of which are water soluble). Thus, in preparations of equal concentration, the potency relationship is ointment → cream → gel → lotion (Table 4-2).

TABLE 4-2.   VEHICLES USED IN DERMATOLOGIC PREPARATIONS

Drying Vehicles

Lotion: A suspension of powder in water. Therapeutic powder remains after aqueous phase evaporates. Useful in hairy areas, particularly the scalp.

Gel: Transparent emulsion that liquifies when applied to skin. Most useful for acne preparations and tar preparations for psoriasis.

Pastes: Combination of powder (usually cornstarch) and ointment; stiffer than ointment.

Moisturizing Vehicles

Creams: Mixture of oil in a water emulsion. More useful than ointments when environmental humidity is high and in naturally occluded areas. Less greasy than ointment.

Ointments: Mixture of water in an oil emulsion. Also has an inert petroleum base. Longer lubricating effect than cream.

FUNGAL INFECTIONS

61. What are useful methods for diagnosing tinea infections?

Although the microscopic examination of **potassium hydroxide (KOH) preparations** is employed in the search for hyphae, the use of **dermatophyte test medium** is reliable, simple, inexpensive, and more definitive. Samples from hair, skin, or nails are obtained by scraping with a scalpel, cotton-tipped applicator, or toothbrush (the latter especially for tinea capitis), and these are inoculated directly onto the test medium. After about 1 to 2 weeks, a color change from yellow to red in the agar surrounding the dermatophyte colony indicates positivity. If the most definitive diagnosis is needed, culture on Sabouraud medium is the test of choice.

KEY POINTS: MAIN FEATURES OF TINEA CAPITIS

1. Scaly alopecia

2. Black-dot hairs often observed

3. Associated with posterior cervical adenopathy

4. Potassium hydroxide test often positive

5. Diagnosis confirmed by positive fungal culture

6. Most common cause: *Trichophyton tonsurans*

62. How does one differentiate between irritant diaper dermatitis and candidal diaper dermatitis?

Both types of dermatitis often present together. *Candidal infection* is a common infection that can be precipitated by the compromise of the cutaneous barrier seen in irritant dermatitis. With candida infection, one typically sees confluent, beefy red plaques involving the groin creases. Scale and satellite papules or pustules are commonly seen at the periphery of the plaque. The diagnosis can be made clinically and with a KOH preparation and yeast culture. Treatment includes a topical anticandidal agent such as clotrimazole and use of a thick barrier cream such as zinc oxide. A few days of a low-potency corticosteroid ointment may reduce the erythema significantly. Remember to consider other causes (such as seborrheic dermatitis, psoriasis, acrodermatitis enteropathica, Langerhans cell histiocytosis, or immunodeficiency) for chronic and refractory diaper dermatitis.

63. Do a scaly scalp and swollen glands qualify a patient to initiate griseofulvin?

No. Scalp scaling and cervical adenopathy are more often caused by seborrheic or atopic dermatitis than tinea capitis.

Williams JV, Eichenfield LF, Burke BL, et al: Prevalence of scalp scaling in prepubertal children, *Pediatrics* 115:e1–e6, 2005.

64. Why is it necessary to culture for tinea capitis?

Tinea capitis can be caused by a variety of dermatophyte fungal organisms, and during the past decade, resistance to commonly used treatments (griseofulvin) has been noted. Children with tinea capitis are requiring longer courses of treatment and higher doses of medication to eradicate the fungal infection. Moreover, other conditions (e.g., alopecia areata, psoriasis of the scalp) may be confused with tinea capitis. Therefore, just like for other pediatric infections, it is important to document the type of infection so that proper treatment may be administered.

65. How can a culture be obtained if fungal culture medium is not available in the office?

The simplest method is to take a cotton swab culturette and moisten it with water. Then take the swab and rub it over the affected areas and all four quadrants of the scalp. The cotton swab can be used to directly inoculate the fungal culture media if you have it in the office or transported back to the laboratory for inoculation.

Friedlander SF, Pickering B, Cunningham BB, et al: Use of the cotton swab method in diagnosing tinea capitis, *Pediatrics* 104:276–279, 1999.

66. What are the clinical presentations of tinea capitis?

Tinea capitis occurs more commonly in Black children in the United States. It can present with scalp scaling, black-dot tinea, inflammation, or a kerion (a boggy, tender mass) (Fig. 4-4). The black-dot presentation occurs when the infected hair shaft breaks at the surface of the scalp, leaving a bald patch with black dots (or lighter dots, depending on hair color). Some patients will have inflammatory papules, pustules, erythema, and scaling or a kerion. Regional adenopathy is common with inflammatory tinea.

Hubbard TW: Predictive value of symptoms in diagnosing childhood tinea capitis, *Arch Pediatr Adolesc Med* 153:1150–1153, 1999.

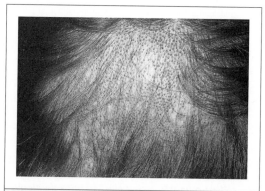

Figure 4-4. Black dot tinea. (From Schachner LA, Hansen RC [eds]: Pediatric Dermatology, 3rd ed. Edinburgh, Mosby, 2003, p 1096.)

67. **Why is topical therapy alone insufficient for tinea capitis?**

The dermatophytes (i.e., fungi) that cause tinea can thrive deep in the hair shaft, beyond the reach of topical therapy alone. Recommended therapy is a combination of oral griseofulvin (microsize or ultramicrosize preparation), which is given after milk, ice cream, or a fatty meal to facilitate absorption, and biweekly shampooing with 1% or 2.5% selenium sulfide or ketoconazole shampoo to decrease the spread of spores.

Pomeranz AJ, Sabnis SS: Tinea capitis: epidemiology, diagnosis and management strategies, *Pediatr Drugs* 4:779–783, 2002.

68. **How should children who are receiving griseofulvin for tinea capitis be monitored?**

The incidence of hepatitis or bone marrow suppression from griseofulvin in children is rare. Children who are undergoing an acute course of treatment (6 to 8 weeks) do not need obligatory blood counts or liver function tests. However, a history of hepatitis or its risk factors would warrant a pretreatment evaluation of liver function and intermittent monitoring. Resistance by tinea to griseofulvin is increasing, and higher, longer dosing may be needed to achieve clinical cure. For those rare cases in which griseofulvin is going to be used for more than 2 months, one should consider obtaining complete blood counts and liver function tests on an every-other-month basis.

69. **What alternatives are available for patients who are not responding to treatment with griseofulvin?**

First, ensure that the patient has been taking an appropriate daily dose of griseofulvin with a fatty meal and that source contacts are treated to minimize the risk of reinfection. If there is bona fide resistance to griseofulvin, oral terbinafine may be considered. Oral terbinafine was recently approved for treatment of tinea capitis in children older than 4 years. Terbinafine granules may be sprinkled on food and administered once a day for 6 weeks. Dosage guidelines are weight based as follows: <25 kg: 125 mg/day; 25-35 kg: 187.5 mg/day; >35 kg: 250 mg/day. When using terbinafine, a complete blood count and hepatic function panel are recommended to be performed at baseline, and patients should be warned about and monitored for evidence of side effects, such as hepatoxicity. Rare cases of hepatic failure and bone marrow suppression have been reported. Fluconazole is another alternative, but it has not been proved more effective than low-dose griseofulvin.

Elewski BE, Cáceres HW, DeLeon L, et al: Terbinafine hydrochloride oral granules versus oral griseofulvin suspension in children with tinea capitis: results of two randomised, investigator-blinded, multicenter, international, controlled trials, *J Am Acad Dermatol* 59:41–54, 2008.

Foster KW, Friedlander SF, Panzer H, et al: A randomized controlled trial assessing the efficacy of fluconazole in the treatment of pediatric tinea capitis, *J Am Acad Dermatol* 53:798–809, 2005.

70. **What is a kerion?**

A *kerion* is a fluctuant and tender mass that occurs in some cases of tinea capitis. It is thought to be primarily an excessive inflammatory response to tinea, and thus initial treatment consists of antifungal agents, principally griseofulvin and selenium sulfide shampoo. Short courses of oral steroids can be considered in those lesions that are exquisitely painful.

Honig PJ, Caputo GL, Leyden JJ, et al: Microbiology of kerions, *J Pediatr* 123:422–424, 1993.

71. **What puts the "versicolor" in tinea versicolor?**

A very common superficial disorder of the skin, tinea versicolor (also known as *pityriasis versicolor*) is caused by the yeast *Malassezia furfur* (formerly known as *Pityrosporum orbiculare*). It appears as multiple macules and patches with fine scales over the upper trunk, arms, and occasionally the face and other areas (Fig. 4-5). Lesions are "versatile" in color (i.e., light tan, reddish, or white) and "versatile" by season (i.e., lighter in summer and darker in winter compared with surrounding skin). The yeast interferes with melanin production, possibly by the disruption of tyrosinase activity, at the involved sites. Diagnosis can be confirmed with a KOH preparation of a scraping from the involved skin, which has characteristic fungal hyphae and a grapelike spore pattern referred to as a "spaghetti and meatball" appearance. Wood light will also display yellow-brown fluorescence.

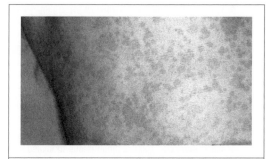

Figure 4-5. Tinea versicolor on the chest. (From Gawkrodger DJ: Dermatology: An Illustrated Colour Text, 3rd ed. London, Churchill Livingstone, 2002, p 38.)

72. **How is tinea versicolor treated?**
    - **Selenium sulfide 2.5% lotion:** The shampoo or lotion is applied over the affected area overnight nightly during the first week, with decreasing frequency over the ensuing weeks.
    - **Ketoconazole 2% shampoo:** The shampoo is applied to wet skin and lathered. Patients are instructed to let the shampoo remain in place without washing for 3 to 5 minutes. Treatment is repeated for 1 to 3 days in a row. Monthly prophylactic treatments are suggested to prevent recurrence.
    - **Oral ketoconazole, fluconazole, and itraconazole:** These treatments, which are sometimes effective after a single one-time dose, may be considered for use in older children and adolescents. However, side effects, including liver toxicity, may occur.

73. **Which rashes resemble tinea pedis (athlete's foot) in children?**
    Other causes of foot dermatitis that mimic tinea pedis include:
    - *Dyshidrotic eczema*: Erythema with microvesicles of interdigital spaces and lateral feet.
    - *Contact dermatitis*: Typically involves dorsum of feet and spares interdigital spaces.
    - *Juvenile plantar dermatosis*: Glazed erythema and fissuring of toes and distal soles. Often pruritic.
    - *Pitted keratolysis*: Small pits that may converge to superficial erosions on sole of foot. Hyperhidrosis and malodor are common. Associated with *Corynebacterium* species or *Micrococcus sedentarius* infections.

HAIR AND NAIL ABNORMALITIES

74. **How fast does hair grow?**
    About 1 cm per month.

75. **On what parts of the skin is hair not normally found?**
    Palms, soles, genitalia, and medial-lateral aspects of toes and fingers.

76. **What causes sparse or absent hair in children?**
    - **Congenital localized:** Nevus sebaceous, aplasia cutis, incontinentia pigmenti, focal dermal hypoplasia, intrauterine trauma (e.g., scalp electrodes), infection (e.g., herpes, gonococcal)

- **Congenital diffuse:** Loose anagen syndrome, Menkes syndrome, trichoschisis, genetic syndromes (e.g., ectodermal dysplasia, lamellar ichthyosis, Netherton syndrome)
- **Acquired localized:** Tinea capitis, alopecia areata, traction alopecia, traumatic scarring (e.g., trichotillomania), androgenic alopecia, Langerhans cell histiocytosis, lupus erythematosus
- **Acquired diffuse:** Telogen effluvium, anagen effluvium, acrodermatitis enteropathica, endocrinopathies (e.g., hypothyroidism)

Datloff J, Esterly NB: A system for sorting out pediatric alopecia, *Contemp Pediatr* 3:53–56, 1986.

77. **Which kind of alopecia simply requires a change in hairstyle as the treatment?**
Traction alopecia. This condition is due to styling with tight braids or ponytails that create tension on the hair shaft. This process contributes to hair thinning and can cause permanent scarring alopecia over time. There are usually no scalp changes, but occasionally an erythematous papular reaction may be seen. Treatment involves loose hairstyles, avoiding chemical processing or heat treatments. With appropriate changes in hairstyling early on, the prognosis is excellent with complete regrowth in time.

Hantash BM, Schwartz RA: Traction alopecia in children, *Cutis* 71:18–20, 2003.

78. **How can alopecia areata be differentiated from tinea capitis clinically?**
In **tinea capitis**, the fungal organism invades the hair shaft but is also present in the epidermis (the top layer of the skin). There are usually changes of scaling and inflammatory lesions that are intermingled with black dots representing broken hairs. In **alopecia areata**, the scalp is smooth, although there may be a pink discoloration. Some hairs within the patch may have a tapered appearance, with the wider end distally and a thinner end at the base of the scalp (i.e., the "exclamation point hair") (Fig. 4-6). There is no lymphadenopathy in patients with alopecia areata, but this is not uncommon in patients with tinea capitis. The gold standard for diagnosis is a positive fungal culture.

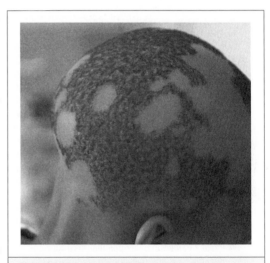

Figure 4-6. Well-demarcated, hairless patches of alopecia areata.

79. **What are poor prognostic indicators for recovery of hair in patients with alopecia areata?**
- Atopy
- Presence of other immune-mediated disease (e.g., thyroid disease, vitiligo)
- Family history of alopecia areata (about 25% of patients)
- Young age at onset
- Nail dystrophy
- Extensive and rapid hair loss

Tosti A, Bellavista S, Iorizzo M: Alopecia areata: a long term follow-up study of 191 patients, *J Am Acad Dermatol* 55:438–441, 2006.

80. **What are treatments for alopecia areata?**
Treatment is based on the extent of disease: patchy, totalis (loss of all scalp hair), or universalis (loss of all body hair). Although the cause is unknown, alopecia areata is generally considered to be a T-cell–mediated autoimmune disorder. Therefore, treatments are directed at suppressing the immune response around the hair follicle. Topical or intralesional corticosteroids are the mainstays of therapy. Systemic corticosteroids are rarely used chronically because of side effects. Anthralin, as an irritant, or other topical sensitizers are designed to cause a mild dermatitis and theoretically alter local immunity to promote hair regrowth. The option of not treating must be reviewed with the family. Support groups should be offered and note that many patients have had improved self-esteem after being fitted with a hair prothesis.

Kos L, Conlon J: An update on alopecia areata, *Curr Opin Pediatr* 21:475–480, 2009.

Children's Alopecia Project: http://www.childrensalopeciaproject.org.

Locks of Love: http://www.locksoflove.org.

National Alopecia Areata Foundation: http://www.naaf.org.

81. **Are most hairs growing or resting?**
Most infants and children have about 90% of scalp hair in the growing (anagen) and about 10% in the resting (telogen) state. On average, a single scalp hair will grow for about 3 years, rest for 3 months, and then, upon falling out, be replaced by a new growing hair.

82. **You are evaluating a healthy 4-year-old with fine, sparse hair who has never had a haircut. What condition do you suspect?**
Loose anagen syndrome is typically seen in 2- to 5-year-old blond girls but may also present in children with darker hair. The hair is of variable lengths and is easily pulled from the scalp. A microscopic examination of a few pulled hairs reveals predominance of anagen hair bulbs with ruffled cuticles. There are no associated nail, skin, or teeth findings in loose anagen syndrome. There is no treatment, but gentle hairstyling should be encouraged. Fortunately, the condition tends to improve over time.

Price VH, Gummer, CL: Loose anagen syndrome, *J Am Acad Dermatol* 20:249–256, 1989.

83. **What is the likely diagnosis in a child who develops diffuse hair loss 3 months after major surgery?**
Telogen effluvium. This is the most common cause of acquired diffuse hair loss in children. In a healthy individual, most hairs are present in a growing (anagen) phase. After a physical or emotional stress such as a significant fever, illness, pregnancy, birth, surgery, or large weight loss, a large number of scalp hairs can convert to the resting (telogen) phase. About 2 to 5 months after the stressful event, the hair begins to shed, at times coming out in large clumps. The condition is temporary and usually does not produce a loss of more than 50% of the hair. When the hair roots are examined, there is a lighter-colored root bulb, which characterizes a telogen hair. The hair loss can continue for 6 to 8 weeks, at which time new, short, regrowing hairs should be visible.
Anagen effluvium, which the loss of growing hairs, is most commonly seen during radiation and chemotherapy treatments for cancer.

84. **What puzzling cause of asymmetrical hair loss in a child will sometimes cause an intern to pull his or her hair out?**
Trichotillomania is hair loss as a result of self-manipulation, such as rubbing, twirling, or pulling. Hair loss is asymmetrical. The most common physical finding is unequal hair lengths in the same region without evidence of epidermal changes of the scalp. Parents often do not

observe the causative behavior, and convincing them of the likely diagnosis may take some effort. Behavior modification, along with the application of petroleum or oil to the hair to make pulling more difficult, is the treatment of choice. Rarely a child will swallow the hair and develop vomiting because of the formation of a gastric trichobezoar (hairball).

85. **What is the "flag sign"?**
The term *flag sign* refers to alternating bands of decreased pigment or structural changes of the hair shaft. It most commonly occurs after nutritional deficiency.

> Wade MS, Sinclair RD: Disorders of hair in infants and children other than alopecia, *Clin Dermatol* 20:16–28, 2002.

86. **What causes green hair?**
Children with blond or light-colored hair can develop green hair after long-term exposure to chlorinated swimming pools. It is the result of the incorporation of copper ions into the hair matrix. Over-the-counter chelating shampoos are available for prevention and treatment.

87. **How should ingrown toenails be managed?**
Soaks, open-toed sandals, properly fitting shoes, topical or systemic antibiotics, incision and drainage, or surgical removal of the lateral portion of the nail may all be used. Control is best obtained by letting the nail grow beyond the free end of the toe. Proper instruction on nail care, including straight rather than arc trimming, is mandatory.

88. **Which pathogens are responsible for paronychia?**
Acute paronychia (inflammation of the nail fold, usually with abscess formation) is most commonly caused by *S. aureus*. The proximal or lateral nail folds become intensely erythematous and tender. If a collection of pus develops at this site, it should be incised and drained. The treatment of acute paronychia includes the oral administration of antistaphylococcal antibiotics.

Chronic paronychia is most often caused by *Candida albicans* and often involves a history of chronic water exposure (e.g., dishwashing, thumb-sucking). Although rarely inflamed, there is edema of the nail folds and separation of the folds from the nail plate. The nails may become ridged and develop a yellow-green discoloration. A bacterial culture may reveal a variety of gram-positive and gram-negative organisms. Therapy includes topical antifungal agents and avoidance of water. There is no place for griseofulvin in the treatment of chronic paronychia.

89. **A healthy 7-year-old child who develops progressive yellowing and increasing friability of all nails over a period of 12 months likely has what condition?**
Twenty-nail dystrophy (trachyonychia). The progressive development of rough nails with longitudinal grooves, pitting, chipping, ridges, and discoloration occurring in isolation in school-aged children has been given this name, although not all nails need be involved. The etiology remains unclear, and most cases resolve spontaneously without scarring. The nail changes, however, may herald other conditions, such as alopecia areata, lichen planus, and psoriasis.

INFESTATIONS

90. **How do lice differ?**
- **Pediculosis capitis** (head lice): *Pediculus capitis,* the smallest and most common of the three human lice, is an obligate human parasite. Spread occurs directly by contact with an infected individual or indirectly through the use of shared combs, brushes, or hats. For unknown reasons, infestation is nearly 35 times more likely among whites than blacks.

- **Pediculosis corporis** (body lice): *Pediculus humanus,* the largest (2 to 4 mm) of the three types, is usually associated with poor hygiene. It does not live on the body but instead in the seams of clothing. It can be a vector for other diseases, such as epidemic typhus, trench fever, and relapsing fever.
- **Pediculosis pubis** (pubic lice): *Phthirus pubis* is also known as the crab louse because it is a broad insect with legs that look like claws. It is sometimes mistaken for a brown freckle. Acquisition is primarily through sexual contact.

91. **What are the clinical findings of head lice infestation?**
Scalp pruritus is most common, but many children are **asymptomatic**. A search for lice should be made in any school-aged child presenting with scalp itching. Nits (lice eggs) are found in greatest density on the parietal and occipital areas.

92. **How is the diagnosis of head lice made?**
On physical examination, an actual louse (wingless, grayish insects about 3 to 4 mm) may be difficult to find, although one should easily be able to find nits. The nits are first attached to the hair close to the surface of the scalp and are oval and flesh colored (Fig. 4-7). They are not easily removed from the hair shaft (compared with hair casts, dandruff, and external debris). Overdiagnosis of head lice is common. Microscopic evaluation of the suspected nit can confirm the diagnosis. When the louse emerges, the empty egg case, or nit, appears white in color and remains firmly attached to the hair shaft as the hair grows out (see Fig. 4-7).

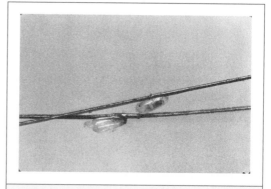

Figure 4-7. Viable head louse egg (*right*) and hatched empty nit (*left*) attached to a child's hair. (From Schachner LA, Hansen RC [eds]: Pediatric Dermatology, 3rd ed. Edinburgh, Mosby, 2003, p 1143.)

Pollack RJ, Kiszewski AE, Spielman A: Overdiagnosis and consequent mismanagement of head louse infestations in North America, *Pediatr Infect Dis J* 19:689–693, 2000.

93. **What types of treatment are available for head lice?**
- **Permethrin:** 1% and 5% (Nix, Elimite)
- **Pyrethrins** (RID, A-200, R&C) (over-the-counter products to which resistance is increasing)
- **Malathion:** 0.5% (Ovide)
- **5% Benzyl alcohol lotion** (prescription recently approved by the FDA for treatment of head lice in children 6 months of age and older)
- **Lindane:** 1% (Kwell) (note "black box warning" regarding serious neurotoxicity)
- **Asphyxiants:** Examples: petroleum jelly (Vaseline), mayonnaise, olive oil (questionable efficacy and messy!)
- **Nit picking** (see question 95)
- **Ivermectin** (off-label use)

Jones KN, English JC 3rd: Review of common therapeutic options in the United States for the treatment of pediculosis capitis, *Clin Infect Dis* 36:1355–1361, 2003.

94. **What precautions should be taken before prescribing malathion 0.5% lotion (Ovide) for head lice?**
Malathion, a weak organophosphate cholinesterase inhibitor, is currently an approved prescription topical treatment for resistant head lice and their eggs. It is approved for use for children age 6 years and older. It is contraindicated for neonates and infants. It is flammable and so should never be used near an open flame or heat source. It should be used in a well-ventilated area given its odor and precautions also include increased absorption through open sores.

95. **Should parents nit pick?**
Once an infestation of lice has been properly treated, the nits are not viable or contagious. Despite this, many schools will not allow children with nits to attend, although this nit-free policy has not been shown to be of benefit for controlling outbreaks. Increasing resistance to therapy may make removal more important to avoid diagnostic confusion. Manual removal (nit picking) is the most effective method, although it is time consuming and tedious. Fine-toothed combs, such as the LiceMeister comb (available through the National Pediculosis Association [http://www.headlice.org]) or other fine-toothed veterinary combs, aid in the removal.

96. **How is a skin scraping for scabies or "scabies prep" done?**
Because the highest percentage of mites are usually concentrated on the hands and feet, the web spaces between digits are the best places to look for the characteristic linear burrows. Moisten the skin with alcohol or mineral oil, scrape across the area of the burrow with a small, rounded scalpel blade (e.g., no. 15 or blunt-edged Foman blade), and place the scrapings on a glass slide with a drop of KOH (or additional mineral oil, if used) and a cover slip. Burrows, if unseen, can be more precisely localized by rubbing a washable felt-tip marker across the web space and removing the ink with alcohol (called the *burrow ink test*). If burrows are present, ink will penetrate through the stratum corneum and outline the site. Under the microscope, mites, eggs, and/or scybala (mite feces) may be seen (Fig. 4-8).

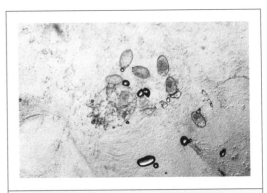

Figure 4-8. Scabies mite and eggs. (From Gates RH [ed]: Infectious Disease Secrets, 2nd ed. Philadelphia, Hanley & Belfus, 2003, p 356.)

97. **What treatment eliminates the scabies babies?**
The treatment of choice for scabies is permethrin 5% cream (Elimite, Acticin). It may be used in children as young as 2 months old. It is more effective than Lindane (the previously accepted treatment for scabies), and it has a much lower risk for neurotoxicity.

The cream is applied from the neck to the toes at night with removal after 8 to 14 hours by bathing or showering. Retreatment in 1 week may be considered. Physicians must make patients aware of the fact that lesions and pruritus may linger for 1 to 2 weeks after effective therapy. One must be supportive during this time to prevent unnecessary retreatment by parents. Antihistamines and low-potency topical steroids may help control symptoms. It must be stressed that all family members and close contacts should be treated simultaneously.

Karthikeyan K: Scabies in children, *Arch Dis Child Educ Pract Ed* 92:ep65–ep69, 2007.

98. **Is there an oral treatment available to treat scabies?**
Yes. Off-label use of *ivermectin* has been reported to treat scabies. It is often considered for patients with a significant dermatitis that precludes the application of topical permethrin. Ivermectin is not recommended for children younger than 5 years or weighing less than 15 kg because it may cross the immature blood-brain barrier.

Currie BJ, McCarthy JS: Permethrin and ivermectin for scabies, *N Engl J Med* 362:717–725, 2010.

99. **What is the "breakfast, lunch, and dinner" sign?**
A series of linear or cluster formation erythematous or urticarial papules (often 3 or more in a row indicative of multiple meals), each with a central pinpoint punctum that occur in response to the bite of a bed bug (*Cimex lactularius*) or other crawling insect.

Stucki A, Ludwig R: Bedbug bites, *N Engl J Med* 359:1047, 2008.

100. **Will getting a new mattress ensure that the bed bugs won't bite?**
No, infestations are not limited to the mattress. Other furniture, clutter in the room, and cracks and crevices in the wall or floor may also harbor bedbugs. They are then attracted to the warm moist carbon dioxide around the sleeping child in the dark of night.

NEONATAL CONDITIONS

101. **What are the most common birthmarks?**
- **Salmon patches** (vascular stains): These are faint, pink-red, macular patches composed of distended dermal capillaries and found on the glabella, eyelids, and the nape of the neck. Seen in 70% of white infants and 60% of black infants. Usually fade, but may persist indefinitely, becoming more prominent during crying.
- **Mongolian spots** (dermal melanosis): These blue-black macules are found on the lumbosacral area and occasionally on shoulders and backs. Seen in 80% to 90% of newborns with darker skin types but only 10% or less of fair-skinned infants. Most of these spots fade by age 2 years and disappear by age 10 years.

102. **How should pustular lesions be evaluated in the newborn period?**
It is important to rule out infectious etiologies because some may be life-threatening. The purulent material should be evaluated with Gram stain, potassium hydroxide (KOH), Tzanck preparation, and bacterial and viral cultures. A Wright stain will reveal the presence of neutrophils or eosinophils (Table 4-3).

TABLE 4-3. COMMON NEONATAL PAPULAR LESIONS

	Neonatal Cephalic Pustulosis	Milia	Erythema Toxicum
Distribution	Face	Face and other areas	Face, trunk, and extremities
Appearance	Papule or pustule	Yellow or white papule	Yellow or white papule
Erythematous	Yes	No	Yes
Contents on smear	Polymorphonuclear cells	Keratin + sebaceous material	Eosinophils
Incidence	Occasional	40%-50% of term infants	30% to 50% of term infants
Course	Last several months	Disappear in 3 to 4 wk	Disappear in 2 wk

103. **What is the differential diagnosis of vesicles or pustules in the newborn?**
See Table 4-4.

TABLE 4-4. DIFFERENTIAL DIAGNOSIS OF VESICLES IN THE NEWBORN	
Noninfectious	**Infectious**
Miliaria	Candidiasis
Erythema toxicum	Staphylococcal folliculitis, impetigo
Transient neonatal pustular melanosis	Herpes simplex virus
Benign cephalic pustulosis (neonatal acne)	Congenital syphilis
Infantile acropustulosis	Varicella
Incontinentia pigmenti	Bacterial sepsis
Langerhans cell histiocytosis	

Adapted from Roberts LJ: Dermatologic diseases. In McMillan JA, DeAngelis CD, Feigin RD, et al (eds): Oski's Pediatrics, Principles and Practice, 3rd ed. Philadelphia, Lippincott Williams & Wilkins, 1999, p 376.

104. **What is the medical significance of cutis marmorata?**
Cutis marmorata is the bluish mottling of the skin often seen in infants and young children who have been exposed to low temperatures or chilling. The reticulated marbling effect is the result of dilated capillaries and venules causing darkened areas on the skin; this disappears with warming. Cutis marmorata is of no medical significance, and no treatment is indicated. However, persistent cutis marmorata is associated with trisomy 21, trisomy 18, and Cornelia de Lange syndromes. There is also a congenital vascular anomaly called *cutis marmorata telangiectatic congenita* that has persistent purple reticulate mottling of the skin. In addition, capillary malformations (port wine stains) may have a reticulated appearance and be mistaken for cutis marmorata.

105. **A healthy infant with scattered reddish nodules on the back skin most likely has what condition?**
Subcutaneous fat necrosis, which consists of sharply circumscribed, indurated nodular lesions usually seen in healthy, term newborns and infants during the first few days to weeks of life. The stony hard areas of panniculitis, which are reddish to violaceous in color, are most often found on the cheeks, back, buttocks, arms, and thighs. Most lesions are self-limited and require no therapy. However, occasionally they may extensively calcify and spontaneously drain with subsequent scarring. Remember that significant hypercalcemia may be present in a small number of patients. Therefore, a serum calcium level should be ordered whenever the disorder is suspected; it should be rechecked periodically until the condition resolves and for several months thereafter.

106. **What should the family of a newborn with a yellow, hairless patch with a cobblestone texture be advised to do?**
The lesion is likely a **nevus sebaceous.** This hamartomatous neoplasm usually presents as a yellow-pink hairless plaque on the scalp or face at the time of birth and is composed primarily of malformed sebaceous glands. Under the influence of androgens at puberty, the glands may hypertrophy and lead to the development of other neoplasms. The exact risk for basal cell carcinoma development is controversial. Some experts advise excision during the preteen, prepubertal years. Careful monitoring of the lesion for new growths or nonhealing ulcerations at all ages is advised, especially during adolescence.

107. **What syndromes are associated with aplasia cutis congenita?**
Aplasia cutis congenita (congenital absence of the skin) presents on the scalp as solitary or multiple well-demarcated ulcerations or atrophic scars. Of variable depth, the lesions may be limited to epidermis and upper dermis or occasionally extend into the skull and dura. Although most children with this lesion are normal without multiple anomalies, other associations include epidermolysis bullosa, placental infarcts, teratogens, sebaceous nevi, and limb anomalies. Aplasia cutis is a feature of trisomy 13, 4p-, oculocerebrocutaneous syndrome, and Adams-Oliver syndrome.

108. **Describe the appearance and distribution of transient neonatal pustular melanosis.**
Consisting of small vesicopustular lesions 2 to 4 mm in size, transient pustular melanosis occurs in almost 5% of African American and less than 1% of white newborns. It may be present at birth or appear shortly after birth. The lesions most often cluster on the neck, chin, palms, and soles, although they may occur on the face and trunk. The pustules rupture easily and progress to brown, pigmented macules with a fine collarette of scale. Microscopic examination of the contents of the pustules reveals neutrophils with no organisms. There are no associated systemic manifestations, and the eruption is self-limited, although the hyperpigmentation may last for months.

109. **Is erythema toxicum neonatorum really toxic?**
Not in the least. Erythema toxicum is a common eruption composed of erythematous macules, papules, and pustules that occur in newborns, usually during the first few days of life. The lesions may start as irregular, blotchy, red macules, varying in size from millimeters to several centimeters. They often develop into 1- to 3-mm, yellow-white papules and pustules on an erythematous base, giving a flea-bitten appearance. They occur all over the body except on the palms and soles, which are spared because the lesions occur in pilosebaceous follicles, which are absent on the palmar and plantar surfaces. The rash is less common in premature infants, with incidence proportional to gestational age and peaking at 41 to 42 weeks. Although it may be seen at birth, it is most common during the first 3 to 4 days of life and is occasionally noted as late as 10 days of life. Erythema toxicum usually lasts 5 to 7 days and heals without pigmentation. Other than the rash, the newborn appears healthy.

110. **For academic purposes (and ICD-10-CM coding), is it possible to be more scientific about the diagnosis of "prickly heat"?**
The scientific name for this condition is *miliaria rubra*. It is due to sweat retention, and its clinical morphology is determined by the level at which sweat is trapped. Sweat trapped at a superficial level produces clear vesicles without surrounding erythema (sudamina or crystallina); miliaria rubra (prickly heat, erythematous papules, vesicles, papulovesicles) is produced by sweat trapped at a deeper level; pustular lesions (miliaria pustulosa) and even abscesses (miliaria profunda) are produced with sweat retention at the deepest of levels (infants rarely develop these types). With the advent of air conditioning, miliaria rarely occurs in newborn nurseries.

111. **What diagnoses should be considered in a neonate born with a sternal cleft malformation?**
Sternal cleft malformations can be associated with *cardiac and vascular defects* (sternal malformation and vascular dysgenesis syndrome). The pediatrician should also evaluate for precursors of infantile hemangiomas of the skin as PHACES syndrome (see question 147) may initially present in this manner. Also, be on the lookout for the development of oral mucosal or airway hemangiomas as well because they have also been reported in patients born with sternal malformations.

Chen YC, Eichenfield LF, Malchiodi J, Friedlander SF: Small facial hemangiomas and supraumbilical raphe: a forme fruste of PHACES syndrome? *Br J Dermatol* 153:1053–1057, 2005.

PAPULOSQUAMOUS DISORDERS

112. **What diseases are associated with the Koebner reaction?**
Koebnerization is a response to local injury whereby skin lesions are found at the sites of trauma (e.g., linear lesions at the sites of scratching). This is seen in patients with psoriasis (Fig. 4-9) as well as those with other conditions including lichen planus and flat warts.

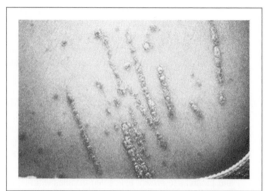

Figure 4-9. Koebner phenomenon in psoriasis with linear plaques at sites of excoriations. (From Cohen BA: Pediatric Dermatology, 2nd ed. St. Louis, Mosby, 1999, p 63.)

113. **What is the typical pattern of lesions in childhood psoriasis?**
Psoriasis presents as well-circumscribed, erythematous plaques with overlying white scale in children and adults. These occur on the scalp, elbows, knees (Fig. 4-10), sacrum, and genitalia. Psoriasis may also present with guttate (droplike) lesions over the trunk and extremities. These children may have group A β-hemolytic streptococcus infection as an underlying precipitating factor. Other triggers include trauma, stress, colder weather, and some medications (e.g., nonsteroidal anti-inflammatory drugs [NSAIDs], antimalarials).

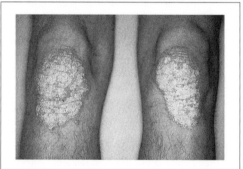

Figure 4-10. Plaques of psoriasis on the knees. (From Gawkrodger DJ: Dermatology: An Illustrated Colour Text, 3rd ed. London, Churchill Livingstone, 2002, p 27.)

114. **What is the likelihood of a child developing psoriasis if one or both parents has the condition?**
The prevalence of psoriasis in the United States is estimated to be 1% to 3%. If one parent has psoriasis, the likelihood of the child having psoriasis is about 8%; if both parents are affected, it increases to 40%.

Nestle FO, Kaplan DH, Barker J: Psoriasis. *N Engl J Med* 361:496–509, 2009.

115. **What percentage of children with psoriasis have nail involvement?**
Nail changes, most commonly pitting, may be the only manifestation of psoriasis. The reported incidence of nail pitting in children with psoriasis is as high as **40%**. Other nail changes include onycholysis (separation of the nail plate from nailbed at the distal margin) and thickening of the nail plate, often with white-yellow discoloration. Subungual debris may occur.

116. **A skin scale that easily bleeds on removal is characteristic of what condition?**
The appearance of punctate bleeding points after removal of a scale is the **Auspitz sign.** It is seen primarily in psoriasis and is related to the rupture of capillaries high in the papillary dermis, near the surface of the skin.

117. **What are treatment modalities for psoriasis?**
Various therapies have been used to treat psoriasis. The choice of treatment will depend on the extent of involvement, previous treatments, and the age of the patient. Topical treatments include topical corticosteroids, calcipotriene (a vitamin D analog), retinoids, and tar. Other treatment modalities include phototherapy and, rarely, systemic retinoids and methotrexate. Etanercept, a soluble tumor necrosis factor receptor, which is approved for use for juvenile idiopathic arthritis, was recently shown to lessen the severity of moderate to severe psoriasis in pediatric patients.

Paller AS, Siegfried EC, Langley RG, et al: Etanercept treatment for children and adolescents with plaque psoriasis, *N Engl J Med* 358:241–251, 2008.

Schön MP, Boehncke W-H: Psoriasis. *N Engl J Med* 352:1899–1912, 2005.

118. **What are the eight Ps of lichen planus?**
- **Papules:** Usually 2 to 6 mm in diameter; often seen in a linear pattern as a result of the Koebner reaction
- **Plaques:** Commonly generated from a confluence of papules with exaggerated surface markings of the overlying skin (Wickham striae)
- **Planar:** Individual lesions, usually flat-topped
- **Purple:** Distinctly violaceous
- **Pruritus:** Often intensely itchy
- **Polygonal:** Borders of papules are often angulated
- **Penis:** Common site of involvement in children
- **Persistent:** Chronic, with remissions and exacerbations for up to 18 months

119. **How is pityriasis rosea distinguished from secondary syphilis?**
Often with difficulty; both are primarily papulosquamous rashes. **Pityriasis rosea** classically consists of oval lesions that organize in parallel fashion on the trunk (the "Christmas tree" distribution) and are preceded in 40% to 80% of cases by a large annular erythematous lesion (herald patch). **Secondary syphilis** lesions occur 3 to 6 weeks after the chancre, and, as compared with pityriasis rosea, they may have more involvement of the palms, soles, and mucous membranes and have accompanying lymphadenopathy. However, because atypical presentations are common, testing for syphilis should be performed in any sexually active individual who is diagnosed with pityriasis rosea.

120. **What is the treatment for pityriasis rosea?**
Pityriasis rosea is a self-limited condition that usually resolves in 6 to 12 weeks. Therefore, treatment is often not required, unless there is significant pruritus or cosmetic disfigurement. A wide range of treatments are reported. Topical corticosteroids help reduce pruritus, but they do not alter the course of the disease. Ultraviolet B phototherapy results in clinical improvement in some individuals. Oral erythromycin has also been shown to be beneficial.

Sharma PK, Yadav TP, Gautam RK, et al: Erythromycin in pityriasis rosea: a double-blind, placebo-controlled clinical trial, *J Am Acad Dermatol* 42:241–244, 2000.

121. **A 5-year-old presents for evaluation of a recent onset of a linear array of pink to hypopigmented papules on the arm. What is the likely diagnosis?**
Although the differential diagnosis may be broad, a common cause of this type of eruption is **lichen striatus.** This eruption is generally asymptomatic, does not require treatment, and usually resolves in about 6 months.

PHOTODERMATOLOGY

122. Why is limiting excessive sun exposure in children important?

Most people experience a significant percentage of their lifetime sun exposure early in life. Years of unprotected sun exposure will lead to freckling, wrinkling, and skin cancer formation, including melanoma. In an era of rising rates of melanoma and squamous and basal cell carcinomas, the use of sun-protection strategies during the pediatric years could lower the risk to an individual. Broad-spectrum sunscreens may attenuate the number of nevi in white children, especially if they have freckles.

Gallagher RP, Rivers JK, Lee TK, et al: Broad-spectrum sunscreen use and the development of new nevi in white children: a randomized clinical trial, *JAMA* 283:2955–2960, 2000.

123. What are good strategies for protection against sun exposure?
- Avoid the sun, if possible, during peak hours (10 AM to 3 PM) or seek shade.
- Wear protective clothing, hats, and sunglasses.
- Apply sunscreen at least 30 minutes before sun exposure.
- Use a broad-spectrum sunscreen with a sun-protection factor (SPF) of 15 to 30 or higher.
- Apply liberal amounts of sunscreen (2 mg/body cm or about 30 mL for an adult or 15 mL for a 7-year-old child).
- Reapply sunscreen every 2 hours, even if it claims to be "waterproof."
- Wear lip protection that has sunscreen in it.

124. What types of sunscreens are available?

Physical sunscreens are composed of zinc oxide or titanium dioxide and function by scattering ultraviolet light. Although they are opaque, newer micronized preparations are easier to apply and more acceptable to patients. **Chemical sunscreens** absorb either ultraviolet A (UVA) or ultraviolet B (UVB) light. Most commercially available sunscreens are combinations of various agents. For sunscreens to function well, they must be applied on all exposed surfaces in adequate quantities and reapplied throughout the day.

125. How is the SPF of a sunscreen determined?

SPF is the level of effectiveness of a sunscreen's ability to protect against UVB light; it is not a measurement of UVA light protection. The SPF rating is a ratio of the dose of ultraviolet light needed to produce minimal redness on sun-protected skin to the dose of ultraviolet light needed to produce minimal redness on unprotected skin.

126. Should sunscreens be avoided in infants?

This is controversial. There are concerns that the skin of infants younger than 6 months has different absorptive characteristics and that biologic systems that metabolize and excrete drugs may not be fully developed. However, there is no evidence that the limited use of sunscreen in infants is problematic. Physical protection (e.g., clothing, hats, shade, sunglasses) is most ideal, but if an infant's skin is not adequately protected, it may be reasonable to apply sunscreen to small areas, such as the face and the back of the hands. Physical sunscreens containing zinc oxide are preferred over chemical sunscreens for use on infant skin.

127. Do we risk developing vitamin D deficiency by using sun protection?

Vitamin D synthesis is a beneficial effect of exposure to ultraviolet light, and several studies suggest an association between low vitamin D levels and the development of cancer. This, however, should not be interpreted as a reason to seek a tan. In most people, adequate amounts of vitamin D can be obtained by ingesting a healthy diet, including foods that naturally contain or are fortified with vitamin D. It is important to note that the American Academy of Pediatrics recently increased their recommended daily intake of vitamin D to prevent rickets and vitamin D deficiency in children.

Wagner CI, Greer FR: AAP Section on Breastfeeding; AAP Committee on Nutrition: Prevention of rickets and vitamin D deficiency in infants, children and adolescents, *Pediatrics* 122:1142–1152, 2008.

128. **Describe causes of pseudoporphyria in children.**
Pseudoporphyria is a phototoxic vesicobullous eruption. It can occur with chronic NSAID use (especially naproxen sodium) and is therefore not uncommon in patients with juvenile idiopathic arthritis. Other medications associated with pseudoporphyria include tetracyclines, dapsone, furosemide, nalidixic acid, retinoids, amiodarone, and voriconazole. It has also been reported in children receiving hemodialysis.

Paller AS, Mancini AJ: Photosensitivity and photoreactions. In Paller AS, Mancini AJ, editors: *Hurwitz Clinical Pediatric Dermatology*, ed 3, Philadelphia, 2006, Elsevier, p 520.

129. **Which "lime" disease is not transmitted by ticks?**
Limes contain psoralens that react with ultraviolet light and that can produce erythema, vesicles, and/or hyperpigmentation on areas of the skin that have come in contact with lime juice. This is known as **phytophotodermatitis** and is seen with other psoralen-containing plants, such as celery and figs. Additionally, berloque dermatitis (*berloque* is French for "pendant," which some lesions can resemble) is an irregularly patterned hyperpigmentation of the neck due to photosensitization by furocoumarins (i.e., psoralens) in perfumes. It is caused by fragrances that contain bergamot oil, an extract from the peel of a type of orange that is grown in southern France and Italy. Bergamot oil contains 5-methoxypsoralen, which enhances the erythematous and pigmentary response of UVA light.

130. **Which conditions are associated with marked sun sensitivity?**
- **Inherited disorders:** Porphyrias, xeroderma pigmentosum, Bloom syndrome, Rothmund-Thomson syndrome, Hartnup disorder
- **Exogenous agents:** Drugs (e.g., tetracyclines, thiazides), photoallergic contact dermatitis (associated with perfumes and para-aminobenzoic acid esters)
- **Systemic disease:** Lupus erythematosus, dermatomyositis
- **Idiopathic disorders:** Polymorphous light eruption, solar urticaria, actinic prurigo, hydroa vacciniforme

Garzon MC, DeLeo VA: Photosensitivity in the pediatric patient, *Curr Opin Pediatr* 9:377–387, 1997.

131. **What is the appearance of polymorphous light eruption?**
The most common pediatric photodermatosis, polymorphous light eruption is characterized by itchy red papules, plaques, or papulovesicles that appear several hours to days after ultraviolet light exposure. It can be diagnosed by phototesting (i.e., the induction of lesions by intentional ultraviolet light exposure) and by skin biopsy. It is usually suggested by the classic history and the exclusion of other photosensitivity disease.

Morison WL: Photosensitivity, *N Engl J Med* 350:1111–1117, 2004.

132. **Is a child with sun sensitivity protected by sitting behind a window?**
Yes and no, depending on the reason for the sensitivity. Ultraviolet light is divided into three wavelength groups: ultraviolet C (UVC), 200 to 290 nm; UVB, 290 to 320 nm; and UVA, 320 to 400 nm. UVC light is cytotoxic and can cause retinal injury, but fortunately it is almost completely absorbed by the ozone layer. UVB light causes sunburn, dermatologic flares (e.g., in patients with lupus erythematosus), and, with chronic exposure, skin cancer. UVA light (which is also emitted from the fluorescent lamps used in most schools) is responsible for psoralen and drug phototoxicity and porphyria flares, and it can cause skin cancer with chronic exposure. Windows block UVB light, but not UVA. Thus, children with UVA-sensitive disorders would not be protected by sitting behind a window unless it has been pretreated with a UVA filter.

PIGMENTATION DISORDERS

133. **What disorders of childhood are associated with areas of hypopigmentation?**
Hypopigmentation is caused by a decrease—not a total absence—of pigmentation or melanin. Conditions that feature hypopigmented lesions include tuberous sclerosis, tinea versicolor, pityriasis alba, nevus depigmentosus, hypomelanosis of Ito, leprosy, and postinflammatory hypopigmentation.

Lio PA: Little white spots: an approach to hypopigmented macules, *Arch Dis Child Educ Pract Ed* 93:98–102, 2008.

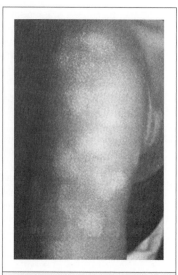

Figure 4-11. Pityriasis alba. Poorly demarcated areas of hypopigmentation in patient with atopic dermatitis. (From Cohen BA: Pediatric Dermatology, 2nd ed. London, Mosby, 1999, p 75.)

134. **Is treatment helpful for children with postinflammatory hypopigmentation?**
In children with **pityriasis alba** (or postinflammatory hypopigmentation associated with atopic dermatitis), very-low-potency topical steroids, emollients, and sun protection measures can make skin color more uniform. Treatment does not appear to help in other cases of postinflammatory hypopigmentation, such as those that occur after infection, abrasions, or burns, but sun protection is advisable (Fig. 4-11).

135. **What treatments are available for vitiligo?**
Vitiligo is a disorder of depigmentation (total absence of pigmentation with sharp demarcations; Fig. 4-12). The etiology is unknown but may be autoimmune in nature. There are rare associations with other autoimmune conditions, including thyroiditis and juvenile-onset diabetes. Treatment is often unsatisfactory. Potent topical steroids have been used for localized areas. Off-label use of topical tacrolimus ointment has been used with some success to treat facial vitiligo in children. Ultraviolet light therapy has been employed for some children with severe, extensive disease. Dyes (including self-tanning agents) and coverage cosmetics are often helpful for camouflaging skin lesions.

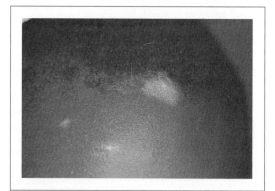

Figure 4-12. Vitiligo. Note well-demarcated areas of total depigmentation.

Isenstein A, Morrell DS, Burkhart CN: Vitiligo: treatment approach in children, *Pediatr Ann* 38:339–344, 2009.

National Vitiligo Foundation: http://www.nvfi.org.

136. **What conditions are associated with congenital depigmentation of the skin?**
Congenital depigmentation, or **albinism,** constitutes a number of genetically inherited syndromes that are characterized by disorders of melanin synthesis and that may affect the skin, hair, and eyes. **Generalized (oculocutaneous) albinism** is often complicated by ocular abnormalities, including visual impairment, photophobia, and nystagmus. Piebaldism is a distinct form of congenital depigmentation that affects segments of skin. Patients with this condition often have a forelock of white hair, which is caused by a genetic mutation that differs from generalized albinism. Localized congenital depigmentation associated with a white forelock, heterochromia irides, and congenital deafness characterizes Waardenburg syndrome.

137. **What is the likely diagnosis if a patient taking trimethoprim-sulfamethoxazole develops a single erythematous, sharply marginated, round lesion that leaves an area of hyperpigmentation upon resolution?**
Fixed drug eruption. These 2- to 10-cm red to violaceous inflammatory plaques are usually solitary and may blister. This hypersensitivity reaction occurs after medication ingestion (commonly antibiotics) especially trimethoprim-sulfamethoxazole and tetracycline. The resultant hyperpigmentation helps to make the distinction.

Morelli JG, Tay YK, Rogers M, et al: Fixed drug eruptions in children, *J Pediatr* 134:365–367, 1999.

138. **Is melanoma in children extremely rare?**
On the contrary, about 1% of all melanoma cases in the United States are diagnosed in patients younger than 20 years. In certain parts of the world, the incidence in pediatric patients is particularly high. Until recently in Sweden, melanoma accounted for 10% of all cancer cases in teenagers.

Downard CD, Rapkin LB, Gow KW: Melanoma in children and adolescents, *Surg Oncol* 16: 215–220, 2007.

Karlsson PM, Fredrikson M: Cutaneous malignant melanoma in children and adolescents in Sweden, 1993–2002: the increasing trend is broken, *In J Cancer* 121:323–328, 2007.

139. **Why are Spitz nevi and malignant melanoma often confused?**
The Spitz nevus can appear suddenly and grow rapidly. Histologically, it has many features that can be mistaken for malignancy. It actually was previously referred to as *benign juvenile melanoma.* "Benign" is the key word for this red to brown, dome-shaped papule, which usually appears on the face or extremity. Clinicopathologic correlation is the key to making this diagnosis. It is essential that an experienced pathologist interpret the biopsy when a Spitz nevus is suspected. Melanoma in childhood has been misdiagnosed as Spitz nevi, and Spitz nevi have been misdiagnosed as melanoma.

140. **What are the clinical features of familial dysplastic nevus syndrome?**
The syndrome, which is also known as the *familial atypical mole syndrome,* is found in families who have acquired nevi that develop into melanoma. These nevi are 5 to 15 mm in diameter and are round to oval in shape. Furthermore, they have irregular and indistinct margins, exhibit variation in color within the same lesion, and have both macular and elevated components. They tend to occur in sun-protected areas.

141. **In children with pigmented nevi, what factors increase the risk of melanoma?**
Melanoma is rare during childhood. If there is a family history of melanoma or atypical moles, a history of severe sunburns before the age of 18 years, or the child has a giant congenital nevus, the risk is greater. Estimated risks vary for different-sized congenital nevi.

The projected lifetime risk for a melanoma developing within a congenital nevus is controversial. For small congenital nevi, the risk is low. For giant congenital nevi, the risk is estimated to be 6% to 8%. Acquired nevi very rarely develop melanomas.

Gibbs NF, Makkar HS: Disorders of hyperpigmentation and melanocytes. In Eichefield LF, Frieden IJ, Esterly NB, editors: *Textbook of Neonatal Dermatology*, ed 2, Philadelphia, 2008, W.B. Saunders, pp 397–421.

142. **What is the differential diagnosis of yellow-brown or orange nodules in children?**
- Nevus sebaceous
- Benign cephalic histiocytosis
- Juvenile xanthogranuloma
- Langerhans cell histiocytosis
- Solitary mastocytoma
- Spitz nevus
- Urticaria pigmentosa
- Connective tissue nevus

143. **What systems should be closely evaluated in a patient presenting with a large segmental café-au-lait patch with jagged borders on an extremity?**
The answers are endocrine and bone. The pigmented lesion of jagged borders resembling the "coast of Maine" is seen in 50% of patients with McCune-Albright syndrome (MAS). Patients with this syndrome also develop polyostotic fibrous dysplasia of bones and propensity for fractures. Hyperactive endocrinopathies also occur and girls may initially present with precocious puberty. The guanine nucleotide-binding protein gene (*GNAS1*) has been found to be mutated inpatients with MAS.

VASCULAR BIRTHMARKS

144. **How are vascular birthmarks classified?**
The updated biologic classification of vascular birthmarks is the most widely accepted classification of vascular birthmarks. It was first proposed in 1982 and was adapted recently to reflect new knowledge. Two broad categories of vascular birthmarks are described: vascular tumors and vascular malformations. There are many types of vascular tumors, but infantile hemangiomas are the most common. Vascular malformations are categorized on the basis of their flow characteristics and types of anomalous channels:
   Vascular tumors (selected):
- Infantile hemangioma
- Congenital hemangioma
- Kaposiform hemangioendothelioma
- Tufted angioma
- Pyogenic granuloma
   Vascular malformations:
- Capillary malformation (port wine stains, salmon patch)
- Venous malformations
- Lymphatic malformation (lymphangioma microcystic, macrocystic)
- Arteriovenous malformations
- Mixed malformations

Enjolras O, Milliken J: Vascular tumors and vascular malformations, new issues, *Adv Dermatol* 13:375–423, 1998.

Mulliken JB, Glowacki J: Hemangiomas and vascular malformations in infants and children, *Plast Reconstr Surg* 69:412–420, 1982.

Vascular Birthmarks Foundation: http://www.birthmark.org.

145. **Describe the life history of infantile hemangiomas.**
Hemangiomas or, more specifically, infantile hemangiomas, are common benign vascular tumors. They are rarely fully developed at birth, but precursor lesions (an area of pallor, telangiectasia, or "bruise") may be detected on close inspection within the first few days of life. They may have superficial and/or deep components. Hemangiomas undergo a growth phase until the child reaches the age of 6 to 12 months, at which time the tumors start to involute. This process of involution occurs over several years. There still may be residual skin changes (e.g., skin redundancy, pallor, atrophy, telangiectasia) after the hemangioma has resolved. Plastic surgical intervention may be considered in selected cases. Because 90% to 95% of these tumors resolve spontaneously, it is important to avoid the temptation of treatments that might result in additional scarring or long-term complication, including cryotherapy, radiation therapy, or sclerosing agents, which can hasten resolution but lead to a higher likelihood of scarring. Management of infantile hemangiomas needs to be individualized as many factors are assessed in the decision to actively treat an infantile hemangioma.

Bruckner AL, Frieden IJ: Hemangiomas of infancy, *J Am Acad Dermatol* 48:477–493, 2003.

146. **What are the major goals of the management of infantile hemangiomas?**
The decisions regarding which hemangiomas require treatment and the best therapeutic modalities may not always be easy ones. The major goals of management are as follows:
- Prevent or reverse life- or function-threatening complications.
- Treat ulcerated hemangiomas.
- Prevent permanent disfigurement caused by a rapidly enlarging lesion.
- Minimize psychosocial stress for the family and the patient.
- Avoid overly aggressive procedures that may result in scarring in lesions that have a good likelihood of involuting without significant residual lesions.

Frieden IJ: Which hemangiomas to treat—and how? *Arch Dermatol* 133:1593–1595, 1997.

147. **Which hemangiomas are especially worrisome?**
- **Multiple cutaneous hemangiomas:** May be associated with visceral hemangiomas (e.g., liver)
- **Large hemangiomas:** May cause significant disfigurement of underlying structures and may be associated with congestive heart failure
- **"Beard" hemangiomas:** May be a marker for underlying laryngeal or subglottic hemangioma that may impair respiratory function
- **Midline spinal hemangiomas:** May be a marker for underlying spinal cord abnormality
- **Head and neck hemangiomas:** Usually larger lesions, may be associated with other congenital anomalies, including central nervous system, cardiac, ocular, and sternal defects (e.g., **p**osterior fossa malformation, **h**emangioma, **a**rterial abnormalities, **c**oarctation, **e**ye abnormalities, **s**ternal defects [PHACE(S)] syndrome).
- **Vulnerable anatomic locations:** Impair vital functions, cause disfigurement (e.g., periocular, neck, lip, nasal tip)
- **Ulcerated hemangiomas:** Increased risk for superinfection, cause pain and lead to scarring

Metry DW, Hebert AA: Benign cutaneous vascular tumors of infancy: when to worry, what to do, *Arch Dermatol* 136:905–914, 2000.

KEY POINTS: WORRISOME HEMANGIOMAS

1. **Multiple cutaneous hemangiomas:** May be associated with visceral hemangiomas (e.g., liver)

2. **Large hemangiomas:** May cause significant disfigurement of underlying structures and may be associated with congestive heart failure

3. **"Beard" hemangiomas:** May be a marker for underlying laryngeal or subglottic hemangioma that may impair respiratory function

4. **Midline spinal hemangiomas:** May be a marker for underlying spinal cord abnormality

5. **Head and neck hemangiomas:** Usually larger lesions, may be associated with other congenital anomalies, including central nervous system, cardiac, ocular, and sternal defects (e.g., **p**osterior fossa malformation, **h**emangioma, **a**rterial abnormalities, **c**oarctation, **e**ye abnormalities, **s**ternal defects [PHACE(S)] syndrome).

6. **Vulnerable anatomic locations:** Impair vital functions, cause disfigurement (e.g., periocular, neck, lip, nasal tip)

7. **Ulcerated hemangiomas:** Increased risk for superinfection, cause pain and lead to scarring

---

148. **What does the typical hemangioma in PHACE syndrome usually look like?**
The infantile hemangiomas associated with PHACE syndrome are typically located on the head and neck area and are often large and plaquelike, covering an area of the skin surface. The term *segmental infantile hemangioma* is used to describe its appearance.

149. **When is treatment indicated for infantile hemangiomas?**
■ Lesions that interfere with normal physiologic functioning (i.e., breathing, hearing, eating, vision), especially periocular hemangiomas (to prevent amblyopia)
■ Recurrent bleeding, ulceration, or infection
■ A rapidly growing lesion that distorts facial features
■ High-output congestive heart failure

Bruckner AL, Frieden IJ: Hemangiomas of infancy, *J Am Acad Dermatol* 48:477–493, 2003.

150. **If intralesional or systemic steroids have failed as options for hemangiomas requiring treatment, what else may be of benefit?**
Several other modalities have been used to manage infantile hemangiomas requiring treatment that fail corticosteroid therapy.
■ **Chemotherapeutic agents (vincristine):** These are usually used for life-threatening hemangiomas for which other modalities have failed.
■ **Embolization**
■ **Surgery**
■ **Interferon-α:** Used subcutaneously, it may act by blocking endothelial cell motility and inhibiting angiogenesis. However, neurotoxicity is a common and severe side effect that has resulted in limiting the use of this drug.
■ **Pulsed dye laser:** This may be used with other modalities but is usually of little benefit in situations in which intralesional or systemic corticosteroids were previously indicated. Limited penetration restricts use to superficial lesions. It can be useful for painful ulcerated hemangiomas that fail to respond to other treatment modalities. Controversy exists regarding its potential to cause scarring.

- **Propranolol:** There have been recent reports that the β-blocker propranolol may be an effective treatment for infantile hemangiomas. Studies are under way to determine the efficacy, safety, and dose regimens of this medication.

151. **Why is an infant with a vascular tumor and new-onset thrombocytopenia so worrisome?**

This can indicate the development of the **Kasabach-Merritt syndrome** (or phenomenon), a life-threatening condition of rapidly enlarging vascular tumors and progressive coagulopathy. Platelets are sequestered within the lesion, forming thrombi and consuming coagulation factors. Ecchymoses may develop initially around the vascular tumor, but a disseminated coagulopathy with anemia can result. Aggressive therapy (systemic steroids, vincristine, interferon-α, and surgery) is frequently needed. Kasabach-Merritt syndrome is not caused by common infantile hemangiomas but rather by two rare vascular tumors (kaposiform hemangioendothelioma and tufted angioma).

152. **How do superficial hemangiomas differ from port wine stains?**

Superficial hemangiomas are superficial, palpable, vascular tumors that usually involute with time. In the past, they were called *strawberry hemangiomas*. **Port wine stains,** which are sometimes called *nevus flammeus*, are flat vascular malformations composed of capillary and postcapillary venule-size vessels that do not involute. Some superficial hemangiomas may mimic port wine stains during the first few weeks of life; observation of their growth pattern is helpful for establishing the correct diagnosis (Table 4-5).

TABLE 4-5. SUPERFICIAL HEMANGIOMAS VERSUS PORT WINE STAINS	
Superficial Hemangiomas	**Port Wine Stains**
Palpable	Flat, macular
Common (4%-10% of children <1 year old)	Less common (0.1%-0.3%)
Often not apparent at birth (more visible at 2-12 wk)	Present at birth
Bright red	Pale pink to blue-red (darkens with age)
Well-defined borders	Borders variable
Pathology: Proliferating angioblastic endothelial cells with variable blood-filled capillaries	Pathology: Dermal capillary dilation
90%-95% involute spontaneously by age 9 yr	No involution: May worsen with darkening and hypertrophy
Rapid growth phase	Proportionate growth (as child grows)
Suggested therapy: Watchful waiting; active treatment for some lesions	Suggested therapy: Flash lamp pulsed-dye laser in children

153. **When are port wine stains associated with other anomalies?**

Sturge-Weber syndrome refers to the association of a facial port wine stain (typically affecting the skin innervated by the first branch of the trigeminal nerve) (Fig. 4-13), an ocular vascular anomaly linked with glaucoma, and a leptomeningeal vascular anomaly associated with seizures and developmental delay.

Klippel-Trenaunay syndrome refers to the association of a limb port wine stain (usually lower extremity) with ipsilateral soft tissue and bony overgrowth and venous varicosities.

154. How are port wine stain–type capillary malformations treated?

Port wine stains are often pink to dark red in color during childhood. With maturity, they often darken and take on their "port wine" color. Treatment of facial capillary malformations is generally recommended during infancy or early childhood when the lesions appear to be more amenable to therapy with the pulsed dye laser.

The pulsed dye lasers that are used for treatment of port wine stains are designed to target oxyhemoglobin and lead to destruction of the blood vessels and subsequent lightening of the stain.

Multiple treatments sometimes requiring general anesthesia or sedation are required to achieve lightening. It is important for patients and families to understand that this treatment often achieves cosmetically acceptable lightening but complete disappearance or removal of the birthmark is not yet possible with the current technologies. In some patients, the stain will redarken after treatment, and touch-up treatments may be required.

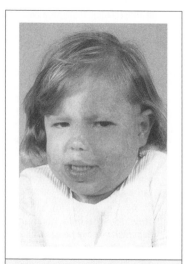

Figure 4-13. Sturge-Weber syndrome. The bilateral port wine stain involves the V_1, V_2, and V_3 regions and the right V_3. (From Sahn EE: Dermatology Pearls. Philadelphia, Hanley & Belfus, 1999, p 225.)

VESICOBULLOUS DISORDERS

155. What is the Nikolsky sign?

This sign demonstrates **epidermal fragility.** Gentle lateral pressure placed on apparently intact skin causes an erosion, especially near preformed vesicles. This sign is positive in several autoimmune, infectious, and inherited blistering conditions, such as bullous pemphigoid, staphylococcal scalded skin syndrome (SSSS), and epidermolysis bullosa.

156. What are causes of skin blistering in childhood?

- **Infectious:** Bacterial (bullous impetigo, SSSS), viral (herpes simplex virus, varicella)
- **Contact dermatitis:** Poison ivy, phytophotodermatitis
- **Inherited disorders:** Epidermolysis bullosa, bullous congenital ichthyosiform erythroderma
- **Autoimmune disorders:** Linear immunoglobulin A disease, bullous pemphigoid, pemphigus vulgaris
- **Other:** Erythema multiforme, toxic epidermal necrolysis, thermal injury (burns)

157. How is SSSS differentiated from toxic epidermal necrolysis (TEN)?

Both are diffuse bullous diseases. **SSSS** commonly arises in children younger than 5 years and develops after a localized staphylococcal infection with diffuse cutaneous disease caused by an exfoliative toxin. The level of blistering includes the superficial levels of the epidermis. **TEN** is believed to be a hypersensitivity reaction (often to a drug) and occurs in all age groups. The level of blistering is deep, and the entire epidermis is necrotic (Table 4-6).

TABLE 4-6. DIFFERENTIATION BETWEEN STAPHYLOCOCCAL SCALDED SKIN SYNDROME AND TOXIC EPIDERMAL NECROLYSIS		
	Staphylococcal Scalded Skin Syndrome	Toxic Epidermal Necrolysis
Etiology	Infectious; group II staphylococci	Immunologic; usually drug related
Morbidity and mortality	Low with treatment	High
Mucous membrane involvement	Rare	Frequent
Nikolsky sign	Present	Absent
Target lesions	Absent	Often present
Level of blister	Upper epidermis (below stratum corneum)	Subepidermal
Histopathology	No epidermal necrosis or dermal inflammation	Full-thickness epidermal necrosis; prominent perivascular dermal inflammation

Adapted from Roberts LJ: Dermatologic diseases. In McMillan JA, DeAngelis CD, Feigin RD, et al (eds): Oski's Pediatrics, Principles and Practice, 3rd ed. Philadelphia, Lippincott Williams & Wilkins, 1999, p 379.

158. **Why are neonates susceptible to SSSS?**
The answer lies in the observation that newborns share their susceptibility to SSSS with older patients in renal failure. It is the *reduced clearance of the exfoliative toxin* by the newborn's immature kidneys that contributes to their increased susceptibility to SSSS.

159. **Where can *S. aureus* be found in patients with SSSS?**
S. aureus commonly colonizes the nasopharynx and the umbilicus. The source of infection may also be present in the urinary tract, a wound, conjunctiva, or blood. The bacteria are not usually present at the site of the skin lesions because they are the result of a systemic toxin-mediated effect.

160. **What is epidermolysis bullosa (EB)?**
EB is a heterogeneous group of inherited disorders characterized by blister formation, either spontaneously or at sites of trauma. There are three general categories of EB: simplex, junctional, and dystrophic. The extent of blistering and the degree of scarring roughly correlate with the level of blister formation in the epidermis or dermis.

Dystrophic Epidermolysis Bullosa Research Association of America: http://www.debra.org.

161. **Should EB blisters be "popped"?**
The answer is **yes.** Because patients with EB have a genetic abnormalities of the proteins that hold their epidermis and dermis intact, the pressure from simple accumulation of fluid within an intact blister can cause the blister to expand. The blister should be drained after a gentle sterile alcohol preparation of the skin, and the blister roof should be left intact.

162. **Is EB a contraindication to routine childhood immunization?**
Although smallpox vaccine is contraindicated, children with EB should otherwise be immunized as per routine. Modifications in the technique may be necessary, such as being more gentle with the sterile skin preparation and not using an adhesive bandage after the immunization. Direct pressure should not be associated with blistering or erosions.
A circumferential nonadherent gauze wrap around the limb may be used after the procedure if a dressing is needed.

163. **What is the likely diagnosis for a 4-year-old who develops a 1-week history of widespread painful and pruritic bullous lesions with crusted lesions around which vesicles are arranged in a string-of-pearls appearance?**
Chronic bullous dermatosis of childhood. This is the most common acquired autoimmune bullous disease of young children. It is characterized on biopsy by immunoglobulin A (IgA) and C3 deposition along the basement membrane (sometimes called *linear IgA bullous dermatosis*). Although the differential diagnosis of bullous diseases is large, the appearance of a new vesicles or bullae in a string of pearls (or cluster-of-jewels) appearance around crusted or erythematous plaques is characteristic.

Sheehan M, Huddleston H, Mousdicas N: Chronic bullous dermatosis of childhood, *Arch Pediatr Adolesc Med* 162:581–582, 2008.

164. **Is steroid therapy beneficial for the treatment of Stevens-Johnson syndrome (SJS) or TEN?**
This is a continuing area of controversy; studies are inconclusive. In SJS, treatment may be considered early during the course if multiple mucosal surfaces are involved, but skin denudation is limited. The potential for steroids to increase medical complications (e.g., hemorrhage, infection) must be taken into account, but a large 2008 study found that it was lower than previously thought. If initiated, clinical response (or lack thereof) should be carefully followed, and steroids should be discontinued if the condition is worsening. Because most cases of SJS will spontaneously resolve, other therapies are vital: skin care, nutritional support, ophthalmologic care, and the treatment of secondary bacterial infections. Steroids have been reported to be associated with an increased mortality rate among patients with TEN.

Koh MJ-A, Yay Y-K: An update on Stevens-Johnson syndrome and toxic epidermal necrolysis in children, *Curr Opin Pediatr* 21:505–510, 2009.

Schneck J, Fagot JP, Sekula P, et al: Effects of treatment on the mortality of Stevens-Johnson syndrome and toxic epidermal necrolysis: a retrospective study on patients included in the EuroSCAR study, *J Am Acad Dermatol* 58:33–40, 2008.

165. **What therapy should be considered for patients with rapidly progressive SJS or TEN?**
Intravenous immunoglobulin should be considered. Caution should be used, especially in patients with poor renal function, hypercoagulable states, and IgA deficiency. Other therapies that have been used include cyclosporine and plasmapheresis.

Mittmann N, Chan B, Knowles S, et al: Intravenous immunoglobulin use in patients with toxic epidermal necrolysis and Stevens-Johnson syndrome, *Am J Clin Dermatol* 7:359–368, 2006.

166. **What infectious agent is most commonly associated with recurrent erythema multiforme?**
Herpes simplex virus.

167. **What common infectious agent should be considered in a child with SJS and a cough?**
Mycoplasma pneumoniae. It is the most common infection associated with SJS.

Bullen LK, Zenel JA: A 15-year-old female who has cough, rash and painful swallow, *Pediatr Rev* 26:176–181, 2005.

ACKNOWLEDGMENT

The editors gratefully acknowledge contributions by Drs. Robert Hayman and Leonard Kristal that were retained from the first three editions of *Pediatric Secrets*.

CHAPTER 5

EMERGENCY MEDICINE

Joan Bregstein, MD, Cindy Ganis Roskind, MD,
and F. Meridith Sonnett, MD

BIOTERRORISM

1. **Why are children more vulnerable to biologic agents than adults?**
   - **Anatomic and physiologic differences:** Thinner dermis, increased surface area-to-volume ratio, smaller relative blood volume, higher minute ventilation
   - **Developmental considerations:** Inability to flee dangerous situations, possible increased risk for posttraumatic stress disorder
   - **Some vaccines not licensed for children:** Anthrax (18 to 65 years), plague (18 to 61 years)
   - **Vaccines more dangerous in children:** Smallpox, yellow fever
   - **Antibiotics less familiar to pediatricians:** tetracyclines, fluoroquinolones

   Cieslak TJ, Henretig FM: Bioterrorism. *Pediatr Ann* 32:145–165, 2003.

   Centers for Disease Control and Prevention: http://www.bt.cdc.gov.

2. **What are the three routes of transmission of anthrax?**
   - **Inhalation:** Most feared; can lead to multiorgan hemorrhagic necrosis
   - **Cutaneous:** Inoculated through wound, causing a black, painless ulcer
   - **Ingestion:** May cause gastrointestinal (GI) or upper respiratory symptoms
   Bacillus anthracis, which is a spore-forming gram-positive rod, can survive for extended periods before entering the body, when it will germinate and proliferate (Fig. 5-1).

   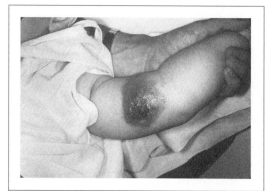

   Figure 5-1. Cutaneous anthrax in a child. (From Schachner LA, Hansen RC [eds]: Pediatric Dermatology, 3rd ed. Edinburgh, Mosby, 2003, p 1033.)

3. **How are the lesions of smallpox distinguished from varicella (chickenpox)?**
   - Smallpox lesions predominate on the face and extremities (centrifugal), whereas varicella lesions are typically heaviest on the trunk (centripetal).
   - The rash of smallpox progresses in similar stages (macules, papules, vesicles, crusting), whereas varicella is seen with multiple crops in differing stages.
   - Smallpox rash develops more slowly than varicella rash.

4. **How can the presenting symptoms of bubonic plague be differentiated from those of plague resulting from bioterrorism?**

Bubonic plague—of "black death" fame—resulted from the bite of fleas, which led to large tender regional adenopathy (the "bubo") with subsequent hematogenous dissemination, multiorgan involvement, and septicemia. In bioterrorism, the organism *Yersinia pestis* would be aerosolized, and inhalation would result in presentations more typical of pneumonic plague, with fever, chills, tachypnea, cough, and bloody sputum; lymphadenitis would likely be a later finding.

Dennis DT, Chow CC: Plague, *Pediatr Infect Dis J* 23:69–71, 2004.

5. **Why should families living near nuclear power plants keep potassium iodide (KI) in their medicine cabinets?**

The American Academy of Pediatrics recommends that families living within 10 miles of a nuclear power plant (or 50 miles in densely populated areas, where evacuations may be more difficult) have KI on hand in the event of a nuclear radiation catastrophe. KI will inhibit the uptake of radioactive iodine (^{131}I) into the thyroid gland. Children are more susceptible than adults to the subsequent development of thyroid cancer if exposed. If KI is administered within 1 hour, 90% of ^{131}I is blocked, but after 12 hours, there is little effect.

Committee on Environmental Health, American Academy of Pediatrics: Radiation disasters and children, *Pediatrics* 111:1455–1466, 2003.

6. **Why are children particularly vulnerable to the terrorism in the form of explosive and blast attacks?**

- Smaller mass results in greater force per unit of body surface from energy released by explosion.
- Children are more susceptible to fractures as a result of incompletely calcified growth plates.
- The chest wall has greater pliability in children, resulting in greater chance of cardiac and pulmonary injury from blast explosives.

Garth RJN: Blast injury of the ear: an overview and guide to management, *Injury* 26:363–366, 1995.

7. **What categories of agents should be considered in the event of a chemical weapons attack?**

- **Nerve:** Nerve agents are similar to organophosphate insecticides and include cholinesterase inhibitors, such as Sarin, Soman, and VX. Nerve agents inhibit the action of acetylcholinesterase at cholinergic neural synapses, where acetylcholine then accumulates. These agents are generally colorless, odorless, tasteless, and nonirritating to the skin. Nerve agent vapors are denser than air and tend to accumulate in low-lying areas, putting children at a higher risk than adults for exposure. The agents used in terrorist attacks are inhaled and absorbed through skin and mucous membranes.
- **Asphyxiants:** Toxic compounds that inhibit cytochrome oxidase, causing cellular anoxia and lactic acidosis (high anion gap). Hydrogen cyanide, the most commonly known toxicant in this class, is a colorless liquid or gas that smells like bitter almonds. Exposure to hydrogen cyanide produces rapid onset of tachypnea, tachycardia, and flushed skin, followed by nausea, vomiting, confusion, weakness, trembling, seizures, and death.
- **Choking and pulmonary agents:** Choking agents include chlorine and phosgene. When inhaled, these agents produce massive mucosal irritation and edema as well as significant damage to lung parenchyma.
- **Blistering and vesicant agents:** Blistering agents include sulfur mustard and Lewisite. Sulfur mustard is an alkylating agent that is highly toxic to rapidly reproducing and poorly differentiated cells; skin, pulmonary parenchyma, and bone marrow are frequently damaged. Lewisite is an arsenical compound that affects skin and eyes immediately on exposure.

8. **What should be the practitioner's initial management when a chemical weapons event occurs?**
The single most important first step for treating all chemical exposures is the **initial decontamination strategy**. Immediate removal of patient clothing can eliminate about 90% of contaminants.

CHILD ABUSE: PHYSICAL AND SEXUAL

9. **What is the most common cause of severe closed head trauma in infants younger than 1 year?**
Shaken impact or shaken baby syndrome. This injury is more likely to occur from severe shaking *and* impact; thus, the dual terminology. Violent shaking of an infant with sudden impact can result in subdural hematomas, subarachnoid hemorrhages, and cerebral infarcts. The diagnosis is suggested by the lack of a corroborating mechanism of injury in the face of a symptomatic child or, rarely, a confession by the perpetrator. In many cases, physical examination reveals retinal hemorrhages (Fig. 5-2). Other signs of trauma are usually lacking. Diagnosis is confirmed by computed tomography (CT) or magnetic resonance imaging (MRI). If a lumbar puncture is performed, the fluid may be bloody or xanthochromic. The prognosis is grim for an infant who is in coma from this abuse: 50% die, and nearly half of the survivors have significant neurologic sequelae.

David TJ: Nonaccidental head injury—the evidence, *Pediatr Radiol* 38:S370–S377, 2008.

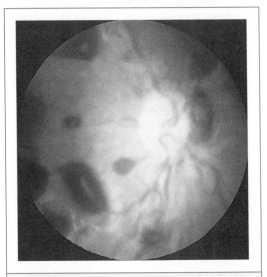

Figure 5-2. Retinal hemorrhages of victim of shaken baby/impact syndrome. (From Zitelli BJ, Davis HW: Atlas of Pediatric Physical Diagnosis, 4th ed. St. Louis, Mosby, 2002, p 181.)

KEY POINTS: RETINAL HEMORRHAGES

1. May be the only sign in an infant of a nonaccidental shaking injury

2. Almost never caused by seizures alone

3. Should always be assessed in an infant whose presenting symptoms include excessive irritability, lethargy, sepsis-like appearance, seizures, or coma

4. Should always be confirmed by an ophthalmologist

5. If found, should be followed by a skeletal series and cranial neuroimaging (computed tomography scanning and/or magnetic resonance imaging)

10. **Why is the diagnosis of shaken baby or impact syndrome often overlooked?**

When an infant is unconscious with respiratory distress, apnea, and/or seizures, the diagnosis of shaken baby syndrome should be considered. However, depending on the degree of shaking and the degree of resulting damage, the symptoms can be mild and nonspecific and may mimic symptoms of a viral illness, feeding disorder or dysfunction, or even colic. Victims may have a history of poor feeding, vomiting, lethargy, and/or irritability that may have gone on for days or weeks.

Jaspan T: Current controversies in the interpretation of nonaccidental head injury, *Pediatr Radiol* 38: S378–S387, 2008.

11. **What diagnostic tests may be contributory if shaken baby or impact syndrome is suspected?**
    - **Head CT:** Good for demonstrating subarachnoid and large extra-axial hemorrhages and mass effect; may be falsely negative, especially early in the presentation
    - **MRI:** Good for diagnosing subdural hemorrhages and intraparenchymal lesions; may miss subarachnoid blood and fractures
    - **Spinal tap:** May yield bloody cerebrospinal fluid
    - **Skeletal survey:** May be normal or may reveal acute or healed rib or other fractures, which are suggestive of abuse
    - **Complete blood count:** May be normal or may show mild to moderate anemia
    - **Prothrombin time and partial thromboplastin time:** May show mild to moderate abnormalities or reveal frank disseminated intravascular coagulation
    - **Amylase:** May show an increase, signifying possible pancreatic damage
    - **Liver function tests:** Abnormalities may signify occult liver injury

    American Academy of Pediatrics, Section on Radiology: Diagnostic imaging of child abuse, *Pediatrics* 123:1430–1435, 2009.

12. **What are important historical indicators of possible child abuse?**
    - Multiple previous hospital visits for injuries
    - History of untreated injuries
    - Cause of trauma not known or inappropriate for age or activity
    - Delay in seeking medical attention
    - History incompatible with injury
    - Parents unconcerned about injury or more concerned about unrelated minor problem (e.g., cold, headache)
    - History of abused siblings
    - Changing or inconsistent stories to explain injury

    Sirotnak AP, Grigsby T, Krugman RD: Physical abuse of children, *Pediatr Rev* 25:264–276, 2004.

    Kottmeier P: The battered child, *Pediatr Ann* 16:343–351, 1987.

13. **What important physical examination findings are indicators of possible child abuse?**
    - Burns, especially cigarette or immersion burns on the buttocks or perineum or burns in a stocking-and-glove distribution
    - Genital trauma or sexually transmitted infection in a prepubertal child
    - Signs of excessive corporal punishment (welts, belt or cord marks, bites)
    - Frenulum lacerations in young infants (associated with forced feeding)
    - Multiple bruises in various stages of resolution
    - Neurologic injury associated with retinal or scleral hemorrhages
    - Fractures suggestive of abuse (e.g., skull fractures in infants, metaphyseal fractures, posterior rib fractures, femur fractures in infants, scapular fractures)

Sirotnak AP, Grigsby T, Krugman RD: Physical abuse of children, *Pediatr Rev* 25:264–276, 2004.

Kottmeier P: The battered child, *Pediatr Ann* 16:343–351, 1987.

14. **If retinal hemorrhages are noted in a child with seizures, how likely are the seizures to have caused the hemorrhages?**
In theory, any seizure might cause retinal hemorrhages through a sudden rise in retinal venous pressure in conjunction with increased central venous and intrathoracic pressure. However, a prospective study of children with seizures who had ophthalmologic evaluation found no evidence of an association of seizures and retinal hemorrhages. Combining their data with some previous studies, the authors determined a prevalence of retinal hemorrhages with a seizure of only about 3 per 10,000—an extremely small likelihood. If retinal hemorrhages are found in a child with seizures, the possibility of nonaccidental injury must be explored.

Curcoy AI, Trenchs V, Morales M, et al: Do retinal haemorrhages occur in infants with convulsions? *Arch Dis Child* 94:873–875, 2009.

15. **When should child abuse be considered in the event of an unexplained death of a child?**
Always. Sudden infant death syndrome (SIDS) should be a diagnosis of exclusion in any unexplained death. Deaths as a result of SIDS usually occur during the first year of life, most commonly (90%) in children less than 7 months old. All children who die suddenly of unclear causes should have a complete physical examination that looks for signs of external trauma (e.g., bruises, injury to the genitalia) and an ophthalmologic examination that looks for retinal hemorrhages.

16. **Which conditions with ecchymoses can be mistaken for child abuse?**
    - **Mongolian spots (dermal melanosis):** These are commonly mistaken for bruises, especially when they occur elsewhere than the classic lumbosacral area; unlike bruises, they do not fade with time.
    - **Coagulation disorders:** In 20% of cases of hemophilia, there is no family history of disease; bruising may be noted in unusual places in response to minor trauma.
    - **Folk medicine:** Southeast Asian practices of spoon rubbing (quat sha) or coin rubbing (cao gio) can produce ecchymoses; the practice of cupping (the inversion of a heated cup on the back) produces circular ecchymoses.
    - **Moxibustion:** This is the Southeast Asian practice of burning an herbal substance on the child's abdomen to cure disease.
    - **Dyes:** Clothing dyes, especially from jeans, sometimes mimic bruising; they are easily removed with topical alcohol.
    - **Vasculitis:** Particularly Henoch-Schönlein purpura with a purpuric rash most commonly on the buttocks and lower extremities

Kaczor K, Pierce MC, et al: Bruising and physical child abuse, *Clin Pediatr Emerg Med* 7:153–160, 2006.

17. **How are fractures dated radiographically in children?**
After a fracture, the following will be seen:
    - **1 to 7 days:** Soft tissue swelling; fat and fascial planes blurred; sharp fracture line
    - **7 to 14 days:** Periosteal new bone formation as soft callus forms; blurring of fracture line; occurs earlier for infants, later for older children
    - **14 to 21 days:** More clearly defined (i.e., hard) callus forming as periosteal bone converts to lamellar bone
    - **21 to 42 days:** Peak of hard callus formation
    - **≥60 days:** Remodeling of bone begins with reshaping of the deformity (up to 1 to 2 years)
    - If the timing of an injury does not correlate with the dating of a fracture or if fractures at multiple stages of healing are present, child abuse should be suspected.

18. **What fractures are suggestive of child abuse?**
Spinal fractures, posterior and anterior rib fractures, skull fractures, metaphyseal chip fractures, and vertebral, femoral, pelvic, or scapular fractures. These are fractures that commonly result from twisting (spiral fractures), throwing, and beating. Metaphyseal chip fractures are the result of the forceful jerking of an extremity. Anterior and posterior rib fractures occur with severe side-to-side compression of the thorax; they are almost never caused by cardiopulmonary resuscitation (CPR). The description and forcefulness of injury should be consistent with the fracture. One should be especially suspicious if such fractures occur in a child who is not yet walking.

Pierce MC, Bertocci G: Fractures resulting from inflicted trauma: assessing injury and history compatibility, *Clin Pediatr Emerg Med* 7:143–148, 2006.

19. **What constitutes the skeletal survey?**
Skeletal injuries, particularly multiple healed lesions, are strong indicators of a pattern of abuse, particularly in the absence of sufficient clinical evidence to justify such a diagnosis. The skeletal survey is a multiple-imaging series that provides multiple views of the following:
- **Appendicular skeleton:** Humeri, forearms, hands, femurs, lower legs, and feet
- **Axial skeleton:** Thorax, pelvis (including mid- and lower lumbar spine), lumbar spine, cervical spine, and skull

"Body grams" (studies that encompass the entire child in one or two exposures) are not thought to be of sufficient sensitivity to be useful. If abuse is highly suspected and the initial study is normal, a follow-up series 2 weeks later will increase the diagnostic yield.

American Academy of Pediatrics, Section on Radiology: Diagnostic imaging of child abuse, *Pediatrics* 123:1430–1431, 2009.

20. **Up to what age should a skeletal survey be ordered?**
If physical abuse is suspected, the American Academy of Pediatrics recommends a mandatory study in children up to the age of 2 years. The yield diminishes after that age and is of little value after age 5 years.

American Academy of Pediatrics, Section on Radiology: Diagnostic imaging of child abuse, *Pediatrics* 123:1432, 2009.

21. **In addition to child abuse, what condition must you consider as a cause of multiple unexplained long bone fractures in a young child?**
Patients with **osteogenesis imperfecta** (OI) are suspected to be victims of child abuse because the history of the injury often does not explain the severity of the fracture. OI is a rare congenital disorder that presents with bone fragility. In addition to frequent fractures, patients with this disorder often present with the following:
- Blue sclera
- Ligamentous laxity
- Osteopenia
- Wormian skull bones
- Dentinogenesis imperfecta
- Family history of OI
- Hearing loss

22. **When are burn injuries suspicious for child abuse?**
Burn injuries account for about 5% of cases of physical abuse. As with other injuries, the description of the incident causing the burn should be consistent with the child's development and the extent and degree of the burn observed. The following types are suspicious for abuse:
- **Immersion burns:** Sharply demarcated lines on the hands and feet (stocking-and-glove distribution), buttocks, and perineum, with a uniform depth of burn; the immersion of a child in a hot bath is a classic example

■ **Geographic burns:** Burns, usually of second or third degree, in a distinct pattern, such as circular cigarette burns or steam iron burns

■ **Splash burns:** Pattern with droplet marks projecting away from the most involved area; splash marks on the back of the body usually require another person and may or may not be accidental

23. **How do you recognize Munchausen syndrome by proxy?**
In this form of child abuse, adults inflict illness on a child or falsify symptoms to obtain medical care for a child. Features include the following:
■ Recurrent episodes of a confusing medical picture
■ Multiple diagnostic evaluations at different medical centers ("doctor shopping")
■ Unsupportive marital relationship, often with maternal isolation
■ Compliant, cooperative, and overinvolved mother
■ Higher level of parental medical knowledge
■ Parental history of extensive medical treatment or illness
■ Conditions resolve with surveillance of the child in the hospital
■ Findings correlate with the presence of the parent

Schreier H: Munchausen by proxy defined, *Pediatrics* 110:985–988, 2002.

Ludwig S: Child abuse. In Fleisher GR, Ludwig S, editors: *Textbook of Pediatric Emergency Medicine*, ed 4, Baltimore, 2000, Lippincott Williams & Wilkins, p 1679.

24. **How often is sexual abuse committed by an individual known previously by the child or adolescent?**
Between 75% and 80% of the time. Relatives are the perpetrators in about one third of cases.

25. **After the documentation of history and a careful physical examination, what evidence should be collected in cases of suspected sexual abuse or assault of a postpubertal female?**
■ **Pregnancy test** if postmenarchal
■ **Evidence of sexual contact,** including two to three swabbed specimens from each area of assault for the following substances: sperm (motile and nonmotile), acid phosphatase (secreted by the prostate; component of seminal plasma), P_{30} (prostate glycoprotein present in seminal fluid), blood group antigens
■ Evidence to document perpetrator: foreign material on clothing, suspected nonpatient hairs; DNA testing (controversial)

American Academy of Pediatrics, Committee on Child Abuse and Neglect: Guidelines for the evaluation of sexual abuse in children, *Pediatrics* 116:506–512, 2005.

26. **If testing is done for sexually transmitted infections (STIs) after postpubertal sexual abuse or assault, which method of collection is preferable: culture or nucleic acid amplification tests (NAATs)?**
Because some courts will only accept positive culture results for gonorrhea and chlamydia (as opposed to NAATs and other indirect tests), **cultures** are preferable over NAATs for any case in which there is likely to be prosecution. However, there may be an advantage to using an NAAT in addition to a culture to detect chlamydia because the high sensitivity makes it more likely to detect before the end of the incubation period.

27. **After the initial emergency department (ED) visit for sexual assault, what kind of follow-up care should the ED physician offer?**
■ HIV follow-up counseling with infectious disease or HIV specialist in 3 to 5 days
■ Follow-up gynecologic examination at 1 to 2 weeks
■ Repeat serologic tests for syphilis and HIV in 6 weeks, 3 months, and 6 months
■ Psychiatric counseling

28. **What is the best predictor of *Neisseria gonorrhoeae* infection in children younger than 12 years who are examined for sexual abuse?**
Vaginal or urethral discharge. Without evidence of discharge, the likelihood of a culture result being positive is near zero. Conversely, the presence of vaginal discharge indicates an increased likelihood of sexual abuse.

> Berkoff MC, Zolotor AJ, Makoroff KL, et al: Has this prepubertal girl been sexually abused? *JAMA* 23:2779–2792, 2008.

> Sicoli RA, Losek, JD, Hudlett JM, et al: Indications for Neisseria gonorrhoeae cultures in children with suspected sexual abuse, *Arch Pediatr Adolesc Med* 149:86–89, 1995.

29. **If a child who is not sexually active is diagnosed with an infection caused by an STI-associated organism, how likely is sexual abuse the reason for acquisition?**
See Table 5-1.

TABLE 5-1. LIKELIHOOD OF SEXUAL ABUSE ACCORDING TO ORGANISM	
Organism	Likelihood of Sexual Abuse
Neisseria gonorrhoeae	Diagnostic
Treponema pallidum (syphilis)	Diagnostic
Chlamydia trachomatis	Diagnostic
Human immunodeficiency virus	Diagnostic
Trichomonas vaginalis	Highly suspicious
Condyloma acuminata	Suspicious
Herpes (genital location)	Suspicious
Bacterial vaginosis	Inconclusive

Adapted from American Academy of Pediatrics: Sexually transmitted diseases. In Pickering LK (ed): 2006 Red Book, 27th ed. Elk Grove Village, IL, American Academy of Pediatrics, 2006, p 172.

30. **Is the size of the hymenal opening an important finding in the diagnosis of sexual abuse?**
The hymenal opening is measured with a child in the supine, frog-leg position, and various studies have attempted to determine a size that most likely correlates with sexual abuse. The upper limit of normal had ranged from 4 to 8 mm, but variations in technique, positioning, and relative relaxation of the patient have rendered such measurements *generally unhelpful and nondiagnostic*. More important as part of the examination is inspection of the posterior hymen and surrounding tissues. Typically, a posterior rim of hymen measuring at least 1 mm is present unless there has been trauma. Complete transaction of the hymen leaves a permanent gap or defect. A full-thickness transaction through the posterior hymen (best visualized in the knee-chest position) is thought to be reliable evidence of trauma. Other variations of hymenal shape or size must be interpreted with caution because there is considerable overlap among abused and nonabused girls.

> Pillai M: Genital findings in prepubertal girls: what can be concluded from an examination? *J Pediatr Adolesc Gynecol* 21:177–185, 2008.

> Berkoff MC, Zolotor AJ, Makoroff KL, et al: Has this prepubertal girl been sexually abused? *JAMA* 23:2779–2792, 2008.

KEY POINTS: SEXUAL ABUSE

1. Most common physical finding: normal examination

2. Perpetrator known to victim in 75% to 80% of cases

3. Diagnostic of abuse: gonorrhea, syphilis, chlamydia, human immunodeficiency virus

4. Culture more medicolegally acceptable than nucleic acid amplification tests

5. Indications for immediate medical examination: alleged assault within 96 hours, ongoing bleeding, or evidence of acute injury

6. Use of accepted or standardized protocols important during evaluative process

31. **What is the most common finding of the physical examination of a child who has been sexually abused?**
A **normal physical examination** is the most common physical finding. It is crucial to know that a normal examination does not rule out sexual abuse.

32. **What are the date-rape drugs?**
Date-rape drugs are substances that render a patient incapable of saying "no" or asserting herself or himself, which makes it easier for a perpetrator to commit rape. The term typically applies to three drugs—*flunitrazepam (Rohypnol)*, *γ-hydroxybutyrate (GHB)*, and *ketamine hydrochloride*—which go by a variety of street names. The effects of these drugs, including somnolence, muscle relaxation, and profound sedation and amnesia, are enhanced by the concurrent use of alcohol.

     Kaufman M: Care of the adolescent sexual assault victim, *Pediatrics* 122:462–470, 2008.

33. **How can you tell whether a patient has been given a date-rape drug?**
Most of these drugs can be detected in blood and/or urine. However, because they are metabolized very quickly, it is important to screen early in your evaluation of the patient. For example, Rohypnol can be detected in blood for 24 hours and in urine up to 48 hours, GHB in urine only for up to 12 hours after ingestion, and ketamine in urine for up to 72 hours. None of these drugs is included in routine drug screen panels.

     Kaufman M: Care of the adolescent sexual assault victim, *Pediatrics* 122:462–470, 2008.

34. **If physical abuse is suspected, are physicians mandated to photograph physical findings?**
No. A good drawing of the physical findings is sufficient. However, if photographs are taken, a card with the patient's name and date of birth and the photographer's name and signature must be included in the photograph so that the patient can be clearly identified. In addition, the body part that is being photographed must be clearly identifiable. If abuse is suspected, it is not necessary to obtain parental consent to take photographs.

ENVIRONMENTAL INJURY

35. **How do fresh- and salt-water drowning differ?**
Fresh water injures the lung primarily by disrupting surfactant, thereby leading to alveolar collapse. Damage to the alveolar membranes leads to the transudation of fluid into the air spaces and pulmonary edema. **Salt water** pulls fluid into the air spaces directly by creating a strong osmotic gradient, and the accumulated water washes away surfactant, thereby leading to alveolar collapse. By either mechanism, patients develop ventilation-perfusion mismatch

and hypoxemia, which may require aggressive mechanical support. Ultimately, management for either fresh- or salt-water drowning is the same.

Harries M: Near drowning. *BMJ* 327:1336–1338, 2003.

Ibsen LM, Koch T: Submersion and asphyxial injury, *Crit Care Med* 30:S402–S408, 2002.

36. **What cardiovascular changes occur as body temperature falls?**
   - **31° to 32°C:** Elevated heart rate, cardiac output, and blood pressure; peripheral vasoconstriction and increased central vascular volume; normal electrocardiogram (ECG)
   - **28° to 31°C:** Diminished heart rate, cardiac output, and blood pressure; ECG irregularities include premature ventricular contractions (PVCs), supraventricular dysrhythmias, atrial fibrillation, and T-wave inversion
   - **<28°C:** Severe myocardial irritability; ventricular fibrillation, usually refractory to electrical defibrillation; often absent pulse or blood pressure; J waves on ECG

37. **What are the physiologic consequences of externally warming a severely hypothermic patient too rapidly?**
   - **Core temperature "after-drop":** The body temperature drops because external rewarming causes peripheral vasodilation and the return of cold venous blood to the core.
   - **Hypotension:** Peripheral vasodilation increases total vascular space, thereby causing a drop in blood pressure.
   - **Acidosis:** Lactic acid returns from the periphery, thereby resulting in rewarming acidosis.
   - **Dysrhythmias:** Rewarming alters acid-base and electrolyte status in the setting of an irritable myocardium.

38. **What are acceptable rewarming methods for the hypothermic child?**
   For patients with mild hypothermia (32° to 35°C), passive rewarming by removing cold clothing and placing the patient in a warm, dry environment with blankets is generally sufficient. Active external rewarming involves the use of heating blankets, hot-water bottles, and overhead warmers and can also be used for patients with acute hypothermia in the 32° to 35°C range. Active external rewarming should not be used for chronic hypothermia (>24 hours). More aggressive core rewarming techniques should be considered for patients with temperatures lower than 32°C. These techniques include gastric or colonic irrigation with warm fluids, peritoneal dialysis, pleural lavage, and extracorporeal blood rewarming with partial bypass. Intravenous and other fluids should be heated to 43°C. Patients should be given warmed, humidified oxygen by face mask or endotracheal tube (ETT).

39. **What organ systems are affected in patients suffering from heat stroke?**
   Heat stroke is a medical emergency of multisystem dysfunction that includes a very high body temperature (usually >41.5°C). The systems that are affected include the following:
   - **Central nervous system (CNS):** Confusion, seizures, and loss of consciousness
   - **Cardiovascular:** Hypotension as a result of volume depletion, peripheral vasodilation, and myocardial dysfunction
   - **Renal:** Acute tubular necrosis and renal failure, with marked electrolyte abnormalities
   - **Hepatocellular:** Injury and dysfunction
   - **Heme:** Abnormal hemostasis, often with signs of disseminated intravascular coagulation
   - **Muscle:** Rhabdomyolysis

   Jardine DS: Heat illness and heat stroke, *Pediatr Rev* 28:249–258, 2007.

40. **How quickly can temperature rise inside a closed automobile as a result of sunlight?**
   In one study in New Orleans, with an outside air temperature at 93°F, temperature reached 125°F in 20 minutes and 140°F in 40 minutes. Leaving the window slightly open

("cracking the window") did not affect the rapid temperature elevation. The dangers of leaving a child unattended in a vehicle for even a few minutes become readily apparent.

Gibbs LI, Lawrence DW, Kohn MA: Heat exposure in an enclosed automobile, *J La State Med Soc* 147:545–546, 1995.

41. **What is the "critical thermal maximum"?**
    42°C. This is the body temperature at which cell death begins as physiologic processes unravel. Enzymes denature, lipid membranes liquefy, mitochondria misfire, and protein production fails.

42. **What are the signs and symptoms of significant upper airway heat exposure in a patient who has been in a house fire?**
    - Carbonaceous sputum
    - Singed nasal hairs
    - Facial burns
    - Respiratory distress
    One should not rely on the presence of respiratory distress as an indicator for prompt endotracheal intubation. The first three signs listed previously represent significant heat exposure to the airway, and progressive swelling can rapidly progress to upper airway obstruction.

43. **What are the signs and symptoms of impeding respiratory failure as a result of mucosal injury and edema from heat exposure during a house fire?**
    - Hoarseness
    - Stridor
    - Increasing respiratory distress
    - Drooling and difficulty swallowing
    An endotracheal tube should be emergently considered for patients with the above signs and symptoms. Upper airway mucosal swelling may make intubation difficult, and the most experienced physician should perform this intervention.

44. **Which laboratory studies are needed for patients with suspected carbon monoxide poisoning?**
    - **Blood carboxyhemoglobin (HbCO) level**
      0% to 1%: Normal (smokers may have up to 5% to 10%)
      10% to 30%: Headache, exercise-induced dyspnea, confusion
      30% to 50%: Severe headache, nausea, vomiting, increased heart rate and respirations, visual disturbances, memory loss, ataxia
      50% to 70%: Convulsions, coma, severe cardiorespiratory compromise
      70%: Usually fatal
    - **Hemoglobin level:** To evaluate correctable anemia
    - **Arterial pH:** To detect acidosis
    - **Urinalysis for myoglobin:** With carbon monoxide poisoning, patients are susceptible to tissue and muscle breakdown with possible acute renal failure resulting from the renal deposition of myoglobin

45. **What are the key aspects of treatment for carbon monoxide poisoning in children?**
    - **100% oxygen** through non-rebreather mask until the carboxyhemoglobin (COHb) level falls to 5%.
      Half-life of COHb is 5 to 6 hours if the patient is breathing room air (at sea level).
      Half-life of COHb is reduced to 1 to 1½ hours if the patient is breathing 100% oxygen (at sea level).
      Half-life of COHb is reduced to under 1 hour with hyperbaric oxygen therapy.
    - **Consider treating for cyanide poisoning**, especially when metabolic acidosis persists after adequate treatment with oxygen.

- Refer for use of **hyperbaric oxygen** for the following conditions:
  History of coma, seizure, or abnormal mental status at the scene or in the ED
  Persistent metabolic acidosis
  Neonate
  Pregnancy (the fetus is more vulnerable to hypoxic effects of CO)
  HbCO level is more than 25%, even if the patient is neurologically intact

46. **Why is carbon monoxide such a deadly toxin?**
    - It is odorless and invisible and can overwhelm a patient without warning.
    - It is ubiquitous as a product of partial combustion (car exhaust emissions, household heating equipment, burning charcoal).
    - In the absence of a clear history, early CO intoxication is often misdiagnosed as a flu-like illness.
    - Intoxication often presents with common symptoms of headache, dizziness, and malaise.
    - CO develops a nearly irreversible bond with hemoglobin (with an affinity 200 to 300 times that of oxygen) that shifts the oxyhemoglobin dissociation curve to the left and changes its shape from sigmoidal to hyperbolic (with greatly diminished O_2 tissue release).
    - CO develops a strong bond with other heme-containing proteins, particularly in the mitochondria, thereby leading to metabolic acidosis and cellular dysfunction (especially in cardiac and CNS tissues).

    Weaver LK: Carbon monoxide poisoning, *N Engl J Med* 360:1217–1225, 2009.

47. **What are the different degrees of burn injuries?**
    See Table 5-2.

TABLE 5-2. CLASSIFICATION OF BURN WOUNDS			
Degree	**Depth**	**Clinical Appearance**	**Cause**
Superficial	Epidermis	Dry, erythematous	Sunburn, scald
Partial	Superficial dermis	Blisters, moist, erythematous	Scald, immersion, contact
	Deep dermis	White eschar	Grease, flash fire
Full thickness	Subcutaneous	Avascular—white/ dark, dry, waxy (yellow)	Prolonged immersion, flame, contact, grease, oil
	Muscle	Charred, skin surface cracked	Flame

Adapted from Coren CV: Burn injuries in children. Pediatr Ann 16:328–339, 1987.

48. **How does the "rule of nines" apply in children?**
    The "rule of nines" is a tool used to estimate the extent of burns in adults. For example, in adults, the entire arm is 9% of the total body surface area (TBSA), the front of the leg is another 9% of the TBSA, and so on. The resulting estimate of the extent of burns is particularly helpful for calculating fluid requirements. Correction for age is necessary with this formula because of differing body proportions. Therefore, for children, use the surface of a patient's palm, which represents about 1% of TBSA, as the tool for estimating the percentage of the TBSA affected by the burn (Fig. 5-3).

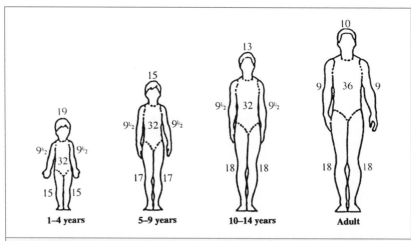

Figure 5-3. Rule of nines as applied to children. (From Carajel HF: Burn injuries. In Behrman RE [ed]: Nelson Textbook of Pediatrics, 14th ed. Philadelphia, WB Saunders, 1992, p 235.)

49. **Which burn injuries are indications for hospitalization?**
   - Partial-thickness burns covering more than 10% of the TBSA
   - Full-thickness burns covering more than 2% of the TBSA
   - Significant burns involving the hands, feet, face, joints, or perineum
   - Burns resulting from suspected child abuse
   - Electrical burns
   - Circumferential burns (which may predispose the patient to vascular compromise)
   - Explosion, inhalation, or chemical burns (in which other organ trauma may be involved)
   - Significant burns in children younger than 2 years

   Rodgers GL: Reducing the toll of childhood burns, *Contemp Pediatr* 17:152–173, 2000.

50. **Why are alkali burns worse than acid burns in the eye?**
   Alkali burns are caused by lye (e.g., Drano, Liquid Plummer), lime, or ammonia, in addition to other agents; they are characterized by liquefaction necrosis. They are worse than acid burns because the damage is ongoing. When spilled in the eye, **acid** is quickly buffered by tissue and limited in penetration by precipitated proteins; coagulation necrosis results, which is usually limited to the area of contact. Alkali, however, has a more rapid and deeper advancement, thereby causing progressive damage at the cellular level by combining with membrane lipids. This underscores the importance of extensive irrigation of the burned eye, particularly in cases of alkali burns.

51. **How do the injuries produced by lightning and high-voltage wires differ?**
   - **Lightning:** Consists of direct current of extremely high voltage (200,000 to 2,000,000,000 volts) delivered over milliseconds. Lightning exposure causes massive electrical countershock with asystole, respiratory arrest, and minimal tissue damage.
   - **High-voltage wires:** Deliver alternating current of lower voltage (rarely exceeding 70,000 volts) over a longer period of time. High-voltage exposure causes ventricular fibrillation and deep tissue injury. The resultant muscle necrosis can lead to substantial myoglobin release and renal failure.

52. **In electrical injury, is alternating or direct current more hazardous?**
At low voltages (e.g., those found in household electrical devices), **alternating current** is more dangerous than direct current. Exposure to alternating current can provoke tetanic muscle contractions so that the victim who has grasped an electrical source is unable to let go, thereby prolonging the exposure and producing greater tissue injury. Direct current or high-voltage alternating current typically causes a single forceful muscular contraction that will push or throw the victim away from the source.

53. **If a toddler suffers a full-thickness burn to the corner of the mouth after biting an electrical cord, what complications might ensue?**
Severe burns of the oral commissure can become markedly edematous within the first several hours. An eschar develops at the site, which can detach and cause significant *bleeding* from the labial artery 1 to 3 weeks later. *Scarring* can be extensive, and plastic surgeons should be consulted early during the management of this kind of injury.

54. **What agents are the most common causes of anaphylaxis seen in U.S. emergency rooms?**
Food. *Peanuts, tree nuts* (e.g., almonds, hazelnuts) and *seafood* head the list and are twice as common as bee stings as a trigger. Severe reactions occur 1 to 2 hours after exposure. Anaphylaxis may occur without a skin reaction, so a high index of suspicion is needed in a child with unexplained sudden bronchospasm, laryngospasm, severe GI symptoms, or poor responsiveness. In some adolescents, certain foods (e.g., wheat, celery, shellfish), if ingested within 4 hours of exercise, can lead to food-dependent, exercise-induced anaphylaxis. Risk factors for fatal anaphylactic reactions include a history of asthma, delayed diagnosis, and delayed administration of epinephrine.

Lack G: Food allergy. *N Engl J Med* 359:1252–1260, 2008.

Liberman DB, Teach SJ: Management of anaphylaxis in children, *Pediatr Emerg Care* 24: 861–866, 2008.

55. **What are important considerations when treating frostbite in children?**
- Rewarm the affected area in water with a temperature of 37° to 43°C (99° to 109°F) for 20 minutes.
- Never attempt to rewarm if there is risk for refreezing.
- Rubbing the affected area may cause further damage to tissue.

KEY POINTS: ENVIRONMENTAL INJURIES

1. Anaphylaxis in children: food (e.g., peanuts, tree nuts, seafood) is twice as common as insect stings as a cause.

2. Carbon monoxide poisoning is often misdiagnosed because the presenting symptoms can be flu-like.

3. Impending upper airway obstruction in house fires is more likely if there is the presence of carbonaceous sputum, singed nasal or facial hairs, or respiratory abnormalities (e.g., hoarseness, stridor).

4. Hospitalization is indicated for significant burns involving the hands, feet, joints, or perineum or if there are circumferential burns.

5. Alkali burns are worse than acid burns because of ongoing liquefaction necrosis.

LACERATIONS

56. What advice should be given over the telephone regarding the transportation of an avulsed digit?

Wrap the severed piece in dry gauze (sterile, if possible). Place the wrapped piece in a small, sealed plastic bag to minimize its contact with water. Place this bag in a container filled with ice. It is incorrect to place the avulsed piece in any liquid because this causes tissue swelling. Direct contact with ice is to be avoided to prevent tissue necrosis.

57. Which lacerations should be referred to a surgeon or an ED physician who is familiar with wound repair?

- Large, complex lacerations
- Stellate or flap lacerations
- Lacerations with questions of tissue viability
- Lacerations involving lip margins (vermilion border)
- Deep lacerations with nerve or tendon damage
- Knife and gunshot wounds
- Strong concern about cosmetic outcome by either the patient or the family
- Lacerations involving open fractures or joint penetration
- Lacerations involving the inner eyelid, owing to the potential of damage to the tear ducts
- Deep lacerations involving the cheek, owing to potential damage to the parotid or facial nerve

58. How many days should sutures remain in place?

Blood supply dictates healing: the more blood, the better and the faster the healing. In general, as the site of laceration proceeds, from head to toe, the length of time of suture placement increases: *eyelids*—3 days; *face, scalp*—5 days; *trunk, upper extremities*—7 to 10 days; and *lower extremities*—8 to 10 days.

59. When should a nerve injury be suspected in a finger laceration?

- **Abnormal testing of sensation** (diminished pain or two-point discrimination)
- **Abnormal autonomic function** (absence of sweat or lack of skin wrinkling after soaking in water)
- **Diminished range of motion of finger** (may also indicate joint, bone, or tendon disruption)
- **Pulsating blood emerging from the wound** (on the flexor aspect, the nerve is superficial to the digital artery, and arterial flow implies nerve damage)

60. What should be done if nerve damage is suspected?

For injuries to major nerves (e.g., the brachial plexus), immediate consultation is necessary. If the digital nerve is injured, immediate repair is not essential, and this is not a true emergency. Delayed nerve repair is very satisfactory, particularly in younger children. If an operating suite and personnel are not poised to proceed, skin closure can be done and the operation deferred (after surgical consultation). Care must be taken to avoid the use of a hemostat or clamp to stop arterial bleeding because this may cause further damage to the nerve. Simple pressure—often for extended periods—generally suffices.

61. Which lacerations should not be sutured?

Lacerations at high risk for infection should be considered for healing by secondary intention or delayed primary closure. As a general rule, these include cosmetically unimportant puncture wounds, human bites, lacerations involving mucosal surfaces (e.g., mouth, vagina), and wounds with a high probability of contamination (e.g., acquired in a garbage bin). Many authorities in the past recommended that wounds untreated for more than 6 to 12 hours on the arms and legs and for 12 to 24 hours on the face not be sutured. However, the type of wound and risk for infection are more important than any absolute time criterion.

For example, a noncontaminated laceration of the face should be considered for suturing even 24 hours after the injury. A good rule of thumb is as follows: If you can irrigate and clean a wound to the point at which it looks "fresh," you are safe to close it primarily. Otherwise, you should let it heal by secondary intention.

KEY POINTS: LACERATIONS

1. The best defense against infection in the setting of wound closure is copious irrigation.

2. Irrigation can be painful and should be done *after* local anesthetic is applied or infiltrated.

3. There is no one universal suture material that is good for all wounds. The material should be chosen based on location, size, and depth of the wound and the tensile strength that is required to easily appose the wound edges.

4. Suspect digital nerve injury if there is abnormal sensation, abnormal autonomic function, diminished range of motion of finger, or pulsating blood emerging from wound.

62. **Which are at greater risk for infection, dog bites or cat bites?**
Generally, infection rates are higher in **cat bites** because of the greater likelihood of a puncture wound rather than a laceration injury. Additionally, *Pasteurella multocida*, which is the most common pathogen responsible for infection, is present in higher concentrations in cat bites. Wounds caused by cat and dog bites usually contain multiple other organisms, including *Staphylococcus aureus*; *Moraxella*, *Streptococcus*, and *Neisseria* species; and anaerobes.

    Kannikeswaran N, Kamat D: Mammalian bites, *Clin Pediatr* 48:145–148, 2009.

    Talon DA, Citron DM, Abrahamian FM, et al: Bacteriologic analysis of infected dog and cat bites, *N Engl J Med* 340:85–92, 1999.

63. **Should antibiotic prophylaxis be given for dog, cat, and human bites?**
This is a controversial topic. Although antibiotics are widely prescribed following mammalian bites, prophylactic antibiotics have been shown to significantly reduce infections in only two settings: bites to the hands and human bites. Some experts recommend treatment for other "high-risk" injuries such as cat bites, foot wounds, puncture wounds, and wounds treated initially after 12 hours. It is important that all such wounds first be irrigated under pressure, cleaned, and débrided as necessary.

    Singer AJ, Dagum AB: Current management of acute cutaneous wounds, *N Engl J Med* 359: 1037–1046, 2008.

64. **Which animals most often carry the rabies virus?**
Although all species of animals are susceptible to rabies virus infection, only a species are important as reservoirs for the disease. In the United States, rabies has been identified most commonly in raccoons, skunks, foxes, coyotes and bats.

    www.cdc.gov/rabies/location/usa/surveillance/domestic_animals.html

65. **Which are more likely to be rabid: cats or dogs?**
During 2000-2004, more cats than dogs were reported rabid in the U.S. This may be due to the fact that there are fewer cat vaccination laws, fewer leash laws with cats and the fact that cats tend to roam more freely than dogs.

    www.cdc.gov/rabies/exposure/animals/domestic.html

66. **If at a local petting zoo a playful 20-month-old child is bitten by a duck, scratched by a rabbit (breaking skin), spit on by a camel, and licked on the face by a horse, should rabies prophylaxis be given?**

In general, no prophylaxis is needed for any of these animal wounds unless the animal is actively rabid. The local health department should be contacted if there is any question. Immediate rabies vaccination and rabies immune globulin are recommended for bites or scratches from bats, skunks, raccoons, foxes, and most other carnivores if these injuries break the skin. Bites from dogs and cats generally do not necessitate prophylaxis if the animal is healthy and can be observed closely for a 10-day period. No case in the United States has been attributed to a dog or cat that has remained healthy for the confinement period of 10 days.

American Academy of Pediatrics: Rabies. In Pickering LK, editor: *2009 Red Book*, ed 28, Elk Grove Village, IL, 2009, American Academy of Pediatrics, pp 552–559.

67. **When is the use of lidocaine with epinephrine contraindicated as a local anesthetic?**

When there is a question of tissue viability and in any instance in which vasoconstriction might produce ischemic injury to an end organ without an alternative blood supply (e.g., tip of the nose, margin of the ear, tip of the finger or toe)

68. **What are methods for decreasing the pain of local lidocaine infiltration?**
   - Infiltration into the subcutaneous layer
   - Infiltration at a slow rate
   - Buffering the anesthetic (e.g., with bicarbonate; there is no magic formula, but one that works is 10 parts lidocaine and 1 part bicarbonate)
   - Warming the anesthetic to body temperature
   - Using a small-gauge needle (e.g., 30 gauge)
   - Distracting the patient or the use of hypnosis or biofeedback

69. **What are some of the ingredients in the alphabet soup of topical anesthetics?**
   - **LET** (**l**idocaine, **e**pinephrine, and **t**etracaine)
   - **TAC** (**t**etracaine, **a**drenaline, and **c**ocaine)
   - **LMX** (4% and 5% lidocaine gel)
   - **V-TAC** (**v**iscous TAC)
   - **PLP** (**p**rilocaine, **l**idocaine, and **p**henylephrine)
   - **EMLA** (**e**utectic **m**ixture of **l**ocal **a**nesthetics, typically lidocaine and prilocaine)

   TAC was among the first of these to be developed, but its higher costs and safety concerns (as a result of the cocaine component) have resulted in others, particularly LET, replacing it as first-line therapy.

Zempsky WT: Pharmacologic approaches for reducing venous access pain in children, *Pediatrics* 122: S140–S153, 2008.

70. **Tissue adhesives: when and when not to consider?**

   Consider tissue adhesives for the following:
   - Wounds with good edge approximation and little wound tension
   - Wounds that are clean and linear
   - Wounds that ordinarily, if sutured, would require sutures 5-0 or smaller (i.e., wounds with little tension)

   Avoid tissue adhesives for the following:
   - Wounds where good edge approximation cannot be achieved (e.g., jagged wounds)
   - Bite or puncture wounds
   - Generally, wounds deeper than 5 mm
   - Hands, feet, or joints, unless the affected area can be immobilized

- Oral mucosa or other mucosal surfaces, or areas with increased amounts of moisture as in the perineum or axilla
- Patients with conditions that may delay wound healing (e.g., diabetes mellitus or patients on long-term steroids)

71. **In which situations might you choose absorbable over nonabsorbable sutures when repairing a pediatric laceration?**
An absorbable suture is generally one that loses most of its tensile strength in 1 to 3 weeks and is fully absorbed within 3 months. Traditionally, absorbable sutures were used only for deep sutures. However, recently, the use of absorbable sutures for percutaneous closure of wounds in adults and children has been advocated. The advantages of absorbable sutures include the elimination of a follow-up visit to remove the patient's sutures and the possibility of decreased scarring and infection. Ideal wound candidates for absorbable sutures include the following:
- Facial lacerations, where skin heals quickly and prolonged intact sutures may lead to a suboptimal cosmetic result
- Percutaneous closure of lacerations under casts or splints
- Closure of lacerations of the tongue or oral mucosa
- Hand and finger lacerations
- Nail bed lacerations

72. **What is the proper fluid to use for wound irrigation?**
Normal saline, sterile water, or even tap water may be used. Betadine surgical scrub solution should be avoided because it is abrasive to tissue.

Bansal BC, Wiebe RA, Perkins SD, Abramo TJ: Tap water for irrigation of lacerations, *Am J Emerg Med* 20:469–472, 2002.

73. **How is conscious sedation best managed in children?**
There is no single best method for the conscious sedation of pediatric patients for diagnostic, radiologic, or minor surgical procedures. Surveys indicate that a wide variety of approaches are used in emergency rooms and radiology suites, including opioids (morphine, fentanyl), benzodiazepines (diazepam, midazolam), barbiturates (pentobarbital, thiopental), and nonbarbiturate anesthetic-analgesic agents (ketamine). Although conscious sedation, by definition, is a state of medically-controlled depressed consciousness with a patent airway, maintained protective reflexes, and appropriate responses to stimulation on verbal command, the potential for rapidly developing problems should be anticipated. These can include hypoventilation, apnea, airway obstruction, and cardiorespiratory collapse. Consequently, pharmacologic agents used for conscious sedation should be administered under supervised conditions and in the presence of competent personnel who are capable of resuscitation, ongoing monitoring (especially pulse oximetry), and sufficient equipment for resuscitation (e.g., positive-pressure oxygen delivery system, suction apparatus). As a rule, few office settings are appropriate for conscious sedation.

Rutman MS: Sedation for emergent diagnostic imaging studies in pediatric patients, *Curr Opin Pediatr* 21:306–312, 2009.

Mandt MJ, Roback MG: Assessment and monitoring of pediatric procedural sedation, *Clin Pediatr Emerg Med* 8:223–231, 2007.

RESUSCITATION

74. **What are the main reasons for out-of-hospital cardiac arrest in pediatric patients?**
In a prospective study of 600 patients, the following were most common (in descending order of frequency):
- SIDS: About 25% of total, no survivors
- Trauma: Pedestrian auto, abuse

- Respiratory failure: Infectious, reactive airways, foreign body aspiration, drowning
- Cardiac abnormalities: Congenital, cardiomyopathy, myocarditis
- CNS abnormalities: Infection, seizure
- Burns

Young KD, Gausche-Hill M, McClung CD, Lewis RJ: A prospective, population-based study of the epidemiology and outcome of out-of-hospital pediatric cardiopulmonary arrest, *Pediatrics* 114: 157–164, 2004.

75. **What are common problems identified in CPR done by professionals?**
A number of studies have demonstrated that for both out-of-hospital and in-hospital arrests:
- CPR is typically not continuous, with chest compressions frequently interrupted as much as 50% of the time.
- Rates of compression are often inadequate (usually slow).
- Chest wall decompression (the relaxation phase) is incomplete.
- Ventilation rates are often too high.

Although most of these results are based on adult data, pediatric studies also indicate poor CPR quality.

Berg MD, Nadkarni VM, Berg RA: CPR—why the new emphasis? *Pediatr Clin N Am* 55:861–872, 2008.

76. **Why is the airway of an infant or child more prone to obstruction than that of an adult?**
- Infants have smaller margins of safety because of their smaller airway diameters. Because airflow is inversely proportional to the airway radius raised to the fourth power (Poiseuille's law), small changes in the diameter of the trachea can result in very large drops in airflow.
- The tracheal cartilage of an infant is softer and can result in collapse more easily if hyperextended.
- In an infant, the lumen of the oropharynx is relatively smaller, owing to the larger size of the tongue and smaller size of the mandible.
- Lower airways are smaller and less developed in children, thus putting them at risk for airway obstruction by small foreign bodies.

77. **How can the correct size of ETTs be estimated for a given patient?**
A guide is that the infant or child's pinky should approximate the internal diameter of the tube. When choosing an uncuffed ETT, the appropriate size may be estimated by the following formula:

$$(Age\ in\ years/4) + 4$$

When choosing a cuffed ETT, the appropriate size may be estimated by the following formula:

$$(Age\ in\ years/4) + 3$$

Because these formulas are estimates, it is advisable to have tubes one half size larger and smaller available before the intubation.

78. **When should cuffed versus uncuffed ETTs be used?**
In the past, uncuffed ETTs were recommended for children younger than 8 years because of concern that the cuff could place excessive pressure on the already narrow portion of the pediatric cricoid cartilage. However, the American Heart Association has advised that in an inpatient setting, a cuffed tube is as safe as an uncuffed tube for all beyond the newborn period. The cuffed tube may even be preferable in patients with poor lung compliance, high airway resistance, and large glottic air leaks.

Bingham RM, Proctor LT: Airway management, *Pediatr Clin N Am* 55:873–886, 2008.

79. **How should the appropriate depth of an ETT be calculated?**
After insertion of an ETT, the appropriate depth (measured from the gum line) may be approximated using the following formula for children older than 1 year:

$$(Age\ in\ years/2) + 12\ cm$$

These measurements should always be confirmed by clinical means and radiography.

80. **How should correct placement of an ETT be confirmed?**
    - Improvement or continued stability of vital signs including oxygen saturation
    - Bilateral chest wall rise
    - Bilateral symmetrical breath sounds
    - Absence of gastric insufflation sounds over the stomach
    - Use of an exhaled CO_2 detector device
    - Direct laryngoscopy
    - Chest radiography

81. **What is a laryngeal mask airway (LMA)?**
An **LMA** is an alternative device that can be used to ventilate children in the ED if an ETT is unable to be placed. It consists of an inflatable silicone mask and rubber connecting tube. It is inserted blindly into the pharynx, forming a low-pressure seal around the laryngeal inlet and permitting gentle positive-pressure ventilation. It does not confer the same protection against aspiration as an ETT, nor is it as stable.

82. **What emergency drugs can be given through an ETT?**
*L*idocaine, *e*pinephrine, *a*tropine, *n*aloxone (**LEAN**). Vasopressin can also be administered through an ETT. However, if available, intraosseous or intravenous administration is always preferable because absorption is more predictable. The optimal dose of most drugs through the endotracheal route is not known. However, recommendations for epinephrine are 10 times the intravenous dose, and for other drugs, 2 to 3 times the intravenous dose. If drugs are being given through the ETT, they should be followed with 5 mL of normal saline and positive-pressure ventilation.

> American Heart Association: *PALS Provider Manual*. Dallas, 2006, American Heart Association, p 164.

83. **What is the Sellick maneuver?**
The **Sellick maneuver** is the application of pressure on the cricoid ring to prevent aspiration. To prevent aspiration, cricoid pressure should be initiated during preparation for intubation from the time sedation is administered or bag-mask ventilation is initiated until the airway is demonstrated to be secure.

84. **What are the potential reasons for acute deterioration in an intubated patient?**
These can be remembered using the **DOPE** acronym:
    - **D**isplacement of the ETT
    - **O**bstruction of the ETT
    - **P**neumothorax
    - **E**quipment failure

> American Heart Association: *PALS Provider Manual*, Dallas, 2006, American Heart Association, p 195.

85. **When is atropine indicated during a resuscitation?**
Atropine may be administered to the child with symptomatic bradycardia with a pulse after other resuscitative measures (i.e., oxygenation, ventilation, and epinephrine) have been initiated. It is useful in breaking the vagally-mediated bradycardia associated with laryngoscopy and may have some benefit during the initial treatment of atrioventricular block.

The deleterious effects of a slow heart rate are more likely to occur in a younger child, whose cardiac output is more dependent on rate changes than volume or contractility changes. Atropine is no longer routinely recommended in the treatment of asystole in children.

American Heart Association: *PALS Provider Manual*, Dallas, 2006, American Heart Association, p 123.

86. **When is the use of calcium indicated during a resuscitation?**
Routine use of calcium is *generally not recommended* in resuscitation protocols because it has not been shown to improve survival until discharge nor to improve neurologic outcome. Calcium use may be justified in certain settings of resuscitation:
- Overdose of a calcium channel blocker
- Hyperkalemia resulting in cardiac dysrhythmia
- Documented hypocalcemia
- Hypermagnesemia
- Hyperkalemia

de Caen AR, Reis A, Bhutta A: Vascular access and drug therapy in pediatric resuscitation, *Pediatr Clin N Am* 55:909–927, 2008.

87. **Why is high-dose epinephrine no longer recommended in pediatric resuscitation?**
Although some studies had suggested an increased rate of return of spontaneous circulation in pediatric patients revived with high-dose epinephrine, a prospective, randomized, blinded trial comparing high-dose epinephrine (100 μg/kg) with standard-dose epinephrine (10 μg/kg) found no benefit. Additional, high-dose epinephrine may be harmful in cardiac arrest secondary to asphyxia.

Perondi MD, Reis AG, et al: A comparison of high-dose and standard-dose epinephrine in children with cardiac arrest, *N Engl J Med* 350:1722–1730, 2004.

88. **What are contraindications to the use of an intraosseous line?**
- Placement into a fractured bone
- Placement through dirty or infected skin
- Use in patients with bone disorders such as osteopetrosis or osteogenesis imperfecta
- Repeat attempt into the same bone (owing to risk for extravasation through the initial puncture site)

Blumberg SM, Gorn M, Crain EF: Intraosseous infusion: a review of methods and novel devices, *Pediatr Emerg Care* 24:50–56, 2008.

89. **Can laboratory tests be obtained from intraosseous lines?**
Compared with venipuncture, there appears to be a good correlation between serum and marrow electrolytes, hemoglobin, drug levels, blood group typing, and renal function tests. Correlation is poorer with liver function tests and arterial blood gas studies (Pco_2 and Po_2). Additionally, the positive correlations appear to worsen after 30 minutes of CPR and/or drug and fluid administration. The most reliable samples on which to base clinical decisions would be those obtained at the time of intraosseous line placement early in the resuscitation.

Blumberg SM, Gorn M, Crain EF: Intraosseous infusion: a review of methods and novel devices, *Pediatr Emerg Care* 24:51, 2008.

90. **What are the complications of intraosseous lines?**
Significant morbidity is very uncommon ($<1\%$). The most common problems are extravasation of fluids and superficial skin infections. Osteomyelitis is rare ($<0.6\%$) and typically only occurs with prolonged infusions. Other rare complications are skin necrosis, bone fractures, and compartment syndrome. Although there is the theoretical risk for

significant bone growth arrest, growth plate damage, and fat embolism, these have not been reported. Obtaining venous access and discontinuing intraosseous infusions as soon as possible after stabilization have been recommended as means to further minimize complications.

Blumberg SM, Gorn M, Crain EF: Intraosseous infusion: a review of methods and novel devices, *Pediatr Emerg Care* 24:51, 2008.

91. **What features indicate that an intraosseous needle has been correctly placed?**
- A soft pop should be felt as you break through the cortex.
- The needle should be very stable.
- There should be free flow of intravenous fluids without infiltration of subcutaneous tissues.
- Bone marrow aspiration, although confirming placement, may not always be possible even when needle placement is correct. Therefore, if you cannot aspirate marrow, you should rely on other signs for determination of placement.

92. **How can a child's weight be estimated?**
Some rules of thumb:
- An average term neonate weighs 3 kg
- An average 1-year-old weighs 10 kg
- An average 5-year-old weighs 20 kg
The following formula may also be used:

$$(Age \times 3) + 7$$

A Broselow tape may also be used.

Luscombe M, Owens B: Weight estimation in resuscitation: is the current formula still valid? *Arch Dis Child* 92:412–415, 2007.

93. **Name the potentially reversible causes of cardiac arrest.**
- **H**s: **H**ypoxemia, **h**ypovolemia, **h**ypothermia, **h**yper/**h**ypokalemia, **h**ypoglycemia, and **h**ydrogen ion (acidosis)
- **T**s: **T**amponade, **t**ension pneumothorax, **t**oxins, and **t**hromboembolism

American Heart Association: *PALS Provider Manual*, Dallas, 2006, American Heart Association, p 178.

94. **What are the typical clinical findings associated with supraventricular tachycardia (SVT)?**
- Sudden onset
- Heart rate generally more than 180 beats per minute in children and more than 220 beats per minute in infants
- Minimal heart rate variability
- Absent, abnormal, or inverted P waves
- Infants: Signs and/or symptoms that are nonspecific or, if SVT for hours or days, suggestive of congestive heart failure or shock (e.g., poor feeding, irritability, vomiting, cyanosis, pallor, cough, respiratory distress, lethargy)
- Verbal children: Palpitations and fluttering in the chest

Salerno JC, Seslar SP: Supraventricular tachycardia, *Arch Pediatr Adolesc Med* 163:268–274, 2009.

95. **If an infant develops SVT, how long before congestive heart failure (CHF) develops?**
It is rare for an infant to develop CHF from SVT in less than 24 hours. When SVT is present for 24 to 36 hours, about 20% develop CHF. At 48 hours, the number increases to 50%.

Salerno JC, Seslar SP: Supraventricular tachycardia, *Arch Pediatr Adolesc Med* 163:268–274, 2009.

96. **What factors are predictive of outcomes after pediatric cardiac arrest?**
See Table 5-3.

TABLE 5-3. PREDICTIVE FACTORS IN PEDIATRIC CARDIAC ARREST

Good Outcome	Poor Outcome
Initiation of prompt CPR	Delayed CPR
Witnessed event	Unwitnessed event
Out-of-hospital arrest	In-hospital arrest
Short interval to EMS survival in out-of-hospital arrests	Prolonged EMS response time
Short duration of CPR	Prolonged resuscitation
Initial rhythm of VT or VF	Initial nonshockable rhythm
	Submersion victims with pulseless VT/VF
	Out-of-hospital traumatic arrest
	In-hospital arrest secondary to septic shock

CPR, cardiopulmonary resuscitation; EMS, emergency medical services; VF, ventricular fibrillation; VT, ventricular tachycardia.

American Heart Association: *PALS Provider Manual*, Dallas, 2006, American Heart Association, p 153.

97. **Are fixed and dilated pupils a contraindication to resuscitation for a patient in cardiac arrest?**
No. Pupillary dilation begins 15 seconds after cardiac arrest and is complete after about 1 minute and 45 seconds. It may only be a sign of transient hypoxia. The only absolute contraindications to resuscitation are rigor mortis, corneal clouding, dependent lividity, and decapitation.

98. **When should a failing resuscitation be stopped?**
Although there are no definitive guidelines, some studies have suggested that when **more than two rounds of epinephrine** have been given and/or **more than 20 minutes** have elapsed since the initiation of resuscitation without clinical cardiovascular or neurologic improvement, the likelihood of death or survival with neurologic devastation greatly increases. Unwitnessed out-of-hospital arrests are almost always associated with a poor outcome. In settings of hypothermia, asystolic patients should be rewarmed to 36°C before resuscitation is discontinued. In patients with acute, reversible conditions such as drug toxicity, extracorporeal cardiac life support may be considered if available.

American Heart Association: *PALS Provider Manual*. Dallas, 2006, American Heart Association, p 182.

Schindler M, Bohn D, Cox PN, et al: Outcome of out-of-hospital cardiac or respiratory arrest in children, *N Engl J Med* 335:1473–1479, 1996.

99. **Why is resuscitation less successful in children than in adults?**
Adults more commonly experience collapse and arrest from primary cardiac disease and associated dysrhythmias—ventricular tachycardia and fibrillation. These are more readily reversible and carry a better prognosis. **Children**, however, have cardiac arrest as a secondary phenomenon from other processes, such as respiratory obstruction or apnea, often associated with infection, hypoxia, acidosis, or hypovolemia. Primary cardiac arrest

is rare. The most common dysrhythmia associated with pediatric cardiac arrest is asystole. It is less frequently reversible, and by the time a child has cardiac arrest, severe neurologic damage is almost always present.

SHOCK

100. **Are all children in shock hypotensive?**
No. Shock is an acute syndrome resulting from cardiovascular dysfunction that renders the circulatory system unable to provide oxygen and substrates to the body. In the initial stages of shock (*compensated shock*), blood pressure is often preserved.

101. **What are the signs and symptoms of early or compensated shock?**
- Unexplained tachycardia
- Mild tachypnea
- Delayed capillary refill
- Orthostatic changes in pressure or pulse
- Irritability

102. **What are the signs and symptoms of late or uncompensated shock?**
- Increased tachycardia
- Increased tachypnea
- Poor peripheral pulses
- Capillary refill markedly delayed
- Cool extremities
- Hypotension
- Altered mental status
- Low urine output

KEY POINTS: SIGNS AND SYMPTOMS OF SHOCK

1. Tachycardia

2. Poor peripheral pulses

3. Slow capillary refill

4. Cool extremities

5. Hypotension

6. Altered mental status

103. **How much blood volume can be lost before hypotension may be seen in an infant?**
The total blood volume in a newborn is 85 mL/kg and in an infant is 65 mL/kg. Seventy percent is contained within the venous side, 12% in the capillary beds, and 8% within the arterial side. A child has significant vasoconstricting abilities, and hypotension may not be seen until to 50% of the blood volume is lost. Thus, in the setting of uncompensated shock, rapid fluid boluses of up to 30 to 40 mL/kg may be necessary to restore intravascular volume.

Carcillo JA, Han K, Lin J, Orr R: Goal-directed management of pediatric shock in the emergency department, *Clin Pediatr Emerg Med* 8:165–175, 2007.

104. **What rule of thumb defines hypotension in children (e.g., systolic blood pressure <5th percentile for age)?**
See Table 5-4.

TABLE 5-4. HYPOTENSION IN CHILDREN	
Age	Systolic Blood Pressure (mm Hg)
<1 month	≤60
1 month to 1 year	≤70
1 to 10 years	≤70 + (2 × age in years)
>10 years	≤90

American Heart Association: *PALS* Provider Manual, Dallas, 2006, American Heart Association.

105. **What types of shock can occur in children?**
   ■ **Hypovolemic:** Decreased circulating volume (most common cause in children)
   ■ **Distributive:** Pooling of blood in peripheral vasculature (septic, anaphylactic, neurogenic)
   ■ **Cardiogenic:** Cardiac dysfunction with decreased cardiac output (e.g., congenital heart disease, dysrhythmia)
   ■ **Obstructive:** Mechanical obstruction of ventricular outflow tract (e.g., cardiac tamponade, tension pneumothorax)

106. **What are the hallmarks of septic shock?**
   ■ Fever or hypothermia
   ■ Metabolic acidosis
   ■ Vasodilation: widened pulse pressure and/or hypotension, bounding pulses

107. **What is the initial management algorithm for septic shock?**
Early recognition of sepsis and initiation of therapy is important to outcome.
   ■ Control and/or maintain airway
   ■ Recognize poor perfusion and shock
   ■ Push 20 mL/kg up to 80 mL/kg of isotonic crystalloid solution as rapidly as possible.
   ■ If there is still evidence of shock or poor perfusion, begin vasoactive therapy, titrating to perfusion status, blood pressure, and mixed venous O_2 saturation.

   American Heart Association: *PALS Provider Manual*, Dallas, American Heart Association, 2006.

108. **Are corticosteroids recommended for the treatment of septic shock?**
There have been some studies in adults suggesting that corticosteroids may be beneficial for the treatment of septic shock. Currently, corticosteroids are recommended only for children who may have *catecholamine-resistant septic shock* or who have a *clear history or evidence of adrenal insufficiency*. Even in these scenarios, use of steroids has not been convincingly shown to impart survival advantage in children.

   Clark L, Preissig C, Rigby MR, et al: Endocrine issues in the pediatric intensive care unit, *Pediatr Clin N Am* 55:805–833, 2008.

   Markovitz BP, Goodman DM, Watson S, et al: A retrospective cohort study of prognostic factors associated with outcome in pediatric severe sepsis: what is the role of steroids? *Pediatr Crit Care Med* 6:270–274, 2005.

109. **What is the most important pharmacologic therapy for anaphylactic shock?**
Epinephrine. Epinephrine should be administered intramuscularly as soon as possible. Plasma concentrations of epinephrine appear to be highest when given intramuscularly in

the thigh compared with subcutaneously or intramuscularly in the arm. If the patient
has severe refractory symptoms and hypotension, epinephrine may be given intravascularly.
Failure to administer epinephrine quickly increases the risk for death from anaphylaxis.

Liberman DB, Teach SJ: Management of anaphylaxis in children, *Pediatr Emerg Med* 24:
861–866, 2008.

110. **What are the possible causes if a 4-day-old infant presents to the ED with
evidence of shock and altered mental status? What is the differential
diagnosis for shock in the newborn period?**
The differential diagnosis is broad, but remember the mnemonic **THE MISFITS**:
- **T**rauma (nonaccidental and accidental)
- **H**eart disease and hypovolemia
- **E**ndocrine (e.g., congenital adrenal hyperplasia)
- **M**etabolic (electrolyte)
- **I**nborn errors of metabolism
- **S**epsis (e.g., meningitis, pneumonia, urinary tract infection)
- **F**ormula mishaps (e.g., underdilution or overdilution)
- **I**ntestinal catastrophes (e.g., volvulus, intussusception, necrotizing enterocolitis)
- **T**oxins and poisons
- **S**eizures

Brousseau T, Sharieff GQ: Newborn emergencies: the first 30 days of life, *Pediatr Clin N Am*
53:69–84, 2006.

111. **A 4-day-old infant presents to the ED in shock with evidence of CHF and
cyanosis. In addition to managing the airway and breathing, what is the first
line of pharmacologic therapy?**
This baby likely has congenital heart disease with a ductal-dependent lesion such as
hypoplastic left heart syndrome or coarctation of the aorta. The baby will require
prostaglandin E_1 infusion to maintain the patency of the ductus arteriosus until corrective
surgery can be performed.

112. **What are the four classes of medications that can be used to support cardiac
output?**
- **Inotropes:** Increase cardiac contractility and often heart rate (e.g., norepinephrine)
- **Vasopressors:** Increase vascular resistance and blood pressure (e.g., higher-dose
dopamine and dobutamine)
- **Vasodilators:** Decrease vascular resistance and cardiac afterload and promote peripheral
perfusion (e.g., sodium nitroprusside)
- **Inodilators:** Increase cardiac contractility and reduce afterload (e.g., milrinone)

113. **What is the likely type of shock for an 8-year-old who, following a head-first
fall into an unfilled swimming pool, presents to the ED with a normal heart
rate of 90 beats per minute, is hypotensive (50/30 mm Hg) despite excessive
fluid resuscitation, and has multiple CT scans that reveal only a small cerebral
contusion?**
This patient is most likely suffering from *neurogenic shock*. Loss of sympathetic tone
prevents the expected tachycardic response. The hallmarks of neurogenic shock are
hypotension with either bradycardia or a normal heart rate despite fluid replenishment. If
the hypotension cannot be corrected with fluid expansion, vasopressor therapy may be
required.

KEY POINTS: SHOCK IN PEDIATRIC TRAUMA

1. Often masked in pediatric patients because the inherent reserve in a child allows for the maintenance of vital signs in the normal range, even in the presence of severe hemodynamic compromise

2. Suspected in patients with tachycardia, a decrease in pulse pressure >20 mm Hg, skin mottling, cool extremities, delayed capillary refill (>2 seconds), and altered mental status

3. Presence of hypotension in a child represents a state of uncompensated shock and indicates severe blood loss of >45% of circulating blood volume

4. Not explainable by head trauma alone, except in the case of an infant with open fontanels and unfused cranial sutures who may have a significant hemorrhage into the subgaleal or epidural space

5. May be associated with long bone (particularly femur) and pelvic fractures

6. Should quickly prompt an evaluation of the child's abdomen for the source of blood loss

TOXICOLOGY

114. **What are the most common poisonings in children younger than 6 years?**
See Table 5-5.

TABLE 5-5. COMMON POISONINGS IN CHILDREN	
Nonpharmaceuticals	Pharmaceuticals
Cosmetics and personal care products	Analgesics
Cleaning substances	Cough and cold preparations
Plants, including mushrooms and tobacco	Topical agents
Battery, toys, and other foreign bodies	Vitamins
Insecticides, pesticides, and rodenticides	Antimicrobials

Bronstein AC, Spyker DA, Cantilena JR, et al: Annual Report of the American Association of Poison Control Centers' National Poison Data System: 25th Annual Report, Clin Toxicol 46:927–1057, 2007, 2008.

115. **Which medications can kill a 10-kg toddler with one or two tablets, capsules, or teaspoonfuls?**
- **Tricyclic antidepressants** (amitriptyline, imipramine, desipramine)
- **Antipsychotics** (thioridazine, chlorpromazine)
- **Antimalarials** (chloroquine, hydroxychloroquine)
- **Antiarrhythmics** (procainamide, flecainide)
- **Calcium channel blockers** (nifedipine, verapamil)
- **Oral hypoglycemics** (glyburide, glipizide)
- **Opioids** (methadone, hydrocodone)
- **Imidazolines** (clonidine, tetrahydrozoline)

Bar-Oz B, Levichek Z, Koren G: Medications that can be fatal for a toddler with one tablet or teaspoonful, *Paediatr Drugs* 6:123–126, 2004.

116. **What medication causes the most overdose deaths in children each year in the United States?**

Acetaminophen. Large numbers of accidental and suicidal intoxications occur each year in part owing to its widespread availability.

> Hanhan UA: The poisoned child in the pediatric intensive care unit, *Pediatr Clin N Am* 55: 669–686, 2008.

KEY POINTS: ACETAMINOPHEN OVERDOSE

1. Significant ingestions may have no initial symptoms.

2. Assess for co-ingestions.

3. Administer charcoal if ingestion was within 4 hours of treatment.

4. Assess plasma acetaminophen level and apply nomogram.

5. Administer the antidote *N*-acetylcysteine if ingestion was within 8 hours of treatment.

117. **Name the toxicology "time bombs."**

Time bombs are medications that lack symptoms early after ingestion but later have a profoundly toxic course.
- **Acetaminophen** (delayed hepatic injury)
- **Iron** (delayed cyanosis and profound metabolic acidosis)
- **Alcohols**—methanol (delayed acidosis), ethylene glycol (delayed nephrotoxicity)
- **Lithium**
- **Anticonvulsants**—phenytoin (Dilantin), carbamazepine
- **Time-release medications**

118. **What empirical drug therapies are indicated for the poisoned child who presents with altered mental status?**

All poisoned patients with depressed mental status should receive oxygen through non-rebreather face mask. Blood glucose should be rapidly evaluated or empirical treatment for hypoglycemia with intravenous glucose, 0.5 g/kg, initiated. Hypoglycemia is associated with ingestion of ethanol, β-blockers, and oral hypoglycemic agents. Naloxone may be given as a diagnostic and therapeutic measure in the event of suspected or known opioid ingestion.

119. **What is gastrointestinal decontamination?**

Gastrointestinal decontamination refers to a variety of medications that may be administered and techniques that may be used to decrease the absorption of ingested poisons. Methods of gastrointestinal decontamination include activated charcoal, whole bowel irrigation, and gastric lavage. The effectiveness of these techniques is difficult to study, and much of the available evidence is based on animal and volunteer studies.

120. **How does single-dose activated charcoal work and when should it be considered?**

Single-dose activated charcoal is prepared as a liquid slurry and given orally to a poisoned patient. As it enters the stomach, it adsorbs toxins, thereby preventing absorption into the circulation. It is most efficacious when given within 1 hour of the time of ingestion.

Single-dose activated charcoal may be considered in patients who have ingested a potentially toxic ingestion that is known to be adsorbed by charcoal within 1 hour of presentation. Charcoal is contraindicated in patients whose airway reflexes are compromised, and it should not be given through nasogastric tube unless the airway is protected with an ETT because of the risk for aspiration.

American Academy of Clinical Toxicology, European Association of Poisons Centres and Clinical Toxicologists: Position statement: single-dose activated charcoal, *J Toxicol Clin Toxicol* 43:61, 2005.

121. **Should activated charcoal be given to a sleepy 2-year-old girl who consumed half a bottle of a liquid antihistamine 2 hours before evaluation?**
No. This child has a potentially compromised airway because of her altered mental status. In addition, the effectiveness of activated charcoal is known to decrease rapidly with time. Therefore, in this clinical scenario, the risks of administering charcoal and potentially causing vomiting and aspiration outweigh the benefits.

American Academy of Clinical Toxicology, European Association of Poisons Centres and Clinical Toxicologists: Position statement: single-dose activated charcoal, *J Toxicol Clin Toxicol* 43:61, 2005.

122. **For what substances is charcoal not recommended?**
■ Hydrocarbons, because of possible increased risk for aspiration
■ Others: acids, alcohols, alkalis, cyanide, iron, heavy metals, and lithium

American Academy of Clinical Toxicology, European Association of Poisons Centres and Clinical Toxicologists: Position statement: single-dose activated charcoal, *J Toxicol Clin Toxicol* 43:61, 2005.

123. **When is gastric lavage indicated?**
Gastric lavage involves the passage of a large orogastric tube (e.g., 24-Fr orogastric for a toddler, 36-Fr orogastric for a teenager) with sequential administration and aspiration of small volumes of normal saline (10 mL/kg in a child; 200-300 mL in an adult) with the intent of removing toxic substances present in the stomach. Efficacy remains unproved, and complications are significant (e.g., laryngospasm, esophageal injury, aspiration pneumonia); it should not be used routinely. However, it may be considered for patients with a life-threatening quantity of a poisonous ingestion occurring within 60 minutes of evaluation whose airway is protected.

American Academy of Clinical Toxicology, European Association of Poisons Centres and Clinical Toxicologists: Position statement: gastric lavage, *J Toxicol Clin Toxicol* 42:933, 2004.

124. **What are the indications for whole bowel irrigation (WBI) in acute ingestions?**
This is a method of gastrointestinal decontamination using a large volume of polyethylene glycol–balanced electrolyte solution such as Go-LYTELY given by mouth or nasogastric tube. These solutions are not known to cause electrolyte imbalance because they are neither significantly absorbed nor do they exert osmotic effect. WBI may be considered for toxic ingestions of sustained-release or enteric-coated medications. It may also be helpful in ingestions of large amounts of iron, or packets of illicit drugs. The most important contraindication to WBI is airway compromise.

American Academy of Clinical Toxicology, European Association of Poisons Centres and Clinical Toxicologists: Position statement: whole bowel irrigation, *J Toxicol Clin Toxicol* 42:843, 2004.

KEY POINTS: TOXICOLOGY

1. Ipecac is no longer routinely recommended for poisoning.

2. Activated charcoal is most efficacious if given within 1 hour of ingestion.

3. Gastric lavage has unproven efficacy for most ingestions.

4. Whole bowel irrigation is indicated for sustained-release or enteric-coated substances.

5. Alkalinization of urine still considered valuable in the management of acute overdoses of salicylates, barbiturates, or tricyclic antidepressants.

125. **How is the manipulation of urinary pH used in treating poisonings?**
Acidification or *alkalinization* of the urine to enhance the excretion of weak acids and bases has been a traditional way to enhance the elimination of toxicologic agents. In recent years, its use has been limited because of the potential complications from fluid overload (e.g., pulmonary and cerebral edema), the risk for acidemia, and the use of other therapeutic advancements (e.g., hemodialysis). However, alkaline diuresis is still considered valuable in the management of acute overdoses of salicylates, barbiturates, or tricyclic antidepressants.

126. **What ingestions and exposures have available antidotes?**
See Table 5-6.

TABLE 5-6. ANTIDOTES

Ingestion or Exposure	Antidote
Acetaminophen	*N*-acetylcysteine (Mucomyst)
Anticholinergics	Physostigmine
Benzodiazepines	Flumazenil
β-Blockers	Glucagon
Carbon monoxide	Hyperbaric oxygen chamber
Calcium channel blocker	Calcium, glucagon
Cyanide	Sodium nitrite, sodium thiosulfate
Digoxin	Digibind (antidigoxin antibody)
Ethylene glycol	Ethanol, fomepizole
Iron	Deferoxamine
Isoniazid	Pyridoxine (vitamin B_6)
Lead	EDTA, DMSA
Mercury	Dimercaprol, DMSA
Methanol	Ethanol
Methemoglobinemic agents	Methylene blue
Opiates	Naloxone, nalmefene
Organophosphates	Atropine, pralidoxime
Phenothiazines (dystonic reaction)	Diphenhydramine
Tricyclics	Bicarbonate
Warfarin (rat poison)	Vitamin K

127. **Narcan is considered an antidote for which kinds of ingestions?**
   Narcan (naloxone) is an antidote for opioid drugs. It reverses the CNS and respiratory depression of morphine and heroin and clears the depressed sensorium in overdoses due to many of the synthetic opioids, including propoxyphene, codeine, dextromethorphan, pentazocine, and meperidine. It is also a known antidote for clonidine.

128. **Which ingestions are radiopaque on abdominal radiograph?**
   The mnemonic **CHIPS** indicates possible suspects.
   - **C**hloral hydrate
   - **H**eavy metals (arsenic, iron, lead)
   - **I**odides
   - **P**henothiazines, psychotropics (cyclic antidepressants)
   - **S**low-release capsules, enteric-coated tablets

   The likelihood of radiopacity depends on numerous factors, including weight of the patient, size of the ingestion, and composition of the pill matrix.

   Barkin RM, Kulig KW, Rumack BH: Poisoning and overdose. In Barkin RM, Rosen P, editors: *Emergency Pediatrics*, ed 4, St. Louis, 1994, Mosby, p 335.

129. **What is a toxidrome?**
   A *toxidrome* is a clinical constellation of signs and symptoms that is very suggestive of a particular poisoning or category of intoxication. For example, patients with salicylate overdose commonly present with fever, hyperpnea and tachypnea, abnormal mental status (ranging from lethargy to coma), tinnitus, vomiting, and sometimes oil of wintergreen odor from methyl salicylate.

   Shannon M: Ingestion of toxic substances by children, *N Engl J Med* 342:186–191, 2000.

130. **What is the toxidrome for anticholinergics?**
   The classic description of anticholinergic toxicity is "mad as a hatter, fast as a hare, red as a beet, dry as a bone, blind as a bat, full as a tick, hot as Hades."
   - The hatter: Delirium, visual hallucinations
   - The hare: Tachycardia, hypertension
   - The beet: Flushed skin, facial flushing
   - The bone: Dry skin, dry mucous membranes
   - The bat: Dilated, sluggish pupils
   - The tick: Urinary retention, decreased GI motility and hypoactive bowel sounds
   - Hades: Hyperpyrexia, inability to sweat

131. **What breath odors may be associated with specific ingestions?**
   See Table 5-7.

TABLE 5-7. BREATH ODORS ASSOCIATED WITH SPECIFIC INGESTIONS	
Characteristic Odor	**Responsible Toxin or Drug**
Wintergreen	Methyl salicylate
Bitter almond	Cyanide
Carrots	Cicutoxin (of water hemlock)
Fruity	Ethanol, acetone (nail polish remover), isopropyl alcohol, chloroform

(continued)

TABLE 5-7. BREATH ODORS ASSOCIATED WITH SPECIFIC INGESTIONS *(continued)*	
Characteristic Odor	Responsible Toxin or Drug
Fishy	Zinc or aluminum phosphide
Garlic	Organophosphate insecticide, arsenic, thallium
Glue	Toluene
Minty	Mouthwash, rubbing alcohol
Mothballs	Naphthalene, *p*-dichlorobenzene, camphor
Peanuts	Vacor rat poison (odor is from a flavoring agent)
Rotten eggs	Hydrogen sulfide, *N*-acetylcysteine, disulfuram
Rope (burned)	Marijuana, opium
Shoe polish	Nitrobenzene

Woolf AD: Poisoning in children and adolescents, Pediatr Rev 14:411–422, 1993.

132. **What are the limitations of the routine toxicology screen?**
Most toxicology screens are intended to detect drugs encountered in substance abuse. Even in larger pediatric hospitals, comprehensive toxicology screens generally include only a fraction of drugs available to children. Most blood screens analyze for acetaminophen, salicylates, and alcohols. Urine is often screened for substances of abuse and other common psychoactive drugs, including antidepressants, antipsychotics, benzodiazepines, sedative-hypnotics, and anticonvulsants. Other potential toxins that can cause mental status changes (carbon monoxide, chloral hydrate, cyanide, organophosphates) or circulatory depression (β-blockers, calcium channel blockers, clonidine, digitalis) may not be included but may be assayed through individual blood tests. In clinical studies, toxicology screens are most valuable in quantitative settings (i.e., assessing drug levels). Additionally, treatment of the acutely poisoned patient must begin long before the results of many toxicology screens are available.

Moeller KE, Lee KC, Kissack JC: Urine drug screening: practical guide for clinicians, *Mayo Clin Proc* 83:66–76, 2008.

133. **After an adolescent's use of marijuana, how long does a urine screen remain positive?**
After first-time single use, the drug screen can be positive for 3 days. A long-term heavy marijuana user can have a positive drug test that may persist 30 days or more after cessation. Two cautions: nonsteroidal medications, including ibuprofen and proton pump inhibitors, have been reported to cross-react with cannabinoid immunoassays. False-negative results can occur if a wily teenager adds Visine to a urine specimen. The chemicals in Visine directly lower the concentrations of the cannabinoids in the urine.

Moeller KE, Lee KC, Kissack JC: Urine drug screening: practical guide for clinicians, *Mayo Clin Proc* 83:66–76, 2008.

134. **How do the types of alcohol ingestions vary?**
All alcohols can cause CNS disturbances ranging from mild mentation and motor abnormalities to respiratory depression and coma. Each alcohol is associated with specific metabolic complications.
- **Ethanol** (present in beverages, colognes and perfumes, aftershave lotion, mouthwash, topical antiseptic, rubbing alcohol)—in infants and toddlers, can cause the classic triad of

coma, hypothermia, and hypoglycemia, and in adolescents, can cause intoxication and mild neurologic findings. At levels higher than 500 mg/dL, it can be lethal.
- **Methanol** (present in antifreeze and windshield washer fluid)—can cause severe, refractory metabolic acidosis and permanent retinal damage leading to blindness.
- **Isopropyl alcohol** (present in jewelry cleaners, rubbing alcohol, windshield deicers, cements, paint removers)—can cause gastritis, abdominal pain, vomiting, hematemesis and CNS depression, moderate hyperglycemia, hypotension, and acetonemia, without acidosis.
- **Ethylene glycol** (present in antifreeze, brake fluid)—causes severe metabolic acidosis. In addition, it is metabolized to oxalic acid, which can cause renal damage by the precipitation of calcium oxalate crystals in the renal parenchyma and can lead to hypocalcemia.

135. **Which alcohol is considered the most lethal?**
Methanol. Deaths can arise from doses as little as 4 mL of pure methanol. Unique to methanol is that it becomes more toxic as it is metabolized. Methanol is broken down by alcohol dehydrogenase to formaldehyde and formic acid. It is the formic acid that causes the refractory metabolic acidosis and ocular symptoms.

136. **What is the treatment for methanol and ethylene glycol ingestions?**
Both methanol and ethylene glycol require the enzyme alcohol dehydrogenase to create their toxic metabolites. Ethanol competitively inhibits the formation of these metabolites by serving as a substrate for the enzyme. However, it is inebriating, it may cause hypoglycemia, and its kinetics are widely variable. Fomepizole is a safer and more effective blocker of alcohol dehydrogenase.

Brent J: Fomepizole for ethylene glycol and methanol poisoning, *N Engl J Med* 360:2216–2223, 2009.

137. **How is the osmolar gap helpful in diagnosing ingestions?**
The osmolar gap is the difference between the measured osmolarity (obtained from freezing point depression) and the calculated osmolarity (calculated = 2 [serum Na] + blood urea nitrogen/2.8 + glucose/18). Normal osmolarity is about 290 mOsm/L. A significant osmolar gap suggests an alcohol poisoning, which typically produces exogenous osmoles.

138. **What is "MUDPILES"?**
MUDPILES is a pneumonic for ingestions associated with a *high anion gap metabolic acidosis.*
- **M**ethanol, metformin
- **U**remia
- **D**iabetic ketoacidosis
- **P**araldehyde
- **I**soniazid, iron, inborn errors of metabolism
- **L**actic acidosis (seen with shock, CO, cyanide)
- **E**thanol, ethylene glycol
- **S**alicylates

139. **How can pupillary findings assist in the diagnosis of toxic ingestions?**
- **Miosis** (pinpoint pupils): Narcotics, organophosphates, phencyclidine, clonidine, phenothiazines, barbiturates, ethanol
- **Mydriasis** (dilated pupils): Anticholinergics (atropine, antihistamines, cyclic antidepressants); sympathomimetics (amphetamines, caffeine, cocaine, LSD, nicotine)
- **Nystagmus:** Barbiturates, ketamine, phencyclidine, phenytoin

140. **If a child has ingested an acetaminophen-containing product, when should the first acetaminophen level be obtained?**
A plasma level obtained **4 hours** after ingestion is a good indicator of the potential for hepatic toxicity. Nomograms are available for determining risk. As a rule, doses under 150 mg/kg are unlikely to be harmful.

141. **When should a "NAC attack" begin?**
N-acetylcysteine (NAC) is a specific antidote for acetaminophen hepatotoxicity by serving as a glutathione substitute in detoxifying the hepatotoxic metabolites. It should be used for any acetaminophen overdose with a toxic serum acetaminophen level within the first 24 hours after ingestion. It is especially effective if used in the first 8 hours after ingestion. If acetaminophen levels are not available on a rapid basis or the time since ingestion is not clear, it is preferable to initiate NAC.

142. **How does NAC prevent hepatotoxicity in acetaminophen overdose?**
Normally, 94% of acetaminophen is metabolized to glucuronide or sulfate form, and 2% is excreted unchanged in urine, both of which are nontoxic. The remaining 4% is conjugated with glutathione (with the help of cytochrome P-450) to form mercaptopuric acid, which is also not hepatotoxic. When a significant acetaminophen overdose occurs, cytochrome P-450 becomes the major system for metabolizing the acetaminophen, leading to depletion of hepatic stores of glutathione. When the glutathione is depleted to less than 70% of normal, a highly reactive intermediate metabolite binds to hepatic macromolecules, causing hepatocellular necrosis. It is presumed that NAC replenishes the glutathione, thus helping the cytochrome P-450 in converting the excess acetaminophen into mercaptopuric acid.

Heard KJ: Acetylcysteine for acetaminophen poisoning, *N Engl J Med* 359:285–292, 2008.

143. **What arterial blood gas pattern is classic for salicylate poisoning?**
Metabolic acidosis and **respiratory alkalosis**. Salicylates directly stimulate the medullary respiratory drive center, causing tachypnea with diminished P_{CO_2} (respiratory alkalosis). They also cause lactic acidosis and ketoacidosis by inhibiting Krebs cycle enzymes, uncoupling oxidation phosphorylation, and inhibiting amino acid metabolism (metabolic acidosis).

144. **What are hidden salicylates?**
These are salicylates that are found in over-the-counter products, such as Pepto-Bismol (bismuth salicylate). Salicylate absorption can be substantial, and in the setting of influenza or chickenpox, Pepto-Bismol use has been discouraged because of the potential for complications such as the development of Reye syndrome.

Szap MD: Hidden salicylates, *Am J Dis Child* 143:142, 1989.

145. **What are the classic ECG findings associated with tricyclic antidepressants?**
Tricyclic antidepressants interfere with myocardial conduction and can precipitate ventricular tachycardias or complete heart block. A QRS interval greater that 0.1 second is predictive of poor outcome in these patients. The presence of a large R wave in lead AVR is also associated with tricyclics. If these findings are noted, treatment with sodium bicarbonate should be initiated. Sodium bicarbonate helps prevent the sodium channel blockade that is caused by these medications. Of note, diphenhydramine (Benadryl), if ingested in high doses, can mimic the ECG findings of tricyclics.

146. **Which clinical and laboratory features correlate with an acutely elevated serum iron?**
Serum iron levels obtained 4 to 6 hours after ingestion correlate with severity of toxicity. Iron levels greater than 300 µg/dL are associated with mild toxicity consisting of local GI symptoms, such as nausea, vomiting, and diarrhea. A serum iron level of 500 µg/dL is associated with serious systemic toxicity, and a level of 1000 µg/dL is associated with death. Other laboratory tests that correlate with an elevated iron level include leukocytosis ($>15,000/mm^3$) and hyperglycemia (>150 mg/dL). Sometimes, radiopaque tablets may be demonstrated on abdominal radiograph.

147. **What are the four clinical stages of iron toxicity and the correlating pathophysiology?**
    - **Stage 1** (0.5 to 6 hours)—During this stage, iron exhibits a direct corrosive effect on the small bowel. Symptoms include nausea, vomiting, abdominal pain, and/or GI hemorrhage.
    - **Stage 2** (6 to 24 hours)—Iron silently accumulates in the mitochondria; patient is relatively symptom free.
    - **Stage 3** (4 to 40 hours)—This phase is characterized by systemic toxicity with shock, metabolic acidosis, depressed cardiac function, and hepatic necrosis.
    - **Stage 4** (2 to 8 weeks)—During this phase, pyloric stenosis and obstruction can develop as a result of earlier local bowel irritation.

148. **When can a toddler who may have swallowed some multivitamins be discharged home?**
    The toxic compound in multivitamin overdose is iron. There are a large variety of children's chewable multivitamins that contain different amounts of elemental iron (0 to 18 mg of elemental iron per tablet). The toxic dose of iron ingestion is at least 20 mg/kg of elemental iron, and the lethal dose of iron reported is in the range of 60 to 180 mg/kg of elemental iron. In a small child, a toxic dose is about 300 mg of elemental iron, which is the equivalent of 20 tablets of multivitamins containing 15 mg/tab of elemental iron. Frequently, the amount of ingestion is not known. Because iron can initially cause nausea, vomiting, or abdominal pain, a child with a suspected but unknown amount of iron poisoning can be observed, and an iron level may be obtained. A child who has no complaints and has a normal physical examination after 4 to 6 hours of observation can be safely discharged home.

149. **Which is more toxic, drinking dishwashing detergent or toilet bowl cleaner?**
    You are better off with the *toilet bowl cleaner*, although both acid (toilet bowl cleaner) and alkali (dishwashing detergent) ingestions may cause severe esophageal burns. Alkalis cause injury by liquefaction necrosis, dissolving proteins and lipids, thereby allowing deeper penetration of the caustic substance and greater local tissue injury. With acids, coagulation necrosis of the tissue occurs. This results in the formation of an eschar that limits the penetration of the toxin into deeper tissues. Compared with acids, alkalis are more typically in solid and paste form, which increases tissue contact time and tissue injury.

150. **Which hydrocarbons pose the greatest risk for chemical pneumonitis?**
    The household hydrocarbons with *low viscosities* pose the greatest aspiration hazard. These include furniture polishes, gasoline and kerosene, turpentine and other paint thinners, and lighter fuels.

151. **What is the differential diagnosis in a child who presents with confusion and lethargy?**
    An altered state or level of consciousness has many causes. The mnemonic **AEIOU TIPS** encompasses the many possible causes:
    - **A**lcohol, abuse of substances
    - **E**pilepsy, encephalopathy, electrolyte abnormalities, endocrine
    - **I**nsulin, intussusception
    - **O**verdose, oxygen deficiency
    - **U**remia
    - **T**rauma, temperature abnormality, tumor
    - **I**nfection
    - **P**oisoning, psychiatric conditions
    - **S**hock, stroke, space-occupying lesion (intracranial)

    Avner JR: Altered states of consciousness, *Pediatr Rev* 27:331–337, 2006.

152. **A patient receiving an antiemetic drug (e.g., promethazine) who develops involuntary, prolonged, twisting, writhing movements of the neck, trunk, and arms likely has what condition?**
Acute dystonia. This dystonic reaction is classically seen as an adverse side effect of antidopaminergic agents such as neuroleptics, antiemetics, or metoclopramide. In children, phenothiazines are the most common culprit. Treatment includes administration of diphenhydramine (Benadryl). Benztropine (Cogentin) is also used in adolescents.

153. **What do "SLUDGE" and "DUMBELS" have in common?**
Both are mnemonics used to remember the problems involved with *organophosphate poisoning*, lipid-soluble insecticides used in agriculture and terrorism ("nerve gas"). Organophosphates inhibit cholinesterase and cause all the signs and symptoms of acetylcholine excess.
- *Muscarinic effects*: Increased oral and tracheal secretions, miosis, salivation, lacrimation, urination, vomiting, cramping, defecation, and bradycardia; may progress to frank pulmonary edema
- *CNS effects*: Agitation, delirium, seizures, and/or coma
- *Nicotinic effects*: Sweating, muscle fasciculation, and, ultimately, paralysis
- The mnemonic **SLUDGE** is: **S**alivation, **l**acrimation, **u**rination, **d**efecation, **G**I cramps, **e**mesis.
- The mnemonic **DUMBELS** is: **D**efecation, **u**rination, **m**iosis, **b**ronchorrhea/bradycardia, **e**mesis, **l**acrimation, **s**alivation.

154. **What metal intoxication can mimic Kawasaki disease?**
Mercury. *Acrodynia* is the term applied to one form of mercury salt intoxication that results in a constellation of signs and symptoms very similar to that currently recognized as Kawasaki disease. The classic presentation of acrodynia was described in children exposed to calomel, a substance used in teething powders, which was essentially mercurous chloride. The symptom complex included swelling and redness of the hands and feet, skin rashes, diaphoresis, tachycardia, hypertension, photophobia, and an intense irritability with anorexia and insomnia. Infants were often very limp, lying in a frog-like position, with impressive weakness of the hip and shoulder girdle muscles. Similar symptoms have been described in children exposed to other forms of mercury, including broken fluorescent lightbulbs or diapers rinsed in mercuric chloride.

155. **Why is cyanide so toxic?**
Cyanide ion binds to the heme-containing cytochrome a_3 enzyme in the electron transport chain of mitochondria, which is the final common pathway in oxidative metabolism. Thus, with a significant exposure, virtually every cell in the body becomes starved of oxygen at the mitochondrial level and is unable to function. The body does have minor routes of cyanide detoxification, including excretion by the lungs and liver through rhodanese, a hepatic enzyme that combines cyanide with thiosulfate to form the less toxic thiocyanate for renal excretion. However, these mechanisms are inadequate in the face of a significant cyanide exposure. As with carbon monoxide poisoning, symptoms tend to be most prominent among the metabolically active organ systems. In particular, the CNS is rapidly affected, causing headache and dizziness, which may progress to prostration, convulsions, coma, and death. Less severe ingestions may be noted initially by burning of the tongue and mucous membranes, with tachypnea and dyspnea due to cyanide stimulation of chemoreceptors.

156. **In what settings should cyanide poisoning be suspected?**
- **Suicidal ingestion**, often involving chemists who have access to cyanide salts as reagents
- **Fires** causing combustion of materials such as wool, silk, synthetic rubber, polyurethane, and nitrocellulose, resulting in the release of cyanide
- Patients who are on **nitroprusside continuous infusion**, an antihypertensive agent that contains five cyanide moieties per molecule

157. **What kinds of plants account for the greatest percentage of deaths due to plant poisonings?**
Mushrooms account for at least 50% of deaths due to plant poisoning. The most dreaded variety is the *Amanita* species, which initially causes intestinal symptoms by one toxin (phallotoxin) and then hepatic and renal failure by a separate toxin (amatoxin). Other mushroom classes can cause a variety of early-onset (<6 hours) symptoms, including muscarinic effects (e.g., sweating, salivation, colic), anticholinergic effects (e.g., drowsiness, mania, hallucinations), gastroenteritis, and Antabuse-type effects if taken with alcohol.

158. **Is mistletoe toxic?**
Mistletoe, the popular Christmas plant, is an evergreen with small white berries. Ingestion of small amounts of the berries, leaves, or stems may result in GI symptoms, including pain, nausea, vomiting, and diarrhea. Rarely, large ingestions have resulted in seizures, hypertension, and even cardiac arrest. In some countries, extracts of mistletoe have been used for illegal abortifacients, brewed in teas that are particularly toxic. In the United States, the typical call to a poison center concerns a child who eats one or two mistletoe berries, which in general is unlikely to produce significant signs or symptoms.

159. **Should swallowed disc batteries be removed?**
Although the concern is that a disc battery may produce corrosive intestinal injury, most traverse the GI tract without incident. An initial radiograph for localization is indicated. If the disc battery is in the esophagus, removal is required. Otherwise, if the battery is in the stomach or beyond and the patient remains asymptomatic, watchful waiting is appropriate with follow-up imaging if the battery is not seen in the stool.

160. **What are the available methods used to remove a foreign body from the esophagus?**
Three methods are used; local custom prevails regarding selection.
- **Esophagoscopy,** the most commonly used method, is done under general anesthesia.
- A **Foley catheter** can be inserted beyond the foreign body, inflated, and then pulled back to remove the object. This extraction method is used by various centers, particularly for coins if the ingestion is less than 24 hours old and no respiratory distress is present. Complications, such as airway obstruction by a displaced coin and esophageal perforation, are possible.
- In **bougienage**, the object is forced into the stomach.

TRAUMA

161. **What are the major signs of a blow-out fracture?**
Traumatic force to the eye can result in a blow-out fracture affecting either the orbital floor or the medial wall. The fracture may result from either a sudden increase in intraorbital pressure or from a direct concussive force to the bony walls. Symptoms and signs can include the following:
- Pain on upward gaze
- Diplopia on upward gaze
- Enophthalmos (i.e., posterior displacement of the globe of the eye)
- Loss of sensation over the upper lip and gums on the injured side
- Compromised upward gaze on the affected side as a result of entrapment of the inferior rectus muscle
- Crepitus over the inferior orbital ridge

162. **When evaluating a patient with an eye injury, when should you suspect a ruptured globe, and how should you handle it?**
The sudden onset of marked visual impairment in the face of eye trauma should raise suspicion for a ruptured globe. The eye will be sunken as a result of decreased intraocular pressure,

and the anterior chamber may be flattened or shallow. You may see a tear-shaped pupil, which is the result of the contents of the iris coming forward and plugging the laceration or puncture. A ruptured globe is a true emergency, and an ophthalmologist should be called immediately. The approach, which is summed up by the acronym **SANTAS**, should be as follows:

- **S**terile dressing and shield should be placed over the eye to protect from further damage.
- **A**ntiemetics should be given to protect against increased pressure.
- **N**PO (nothing by mouth) to prepare for surgery.
- **T**etanus shot should be given.
- **A**nalgesics, either parenteral or oral (avoid topical), should be administered.
- **S**edation, if not contraindicated by other injuries, should be given.

Rahman WM, O'Connor TJ: Facial trauma. In Barkin RM, editor: *Pediatric Emergency Medicine, Concepts and Clinical Practice*. St. Louis, 1997, Mosby, pp 252–283.

163. **In the setting of facial trauma, when are drops for pupillary dilation contraindicated?**
These drops should not be used in patients who require sequential neurologic examinations (e.g., after severe head trauma), in whom increasing intracranial pressure with herniation is possible. They are also contraindicated in the setting of acute-angle glaucoma. The risk for inducing glaucoma is very low in children, but if symptoms of glaucoma (e.g., moderate eye pain, decreased vision, cloudy cornea, asymmetric pupil size, poor pupillary reaction) are present, dilation should be deferred. All these drops can have side effects, which can be minimized by applying pressure over the medial canthus to avoid systemic absorption.

164. **When should an avulsed tooth be reimplanted?**
Avulsion is the complete displacement of the tooth from its socket. Primary teeth (i.e., baby teeth) should not be reimplanted because nerve root damage or dental ankylosis may result. Secondary teeth should be repaired as soon as possible to maximize the chance of tooth viability. Thus, early insertion after gently rinsing the tooth is preferable (even if this does not result in a perfect fit, reimplantation may prevent the root from drying). It is important to disturb the root as minimally as possible. If not reimplantable (e.g., in the case of an uncooperative patient), a dislodged tooth should be gently rinsed, transported in cold milk or saliva or under a parent's tongue, and reimplanted temporarily until definitive dental care can be obtained.

Bernius M, Perlin D: Pediatric ear, nose and throat emergencies, *Pediatr Clin N Am* 55:209–210, 2006.

165. **What are the three most important considerations when evaluating nasal trauma?**
- **Bleeding:** If persistent, bleeding should be controlled with pressure, topical vasoconstrictors, cauterization, and anterior or posterior nasal packing.
- **Septal hematoma:** If the nasal septum is bulging into the nasal cavity, there is likely a hematoma that must be drained. If drainage is not performed, abscess formation or pressure necrosis can result and lead to a saddle-nose deformity.
- **Watery rhinorrhea:** This may be a sign of cribriform plate, suborbital ethmoid, sphenoid sinus, or frontal sinus fracture with cerebrospinal fluid leak. Radioisotope scans or CT scans with metrizamide dye can confirm the fracture; hospitalization is warranted if this is positive. More extensive facial trauma requires evaluation for many items, especially mid-face fractures and eye damage. Determining whether the nose is fractured is a lower priority item because fracture reduction is done only if there is distortion of the nose. Furthermore, such distortion cannot be properly assessed acutely because of swelling.

166. **How does one distinguish nasal mucosal drainage from cerebrospinal fluid leakage?**
This often becomes an issue when children have nasal rhinorrhea after trauma. The simplest test is to check the glucose concentration. The glucose level of cerebrospinal fluid is normally 40 to 80 mg/dL, whereas the glucose concentration of nasal mucus is normally near 0 mg/dL.

167. **How long can you wait before a broken nose in a child must be reduced?**
If a nasal bone fracture causes asymmetry (which is noted as the swelling from acute trauma subsides), the fracture should be reduced within 4 to 5 days; a longer delay may result in malunion.

168. **After a motor vehicle collision, an 8-year-old presents with right-sided pain, a heart rate of 150 beats per minute, a blood pressure of 110/80 mm Hg, and capillary refill time of 3.5 seconds. How should his initial fluid therapy be managed?**
It is important to recognize that this child is in shock, despite a normal blood pressure for age. For children in shock, changes in blood pressure are often late and precipitous. Findings of tachycardia, prolonged capillary refill, and diminished pulses are indicative of intravascular *hypovolemia* in this patient, requiring aggressive fluid resuscitation. Isotonic crystalloid (saline or lactated Ringer solution) should be given in boluses of 20 mL/kg over 5 to 10 minutes. If, after 40 mL/kg of crystalloid, hemodynamic measures have not improved or have worsened, blood products should be given in 10-mL/kg boluses.

169. **What are the signs and symptoms of a tension pneumothorax?**
A *tension pneumothorax* presents with hypotension, respiratory distress, diminished breath sounds on the affected side, and tracheal deviation. Treatment begins with emergent needle decompression in the second intercostal space at the mid-clavicular line followed by a chest tube.

170. **Which children with acute minor blunt head trauma require emergency CT scans?**
The largest prospective study of children younger than 18 years (>42,000 patients) with head trauma was designed to determine which patients might be at very low risk for clinically important traumatic brain injury for whom CT might be unnecessary. Derived and validated prediction rules were developed based on age. Negative predictive values (i.e., the likelihood of something not being present, in this case significant brain injury) were 100% for the younger group and 99.95% for the older group (and thus CT was thought to be unnecessary) if the following were characteristics were seen on evaluation:
- **Younger than 2 years:** Normal mental status, no scalp hematoma except frontal, no loss of consciousness or loss of consciousness for less than 5 seconds, nonsevere injury mechanism (e.g., fall of less than 3 feet, motor vehicle collision without patient ejection or death of another passenger, no head injury by high-impact object), no palpable skull fracture, acting normally according to parents
- **Aged 2 years and older:** Normal mental status, no loss of consciousness, no vomiting, nonsevere injury mechanism, no signs of basilar skull fracture, no severe headache

   Kuppermann N, Holmes JF, Dayan PS, et al: Identification of children at very low risk of clinically-important brain injuries after head trauma: a prospective cohort study, *Lancet* 374:1160–1170, 2009.

171. **What is the risk associated with CT scans in children?**
The ionizing radiation of CT scans may be implicated as the cause of lethal malignancies. Using data from the cancer rates after the atomic bomb blasts in Japan in World War II and comparing that degree of radiation and sequelae to CT radiation, it is estimated that the

potential rate of lethal malignancies from pediatric cranial CT may be between 1 in 1000 and 1 in 1500. This highlights the need to obtain CT studies with appropriate clinical indications and to limit the amount of radiation as low as possible during the procedure.

Brenner DJ, Hall EJ: Computed tomography—an increasing source of radiation exposure, *N Engl J Med* 35:2277–2284, 2007.

172. **When intracranial pressure is acutely elevated, how long is it before papilledema develops?**
Generally, 24 to 48 hours.

173. **What are the components of the Glasgow Coma Scale?**
Developed in 1974 by the neurosurgical department at the University of Glasgow, the scale was an attempt to standardize the assessment of the depth and duration of impaired consciousness and coma, particularly in the setting of trauma. The scale is based on eye opening, verbal responses, and motor responses, with a total score that ranges from 3 to 15 (Table 5-8).

TABLE 5-8. GLASGOW COMA SCALE

Best Verbal Response*

5	Oriented, appropriate conversation
4	Confused conservation
3	Inappropriate words
2	Incomprehensible sounds
1	No response

Best Motor Response to Command or to Pain (e.g., rubbing knuckles on sternum)

6	Obeys a verbal command
5	Localizes
4	Withdraws
3	Abnormal flexion (decorticate posturing)
2	Abnormal extension (decerebrate posturing)
1	No response

Eye Opening

4	Spontaneous
3	In response to verbal command
2	In response to pain
1	No response

*Children <2 years old should receive full verbal scores for crying after stimulation.

174. **How do the signs of different types of CNS herniation differ?**
- **Tentorial herniation** (unilateral herniation of the temporal lobe from the middle to the posterior fossa through rigid tentorium): Ipsilateral third nerve findings (dilated pupil, ptosis, loss of medial gaze) and contralateral hemiparesis and decerebrate posturing
- **Cerebellar tonsils through foramen magnum:** Abnormalities of tone, bradycardia, hypertension, and progressive respiratory distress (Cushing triad)

- **Subfalcine herniation** (herniation of one cerebral hemisphere beneath the falx cerebri to the opposite side): Leg weakness and bladder abnormalities

These clinical findings tend to overlap, and an altered state of consciousness is often the initial symptom.

175. **How, when, and where are car seats to be used?**

All 50 states require that children riding in cars be restrained in an approved safety seat based on weight, height, and age. Previous recommendations involved the use of rear-facing seats until 20 to 22 pounds. Data now support rear-facing seats for older toddlers up to 30 to 35 pounds. With rear-facing seats, older toddlers are one fifth as likely to die or sustain serious injuries compared with those in forward-facing seats. All children younger than 13 years should ride in the back seat. For children younger than 3 years, the center rear seat is the safest location. Despite these recommendations, in 2006, 45% of children killed in motor vehicle collisions were unrestrained.

- Up to 30 to 35 pounds: Rear-facing infant or convertible seat
- >35 to 65 pounds: Forward-facing convertible seat
- 35 to 100 pounds or less than 4 feet, 9 inches tall: Belt-positioning booster seat
- >4 feet, 9 inches tall: Shoulder strap with belt

Agran PF, Hoffman B: Child passenger safety: direction, selection, location, installation, *Pediatr Ann* 37:614–621, 2008.

Bull MJ, Durbin DR: Rear-facing car safety seats: getting the message right, *Pediatrics* 121:619–620, 2008.

176. **How does the location of cervical spine fractures vary between younger children and older children and adults?**

Younger children tend to have fractures of the upper cervical spine, whereas older children and adults have fractures more often involving the lower cervical spine, for the following reasons:

- Changing fulcrum of the spine: In an infant, the fulcrum of the cervical spine is at approximately C2-C3; in a child who is 5 to 6 years old, the fulcrum is at C3-C4; from 8 to adulthood, it is at C5-C6. These changes are in large part the result of the relatively large head size of a child compared with that of an adult.
- Younger children have relatively weak neck muscles.
- Younger children have poorer protective reflexes.

Woodward GA: Neck trauma. In Fleisher GR, Ludwig S, editors: *Textbook of Pediatric Emergency Medicine*, ed 4, Baltimore, 2000, Williams & Wilkins, p 1318.

177. **Which patients may have SCIWORA?**

Up to two thirds of children with spinal cord injuries have **SCIWORA** (**s**pinal **c**ord **i**njury **w**ithout **r**adiographic **a**bnormality). Most of these patients are younger than 8 years and have signs and symptoms that are consistent with spinal cord injury, but radiographic and CT studies reveal no bony abnormalities. It is postulated that the highly malleable pediatric spine allows the cord to sustain injury from flexion-extension forces without causing bony disruption. The more recent use of MRI among these children may help to clarify the causes. The initial neurologic complaints of these children should be taken seriously. Even with normal radiographs, a patient with an altered sensorium or with neurologic abnormalities that are consistent with cervical cord injury (e.g., motor or sensory changes, bowel and bladder problems, vital sign instability) requires continued neck immobilization and more extensive evaluation.

178. **Are single lateral cervical spine radiographs sufficient to "clear" a patient after neck injury?**

No. In some studies, the sensitivity of a single view for fractures is only 80%. The American College of Radiology guidelines recommend at least three views: (1) anteroposterior (including the C7-T1 junction, C1-C7); (2) lateral; and (3) open mouth (odontoid). The last view is often difficult to obtain in younger children. CT and MRI are reserved for more extensive evaluation for spinal cord injury when the initial three views are negative in symptomatic patients. The use of oblique films is controversial.

Eubanks JD, Gilmore A, Bess S, et al: Clearing the pediatric cervical spine following injury, *J Am Acad Orthop Surg* 14:552–564, 2006.

179. **If the abdominal CT scan is negative in a patient with blunt abdominal trauma, can you be certain that there is no intra-abdominal injury?**
No. CT scans may miss some bowel, diaphragmatic, and pancreatic injuries. If the CT shows free fluid in the abdominal cavity but no obvious organ injury, there may be injury to the gastrointestinal tract or the mesentery. Worsening abdominal pain or persistent emesis requires serial examinations, possible repeat CT scan, and at the discretion of the surgeon, exploratory laparotomy.

Wegner S, Colletti JE, Van Wie D: Pediatric blunt abdominal trauma, *Pediatr Clin N Am* 53: 243–256, 2006.

180. **Why is left shoulder pain after abdominal trauma a worrisome sign?**
This may represent blood accumulating under the diaphragm, resulting in pain referred to the left shoulder (*Kehr sign*). The sign can be elicited by left upper quadrant palpation or by placing the patient in the Trendelenburg position. The finding is worrisome because it suggests possible solid organ abdominal injury—most commonly the spleen—and requires surgical consultation and radiographic studies (usually CT or ultrasound) to grade the extent of injury.

Powell M, Courcoulas A, Gardner M, et al: Management of blunt splenic trauma: significant differences between adults and children, *Surgery* 122:654–660, 1997.

181. **A 5-year-old child has ecchymosis of the lower abdomen after a motor vehicle collision. What should you immediately suspect?**
This child's injuries should immediately key you in to the possibility of a **lap-belt injury**. In children who are either too young (<8 years old) or too small, the lap belt of a car rests abnormally high on the child's body and, instead of crossing the lap at the hips, crosses the lap at the lower abdomen. The most common injuries to suspect are lumbar spine injuries, particularly a flexion disruption (Chance) fracture and bowel or bladder perforations or disruptions.

Sivit CJ, Taylor GA, Newman KD, et al: Safety-belt injuries in children with lap-belt ecchymosis: CT findings in 61 patients, *Am J Radiol* 157:111–114, 1991.

182. **In a 7-year-old boy with a radiographically proven pelvic fracture, what diagnostic procedure should be done?**
The urethra, as it passes through the prostate, is very close to the pubic bone and is thus susceptible to injury from a pelvic fracture. Urethral damage should be suspected in all patients with pelvic fractures, even those without hematuria. The recommended diagnostic procedure is a **retrograde urethrogram**.

183. **In this same patient as in question 182, blood at the tip of the penis is noted. Why is catheterization contraindicated?**
A boggy, high-riding prostate found on rectal examination and blood seen at the urethral meatus are clinical signs of possible urethral disruption; these two findings are contraindications for passing a Foley catheter. A partial urethral disruption could potentially be made into a complete one with the passing of the catheter.

184. **What is the focus of the FAST examination?**

    FAST stands for **f**ocused **a**ssessment with **s**onography in **t**rauma. It is used as a screen for abdominal bleeding as blood appears black (hypoechoic) against the bright (hyperechoic) background of the internal organs. It was originally designed to replace diagnostic peritoneal lavage as a screen for abdominal bleeding, but the procedure can also can evaluate the pericardium and pleural spaces ("enhanced FAST"). A FAST exam evaluates four principal areas for bleeding: the pericardial sac, the hepatorenal fossa (Morrison pouch), the splenorenal fossa, and the pelvis (pouch of Douglas). This noninvasive tool provides clinicians with rapid information about potentially life-threatening thoracic and abdominal injury. In victims of blunt abdominal trauma who are unstable, a positive FAST examination can be an indication that the patient needs urgent surgical intervention.

    Levy JA, Bachur RG: Bedside ultrasound in the pediatric emergency department, *Curr Opin Pediatr* 20:235–242, 2008.

ACKNOWLEDGMENT

The editors gratefully acknowledge contributions by Drs. Jane M. Lavelle and Fred Henretig that were retained from previous editions of *Pediatric Secrets*.

CHAPTER 6

ENDOCRINOLOGY

Sharon E. Oberfield, MD, Mary Pat Gallagher, MD, and Daniel Esten Hale, MD

ADRENAL DISORDERS

1. **What are the symptoms of adrenal insufficiency?**
   - **Newborns:** Nonspecific findings of vomiting, irritability, and poor weight gain; may progress to cardiovascular shock
   - **Children:** Lethargy, easy fatigability, poor weight gain, and vague abdominal complaints; hyperpigmentation (primary insufficiency); symptoms of hypoglycemia (primary or secondary insufficiency); may also have vascular collapse with intercurrent illness

2. **What distinguishes primary and secondary adrenal insufficiency?**
   - **Primary:** Abnormality of the adrenal gland, low cortisol accompanied by an elevated adrenocorticotrophic hormone (ACTH) level; may also have mineralocorticoid deficiency
   - **Secondary:** Hypothalamic or pituitary dysfunction, low cortisol accompanied by an inappropriately normal or low ACTH level; normal mineralocorticoid production; often associated with multiple pituitary deficiencies

3. **What is the differential diagnosis of primary adrenal insufficiency?**
   - **Inherited enzymatic defects:** Congenital adrenal hyperplasia (multiple enzymatic defects are known), congenital adrenal hypoplasia
   - **Autoimmune disease:** Isolated, autoimmune polyendocrinopathy syndromes (APS) I and II, Schmidt syndrome
   - **Infectious disease:** Tuberculosis, meningococcemia, disseminated fungal infections
   - **Trauma:** Bilateral adrenal hemorrhage
   - **Adrenal hypoplasia**
   - **Iatrogenic:** Use of exogenous steroids

4. **What are the most common causes of secondary adrenal insufficiency?**
   Secondary causes can include failure of the hypothalamic and/or pituitary gland axis to develop in the embryonic stage or disruption of the axis as a result of tumor, central nervous system (CNS) trauma, irradiation, infection, or surgery.

5. **Can clinical clues suggest that adrenal insufficiency is a primary rather than secondary problem?**
   - **Primary adrenal insufficiency:** ACTH levels will rise as a result of disruption of the hormonal feedback loop, and these elevated levels often cause hyperpigmentation. Primary deficiency commonly leads to hyponatremia and hyperkalemia. This can present as salt craving or muscle cramping. Mild hypercalcemia may also be found.
   - **Secondary adrenal insufficiency:** ACTH levels are low; therefore, no hyperpigmentation occurs. Furthermore, in secondary insufficiency, the zona glomerulosa of the adrenal gland (responsible for aldosterone secretion) remains intact. Therefore, hyperkalemia and volume depletion are distinctly uncommon, but dilutional hyponatremia may occur as a result of decreased capacity to excrete a water load. The most important clinical clues come from the history; that is, has the child been exposed to exogenous steroids, or is there a history of CNS insult?

6. **What is the most common form of congenital adrenal hyperplasia (CAH)?**
CAH refers to a group of autosomal recessive disorders that result from various enzymatic defects in the biosynthesis of cortisol. Depending on the enzyme involved, the blockade can result in excesses or deficiencies in the other steroid pathways (i.e., mineralocorticoids and androgens). 21-Hydroxylase deficiency accounts for more than 90% of cases; the complete (salt-losing, about two thirds of cases) and partial (simple virilizing) forms occur in about 1 in 12,000 births and have an equal sex distribution. There are substantial differences in prevalence in various racial and ethnic groups. A late-onset or attenuated form (mild deficiency) manifests in adolescent girls with hirsutism and menstrual irregularities.

Zoltan A, Zhou P: Congenital adrenal hyperplasia: diagnosis, evaluation, management, *Pediatr Rev* 30: e49–e57, 2009.

7. **In newborns with CAH, why are girls likely to be diagnosed earlier than boys?**
The most obvious clinical feature of CAH in the newborn period is ambiguous genitalia as a result of the effects of excess androgen on the clitoris and labia majora. In boys, androgen excess does not cause any clearly abnormal appearance of the external genitalia. In girls, however, ambiguous genitalia are common. CAH should always be considered in the differential diagnosis of ambiguous genitalia, particularly in infants with a 46,XX karyotype.

8. **How do the major steroid preparations vary in potency?**
See Table 6-1.

TABLE 6-1. POTENCY OF COMMON STEROID PREPARATIONS

Name	Relative Glucocorticoid Potency	Relative Dosing (mg)	Relative Mineralocorticoid Potency
Cortisone	1	100	+
Hydrocortisone	1.25	80	++
Prednisone	5	20	+
Prednisolone	5	20	+
Methylprednisolone	6	16	0
9a-Fluorocortisol	20	5	+++++
Dexamethasone	50	1	0

Adapted from Donohoue PA: The adrenal cortex. In McMillan JA, DeAngelis CD, Feigin RD, Warshaw JB (eds): Oski's Pediatrics, Principles and Practice, 3rd ed. Philadelphia, JB Lippincott, 1999, p 1814.

9. **How do physiologic, stress, and pharmacologic doses of hydrocortisone differ?**
   - **Physiologic:** Careful studies have shown that adrenal glucocorticoid production in the normal individual is about 7 to 8 mg/m^2 per 24 hours. Because 50% to 60% of oral hydrocortisone is absorbed, the recommended oral physiologic replacement is about 12 to 15 mg/m^2 per 24 hours.
   - **Stress:** On the basis of studies performed before the development of high-quality radioimmunoassays, a consensus developed that production of glucocorticoid increased about threefold when individuals were physiologically stressed. Hence, when the term *stress dose* is used, it generally means that the dose is at least three times above physiologic replacement, that is, 50 to 100 mg/m^2 per 24 hours of hydrocortisone.

■ **Pharmacologic:** Glucocorticoids are extensively used in pharmacologic doses for the treatment of various inflammatory processes and in surgery or trauma to reduce or prevent swelling and inflammation. Doses of glucocorticoid higher than 50 mg/m^2 per 24 hours of hydrocortisone that are being used to treat these conditions are referred to as *pharmacologic doses*; that is, the medication is not being used for adrenal replacement or stress dosing.

10. **When does adrenal-pituitary axis suppression occur in prolonged glucocorticoid treatment?**
As a general rule, the longer the duration of treatment and the higher the dose of glucocorticoid, the greater the risk for adrenal suppression. If pharmacologic doses of glucocorticoids are used for less than 10 days, there is a relatively low risk for permanent adrenal insufficiency, whereas daily use for more than 30 days carries a high risk for prolonged or permanent adrenal suppression. The reason for glucocorticoid treatment must also be considered; that is, a child with severe head trauma may have initially been on treatment with glucocorticoids to reduce brain swelling but is also at significant risk for secondary pituitary deficiencies.

CALCIUM METABOLISM AND DISORDERS

11. **What are the causes of hypercalcemia?**
Remember the "**High 5-Is**" mnemonic: **H** (**h**yperparathyroidism) plus the five **I**s (**i**diopathic, **i**nfantile, **i**nfection, **i**nfiltration, and **i**ngestion) and **S** (**s**keletal disorders).
Hyperparathyroidism:
■ Familial
■ Isolated
■ Syndromic
Idiopathic:
■ Williams syndrome
Infantile:
■ Subcutaneous fat necrosis
■ Secondary to maternal hypoparathyroidism
Infection:
■ Tuberculosis
Infiltration:
■ Malignancy
■ Sarcoidosis
Ingestion:
■ Milk-alkali syndrome
■ Thiazide diuretics
■ Vitamin A intoxication
■ Vitamin D intoxication
Skeletal disorders:
■ Hypophosphatasia
■ Immobilization
■ Skeletal dysplasias

12. **An 8-year-old in a spica cast after hip surgery develops vomiting and a serum calcium concentration of 15.3 mg/dL. What should be the level of concern?**
A serum calcium concentration of more than 15 mg/dL or the presence of significant symptoms (i.e., vomiting, hypertension) constitutes a medical emergency and requires immediate intervention to lower the calcium level. The initial mainstay of treatment is isotonic

saline at two to four times maintenance rates and furosemide, 1 mg/kg intravenously every 6 hours. Furosemide is a potent diuretic and calciuric agent. Meticulous monitoring of input and output and of serum and urinary electrolytes (including serum magnesium) is vital. Electrocardiogram (ECG) monitoring is mandatory because hypercalcemia can be associated with conduction disturbances including premature ventricular contractions, ventricular tachycardia, prolonged PR interval, prolonged QRS duration, and atrioventricularblock. Additional treatment with glucocorticoids and antihypercalcemic agents may also be needed. Quicker results may be obtained using an ionized calcium. Serious consideration should be given to intensive care unit treatment and careful monitoring of inputs and outputs.

13. **Is it the Chvostek or Trousseau sign that gets the tap?**
    - **Chvostek:** Both are clinical manifestations of hypocalcemia or hypomagnesemia that occur because of neuromuscular irritability.
    - **Chvostek sign:** Tapping on the facial nerve in front of the ear results in movement of the upper lip.
    - **Trousseau sign:** Inflating a blood pressure cuff at pressures greater than systolic for 2 to 5 minutes results in carpopedal spasm.
      An easy way to remember the difference is that the **C**hvostek sign affects part of the **c**heek.

14. **What is hypoparathyroidism?**
    Parathyroid hormone (PTH) is a calcium regulatory hormone that increases serum calcium by increasing the resorption of Ca^{2+} from bone and by increasing gastrointestinal and urinary absorption of calcium through the increasing synthesis of calcitriol. Hypoparathyroidism can result from anomalies of the gland, destruction by surgery or autoimmune processes, biosynthetic abnormalities, or decreased distal cellular responsiveness to the hormone. The result can be acute and chronic hypocalcemia. The assays for intact PTH are now widely available, and a level should be obtained in a child found to be hypocalcemic. The result should be interpreted in light of the calcium level; that is, is the PTH appropriately elevated for the degree of hypocalcemia?

    Shoback D: Hypoparathyroidism, *N Engl J Med* 359:391–403, 2008.

15. **In what clinical circumstances should hypoparathyroidism be suspected?**
    - Manifestations of hypocalcemia (e.g., carpopedal spasm, bronchospasm, tetany, seizures)
    - Lenticular cataracts (these can also occur with other causes of long-standing hypocalcemia)
    - Changing behaviors, ranging from depression to psychosis
    - Mucocutaneous candidiasis (seen in familial form)
    - Dry and scaly skin, psoriasis, and patchy alopecia
    - Brittle hair and fingernails
    - Enamel hypoplasia (if hypocalcemia present during dental development)

16. **What are the main causes of hypocalcemia in children?**
    - **Nutritional:** Inadequate intake of vitamin D and in rare instances severely inadequate intake of calcium and/or excessive intake of phosphate may cause this condition.
    - **Renal insufficiency:** This may be the result of the following: (1) increased serum phosphorus from a decreased glomerular filtration rate with depressed serum calcium and secondary hyperparathyroidism, or (2) decreased activity of renal α-hydroxylase, which converts 25-hydroxyvitamin D into the biologically active form, $1,25\text{-}(OH)_2$ D.
    - **Nephrotic syndrome:** With lowered serum albumin, total calcium levels are reduced. Additionally, intestinal absorption of calcium is decreased, urinary losses of cholecalciferol-binding globulin are increased, and urinary losses of calcium are increased with prednisone therapy.

- **Hypoparathyroidism:** In infants, this may result from a developmental defect during embryogenesis (aplasia or hypoplasia) and may occur in the context of a syndrome such as DiGeorge syndrome. In older children, it may occur in the context of autoimmune polyglandular disease or mitochondrial myopathy syndromes.
- **Pseudohypoparathyroidism:** This is a group of peripheral resistance syndromes in which resistance to PTH results in elevated parathyroid hormone levels in the setting of normal renal function.
- **Disorders of calcium sensor genes**

Umpaichitra V, Bastian W, Castells S: Hypocalcemia in children: Pathogenesis and management, *Clin Pediatr* 40:305–312, 2001.

17. **In what syndrome of hypocalcemia is a short fourth metacarpal seen?**
    Albright hereditary osteodystrophy (AHO), a type of pseudohypoparathyroidism, is characterized by short stature, obesity, developmental delay, and brachydactyly (the shortening of hand bones).

CLINICAL SYNDROMES

18. **How does the syndrome of inappropriate secretion of antidiuretic hormone (SIADH) develop?**
    Antidiuretic hormone (ADH) is released from the posterior pituitary gland and serves as a regulator of extracellular fluid volume. The secretion of ADH is regulated by changes in osmolality sensed by the hypothalamus and alterations in blood volume detected by carotid and left atrial stretch receptors. Intracranial pathology can increase the secretion of ADH directly by local CNS effects, and intrathoracic pathology can increase secretion by stimulating volume receptors. Medications can directly promote ADH release and enhance its renal effects. SIADH is usually asymptomatic until symptoms of water intoxication and hyponatremia develop. Nausea, vomiting, irritability, personality changes, progressive obtundation, and seizures can result. An individual with hyponatremia that has developed over a prolonged period of time is less likely to have symptoms than one in whom the hyponatremia has developed acutely.

19. **What is cerebral salt wasting and how is it separated from SIADH?**
    Cerebral salt wasting (CSW) is defined as excessive urinary sodium and subsequent hyponatremia and dehydration in individuals with intracranial disease. The mechanism is not clear. CSW typically develops in the first week after brain injury and generally resolves over time. Both CSW and SIADH are associated with hyponatremia. However, individuals with CSW have signs of intravascular volume depletion (e.g., rapid pulse, low blood pressure), whereas children with SIADH have evidence of intravascular volume overload. In SIADH, fluid restriction often leads to an increase in the serum sodium. In contrast, fluid restriction in CSW does not result in an increase in serum sodium and may be dangerous and can result in cardiovascular compromise.

20. **What are the five criteria for the diagnosis of SIADH?**
    1. Hyponatremia with reduced serum osmolality
    2. Urine osmolality elevated compared with serum osmolality (a urine osmolality <100 mOsm/dL usually excludes the diagnosis)
    3. Urinary sodium concentration excessive for the extent of hyponatremia (usually >20 mEq/L)
    4. Normal renal, adrenal, and thyroid function
    5. Absence of volume depletion

21. **What clinical features suggest diabetes insipidus (DI)?**
    Because DI is caused by an insufficiency of ADH or the inability to respond to ADH, the signs and symptoms tend to be directly related to excessive fluid loss. The clinical spectrum

may vary depending on the child's age. The infant may present with symptoms of failure to thrive as a result of chronic dehydration, or there may be a history of repeated episodes of hospitalizations for dehydration. There may also be a history of intermittent low-grade fever.

Often, caretakers report a large-volume intake or an inability to keep a dry diaper on the infant. In the young child, DI may appear to be difficulty with toilet training. In the older child, the reappearance of enuresis, increasing frequency of urination, nocturia, or dramatic increases in fluid intake may herald the diagnosis. Frequent urination with large urinary volumes should lead to the suspicion of DI, and the absence of glucosuria is sufficient to rule out diabetes mellitus.

22. **How is the diagnosis of DI made?**
Deprivation of water intake for a limited time and judicious monitoring of physical and biochemical parameters may be required. The diagnosis of DI rests on the demonstration of the following: (1) an inappropriately dilute urine in the face of a rising or elevated serum osmolality; (2) urine output that remains high despite the lack of oral input; and (3) changes in physical parameters that are consistent with dehydration (weight loss, tachycardia, loss of skin turgor, dry mucous membranes). A child who, with water deprivation, appropriately concentrates urine (>800 mOsm/L) and whose serum osmolality remains constant (<290 mOsm/L) is unlikely to have DI. When DI is considered, a pediatric endocrinology consult is strongly recommended.

If a child meets the criteria for the diagnosis of DI, the water-deprivation test is usually ended with the administration of some form of ADH, such as desmopressin, and the provision of fluids. If the urine subsequently becomes appropriately concentrated, this confirms the diagnosis of ADH deficiency (central DI). Failure to concentrate suggests renal resistance to ADH (nephrogenic DI). DI may often be the first clinic sign of tumor of the hypothalamus or base of the skull (e.g., Wegener granulomatosis). Magnetic resonance imaging (MRI) of the brain is recommended if a diagnosis of DI is confirmed.

Linshaw MA: Congenital nephrogenic diabetes insipidus, *Pediatr Rev* 28:372–379, 2007.

Cheetham T, Baylis PH: Diabetes insipidus. *Paediatr, Drugs* 4:785–796, 2002.

DIABETIC KETOACIDOSIS

23. **What is diabetic ketoacidosis (DKA)?**
This is a state of severe metabolic derangement that results from both insulin deficiency and increased amounts of counterregulatory hormones (catecholamines, glucagon, cortisol, and growth hormone). Its main features are hyperglycemia (glucose usually >300 mg/dL), ketonemia (serum ketones >3 mmol/L with ketonuria), and acidosis (venous pH <7.30 or serum HCO_3 <15 mEq/L).

24. **What percentage of newly diagnosed diabetic patients present with symptoms of DKA?**
30%, although this is quite variable from location to location, dependent on access to care, economic status of the community, and other factors. The early symptoms of DKA are more likely to be missed or misinterpreted in young children. In one study of 247 children younger than 6 years with new-onset type 1 diabetes mellitus, 44% presented with DKA.

Rewers A, Klingensmith G, Davis C, et al: Presence of diabetic ketoacidosis at diagnosis of diabetes mellitus in youth: the Search for Diabetes in Youth Study, *Pediatrics* 121:e1258–e1266, 2008.

Quinn M, Fleischman A, Rosner B, et al: Characteristics at diagnosis of type 1 diabetes in children younger than 6 years, *J Pediatr* 148:366–371, 2006.

25. **What are the mainstays of therapy for DKA?**
■ Adequate initial supportive care (airway maintenance, supplemental oxygen as needed)
■ Volume resuscitation (which begins before starting insulin therapy)

■ Insulin administration
■ Frequent monitoring of vital signs, electrolytes, glucose, and acid-base status

Koul PB: Diabetic ketoacidosis: a current appraisal of pathophysiology and management, *Clin Pediatr* 48:135–144, 2009.

26. **What should be the initial fluid management in DKA?**
The association of the rate of sodium and fluid administration in DKA and development of cerebral edema remains controversial. The concern is that too rapid a rehydration with falling osmolarity might contribute to edema. The International Society for Pediatric and Adolescent Diabetes (ISPAD) recommends the following:
Initial:
■ In the rare patient who presents in shock, circulatory volume should be rapidly restored with isotonic saline (or Ringer lactate) in 20 mL/kg boluses with reassessment after each bolus.
■ In patients who are severely volume depleted but not in shock, the initial volume is typically 10 mL/kg given over 1 to 2 hours.
Subsequent: Rehydration is given evenly spaced over 48 hours. Because the severity of dehydration is often difficult to accurately assess, fluid is usually infused at a rate rarely in excess of 1.5 to 2 times the usual maintenance fluid for weight.
Next 4 to 6 hours: Initiation of deficit fluid replacement continued with isotonic saline (or Ringer lactate)
Thereafter: Change to a solution with tonicity >0.45% saline with added potassium.

Wolfsdort J, Craig ME, Daneman D, et al: Diabetic ketoacidosis in children and adolescents with diabetes, *Pediatr Diabetes* 10(Suppl 12):118–133, 2009.

27. **Why is a falling serum sodium concentration during the treatment of DKA of concern?**
Most patients with DKA have a significant sodium deficit of 8 to 10 mEq/kg, which needs to be replaced. After initial fluid boluses, fluids containing 0.5% normal saline or greater may be required. As a general rule, the serum sodium is low at the outset and rises throughout the course of treatment. "Corrected" serum sodium should be followed throughout treatment. An initial sodium of more than 145 mEq/L suggests severe dehydration or hyperosmolarity. An initial sodium that is normal or low and begins to fall with treatment merits prompt attention because it indicates either inappropriate fluid management or the onset of inappropriate diuretic hormone secretion (SIADH) and can signal impending cerebral edema.

28. **What is the typical potassium status in children with DKA?**
In almost all children with DKA, there is a depletion of intracellular potassium and a **substantial total body potassium** deficit of 3 to 6 mmol/kg, although the initial serum potassium value may be normal or high, in large part due to acidosis. Replacement therapy will be needed. If the patient is hypokalemic, potassium should be begun with the initial volume expansion and before insulin administration. Insulin administration results in potassium transport into cells with a further decrease in serum levels. If the initial potassium level is within a normal range, begin potassium replacement (with the concentration in the infusate at 40 mEq/L) after the initial volume expansion and concurrent with starting insulin therapy. If the initial potassium measurement is elevated, defer potassium replacement until urine output has been documented or the hyperkalemia abates. Of note, if rapid serum potassium levels are not available, an ECG to look for changes of hypokalemia or hyperkalemia (e.g., T-wave changes) can be valuable in guiding management.

Wolfsdort J, Craig ME, Daneman D, et al: Diabetic ketoacidosis in children and adolescents with diabetes, *Pediatr Diabetes* 10(Suppl 12):118–133, 2009.

29. **Why do potassium levels fall during the management of DKA?**
    - Dilutional effects of rehydration
    - Correction of acidosis (less K^+ exchanged out of cell for H^+ as pH rises)
    - Insulin administration (increases cellular uptake of K^+)
    - Ongoing urinary losses

    Most patients are potassium depleted, although the serum K^+ is usually normal or elevated. A low K^+ is particularly worrisome because it suggests severe potassium depletion.

30. **Should bicarbonate be used for the treatment of children with DKA?**
    See Table 6-2.

TABLE 6-2. FACTORS DETERMINING USE OF BICARBONATE TREATMENT IN DIABETIC KETOACIDOSIS	
Pros	**Cons**
Improved pH enhances myocardial contractility and response to catecholamines	Cardiac function problems rare in children
Ventilatory response to acidosis blunted when pH is <7.0	Ventilatory response well maintained in children
No adverse effect of bicarbonate on oxygenation has been demonstrated clinically	May alter oxygen-binding of hemoglobin, potentially decreasing tissue oxygenation
Questionable relevance of central nervous system acidosis	Paradoxical central nervous system acidosis documented in humans
May be useful in the rare patient with hyperkalemia	Hypokalemia may result from uptake of K^+ as acidosis is corrected; low serum K is six times more common after bicarbonate treatment
	May be associated with increased hyperosmolarity and cerebral edema

31. **Are there any indications for the use of bicarbonate?**
    Bicarbonate administration for the acidosis in DKA has not been shown to be beneficial in controlled trials. The establishment of an adequate intravascular volume and the provision of sufficient quantities of insulin are far more important in the treatment of DKA than bicarbonate. The decision to initiate bicarbonate therapy should be based on an arterial blood gas level and not a venous blood gas level. Two indications include:
    - **Profound acidosis** (arterial pH <6.9), which may be compromising cardiac contractility and/or adversely affecting the action of epinephrine during resuscitation
    - **Life-threatening hyperkalemia** with bradycardia, severe muscle weakness

    If administered, bicarbonate should be given cautiously at a rate of 1 to 2 mEq/kg over 60 minutes.

    Wolfsdort J, Craig ME, Daneman D, et al: Diabetic ketoacidosis in children and adolescents with diabetes, *Pediatr Diabetes* 10(Suppl 12):125, 2009.

    Green SM, Rothrock SG, Ho JD, et al: Failure of adjunctive bicarbonate to improve outcome in severe pediatric diabetic ketoacidosis, *Ann Emerg Med* 31:41–48, 1998.

32. **When should glucose be added to the infusate in patients with DKA?**
When the glucose level approaches 300 mg/dL. It is usually wise to order the appropriate glucose-containing fluid in advance because it is not desirable to have a child become hypoglycemic. Many centers now use the "two-bag" method: they order two bags of intravenous fluid, with identical electrolyte content except for the glucose concentration. One contains 10% glucose, and the other contains no glucose. As the blood sugar approaches 300 mg/dL, glucose is added to the infusate (through a Y tube). With the two-bag system, it is possible to alter the concentration of glucose anywhere between 0% and 10%, with a goal of maintaining the blood sugar in the 100- to 200-mg/dL range, thereby avoiding hypoglycemia. It is important to note that if the blood glucose is decreasing too quickly or is too low before the resolution of acidosis, an increased serum glucose should be attained by increasing glucose in the infusate rather than by decreasing the insulin.

KEY POINTS: DIABETIC KETOACIDOSIS

1. Triad of metabolic derangement includes hyperglycemia, ketonemia, and acidosis.

2. Abdominal pain can mimic appendicitis; hyperventilation can mimic pneumonia.

3. Initial bolus of insulin is no longer recommended.

4. Total-body potassium is usually significantly diminished.

5. Cerebral edema is the most common cause of death.

6. If the sodium level begins to fall with fluid replenishment, beware of secretion of antidiuretic hormone and possible cerebral edema.

7. Bicarbonate therapy is usually not indicated for acidosis.

33. **In the past a bolus of insulin was given at the start of therapy for DKA. Is that still recommended?**
No. An initial bolus (traditionally 0.1 U/kg) was previously given before any subsequent insulin. This has been found to be unnecessary and may increase the risk for cerebral edema.

Wolfsdorf J, Glaser N, Sperling MA: Diabetic ketoacidosis in infants, children, and adolescents: a consensus statement from the American Diabetes Association, *Diabetes Care* 29:1150–1159, 2006.

34. **Is continuous or bolus insulin better for the initial treatment of DKA?**
Extensive evidence demonstrates that **continuous** "low-dose" intravenous (IV) insulin (0.1 unit/kg/hr) should be the standard of care. Therapy should be begun 1 to 2 hours after starting fluid replacement therapy. Beginning insulin at the start of fluid therapy increases the risk for severe hypokalemia and of rapidly decreasing the serum osmolarity. In general, this infusion should be maintained until the acidosis has significantly improved (pH >7.30, bicarbonate >15 mmol/L, and/or closure of the anion gap). If continuous IV administration of insulin is not possible, short- or rapid-acting insulin (insulin lispro or insulin aspart) can be given subcutaneously (SC) or intramuscularly (IM) every 1 to 2 hours if peripheral circulation is not impaired. A recommended initial dose is 0.3 unit/kg SC followed 1 hour later by SC insulin at 0.1 unit/kg every hour or 0.12 to 0.2 unit/kg every 2 hours.

Wolfsdorf J, Craig ME, Daneman D, et al: Diabetic ketoacidosis in children and adolescents with diabetes, *Pediatr Diabetes* 10(Suppl 12):123–124, 2009.

Wolfsdorf J, Glaser N, Sperling MA: Diabetic ketoacidosis in infants, children, and adolescents: a consensus statement from the American Diabetes Association, *Diabetes Care* 29:1153–1154, 2006.

35. **What risk factors are associated with the development of cerebral edema?**
    Cerebral edema occurs in 0.5% to 1% of pediatric patients and accounts for most case fatalities that occur in cases of DKA. Its pathogenesis is incompletely understood. It is unpredictable, often occurring as biochemical abnormalities are improving. It may be sudden in onset or occur gradually, but it typically occurs during the first 5 to 15 hours after therapy begins. Risk factors identified include the following:
    - Younger age
    - Newly diagnosed patients
    - Attenuated rise in serum sodium during therapy
    - Greater hypocapnia (after correcting for acidosis)
    - Increased blood urea nitrogen (BUN)
    - Bicarbonate therapy for acidosis
    - Administration of insulin in first hour of fluid treatment
    - Higher volumes of fluid given during the first 4 hours

      Wolfsdort J, Craig ME, Daneman D, et al: Diabetic ketoacidosis in children and adolescents with diabetes, *Pediatr Diabetes* 10(Suppl 12):126, 2009.

      Levin DL: Cerebral edema in diabetic ketoacidosis, *Pediatr Crit Care Med* 9:320–329, 2008.

36. **What signs and symptoms suggest worsening cerebral edema during the treatment of DKA?**
    - Headache
    - Vomiting, recurrent
    - Change in mental status: increased drowsiness, irritability, restlessness
    - Change in neurologic status: cranial nerve palsy, abnormal papillary responses, abnormal posturing
    - Incontinence
    - Rising blood pressure
    - Inappropriate heart rate slowing
    - Decreased oxygen saturation

      Wolfsdort J, Craig ME, Daneman D, et al: Diabetic ketoacidosis in children and adolescents with diabetes, *Pediatr Diabetes* 10(Suppl 12):126, 2009.

DIABETES MELLITUS

37. **What are the risks of a child developing insulin-dependent diabetes mellitus (IDDM, type 1) if one sibling or parent is affected?**
    - Overall (sibling has IDDM): 6%
    - Identical twins: 50%
    - HLA identical: 15%
    - HLA haploidentical: 6%
    - HLA nonidentical: 1%
    - Father has IDDM: 6%
    - Mother has IDDM: 2%

      Cooke DW, Plotnick L: Type 1 diabetes mellitus in pediatrics, *Pediatr Rev* 29:374–384, 2008.

38. **How long does the "honeymoon" period last in newly diagnosed insulin-dependent diabetic patients?**
    - The honeymoon usually begins within 1 to 2 weeks after the initiation of insulin treatment. It is a period of falling or minimal exogenous insulin requirements that reflects continued residual endogenous insulin production. The duration of the honeymoon in a particular individual may last for a few weeks or months, but this is not predictable. However,

evidence is accumulating that it may be prolonged by the maintenance of excellent control. Cessation of the honeymoon is often heralded by elevated fasting blood glucose levels before breakfast or by an increasing insulin requirement.

39. **How do the types of insulin vary in their timing and duration of action?**
See Table 6-3.

TABLE 6-3. PHARMACOKINETICS OF INSULIN AND INSULIN-LIKE AGENTS			
Insulin*	Onset	Peak	Effective Duration
Rapid Acting			
Lispro (Humalog)	5-15 min	30-90 min	3-5 hr
Aspart (NovoLog)			
Short Acting			
Regular U100	30-60 min	2-3 hr	4-8 hr
Regular U500 (concentrated)			
Buffered regular (Velosulin)			
Intermediate Acting			
Isophane insulin (NPH, Humulin N/Novolin N)	2-4 hr	4-10 hr	10-16 hr
Insulin detemir	2-4 hr	3-8 hr	10-24 hr
Long-Acting			
Insulin zinc extended (Ultralente, Humulin U)	6-10 hr	10-16 hr	18-24 hr
Glargine (Lantus)	2-4 hr[†]	No peak	20-24 hr

NPH = neutral protamine Hagedorn insulin lispro protamine (neutral protamine lispro).
*Assuming 0.1-0.2 U/kg per injection. Onset and duration vary significantly by injection site.
[†]Time to steady state.
Adapted from American Diabetes Association: Practical Insulin: A Handbook for Prescribing Providers, 2002.

40. **When should the Somogyi phenomenon be suspected?**
The *Somogyi phenomenon* is rebound hyperglycemia after an incident of hypoglycemia. This rebound is secondary to the release of counterregulatory hormones, which is the natural response to hypoglycemia. As tighter glucose control is maintained, there is an increased likelihood of hypoglycemia and, therefore, of the Somogyi phenomenon. If the hypoglycemia is recognized and treated promptly, rebound hyperglycemia is less likely to occur. Thus, the Somogyi phenomenon is commonly reported more frequently at night because there is the greater likelihood of unrecognized and untreated hypoglycemia when the child is asleep. The Somogyi phenomenon should be suspected when a child whose blood sugar is in excellent control begins to have intermittent high blood glucoses in the morning. If that pattern is noted, blood glucose should be checked between 2:00 and 3:00 AM on several nights to determine whether hypoglycemia is occurring. If hypoglycemia can be documented, the dose or type of evening insulin may need to be altered, or the time that the dose is given may need to be changed.

41. **What causes the "dawn phenomenon"?**

The term *dawn phenomenon* describes a rise in blood glucose that occurs during the early morning hours (between 5:00 and 8:00 AM), particularly among patients who have normal glucose levels throughout most of the night. The rise in glucose is thought to be due to several factors, including the following:

- The normal increase in the morning cortisol level
- The cumulative effect of increased nocturnal growth hormone
- Insulinopenia as a result of the length of time since the last injection

Strategies for managing the dawn phenomenon include shifting more aggressive insulin use to the evening and pre-bedtime hours, using a type of insulin that has a longer duration or peak of action, initiating insulin pump therapy, not eating a carbohydrate snack at bedtime, or increasing the amount of vigorous physical activity in the evening hours. The specific strategy or combination of strategies must be tailored to the individual child.

KEY POINTS: DIABETES MELLITUS TYPE 1

1. Destruction of pancreatic islet cells causes an absolute insulin deficiency.

2. Classic triad of symptoms includes polyuria, polydipsia, and polyphagia.

3. Tighter glucose control substantially lowers complication rates of retinopathy, nephropathy, and neuropathy.

4. Obtaining a hemoglobin A_1C (glycosylated) level is a way to assess average control during the previous 2 to 3 months.

5. Puberty is a time of increased insulin resistance, thereby requiring increased dosing.

42. **How rapidly can renal disease develop after the onset of diabetes mellitus?**

Microscopic changes in the glomerular basement membrane may be present by 2 years after the diagnosis of diabetes. Microalbuminuria is often present within 10 to 15 years. Retrospective studies suggest that as many as 50% of patients with IDDM diagnosed before the age of 30 years will ultimately develop end-stage renal disease. Patients with diabetic nephropathy account for more than 25% of those receiving long-term renal dialysis in the United States. Progression can be substantially delayed by meticulous attention to glycemic control.

Joslin Diabetes Center: http://www.joslin.org.

43. **How is hemoglobin A_1C helpful for monitoring diabetic control?**

Glycohemoglobin, also known as glycosylated hemoglobin or hemoglobin A_1C, is a hemoglobin-glucose combination formed nonenzymatically within the cell. Initially, an unstable bond is formed between glucose and the hemoglobin molecule. With time, this bond rearranges to form a more stable compound in which glucose is covalently bound to the hemoglobin molecule. The amount of the unstable form may rise rapidly in the presence of a high blood glucose level, whereas the stable form changes slowly and provides a time-average integral of the blood glucose concentration through the 120-day life span of the red blood cell. Thus, glycohemoglobin levels provide an objective measurement of averaged diabetic control over time.

Cooke DW, Plotnick L: Type 1 diabetes mellitus in pediatrics, *Pediatr Rev* 29:374–384, 2008.

Rewers M, Pihoker C, Donaghue K, et al: Assessment and monitoring of glycemic control in children and adolescents with diabetes, *Pediatr Diabetes* 8:408–418, 2007.

44. **What are the goals for hemoglobin A₁C?**
The American Diabetic Association recommends different target HbA₁C goals for type 1 diabetics based on age. The higher goals for younger children are based on the increased vulnerability of that age group to hypoglycemia (Table 6-4).

TABLE 6-4. HEMOGLOBIN A₁C GOALS	
Age	HbA₁C Goal
<6 yr	7.5%-8.5%
6-12 yr	<8.0%
12-19 yr	<7.5%
>19 years	<7.0%

Djedjos CS, Cooke DW: New tools for managing type 1 diabetes, Contemp Pediatr 26:44–54, 2009.

45. **What pathophysiologic process characterizes type 2 diabetes?**
The key characteristic of type 2 diabetes is resistance to insulin action. There may also be insulin secretory defects.

46. **Is the incidence of type 2 diabetes increasing?**
Dramatically. Previously rare in pediatrics, type 2 diabetes in children has been called an emerging epidemic. It has increased 10-fold over the past 15 years and accounts for up to one half of new-onset diabetes cases in some centers in the United States. Some estimates expect that one of every three children born in the year 2000 will develop diabetes. The reason for the increase is unclear, but it is likely related in part to current trends of increasing childhood obesity, poor dietary habits, and sedentary behavior.

Amed S, Daneman D, Mahmud FH, et al: Type 2 diabetes in children and adolescents, *Exp Rev Cardiovasc Ther* 8:393-406, 2010.

47. **What historical and clinical features suggest type 2 rather than type 1 diabetes?**
- **Obesity** is the hallmark of type 2 diabetes, whereas it may or may not be present in children with type 1 diabetes at diagnosis.
- **Racial and ethnic minority groups,** particularly African Americans, Mexican Americans, and Native Americans, are often affected.
- **Family history** is usually strongly positive; more than 50% of affected children have one or more first-degree relative with type 2 diabetes.
- **Acanthosis nigricans,** a marker of insulin resistance, is present in 90% of cases, most commonly on the posterior neck.
- **Hyperandrogenism** in girls is another disorder that is associated with insulin resistance and obesity.
- **Puberty** increases insulin resistance in all adolescents as a result of high levels of growth hormone.
- **Differing symptoms:** Unlike patients with type 1 diabetes, most youths with type 2 diabetes have little or no weight loss and absent or mild polyuria or nocturia, and most have glycosuria without ketonuria (although up to 33% can have ketonuria).

Liu L, Hironaka K, Pihoker C: Type 2 diabetes in youth, *Curr Probl Pediatr Adolesc Health Care* 34:254–272, 2004.

48. **What is acanthosis nigricans?**
Acanthosis nigricans is hyperpigmented and often highly rugated patches that are found most prominently in intertriginous areas, especially on the nape of the neck (Fig. 6-1). This is a marker of insulin resistance.

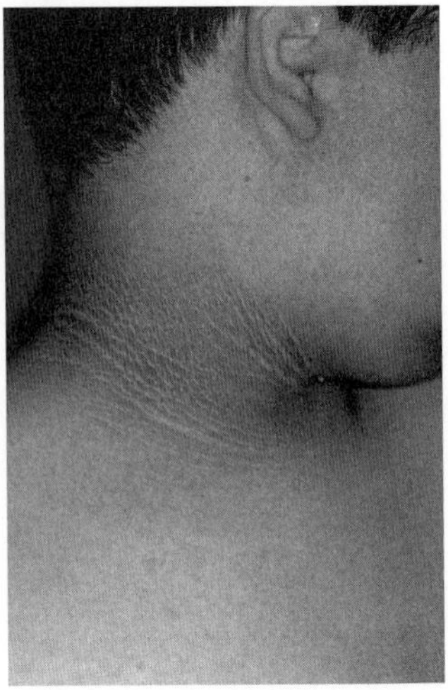

49. **How is type 2 diabetes diagnosed?**
■ Random glucose concentration of 200 mg/dL or higher (if polyuria, polydipsia, weight loss)
■ Fasting (>8 hours) glucose concentration of more than 125 mg/dL
■ Abnormal oral glucose tolerance test defined as a 120-minute glucose concentration of more than 200 mg/dL after drinking 1.75 g/kg of glucose (with a maximal dose of 75 g)

Although classification can usually be made on the basis of clinical characteristics, measurement of levels of fasting insulin and C-peptide (low in type 1; normal or elevated in type 2) or islet cell autoantibodies (present in type 1; generally absent in type 2) can be useful.

Fig. 6-1. Acanthosis nigricans in an adolescent male. (From Schachner LA, Hansen RC [eds]: Pediatric Dermatology, 3rd ed. Edinburgh, Mosby, 2003, p 915.)

American Diabetes Association: Report of the expert committee on the diagnosis and classification of diabetes mellitus, *Diabetes Care* 28(Suppl 1):S37–S42, 2005.

American Diabetes Association: http://www.diabetes.org.

50. **Which pediatric patients should be screened for type 2 diabetes?**
Beginning at 10 years of age (or earlier if puberty initiates before age 10 years), a fasting blood sugar should be obtained for patients with the following:
■ Body mass index more than 85th percentile for age and sex, *plus*
■ Any two of following risk factors: positive family history in first- or second-degree relative; Native American, African American, Hispanic, or Asian or Pacific Islander; presence of associated conditions (acanthosis nigricans, hypertension, dyslipidemia, polycystic ovarian syndrome)

American Diabetes Association: Type 2 diabetes in children and adolescents, *Diabetes Care* 23:381–389, 2000.

Juvenile Diabetes Research Foundation: http://www.jdrf.org.

KEY POINTS: DIABETES MELLITUS TYPE 2

1. Pathophysiology includes tissue-level insulin resistance.

2. Incidence is rising rapidly in association with increased rate of pediatric obesity.

3. In acanthosis nigricans, altered skin pigmentation and texture are associated with insulin resistance, which is found in 90% of cases.

4. Diagnosis is based on detecting hyperglycemia: fasting ($\geq$126 mg/dL), random ($\geq$200 mg/dL), or postprandial glucose challenge ($\geq$200 mg/dL).

5. Screen patients based on known risk factors (obesity, ethnicity, family history).

51. **When should oral hypoglycemic agents be considered as part of therapy?**
If glucose control is not achieved with dietary adjustments and exercise within 2 to 3 months, oral hypoglycemic agents should be considered. Data on children and adolescents are limited. Metformin (Glucophage) is the best studied and is recommended as initial therapy by many experts, but four category types of oral agents for use in type 2 diabetes are available.

Liu L, Hironaka K, Pihoker C: Type 2 diabetes in youth, *Curr Probl Pediatr Adolesc Health Care* 34:254–272, 2004.

GROWTH DISTURBANCES

52. **How do the growth rates of boys and girls differ?**
In both boys and girls, the rate or velocity of linear growth begins to decelerate right after birth. In girls, this deceleration continues until the age of about 11 years, at which time the adolescent growth spurt begins. For boys, the deceleration continues until the age of about 13 years. The peak rate of increase in boys occurs at 14 years of age. Growth and growth rate charts are readily available from the Centers for Disease Control and Prevention website (http://www.cdc.gov/growthcharts/).

53. **What is the best predictor of a child's eventual adult height?**
Mid-parental height. This is an estimate of a child's expected genetic growth potential based on parental heights (preferably measured rather than by history).
For girls: ([father's height – 13 cm] + [mother's height])/2.
For boys: ([mother's height + 13 cm] + [father's height])/2.

This gives the range (±5 cm) of expected adult height. The predicted height can be compared with the present height percentile, and any significant deviation can be a clue to an abnormal growth pattern in a child. It is important to remember that some forms of growth hormone deficiency are inherited, so one should not automatically assume that the short child with short parents has familial short stature.

54. **When have most children achieved the height percentile that is consistent with parental height?**
By the age of 2 years. Rough estimates of ultimate adult height can be obtained by taking a boy's length at age 2 years and a girl's length at age 18 months and doubling them.

55. **Name the major categories of causes of short stature.**
- *Familial* (for short children, ≤ 3 standard deviations, with very short parents, consider genetic forms of short stature)
- *Constitutional delay* ("late bloomer")
- *Chronic disease/treatment* (e.g., inflammatory bowel disease, chronic renal failure, renal tubular acidosis, cyanotic congenital heart disease)
- *Chromosomal/syndromic* (e.g., Turner [45,X], 18q-, Down, achondroplasia)
- *Endocrine* (e.g., hypothyroidism, growth hormone deficiency, hypopituitarism, hypercortisolism [endogenous and exogenous])
- *Psychosocial* (e.g., chaotic social situation, orphanage)
- *Intrauterine* (e.g., small for gestational age)
  Genetic patterns and constitutional delay account for the largest percentage of known causes.

56. **In a child with short stature, what rate of growth makes an endocrinologic cause unlikely?**
In general, heights should be measured over at least a 6-month interval to calculate an accurate rate because growth rates are not completely linear, and measurement is relatively imprecise. Rates of growth are also highly dependent on the age and pubertal status of the

child. Growth velocity charts are available at http://www.cdc.gov/growthcharts. Growth rates that are consistently below the 25th percentile or crossing percentiles downward after the age of 2 years warrant careful consideration and possibly investigation.

57. **When evaluating a short child, why should you ask when the parents reached puberty?**
The age at which puberty occurred in other family members may help identify children with constitutional delay because this entity tends to run in families. Most women will remember their age at menarche, and this age can be used as a reference for the age at which other pubertal events occurred. The strongest association for pubertal delay is between father and son. The most useful reference point for adult males is the age at which they reached adult height because almost all normal males will have reached their adult height by the age of 17 years (before high school graduation). Significant growth beyond this age suggests a history of pubertal delay.

58. **When does the pubertal growth spurt occur?**
For children with an average growth rate, pubertal growth begins earlier in girls. Mean age at the initiation of this spurt is 11 years for boys and 9 years for girls. Peak height velocity occurs at 13.5 years for boys and 11.5 years for girls. Peak velocity occurs at Tanner breast stage II to III for girls and Tanner testis stage III to IV for boys. Girls generally stop growing at an average of 14 years of age, but boys continue to grow until 17 years of age. The major hormone affecting growth cessation is estradiol in both girls and boys. The timing of the pubertal growth spurt may be earlier in certain ethnic groups and in very obese children.

Rogol AD, Roemmich JN, Clark PA: Growth at puberty, *J Adolesc Health* 31(Suppl):192–200, 2002.

59. **Are upper to lower body ratios helpful for the diagnosis of growth problems?**
Disproportionate short stature generally refers to an inappropriate ratio between truncal length and limb length (upper to lower segment ratio). Lower segment (limb length) is the distance from the superior border of the pubic bone to the floor surface. Height minus the lower segment gives the height of the upper segment (truncal length). In an infant, the head and trunk are quite long relative to the limbs, so the ratio of truncal length to limb length is about 1.7. Throughout childhood, this ratio declines, so that by 7 to 10 years of age this ratio is about 1.0. The adult ratio is 0.9.

An increased ratio is seen in bony dysplasias (e.g., achondroplasia, hypochondroplasia), hypothyroidism, gonadal dysgenesis, and Klinefelter syndrome (the patients are then tall in adolescence). Decreased ratios are seen in certain syndromes (e.g., Marfan syndrome), spinal disorders (e.g., scoliosis), and children who have been exposed to specific types of therapy (e.g., spinal irradiation).

Halac I, Zimmerman D: Evaluating short stature in children, *Pediatr Ann* 33:170–176, 2004.

60. **What laboratory studies should be obtained when evaluating short stature?**
Extensive laboratory tests are generally not indicated unless the growth velocity is abnormally low. Laboratory testing may include any or all of the following: complete blood count, urinalysis, chemistry panel, sedimentation rate, thyroxine, thyroid-stimulating hormone, insulin-like growth factor-1 (IGF-1), and IGF-binding protein-3 (IGFBP-3). Depending on the ethnic background of the child or the clinical history, testing might also be done for celiac disease, inflammatory bowel disease, renal tubular acidosis, or other occult conditions.

Random growth hormone levels are of little value because they are generally low in the daytime, even in children of average height. IGF-1 (or somatomedin C) mediates the anabolic effects of growth hormone, and levels correlate well with growth hormone status. However, IGF-1 can also be low in nonendocrine conditions (e.g., malnutrition, liver disease), and the assays are somewhat inconsistent from laboratory to laboratory.

IGFBP-3, which is the major binding protein for IGF-1 in serum, is also regulated by growth hormone. IGFBP-3 levels generally indicate growth hormone status and are less affected by nutritional factors than IGF-1. Many endocrinologists now use IGF-1 and IGFBP-3 as their initial screening tests for growth hormone deficiency.

Dattani M, Preece M: Growth hormone deficiency and related disorders: insights into causation, diagnosis, and treatment, *Lancet* 363:1977–1987, 2004.

61. **In a very obese child, how does height measurement help to determine whether an endocrinopathy might be the cause?**
In children with simple obesity (e.g., familial), linear growth is typically enhanced; in children with endocrinopathies, it is usually impaired. If the height of a child is at, or greater than, the mid-parental height percentile, an endocrine cause of the obesity is unlikely. In some children with craniopharyngiomas, significant obesity with good linear growth can be seen despite documented growth hormone deficiency.

62. **How does a growth chart help determine the diagnosis of failure to thrive?**
If an infant is demonstrating deceleration of a previously established growth pattern or growth that is consistently less than the fifth percentile, the pattern of growth of head circumference, height, and weight can help establish the likely cause (Fig. 6-2). There are three main types of impaired growth:
- **Type I:** Retardation of weight with near-normal or slowly decelerating height and head circumference; most commonly seen in undernourished patients.
- **Type II:** Near-proportional retardation of weight and height with normal head circumference; most commonly seen in patients with constitutional growth delay, genetic short stature, endocrinopathies, and structural dwarfism.
- **Type III:** Concomitant retardation of weight, height, and head circumference; seen in patients with in utero and perinatal insults, chromosomal aberrations, and central nervous system abnormalities.

63. **How can one track growth in children who have spinal cord abnormalities or severe scoliosis?**
There is an excellent 1:1 correlation between span (longest fingertip to longest fingertip measured across the nape of the neck) and height. Thus, span is a useful proxy measure for height/length if it is not possible to get an accurate height. Height and rate of growth, when determined in this way, can be plotted on standard growth and velocity charts.

64. **What is bone age?**
A measure of *somatic maturity* and *growth potential*. Standards of normal skeletal radiographic maturation are available, and these are based on the progression of ossification centers that occur at particular ages. A radiograph of the left hand and wrist is taken and compared with those standards to determine a patient's bone age. This result can be compared with chronologic age to gauge the remaining potential for growth. The interpretation of bone ages can be somewhat difficult and dependent on the pediatric experience of the radiologist.

65. **Why is a bone age determination helpful for evaluating short stature?**
A single bone age is of value for differentiating familial short stature and genetic diseases, in which bone age is normal, from other causes of short stature. A delayed bone age (>2 standard deviations below the mean) that correlates with the child's height age (age on growth chart at which child's height would be at the 50th percentile) is suggestive of constitutional delay, whereas a markedly delayed bone age is suggestive of endocrine disease. Serial bone ages determined every 6 to 12 months are often helpful because, in

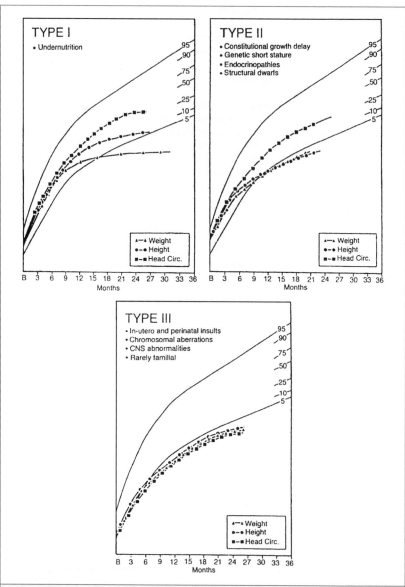

Fig. 6-2. Types I, II, and III of impaired growth. (From Roy CC, Silverman A, Alagille DA: Pediatric Clinical Gastroenterology, 4th ed. St. Louis, Mosby, 1995, pp 4-8.)

both the normal child and the child with constitutional delay, the bone age will advance in parallel with the chronologic age. In endocrine disease, the bone age falls progressively further behind the chronologic age. Bone age may be normal or delayed in patients with chronic disease, depending on the severity of disease, its duration, and the type of treatment used.

66. **What features suggest constitutional delay as a cause of short stature?**
    - No signs or symptoms of systemic disease
    - Bone age delayed up to 2 to 4 years but consistent with height age (age at which individual's height would plot on the 50th percentile)
    - Period of poorest growth often occurring between the ages of 18 and 30 months, with steady linear growth thereafter (i.e., normal rate of growth for bone age)
    - Parental or sibling history of delayed physical development
    - Height prediction consistent with family characteristics

KEY POINTS: GROWTH DISTURBANCES

1. Bone age is used as a diagnostic key: genetically determined short stature (bone age = chronologic age) versus constitutional delay (bone age < chronologic age).

2. Midline defects (e.g., single maxillary incisor, cleft lip/palate) and short stature suggest hypopituitarism.

3. Random growth hormone levels are usually not helpful (due to pulsatile delivery during sleep); provocative testing is more reliable.

4. Family history is key. Use growth data about family—especially siblings—to establish a pattern.

5. Short stature with overweight suggests endocrinopathy (adrenal, thyroid) and growth hormone deficiency.

6. Growth hormone deficiency that appears during the first year of life is associated with hypoglycemia; after the age of 5 years, it is associated with short stature.

67. **How is constitutional delay managed?**
    If the results of history, physical examination, and clinical laboratory evaluation are unremarkable, the child is seen once every 3 to 6 months for accurate height measurements and determination of growth velocity. A bone age test may be done yearly to assess the progression of bony maturation. In patients with constitutional delay, the rate of bone maturation should keep pace with the chronologic age. In children who are of mid- to late pubertal ages (girls >13 years; boys >14 years) but showing minimal or no signs of puberty, selective use may be made of estrogen or testosterone supplementation to initiate puberty, or additional assessment may be indicated.

68. **Should growth hormone therapy be given to the normal short child?**
    This is an area of controversy in pediatric endocrinology. Opponents argue that short stature is not a disease, that current height velocity may not be predictive, and that what constitutes growth hormone sufficiency and insufficiency is not clearly defined. Long-term safety remains under study, and some recent studies suggest impairment of testicular function in treated males. Proponents counter that the treatment is safe and does improve height in 50% of treated patients to at least 5 cm greater than pretreatment predictions. Surveys have indicated that most pediatric endocrinologists support growth hormone use in patients with short stature, normal growth hormone stimulation tests, and subnormal growth velocity.

Allen DB: Growth hormone therapy for short stature: is the benefit worth the burden? *Pediatrics* 118:343–348, 2006.

Bridges N: New indications for growth hormone, *Arch Dis Child Educ Pract Ed* 90:ep7–ep9, 2005.

69. **What are the clinical manifestations of growth hormone excess?**
    Before puberty, the cardinal manifestations are an increase in growth velocity with minimal bone deformity and soft tissue swelling—a condition called *pituitary gigantism*. Hypogonadotropic hypogonadism and delayed puberty often coexist with growth hormone excess, and affected children exhibit eunuchoid body proportions. If the growth hormone excess occurs after puberty (after epiphyseal closure), the more typical features of acromegaly occur, including coarsening of the facial features and soft tissue swelling of the feet and hands. Growth hormone excess is rare in children.

HYPOGLYCEMIA

70. **How is hypoglycemia defined?**
    A **serum glucose of less than 50 mg/100 mL** is defined as hypoglycemia in childhood. Some argue for lower levels being used for term and preterm infants; however, these arguments are based on population sampling data rather than on physiology. Hypoglycemia is a laboratory finding, and its presence should always lead to a diligent search for the underlying pathology. A common cause of a falsely reported abnormal glucose is that the plasma is not quickly separated from the red blood cells. The red cells continue to metabolize glucose, thus lowering the glucose, often into the abnormal range. This should be suspected when the glucose result is reported as part of a chemistry panel, especially if the child was reported to be asymptomatic.

71. **Describe the clinical findings associated with hypoglycemia.**
    Neuroglycopenic symptoms include irritability, headache, confusion, unconsciousness, and seizure. **Adrenergic** signs include tachycardia, tremulousness, diaphoresis, and hunger. Any combination of the above signs and symptoms should lead to the measurement of the blood glucose level.

72. **What are the causes of childhood hypoglycemia?**
    No single cause predominates in any age group. Therefore, the entire differential diagnosis must be considered in any child who presents symptoms of hypoglycemia. Hypoglycemia often occurs as a result of a combination of two or more of the problems listed in Table 6-5 (e.g., prolonged fasting during an illness coupled with fever in medium-chain acyl-CoA dehydrogenase deficiency). Specific genetic testing is now available for a number of these entities.

73. **An unconscious 3-year-old girl is brought to the emergency department with a serum glucose concentration of 26 mg/dL. What other laboratory tests should be performed?**
    The critical action is to be sure to gather the correct samples at this time, including both blood and urine. It is strongly recommended that an extra purple top and red top tube of blood be drawn, if at all possible. The first urine specimen obtained after the presentation of the child, even if this cannot be gotten for several hours after the acute event, is of significant value. The principal laboratory evaluations should include the measurement of the following: (1) the metabolic compounds associated with fasting adaptation; (2) the hormones that regulate these processes; and (3) drugs that can interfere with glucose regulation. The extra tubes of blood should be kept for additional analyses once the first battery of tests described below are available or after specific recommendations by a metabolic specialist.
    The **blood** can be sent for the measurement of the following:
    - Markers of the principal regulatory hormones: insulin, growth hormone, and cortisol
    - Markers of fatty acid metabolism: ketones (β-hydroxybutyrate and acetoacetate), free fatty acids, and total and free carnitine

TABLE 6-5. DIFFERENTIAL DIAGNOSIS OF CHILDHOOD HYPOGLYCEMIA

Decreased Glucose Utilization

Hyperinsulinism: Islet-cell adenoma or hyperplasia (nesidioblastosis), oral hypoglycemic
    agents, exogenous insulin

Decreased Glucose Production

Inadequate glycogen reserves: Enzymatic defects in glycogen synthesis and glycogenolysis

Ineffective glyconeogenesis: Inadequate substrate (e.g., ketotic hypoglycemia), enzymatic
    defects

Diminished Availability of Fats

Depleted fat stores

Failure to mobilize fats (e.g., hyperinsulinism)

Defective use of fats: Enzymatic defects in fatty acid oxidation (e.g., medium-chain acyl
    CoA dehydrogenase deficiency)

Decreased Fuels and Fuel Stores

Fasting, malnutrition, prolonged illness, malabsorption

Increased Fuel Demand

Fever, exercise

Inadequate Counterregulatory Hormones

Growth hormone or cortisol deficiency, hypopituitarism

- Markers of gluconeogenic pathways: lactate, pyruvate, and alanine
  Urine can be tested for the following:
- Ketones
- Metabolic byproducts associated with known causes of hypoglycemia (e.g., organic acids,
  amino acids)
- Toxicology screen, especially for alcohol and salicylates

Taken together, these tests provide valuable clues as to the cause. For example, low
levels of ketones and free fatty acids suggest that fat was not appropriately mobilized.
As a consequence, ketones were not formed by the liver. Those biochemical abnormalities
are seen in hyperinsulinemic states and can be confirmed by documenting a high level of
circulating insulin. Low urinary ketones also suggest an enzymatic defect in fatty acid oxidation.

Pershad J, Monroe K, Atchison J: Childhood hypoglycemia in an urban emergency department: epidemiology and diagnostic approach to the problem, *Pediatr Emerg Care* 14:268–271, 1998.

74. **In patients with acute hypoglycemia, what are the treatment options?**
    The principal acute treatment is the provision of glucose orally or intravenously. If the patient
    is alert, 4 to 8 ounces of a sugar-containing liquid (e.g., orange juice, cola) may be given.
    If the patient is obtunded, intravenous glucose (2 to 3 mL/kg of $D_{10}W$ or 1 mL/kg of $D_{25}W$)
    should be administered rapidly. If venous access cannot be achieved promptly, glucose can
    be provided through a nasogastric tube because glucose is rapidly absorbed from the gut.
    The risk for prolonged hypoglycemia far outweighs the risk associated with the passage of a
    nasogastric tube in an obtunded patient. Subsequently, the blood sugar should be monitored
    closely and, if necessary, maintained by the constant infusion of glucose (6 to 8 mg/kg/min).
    D_{10} in an electrolyte solution given at about 1.5 times maintenance dose approximates that
    glucose rate. Larger quantities may be necessary, and the blood sugar should be closely
    followed.

Glucagon promotes glycogen breakdown. In settings in which glycogen stores have not been depleted (e.g., insulin overdose), 1 mg of glucagon IM or SC will raise blood glucose levels.

Glucocorticoids should not be used routinely. Their only clear indication is in known primary or secondary adrenal insufficiency. In other settings, they have little acute value and may cloud the diagnostic process. The decision to use glucocorticoids is somewhat dependent on the child's medical history (e.g., reasonable to use in the context of a history of prior central nervous system irradiation).

HYPOTHALAMIC AND PITUITARY DISORDERS

75. **What clinical signs or symptoms suggest hypothalamic dysfunction?**
The signs and symptoms of hypothalamic dysfunction are as variable as the processes controlled by the hypothalamus, ranging from disorders of hormonal production to disturbances of thermoregulation. Precocious or delayed sexual maturation represent the most common presentations of a hypothalamic endocrine abnormality in childhood. Diabetes insipidus, behavioral and cognitive disturbances, and excessive sleepiness are found in about one third of all patients with hypothalamic dysfunction and may be the first manifestation of disease. Eating disorders (obesity, anorexia, bulimia) and convulsions are also reported. Dyshidrosis and disturbances of sphincter control (e.g., encopresis, enuresis) are occasionally seen.

76. **List the intracranial processes that can interfere with hypothalamic-pituitary function.**
    - **Congenital:** Inherited deficiencies of gonadotropin-releasing factor, growth hormone–releasing hormone; syndromic (Laurence-Moon-Biedl and Prader-Labhart-Willi syndromes)
    - **Structural:** Craniopharyngioma, Rathke pouch cyst, hemangioma, hamartoma
    - **Infectious:** Meningitis and encephalitis
    - **Tumors:** Glioma, dysgerminoma, ependymoma, Wegener granulomatosis, histiocytosis X
    - **Idiopathic**

77. **What is the significance of an enlarged sella turcica on a skull film?**
The sella turcica derives its name from the Latin words for *Turkish saddle*. The name reflects the anatomic shape of the saddle-like prominence on the upper surface of the sphenoid bone in the middle cranial fossa, above which sits the pituitary gland. A variety of conditions can lead to sellar enlargement, including tumors of the pituitary or functional hypertrophy of the pituitary, which may occur in primary hypothyroidism or primary hypogonadism. Modern imaging techniques have supplanted the skull series as a tool for searching for pituitary or hypothalamic disease; however, an enlarged sella may be noted on children in whom skull series are obtained for other reasons (e.g., head trauma).

78. **Which tests are useful for studying suspected hypothalamic and pituitary malfunction?**
Either MRI or computed tomography (CT) is required to rule out structural pathology before searching for functional abnormalities. Studies of the pituitary-hypothalamus may include any or all of the following:
    - **Prolactin:** Random levels tend to be elevated in the presence of hypothalamic lesions. A normal level does not rule out CNS pathology. An elevated level may occur in an anxious or stressed child during venipuncture.
    - **Thyrotropin-releasing hormone (TRH) provocative test:** TRH normally promotes the rapid release of thyroid-stimulating hormone (TSH) by the pituitary. In the presence of pituitary or hypothalamic dysfunction, the release of TSH is often blunted and delayed.

TRH also promotes the release of prolactin. In patients with hypothalamic dysfunction, the prolactin response is often altered as well. TRH has not been available in a U.S. Food and Drug Administration–approved formulation since 2002.

■ **Growth hormone production tests** (see question 60): These tests are generally indicated only if the child's growth rate is subnormal. Growth hormone–releasing factor is now available for testing pituitary responsiveness. It has proved useful, in some instances, for delineating pituitary causes of growth hormone underproduction from primary hypothalamic disease.

■ **Gonadotropin-releasing hormone (GnRH) provocative test:** Random levels of leuteinizing hormone and follicle-stimulating hormone are not generally helpful if one is searching for pituitary hypofunction. The results of the GnRH test must be correlated with the age of the child because there are developmental changes in the response to GnRH. GnRH is not available for use in testing.

■ **ACTH stimulation testing (Cortrosyn):** This test of adrenal production of cortisol is often used in determining whether there has been adrenal destruction or to demonstrate more subtle abnormalities in adrenal steroid hormonogenesis. The hypothalamic-releasing hormone, corticotrophin-releasing factor, is also available and can be used to examine the production of ACTH by the pituitary.

■ **Simultaneous urine and serum osmolalities:** A normal serum osmolality and a concentrated urine osmolality tend to rule out diabetes insipidus. If these results are equivocal, a water deprivation test may be required.

SEXUAL DIFFERENTIATION AND DEVELOPMENT

79. **An infant is born with ambiguous genitalia. What features of the history and physical examination are key in the evaluation?**
Of note, the term *ambiguous genitalia* is largely antiquated. The contemporary terminology is *disorder of sexual differentiation* (DSD). This term is thought to more accurately suggest causation rather than consequence and to be less pejorative in discussions with families and nonmedical lay people.

History: One should search for evidence of maternal androgen excess (hirsutism during pregnancy) or androgen ingestion (rare now, but common in the 1960s with certain progestational agents), other hormonal use (e.g., for infertility or endometriosis), alcohol use, parental consanguinity, previous neonatal deaths, or a family history of previously affected children.

Physical examination: The presence of a gonadal structure in the labioscrotal fold strongly implies the presence of some Y chromosomal material. Gonads containing both ovarian and testicular components (ovotestes) have been found in the inguinal canal. However, it is rare to find an ovary in the inguinal canal. In the absence of a palpable gonad, no conclusions can be drawn regarding probable chromosomal sex. The size of the phallic structure and the location of the urethral meatus provide no information about genetic or chromosomal make up. However, phallic size and function are important considerations when determining the sex the child will be reared.

The presence of *midline abnormalities* (e.g., cleft palate) suggests hypothalamic or pituitary dysfunction, whereas congenital anomalies such as imperforate anus suggest structural derangements. A digital rectal examination will confirm the patency of the anus and may allow palpation of the uterus. In infants and young children, ultrasound is the more definitive approach to exploring intra-abdominal structures and can often be helpful in confirming the presence or absence of müllerian structures and gonads. Other anomalies should be noted because ambiguous genitalia can be a feature of numerous syndromes.

Shomaker K, Bradford K, Key-solle M: Ambiguous genitalia, *Contemp Pediatr* 26:40–56, 2009.

Wolfsdorf J, Padilla A: Goodbye intersex ... hello DSD, *Int Pediatr* 23:120–121, 2008.

80. **What are the causes of a DSD?**

Undervirilized male (XY karyotype):
- Androgen resistance: Complete (testicular feminization), partial
- Defects of androgen synthesis: 3-β-hydroxysteroid dehydrogenase deficiency, 5-α-reductase deficiency

Virilized female (XX karyotype):
- Excess androgen: Congenital adrenal hyperplasia, 21-hydroxylase deficiency, 3-β-hydroxysteroid dehydrogenase deficiency
- Maternal androgen exposure: Medication, virilizing adrenal tumor

Intersex (mosaic karyotypes; e.g., XO/XY)

Structural abnormalities

Houk CP, Lee PA: Consensus statement on terminology and management: disorders of sex development, *Sex Dev* 2:172–180, 2008.

MacLaughlin DT, Donahoe PK: Sex determination and differentiation, *N Engl J Med* 350:367–378, 2004.

81. **Which studies are essential for the evaluation of a DSD?**
- **Ultrasonography:** This test is the most helpful for identifying internal structures, particularly the uterus and occasionally the ovaries. The absence of a uterus suggests that testes were present early in gestation and produced müllerian-inhibiting factor, thereby causing regression of the müllerian-derived ducts and thus the uterus. The injection of contrast medium into the urethrovaginal openings will often demonstrate a pouch posterior to the fused labioscrotal folds. Occasionally, the cervix and cervical canal will be highlighted by this study as well.
- **Chromosomal analysis:** Obviously, this is useful for predicting gonadal content. Buccal smears searching for clumps of the nuclear membrane chromatin (Barr bodies, which represent the inactive X chromosome in girls) should not be used (even preliminarily) because of their high rates of inaccuracy. There are now a number of highly specialized and sensitive genetic tests to confirm the presence or absence of X or Y chromosomal material. A geneticist should always be consulted in infants with a DSD.
- **Measurement of adrenal steroids** (17-hydroxyprogesterone, 11-deoxycortisol, 17-hydroxypregnenolone): 17-Hydroxyprogesterone is the precursor that is elevated in the most common variety of congenital adrenal hyperplasia associated with ambiguous genitalia (21-hydroxylase deficiency).
- **Measurement of testosterone and dihydrotestosterone**

As important and useful as the testing is, it is also useful to have input from staff with expertise in this area, including a geneticist, a pediatric endocrinologist, and a pediatric urologist. It is also essential that information be synthesized by this group after all data are available and that it be communicated to the family by a single spokesperson.

Lee PA, Houk CP, Ahmed SF, Hughes IA: Consensus statement on management of intersex disorders, *Pediatrics* 118:e488–e500, 2006.

82. **What major criteria are used to define a micropenis?**

To be classified as a micropenis, the phallus must meet two major criteria:
1. The phallus must be normally formed, with the urethral meatus located on the head of the penis and the penis positioned in an appropriate relationship to the scrotum and other pelvic structures. If these features are not present, then the term *micropenis* should be avoided.
2. The phallus must be more than 2.5 standard deviations below the appropriate mean for age. For a term newborn, this means that a penis less than 2 cm in stretched length is classified as a micropenis.

It is essential that the phallus be measured appropriately. This entails the use of a rigid ruler pressed firmly against the pubic symphysis, depressing the suprapubic fat pad as much as possible. The phallus is grasped gently by its lateral margins and stretched. The measurement is taken along the dorsum of the penis. Note should also be made of the breadth of the phallic shaft. Micropenis must be recognized early in life so that appropriate diagnostic testing can be done.

Lee PA, Mazur T, Danish R, et al: Micropenis. I. Criteria, etiologies and classification, *Johns Hopkins Med J* 146:156–163, 1980.

83. **Outline the three main concerns to be addressed during the initial evaluation of a 1-month-old infant with micropenis.**
    1. **Is there a defect in the hypothalamic-pituitary-gonadal axis?** Specific tests include the measurement of testosterone, dihydrotestosterone, luteinizing hormone, and follicle-stimulating hormone. Because circulating levels of these hormones are normally quite high during the neonatal period, the measurement of random levels during the first 2 months of life may be useful for identifying diseases of the testes and pituitary. Beyond 3 months of age, the tests are generally not useful because the entire axis becomes quiescent and remains so until late childhood. Depending on the patient's age, provocative tests may be necessary, including the following: (1) repetitive testosterone injection to evaluate the ability of the penis to respond to hormonal stimulation; (2) the use of human chorionic gonadotropin as a stimulus for testosterone production by the testes; and (3) leuprolide administration to examine the responsiveness of the pituitary to stimulation. The trial of testosterone therapy is especially important because it indicates whether phallic growth is possible. If it is not, gender reassignment may become a consideration.
    2. **Does a possible pituitary deficiency involve other hormones?** Isolated growth hormone deficiency, gonadotropin deficiency, and panhypopituitarism have been associated with micropenis. The presence of hypoglycemia, hypothermia, or hyperbilirubinemia (e.g., associated with hypothyroidism) in a child with micropenis should lead one to search for other pituitary hormone deficits and structural abnormalities of the CNS (e.g., septo-optic dysplasia).
    3. **Is there a renal abnormality?** Because of the association of genital and renal abnormalities and nature's endless variations, it may be important in some cases to obtain an abdominal and pelvic ultrasound to better define the internal anatomy.

84. **Discuss the terms that denote aspects of precocious sexual development.**
    The terms used to describe precocious puberty reflect the fact that normal puberty is an orderly process by which female children are feminized and male children masculinized. The development of breast tissue without pubic hair is called *premature thelarche*. If pubic hair subsequently develops, the term *precocious puberty* is used. If pubic hair develops without breast tissue, it is *premature pubarche*. Because pubic hair development in the female is thought to be the result of adrenal androgens, the term *premature adrenarche* is commonly used. If the pubertal changes are early and appear to proceed in the orderly fashion of breast budding, pubic hair development, growth spurt, and, finally, menstruation, the term *true precocious puberty* is used. When some of the changes of puberty are present but their appearance is isolated or out of normal sequence (e.g., menses without breast development), the term *pseudoprecocious puberty* is used.

85. **If a 7.2-year-old girl develops breast buds and pubic hair, is this normal or precocious?**
    Precocious puberty is the appearance of physical changes associated with sexual development earlier than normal. Traditionally this has been the development of feminine characteristics in girls who are younger than 8 years and masculine characteristics in boys who are younger than 9 years. In 1997, an office-based study of 17,000 healthy

3- to 12-year-old girls revealed that puberty was occurring on average 1 year earlier in white girls and 2 years earlier in black girls and suggested a revision of guidelines for the ages at which precocious puberty should be investigated. Many experts now recommend that an evaluation for precocious puberty of girls need not be undertaken for white girls older than 7 years or black girls older than 6 years with breast and/or pubic hair development. However, this remains controversial and a subject of ongoing debate and data collection. The recommendations for boys remain that investigations for pathologic etiologies be undertaken if pubertal changes begin before the age of 9 years.

Kaplowitz PB, Oberfield SE: Reexamination of the age limit for defining when puberty is precocious in girls in the United States: implications for evaluation and treatment, *Pediatrics* 104:936–941, 1999.

Herman-Giddens ME, Slora EJ, Wasserman RC, et al: Secondary sexual characteristics and menses in young girls seen in office practice: a study from the Pediatric Research in Office Settings network, *Pediatrics* 99:505–512, 1997.

86. **Breast buds are noted on a 2-year-old girl. Is this worrisome?**
Premature thelarche, or the development of breast buds, is the most common variation of normal pubertal development. A form of mild estrogenization, it typically occurs between the ages of 1 and 3 years. It is usually benign and should not be associated with the onset of other pubertal events. Precocious puberty, rather than simple premature thelarche, should be suspected if the following occur:
- Breast, nipple, and areolar development reach Tanner stage III (i.e., continued progression is of concern).
- Androgenization with pubic and/or axillary hair begins.
- Linear growth accelerates.
- Ongoing parental observation and periodic reexamination are all that are required if there are no signs of progression.

87. **Which aspects of the physical examination are particularly important when evaluating a patient with precocious puberty?**
- **Evidence of a CNS mass:** Examination of optic fundus for possible increased intracranial pressure; visual field testing for evidence of optic nerve compression by a hypothalamic or pituitary mass
- **Evidence of androgenic influence:** Presence of acne and facial and axillary hair; increased muscle bulk and definition; extent of other body or pubic hair; in boys, increased scrotal rugation accompanied by thinning and pigmentation and penile elongation; in girls, clitoromegaly
- **Evidence of estrogenic influence:** Size of breast tissue and nipple and areolar contouring; vaginal mucosa color (increased estrogen causes cornification of vaginal epithelium with a color change from prepubertal shiny red to a more opalescent pink); labia minor (become more prominent and visible between the labia majora as puberty progresses)
- **Evidence of gonadotropic stimulation:** Testicular enlargement of greater than 2.5 cm in length or more than 4 mL in volume (preferably measured using a Prader orchidometer of labeled volumetric beads); pubertal development without testicular enlargement usually suggests adrenal pathology
- **Evidence of other mass:** Asymmetrical testicular enlargement; hepatomegaly; abdominal mass

88. **Which radiologic and laboratory tests are indicated for the evaluation of precocious puberty?**
Radiologic evaluation
- *Bone age*: This study helps to determine the duration of exposure to the elevated sex hormone. A significantly advanced bone age compared with the chronologic age suggests long-term exposure.

- *Abdominal and pelvic ultrasound:* In boys, this test identifies possible adrenal or hepatic masses; in girls, it identifies adrenal masses, ovarian masses, or cysts. Increased uterine size and echogenicity suggest endometrial proliferation in response to circulating estrogen.
- *Head CT or MRI:* This evaluation is useful in identifying pituitary or hypothalamic abnormalities.

Laboratory evaluation

- Luteinizing hormone, follicle-stimulating hormone, estradiol, testosterone
- Adrenal steroid levels (17-hydroxyprogesterone, androstenedione, cortisol): More extensive testing may be needed in a virilized child if the initial studies are normal.
- Provocative testing of the hypothalamic-pituitary axis (using a synthetic GnRH) or of the adrenal gland using a synthetic ACTH, especially in the child with slight but progressive pubertal changes

89. **Boys or girls: Who is more likely to have an identifiable cause for precocious puberty?**
Although precocious puberty occurs much more frequently in girls (80% of cases are girls), boys are more likely to have identifiable pathology. As a second general rule, the younger the child and the more rapid the onset of the condition, the greater the likelihood of detecting pathology.

90. **When along the pubertal spectrum does the male voice begin to crack?**
Voice "breaking" has traditionally been regarded as one of the harbingers of puberty. However, sequential voice analysis reveals that it is usually a late event in puberty, typically occurring between Tanner stages III and IV.

Harries ML, Walker JM, Williams DM, et al: Changes in the male voice at puberty, *Arch Dis Child* 77:445–447, 1997.

THYROID DISORDERS

91. **Which thyroid function tests are "standard"?**
Diseases of the thyroid represent a heterogeneous group of disorders. As such, there are no "standard" thyroid function studies that are appropriate for all children with suspected thyroid disease. The choice of laboratory tests is based on the results of a careful history and physical examination.
  Clinical findings that suggest hyperthyroidism: A TSH level and a thyroxine level (total T_4 or free T_4) should be obtained. Compared to total T_4, the free T_4 is the biologically active component and theoretically is a better measure of thyroid function. TSH suppression is probably the most sensitive indictor of hyperthyroid status. If the patient is symptomatic and has a suppressed TSH level with a normal T_4 level, it will be necessary to obtain a triiodothyronine (T_3) radioimmunoassay because cases of T_3 thyrotoxicosis do occur. If the patient is asymptomatic but has an elevated T_4 level, some measure of binding capacity should be obtained (e.g., a T_3 uptake).
  Clinical findings that suggest hypothyroidism: The laboratory evaluation consists of the quantitation of T_4 (total T_4 or free T_4) and TSH. A low T_4 level and an elevated TSH level are diagnostic of hypothyroidism.

92. **How do antiepileptic medications affect thyroid function tests?**
Medications that bind to albumin, such as phenytoin (Dilantin), can cause changes in thyroid assays because some will displace T_4. Thus, the total T_4 will be low. The confusion that this can cause has been ameliorated somewhat by the wide availability of reliable free T_4 assays.

93. **Of what value is the T_3 resin uptake (T_3RU) test?**
The T_3RU test is a measure of serum thyroid-binding capacity. Because T_4 is primarily protein bound, only a small amount exists in the unbound (free) state. Physiologically, the

free T_4 is the metabolically active compound, but historically it was technically complex to assay directly. For many years, the primary strategy for determining the free T_4 was simply to measure T_3RU and total T_4 and calculate the unbound T_4 (free T_4). Contemporary assays for free T_4 are fairly consistent and reliable. As a consequence, T_3RU is less frequently measured. In patients with primary thyroidal disease, the T_3RU and the T_4 should go in the same direction (i.e., both increase or both decrease). If they go in opposite directions, it is probably a binding problem.

94. **What signs and symptoms in an infant suggest congenital hypothyroidism?**
    See Table 6-6.

TABLE 6-6. SYMPTOMS AND SIGNS OF HYPOTHYROIDISM IN INFANCY

Symptoms	Signs
Lethargy	Hypotonia, slow reflexes
Poor feeding	Poor weight gain
Prolonged jaundice	Jaundice
Constipation	Distended abdomen
Mottling	Acrocyanosis
Cold extremities	Coarse features
	Large fontanels, wide sutures
	Hoarse cry
	Goiter

95. **What causes congenital hypothyroidism?**
    - Primary: Agenesis or dysgenesis, ectopic, dyshormonogenesis
    - Secondary: Hypopituitarism, hypothalamic abnormality
    - Other: Transient, maternal factors (e.g., goitrogen ingestion, iodide deficiency)

96. **How common is goiter (thyroid enlargement) in newborns with congenital hypothyroidism?**
    Congenital goiter is seen in only 20% of newborns with congenital hypothyroidism. Maternal ingestion of antithyroid medications, iodides, and goitrogens; congenital thyroid dyshormonogenic defects; and congenital hyperthyroidism are associated with palpable thyromegaly. Goiter in the newborn is difficult to recognize because of the infant's relatively short neck and increased subcutaneous fat. Palpation of the neck is often overlooked during newborn examinations. On occasion, there may be sufficient posterior extension of the goiter to cause airway obstruction in infants, especially in a mother on goitrogens (e.g., propylthiouracil).

97. **How effective are screening programs for congenital hypothyroidism?**
    Screening programs correctly identify 90% to 95% of children who are affected with congenital hypothyroidism. Screening programs are most likely to miss infants with large ectopic glands, those with partial defects in thyroidal hormone biosynthesis, and those with secondary (pituitary or hypothalamic) disease. If an infant presents with a clinical picture of hypothyroidism and has had a normal newborn screen, it is important to realize that the false-negative rate of the screening is up to 10%.

98. **Discuss the risks of delaying treatment for congenital hypothyroidism.**
Therapy should begin as early as possible because outcome is related to the time treatment is started. Because less than 20% of patients will have distinctive clinical signs at 3 to 4 weeks of age, screening is now performed on all newborns in the United States at 2 to 3 days of age, and most affected children are started on therapy before they are 1 month old. Many pediatricians and screening programs undertake a second screen at 2 weeks of age to ensure that children with treatable conditions are not missed. The prognosis for intellectual development is directly related to the amount of time from birth to the initiation of therapy. Children begun on hormone replacement before 30 days of age have a mean intelligence quotient of 106, but those whose treatment started at 3 to 6 months have a mean intelligence quotient of 70.

99. **A suspected goiter (diffuse enlargement of the thyroid gland) is noted during a routine examination of an asymptomatic 7-year-old boy. What should be the course of action?**
The evaluation of a child with goiter is generally simple. In the absence of signs of thyroidal disease, history should be obtained regarding recent exposure to iodine or other halogens. A family history should be obtained regarding thyroidal disease because thyroiditis tends to run in families. The initial laboratory evaluation typically includes T_4, TSH, and antithyroidal antibodies. If there is discrete nodularity within the thyroid or the gland is rock hard or tender, further diagnostic evaluation (ultrasound, CT) may be indicated. Parathyroid enlargement or lymphoma may be misdiagnosed as goiter.

100. **What is the most common cause of acquired hypothyroidism in childhood?**
The most common cause is **chronic lymphocytic thyroiditis**, also called *Hashimoto thyroiditis* or *autoimmune thyroiditis*. Its incidence during adolescence is about 1% to 2%. The female-to-male ratio is 2:1.

   Counts D, Varma SK: Hypothyroidism in children, *Pediatr Rev* 30:251–257, 2009.

101. **What is the most common clinical presentation of symptoms of Hashimoto thyroiditis?**
Although symptoms of hypothyroidism or hyperthyroidism may be present, most pediatric patients are asymptomatic, and the condition is detected by the presence of goiter. The diagnosis of Hashimoto thyroiditis is primarily based on the demonstration of antithyroidal antibodies.

   Pearce EN, Farwell AP, Braverman LE: Thyroiditis, *N Engl J Med* 348:2646–2655, 2003.

102. **What should a parent be told about the prognosis of a child who has euthyroid goiter caused by chronic lymphocytic thyroiditis?**
About 50% of all children who present with symptoms of euthyroid goiter will have resolution of the goiter over several years, regardless of whether thyroxine replacement is given. It is difficult to predict which children will recover completely, which will remain euthyroid with goiter, and which will become hypothyroid. Large goiters and increased thyroglobulin at presentation, together with an increase over time in thyroid peroxidase antibody and TSH levels, are the most significant predictors for the development of hypothyroidism. Any child identified with thyroid disease should have T_4 and TSH values monitored every 4 to 6 months.

   Radetti G: The natural history of euthyroid Hashimoto's thyroiditis in children, *J Pediatr* 149: 827–832, 2006.

103. **What other autoimmune endocrine diseases are associated with chronic lymphocytic thyroiditis?**
Adrenal insufficiency (Schmidt syndrome), diabetes mellitus, juvenile idiopathic arthritis, systemic lupus erythematosus, and autoimmune polyendocrine syndrome (type II)

104. **What does a normal T_4 and an elevated TSH suggest?**
The diagnosis of hypothyroidism is based on finding both a low T_4 level and an elevated TSH level. However, on occasion, the T_4 level can be maintained in a normal range by increased stimulation of the thyroid gland by TSH. This combination of laboratory values is suggestive of a failing thyroid and is referred to as *compensated hypothyroidism*. Because TSH is the most useful physiologic marker for the adequacy of a circulating level of thyroid hormone, an elevated TSH level is an indication for thyroid replacement therapy. If the TSH level is only minimally elevated and the child is asymptomatic, it is worthwhile to wait 4 to 6 weeks and repeat the T_4 and TSH tests before instituting therapy.

105. **What is the most common cause of hyperthyroidism in children?**
Graves disease is a multisystem disease that is characterized by hyperthyroidism, infiltrative ophthalmopathy, and occasionally, an infiltrative dermopathy. The features of this disease may occur singly or in any combination. In children, the ophthalmopathy appears to be less severe, and the dermopathy is rare; the full syndrome may never develop. There has been a tendency to use the terms *Graves disease*, *thyrotoxicosis*, and *hyperthyroidism* interchangeably, but there are other causes of hyperthyroidism in childhood (e.g., factitious).

106. **In addition to Graves disease, what conditions may cause hyperthyroidism?**
   - *Excess TSH:* TSH-producing tumor (these are extraordinarily rare in children)
   - *Abnormal thyroid stimulation:* TSH receptor antibody
   - *Thyroid autonomy:* Adenoma, multinodular goiter, activating mutations of G proteins (e.g., McCune-Albright syndrome)
   - *Thyroid inflammation:* Subacute thyroiditis, Hashimoto thyroiditis
   - *Exogenous hormone:* Ingestion, ectopic thyroid tissue

107. **Describe the typical features of hyperthyroidism that occurs as a result of Graves disease.**
History: The onset of symptoms is usually gradual, with increasing emotional lability and deteriorating school performance. Sleep disturbances, nervousness, and weight loss may be noted, as may easy fatigability and heat intolerance. Observation of the child's behavior while the history is being obtained from the parent is often instructive.
   Physical examination: Weight may be low for height, and many children will be tall for age and genetic potential. Some children will have experienced an acceleration in growth rate at the same time that their behavior began to deteriorate. The pulse rate is usually inappropriately high for age. A widened pulse pressure or an elevated blood pressure is often noted, although this is a more variable finding in children than in adults.

108. **What causes Graves disease?**
Graves disease is an autoimmune disorder in which TSH receptor antibodies bind to the TSH receptor, thereby resulting in the stimulation of thyroid hormone production and subsequent hyperthyroidism. Most thyroid receptor antibodies belong to the IgG class. The general name used for these antibodies is **human thyroid-stimulating immunoglobulins** (HTSI or TSI). These were formerly called *long-acting thyroid stimulator* (LATS).

KEY POINTS: THYROID DISORDERS

1. Midline neck masses usually involve the thyroid gland or thyroid remnants, such as a thyroglossal duct cyst.

2. Neck extension improves visualization and palpation of thyroid masses, especially with swallowing.

3. About 20% to 40% of solitary thyroid nodules in adolescents are malignant; expedited evaluation is needed.

4. Chronic lymphocytic thyroiditis is the most common cause of pediatric goiter in the United States.

5. Chronic lymphocytic thyroiditis most commonly appears as an asymptomatic goiter, thereby reinforcing the need for thyroid palpation (an often overlooked examination feature).

6. The best initial screening studies for hypothyroidism and hyperthyroidism are those measuring total T_4 and thyroid-stimulating hormone.

---

109. **Why does exophthalmos occur in Graves disease?**
The reason is unknown, but several facts suggest an autoimmune process:
- Histologic studies reveal lymphocytic infiltration of the retrobulbar muscles.
- Circulating lymphocytes are sensitized to an antigen that is unique to the retrobulbar tissues.
- The thyroglobulin-antithyroglobulin antibody complexes found in patients with Graves disease bind specifically to the extraorbital muscles. There may be a separate class of antibodies that is responsible for changes in the retrobulbar muscles.

Bahn RS: Graves' opthalmopathy, *New Engl J Med* 362:726–738, 2010.

110. **What treatment options are available for children with Graves disease?**
The three types of therapy are antithyroid medication, radioactive (^{131}I) ablation, and subtotal thyroidectomy.

Cheetham TD, Hughes IA, Barnes ND, Wraight EP: Treatment of hyperthyroidism in young people, *Arch Dis Child* 78:207–209, 1998.

Rivkees SA, Dinauer C: An optimal treatment for pediatric Graves disease is radioiodine, *J Clin Endocrinol Metab* 92:797–800, 2007.

111. **Describe the principal modes of actions and the side effects of medications used to treat Graves disease.**
The thioamide derivatives—propylthiouracil and methimazole—have historically been the keystones of long-term management. However, their effective onset of action is slow because they block the synthesis but not the release of thyroid hormone. Propranolol is useful for treating many of the β-adrenergic effects of hyperthyroidism. It is used during the acute management of Graves disease but should be discontinued when the thyroid disease is controlled. Iodide (which can transiently block thyroid hormone release) and glucocorticoids are useful stopgap medications while awaiting the inhibitory effects of the thioamide; they are generally used only when the patient is acutely symptomatic (i.e., thyroid storm). The thioamides are associated with some side effects, the most serious of which have been a lupus-like syndrome involving the lungs or liver, neutropenia, and elevated transaminase levels.

Brent GA: Graves' disease, *N Engl J Med* 358:2594–2605, 2008.

Dotsch J, Rascher W, Dorr HG: Graves' disease in childhood: a review of the options for diagnosis and treatment, *Paediatr Drugs* 5:95–102, 2003.

112. **Has radioactive iodide fallen into disfavor as a treatment option for Graves disease?**
On the contrary, radioactive iodide (^{131}I) is increasing in popularity. In some pediatric endocrinology centers, this is now considered the first line of therapy. Concern had been voiced about the possible risk for thyroid carcinoma, leukemia, thyroid nodules, or genetic mutations, but as the individuals treated with ^{131}I during childhood have been followed for prolonged periods, experience suggests that children are not at a significantly increased risk for developing these conditions.

Rivkees SA, Sklar C, Freemark M: The management of Graves' disease in children, with special emphasis on radioiodine treatment, *J Clin Endocrinol Metab* 83:3767–3776, 1998.

113. **During a routine physical examination, a solitary thyroid nodule is palpated on an asymptomatic 10-year-old child. Can a wait-and-see approach be taken?**
Absolutely not. In children with a solitary nodule, about 30% to 40% have a carcinoma, 20% to 30% have an adenoma, and the remainder will have thyroid abscess, thyroid cyst, multinodular goiter, Hashimoto thyroiditis, subacute thyroiditis, or nonthyroidal neck mass. Given the relatively high incidence of carcinoma, a thyroidal mass demands prompt evaluation. Previous irradiation to the head or neck is associated with a significantly increased incidence of thyroid carcinoma. A family history of thyroid disease increases the likelihood of chronic lymphocytic thyroiditis or Graves disease. The presence of tenderness on palpation or high titers of antithyroid antibodies points away from a malignant process. However, in all cases, radiologic studies should be undertaken; in many cases, surgical exploration is required.

114. **How should this solitary thyroid nodule be investigated?**
The principal tools used in the investigation of a thyroid mass are ^{123}I **scanning** and ultrasound. **Ultrasound** is useful for delineating the size of the mass, its anatomic relationship to the rest of the thyroid, and the presence of cystic structures. ^{123}I imaging that reveals a single nonfunctioning mass ("cold" nodule) suggests a carcinoma or adenoma and is a clear indication for surgery. Patchy uptake is more characteristic of chronic lymphocytic thyroiditis, whereas a poorly functioning lobe may be found in a subacute thyroiditis. **Fine-needle biopsy** is another approach to the investigation of a thyroid mass but is not widely used in pediatric practice.

Mehanna HM, Jain A, Morton RP, et al: Investigating the thyroid nodule, *BMJ* 338:705–709, 2009.

115. **How is the euthyroid sick syndrome diagnosed?**
This syndrome is an adaptive response to slow body metabolism. It is also called the low T_3 syndrome because the most consistent finding is a depression of serum T_3. Reverse T_3, a metabolically inactive metabolite, is increased, although this is rarely measured. T_4 and thyroid binding globulin levels may be low or normal; free T_4 and TSH levels are normal. In sick preterm infants, the clinical picture is often confusing because levels of T_4, free T_4, and T_3 are naturally low. Infants and children with the euthyroid sick syndrome generally revert to normal as the primary illness resolves.

Shih JL, Agus MSD: Thyroid function in the critically ill newborn and child, *Curr Opin Pediatr* 21:356–540, 2009.

CHAPTER 7

GASTROENTEROLOGY

Andrew B. Grossman, MD, and Chris A. Liacouras, MD

CLINICAL ISSUES

1. **What are the causes of pancreatitis in children?**
   - **33%: Systemic disorders** (sepsis and shock, vasculitis, and viral infections, including mumps, influenza, and Epstein-Barr virus)
   - **25%: Idiopathic**
   - **15%: Trauma**
   - **10%: Anatomic and structural anomalies** (pancreatic divisum, duct anomalies, choledochal cyst, and cholelithiasis)
   - **5%: Metabolic disorders** (cystic fibrosis, hypercalcemia, hyperlipidemia, α_1-antitrypsin deficiency, and organic acidemias)
   - **5%: Drugs and toxins** (certain chemotherapeutic agents, valproic acid, thiazides, and alcohol)
   - **2%: Hereditary** (familial)

   Durie PR: Disturbances of exocrine pancreatic dysfunction. In Rudolph CD, Rudolph AM editors: *Rudolph's Pediatrics*, ed 21, New York, McGraw-Hill, 2003, p 1467.

2. **What are the potential pitfalls of relying solely on serum amylase to diagnose pancreatitis?**
   Although serum amylase is the most widely used test for diagnosis, it may not be the most sensitive or specific. It is usually elevated during the first 12 hours of the condition, but it may return to normal within 24 to 72 hours. A child can have severe pancreatitis with a normal serum amylase level.

   Falsely elevated serum amylase can occur if amylase is released from other injured areas (e.g., salivary glands in mumps, intestines in Crohn disease, ovaries and fallopian tubes in salpingitis). Isoenzyme determinations can help to identify the source if the clinical picture is confusing.

   The serum lipase remains elevated for longer periods. Other blood tests that should be considered include cationic trypsinogen, hepatic transaminases, blood glucose, and calcium.

3. **How is ascites diagnosed by physical examination?**
   Severe ascites is commonly diagnosed by observation of the child in a supine and then an upright position. Bulging flanks, umbilical protrusion, and scrotal edema (in males) are generally evident. Three main techniques are used when the diagnosis is not obvious:
   - **Fluid wave:** This sign can be elicited in a cooperative patient by tapping sharply on one flank while receiving the wave with the other hand. The transmission of the wave through fatty tissue should be blocked by a hand placed on the center of the abdomen.
   - **Shifting dullness:** With the patient supine, percussion of the abdomen will demonstrate a central area of tympany at the top that is surrounded by flank percussion dullness. This dullness shifts when the patient moves laterally or stands up.
   - **"Puddle sign":** A cooperative and mobile patient may be examined in the knee-chest position. The pool of ascites is tapped while you listen for a sloshing sound or change in sound transmission with the stethoscope.

Small amounts of ascites can be extremely difficult to detect with physical examination in children. Although ascites can be demonstrated on radiographs, the most sensitive and specific test is an abdominal-pelvic ultrasound, which can detect as little as 150 mL of ascitic fluid.

4. **How does the major cause of ascites in neonates differ from that of older children?**
   Older children: Portal hypertension as a result of hepatic (e.g., chronic liver disease of multiple etiologies), prehepatic (e.g., portal vein thrombosis), or posthepatic (e.g., congestive heart failure, constrictive pericarditis) conditions
   Infants: Urinary ascites most commonly as a result of obstructive renal disease (e.g., posterior urethral valves)

5. **In what clinical settings is rectal prolapse most commonly seen?**
   - Constipation
   - Celiac disease
   - Malnutrition
   - Severe coughing (e.g., pertussis)
   - Cystic fibrosis
   - Enterobius vermicularis (pinworm) infestation
   - Colonic polyps
   - Myelomeningocele
   - Abnormalities of sacrum or coccyx
   - Ehlers-Danlos syndrome

6. **How is the diagnosis of pinworms made?**
   Direct visualization of larger adult worms in the perianal region of a child can sometimes be successful, with the best examination time 2 to 3 hours after the child is asleep. Additionally, **transparent adhesive tape** can be applied to the perianal region to collect eggs; the tape can be examined under low-power microscopy (Fig. 7-1). These specimens are best obtained in the morning.

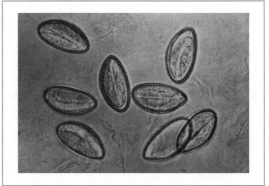

Figure 7-1. Pinworm eggs as collected on adhesive tape. (From the Public Health Image Library, Centers for Disease Control and Prevention: http://phil.cdc.gov.)

Because few pinworm ova are present in stool, examination of stool specimens for ova and parasites (for pinworms) is not recommended.

American Academy of Pediatrics: Pinworm infection. In Pickering LK, editor: *2009 Red Book: Report of the Committee on Infectious Diseases*, ed 28, Elk Grove Park, IL, 2009, American Academy of Pediatrics, p 520.

7. **What is the likely diagnosis of an infant with excessive secretions and choking episodes in whom a nasogastric tube cannot be passed into the stomach?**
   Esophageal atresia with tracheoesophageal fistula. This congenital anomaly is usually diagnosed during the newborn period, often when a chest radiograph reveals the intended nasogastric tube coiled in the blind upper esophageal pouch with the stomach distended with air. Treatment is surgical. The possible variations are shown in Fig. 7-2.

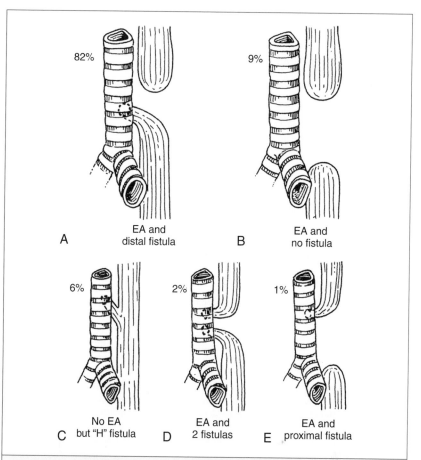

Figure 7-2. A, Esophageal atresia with distal esophageal communication with the tracheobronchial tree (most common type: 80%). **B,** Esophageal atresia without a distal communication. **C,** H-type fistulas between otherwise intact trachea and esophagus. **D,** Esophageal atresia with both proximal and distal communication with the trachea. **E,** Esophageal atresia with proximal communication. (From Blickman H [ed]: The Requisites: Pediatric Radiology, 2nd ed. Philadelphia, Mosby, 1998, p 93.)

8. **What would be the most common condition that might present as a food impaction in an adolescent?**

   Eosinophilic esophagitis. Occurring in children and adults, eosinophilic esophagitis is characterized by multiple symptoms that are suggestive of gastroesophageal reflux (GER), including heartburn, emesis, regurgitation, epigastric pain, and feeding difficulties, which are typically unresponsive to acid suppression therapy. Pathologically, this is characterized by eosinophilic inflammation of the esophagus and is almost always related to food antigens. In adolescents and adults, eosinophilic esophagitis often presents with symptoms of dysphagia or, occasionally, food impaction.

   Furuta GT, Liacouras CA, Collins MH, et al: Eosinophilic esophagitis in children and adults: a systematic review and consensus recommendations for diagnosis and treatment, *Gastroenterology* 133:1342–1363, 2007.

9. **List the indications for lower gastrointestinal (GI) colonoscopy or endoscopy in children.**
   - Hematochezia in the absence of an anal source
   - History of familial polyposis
   - Chronic diarrhea of unclear etiology
   - Persistent severe unexplained mid- to lower abdominal pain
   - Colitis of unclear etiology
   - Diagnosis and management of inflammatory bowel disease
   - Removal of foreign body
   - Ureterosigmoidostomy, surveillance
   - Abnormality on barium enema
   - Dilation of a colonic stricture

10. **When is colonoscopy contraindicated?**
    - Suspected perforation
    - Toxic megacolon
    - Recent abdominal surgery
    - Unstable medical illness (abnormal vital signs or severe anemia)
    - Inadequate bowel preparation
    - Coagulopathy
    - Massive lower GI bleeding

    Fox VL: Colonoscopy. In Walker WA, Durie PR, Hamilton JR, et al, editors: *Pediatric Gastrointestinal Disease*, ed 2, St. Louis, 1996, Mosby, pp 1533–1541.

11. **What characterizes functional abdominal pain in children?**
    Previously called *recurrent abdominal pain*, this entity is common in pediatric practice and refers to children without evidence of inflammatory, anatomic, infectious, allergic, metabolic, or neoplastic processes that explain the symptoms. The cause is likely multifactorial, including abnormalities in the enteric nervous system with possible visceral hyperalgesia, or a decreased threshold for pain in response to changes in intraluminal pressure secondary to physiologic stimuli. This combination of biopsychosocial mechanisms (physiologic, psychological, and behavioral) results in a broad range of management approaches.

12. **In children with abdominal pain, what historic features suggest a possible organic or serious cause?**
    - Involuntary weight loss
    - Deceleration of linear growth
    - GI blood loss
    - Significant vomiting (e.g., bilious emesis, hematemesis, protracted vomiting, cyclical vomiting, pattern concerning to physician)
    - Chronic severe diarrhea
    - Alarm signs on abdominal examination (right upper or lower quadrant tenderness, localized fullness or mass effect, peritoneal signs, hepatomegaly, splenomegaly, costovertebral angle tenderness)
    - Unexplained fevers
    - Family history of inflammatory bowel disease or other significant GI illnesses
    - Presentation of symptoms before 4 years or after 15 years of age

    Rasquin A, DiLorenzo C, Forbes D, et al: Childhood functional gastrointestinal disorders: child/adolescent, *Gastroenterology* 130:1527–1537, 2006.

    Chronic abdominal pain in children: a clinical report of the American Academy of Pediatrics and North American Society for Pediatric Gastroenterology, Hepatology, and Nutrition, *J Pediatr Gastoenterol Nutr* 40:245–248, 2005.

13. **What treatments are used for functional abdominal pain in children?**
    - **Dietary:** Low-lactose diets, dietary fiber, low-fructose diets, probiotics
    - **Pharmacologic:** Antidepressants, antispasmodics, prokinetic agents, H_2-receptor antagonists, leukotriene-receptor antagonists
    - **Psychological:** Cognitive behavioral therapy, family intervention, relaxation and distraction techniques
    - **Complementary and alternative medicine:** Herbal medicine, peppermint oil, biofeedback, hypnotherapy, massage therapy, acupuncture

    Whitfield KL, Shulman RJ: Treatment options for functional gastrointestinal disorders, *Pediatr Ann* 38:288–294, 2009.

    Banez GA: Chronic abdominal pain in children: what to do following the medical evaluation, *Curr Opin Pediatr* 20:571–575, 2008.

14. **What distinguishes the irritable bowel syndrome in children?**
    Another functional GI disorder, *irritable bowel syndrome* is a chronic pain syndrome similar to functional abdominal pain but associated at least 25% of the time with at least two of the following: improvement with defecation, onset of pain associated with a change in frequency of stool, or onset associated with a change in the form or appearance of stool.

    Sood MR: Treatment approaches to irritable bowel syndrome, *Pediatr Ann* 38:272–276, 2009.

    Mayer EA: Irritable bowel syndrome, *N Engl J Med* 358:1692–1699, 2008.

15. **How does the average volume of the swallow of a child compare with that of an adult?**
    - Child (age 1¼ to 3½ years): 4.5 mL
    - Adult male: 21 mL
    - Adult female: 14 mL
    - Average: 0.27 mL/kg

    Jones DV, Work CE: Volume of a swallow, *Am J Dis Child* 102:427, 1961.

16. **What is intractable singultus?**
    Persistent hiccups.

17. **What is the most commonly ingested foreign body?**
    Coins account for more than 20,000 visits yearly to emergency rooms in the United States. Symptomatic patients are more likely to have the coin lodged in the esophagus, although a significant portion of these patients may be asymptomatic. Coins lodged in the esophagus should be removed endoscopically within 24 hours because of the risk for ulceration and perforation.

18. **Which is potentially more dangerous after ingestion: a penny made in 1977 or one made in 1987?**
    The penny from 1987. In 1982, the composition of pennies changed. Coins minted after that date have higher concentrations of zinc, which is more corrosive and potentially more harmful after prolonged contact with stomach acid.

19. **What is the difference radiographically between a coin in the esophagus and a coin in the trachea?**
    A coin in the esophagus appears *en face* in the anteroposterior view (sagittal plane), whereas a coin in the trachea appears *en face* on the lateral view (coronal plane). This occurs because the cartilaginous ring of the trachea is open posteriorly, but the opening of the esophagus is widest in the transverse position.

20. **A teenage girl has symptoms of swallowing difficulties improved by positional head and neck changes, nocturnal regurgitation, and halitosis. What is the likely diagnosis?**

    Achalasia. The cardinal symptom of this motility disorder of the esophagus is dysphagia. The diagnosis is made by barium swallow and esophageal manometry. The barium swallow will usually show a dilated esophagus that tapers at the level of the gastroesophageal junction, commonly referred to as a "bird's beak" (Fig. 7-3). The manometric findings are diagnostic, including elevated basal lower esophageal sphincter pressure with failure to relax and the absence of peristalsis throughout the esophageal body during the swallow.

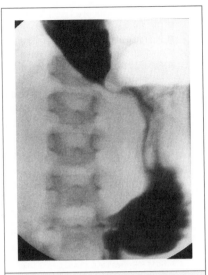

Figure 7-3. Barium swallow in a child with achalasia showing esophageal dilation and rapid tapering in a beak-like appearance. (From Wyllie R, Hyams JS, Kay M [eds]: Pediatric Gastrointestinal and Liver Disease, 3rd ed. Philadelphia, Saunders, 2006, p 330.)

CONSTIPATION

21. **When is the first stool of a neonate normally passed?**

    Ninety-nine percent of infants pass a stool within the first 24 hours of life, and 100% do so within 48 hours of birth. Failure to pass a stool can be an indication of intestinal obstruction or anatomic abnormality. About 95% of patients with Hirschsprung disease and 25% of patients with cystic fibrosis do not pass their first stool during the first 24 hours. The rule of early passage does not apply to premature babies, in whom delayed evacuation (>24 hours) is common, particularly with extreme prematurity.

22. **What constitutes constipation in childhood?**

    Constipation is defined as a delay or difficulty in defecation, present for 2 or more weeks and sufficient to cause distress in the patient. Normal stool frequency varies from several times a day to three stools per week. In children, constipation should be considered when the normal stooling pattern becomes more infrequent, when stools become hard or are difficult to expel, or when the child exhibits withholding patterns or behavioral changes toward moving his or her bowels. Soiling (encopresis) can be a sign of constipation.

    Biggs WS, Dery WH: Evaluation and treatment of constipation in infants and children, *Am Fam Physician* 73:469–482, 2006.

23. **What features suggest an organic etiology for constipation?**
    - History of weight loss and inadequate weight gain
    - Lumbosacral nevi or sinus
    - Multiple café-au-lait spots
    - Abnormal neurologic examination (decreased tone, strength; abnormal reflexes)

- Anal abnormalities (anteriorly displaced, patulous, or tight)
- Gross or occult blood in stool
- Abdominal distention with or without vomiting

Croffie JM, Fitzgerald JF: Constipation and irritable bowel syndrome. In Liacouras CA, Piccoli DA, editors: *Pediatric Gastroenterology: The Requisites in Pediatrics*, Philadelphia, 2008, Mosby Elsevier, p 33.

24. **What is the most important component of the physical examination when evaluating constipation?**
The rectal examination. The presence of large amounts of stool in the rectal vault almost always indicates functional constipation. Lack of stool in the rectal vault could indicate recent evacuation; if expulsion of stool occurs after removal of the examining finger, Hirschsprung disease should be considered. Failure to perform a rectal examination is a common omission during the evaluation of children, and impaction in chronic constipation often goes undetected.

Safder S: Digital rectal examination and the primary care physicians: a lost art? *Clin Pediatr* 45:411–414, 2006.

Gold DM, Levine J, Weinstein TA, et al: Frequency of digital rectal examination in children with chronic constipation, *Arch Pediatr Adolesc Med* 153:377–379, 1999.

KEY POINTS: CONSTIPATION

1. Ninety-nine percent of full-term infants pass stool less than 24 hours after birth. Failure to pass stool within the first 48 hours of life should be considered pathologic until proved otherwise.

2. The rectal examination is a common omission among patients undergoing an evaluation for constipation. Tone, the amount of stool, and the size of the rectal vault should be assessed.

3. Fecal soiling is almost always associated with severe functional constipation and not Hirschsprung disease.

4. Treatment of functional constipation is multimodal and includes medications.

5. Organic causes are suggested by weight loss, lumbosacral nevi, anal abnormalities, blood in stool, and abdominal distention.

25. **Which clinical features differentiate chronic retentive constipation from Hirschsprung disease?**
See Table 7-1.

26. **How is Hirschsprung disease diagnosed?**
Hirschsprung disease results from the failure of normal migration of ganglion cell precursors to their location in the GI tract during gestation. The diagnosis can be made by obtaining an unprepped **barium enema**, which will demonstrate a change in the caliber of the large intestine at the site where normal bowel meets aganglionic bowel (transition zone). An unprepped barium enema is required because the use of cleansing enemas can dilate the abnormal portion of the colon and remove some of the distal impaction, thereby resulting in a false-negative result. After the study, the retention of barium for 24 or more hours is

TABLE 7-1. CLINICAL DISTINCTIONS BETWEEN CHRONIC RETENTIVE CONSTIPATION AND HIRSCHSPRUNG DISEASE

Clinical Feature	Functional Constipation	Hirschsprung Disease
Age of onset	>1 yr	<1 yr
Passage of meconium	Within 24 hr	Meconium passes after 24 hr
Abdominal pain	Frequent, colicky	Rare
Stool size	Large	Small, ribbon-like
Stool withholding behavior	Present	Absent
Encopresis (soiling)	Present	Very rare
Rectum	Filled with stool	Empty
Rectal examination	Stool in rectum	Explosive passage of stool
Growth	Normal	Poor

suggestive of Hirschsprung disease or a significant motility disorder. This study is less reliable in a child younger than 6 months. **Rectal suction biopsies** or **full-thickness surgical biopsies** will confirm the absence of ganglion cells. Anal manometry is less reliable in children; in small infants, it requires specialized equipment.

27. **How is encopresis defined?**
Encopresis, or fecal soiling, may be defined as the involuntary passage of fecal material in an otherwise healthy and normal child. Children with encopresis typically sense no urge to defecate. Fecal soiling is almost always associated with severe functional constipation.

28. **How should children with chronic constipation and encopresis be managed?**
   - The rectosigmoid colon should be **aggressively cleansed** of fecal material. Multiple enemas over 3 to 9 days are commonly needed. Adult enemas should be used in children who are older than 3 years.
   - Medications that act as an **osmotic laxative** by drawing fluid into the intestine to promote the passage of soft stools include polyethylene glycol powder and lactulose (a nonabsorbable sugar). For cases of long-standing functional constipation, osmotic laxatives should be continued for a minimum of several months while the dilated rectum returns to normal size.
   - An **oral lubricant**, such as mineral oil or Kondremul, can help promote the continued passage of stool but can contribute to accidental soiling. In difficult cases, **stimulant medications**, such as milk of magnesia or Senokot, can be substituted for short-term use.
   - It is extremely important to **educate** patients and parents about the mechanics of the disorder. A high-fiber diet, possible limitation of dairy and complex carbohydrates, defined periods of toilet sitting, and a behavior modification system that rewards normal bowel movements are essential for eventual success. Integrative approaches of biofeedback, relaxation strategies, and mental imagery have been used for children who have severe "defecation anxiety." A goal is one to two soft bowel movements a day. Relapses are common.

Candy D, Belsey J: Macrogol (polyethylene glycol) laxatives in children with functional constipation and faecal impaction: a systematic review, *Arch Dis Child* 94:156–160, 2009.

Culbert TP, Banez GA: Integrative approaches to childhood constipation and encopresis, *Pediatr Clin N Am* 54:927–947, 2007.

Evaluation and Treatment of Constipation in Infants and Children; Recommendations of the North American Society for Pediatric Gastroenterology, Hepatology, and Nutrition, *J Pediatr Gastroenterol Nutr* 43:e1–e13, 2006.

29. **What tests, in addition to those ruling out Hirschsprung disease, are commonly considered for refractory cases of constipation?**
Laboratory testing will include serum calcium, thyroid-stimulating hormone, lead, and celiac disease panel. A sweat test might be considered. Magnetic resonance imaging of the spine to rule out spina bifida occulta or tethered cord is sometimes helpful. Anorectal manometry can help diagnose a motility disorder.

DIARRHEA AND MALABSORPTION

30. **Which historical questions are key when seeking the cause of diarrhea?**
■ Recent medications, especially antibiotics
■ History of immunosuppression (e.g., recurrent major infections, history of malnutrition, acquired immunodeficiency syndrome, immunosuppressive medications)
■ Illnesses in other family members or close contacts
■ Travel outside of the United States
■ Travel to rural or seacoast areas (i.e., involving the consumption of untreated water, raw milk, or raw shellfish)
■ Attendance in day care
■ Recent foods; particularly focus on juice and fructose consumption
■ Presence of family pets
■ Food preparation and water source

Thielman NM, Guerrant RL: Acute infectious diarrhea, *N Engl J Med* 350:38–47, 2004.

31. **Which children should be seen for the medical evaluation of acute diarrhea?**
■ Young age (<6 months or weighing <8 kg)
■ History of premature birth, chronic medical conditions, or concurrent illness
■ Fever ≥38°C for infants <3 months old or ≥39°C for children 3 to 36 months old
■ Visible blood in stool
■ High output, including frequent and substantial volumes of diarrhea
■ Persistent vomiting
■ Caregiver's report of signs that are consistent with dehydration
■ Change in mental status
■ Suboptimal response to oral rehydration therapy or inability of caregiver to administer this therapy

King CK, Glass R, Bresee JS, Duggan C, Centers for Disease Control and Prevention: Managing acute gastroenteritis among children: oral rehydration, maintenance, and nutritional therapy, *MMWR Recomm Rep* 52:1–16, 2003.

32. **In what settings can diarrhea be a severe, life-threatening illness?**
Severe diarrhea of any cause can lead to dehydration, which can cause significant morbidity and mortality. However, diarrhea can be a sign of a serious associated illness, which in itself can be life-threatening:
■ Intussusception
■ *Salmonella* gastroenteritis (neonatal or compromised host)
■ Hemolytic-uremic syndrome
■ Hirschsprung disease (with toxic megacolon)
■ Pseudomembranous colitis
■ Inflammatory bowel disease (with toxic megacolon)

Fleisher GR: Diarrhea. In Fleisher GR, Ludwig S, editors: *Textbook of Pediatric Emergency Medicine*, ed 4, Baltimore, 2000, Lippincott Williams & Wilkins, p 204.

33. **Why is true diarrhea during the first few days of life especially concerning?**
In addition to the greater potential for dehydration in a newborn, diarrhea in this age group is more commonly associated with major congenital intestinal defects involving electrolyte transport (e.g., congenital sodium- or chloride-losing diarrhea), carbohydrate absorption (e.g., congenital lactase deficiency), immune-mediated defects (e.g., autoimmune enteropathy), or those characterized by villous blunting (e.g., microvillus inclusion disease). Although viral enteritis can occur in the nursery, any newborn with true diarrhea warrants thorough evaluation and possible referral to a tertiary center.

Sherman PM, Mitchell DJ, Cutz E: Neonatal enteropathies: defining causes of protracted diarrhea in infancy, *J Pediatr Gastroenterol Nutr* 30:16–26, 2004.

34. **What are the most useful stool tests for diagnosing fat malabsorption?**
Measurement of 72-hour fecal fat is the gold standard test for fat malabsorption. The patient must ingest a high-fat diet for 3 to 5 days (100 g daily for adults), and all stool is collected for the final 72 hours. A complete and accurate dietary history should be obtained concomitantly so the coefficient of fat absorption can be calculated. Steatorrhea is present if more than 7% of dietary fat is malabsorbed. In normal infants, up to 15% of fat can be malabsorbed. Other tests include Sudan staining of stool for fat globules (a qualitative test that, if positive, indicates gross steatorrhea), the steatocrit, and monitoring absorbed lipids after a standardized meal.

35. **What stool test is most useful for helping diagnose GI protein loss?**
Fecal α_1-antitrypsin measurement is the most useful stool marker of protein malabsorption. It is important to concomitantly measure serum α_1-antitrypsin to ensure that the patient does not have α_1-antitrypsin deficiency, which could result in a false-negative stool study.

36. **How do patterns of secretory or enterotoxigenic and inflammatory diarrhea vary?**
Secretory or enterotoxigenic disease is characterized by watery diarrhea and the absence of fecal leukocytes. Inflammatory disease is characterized by dysentery (i.e., symptoms and bloody stools) as well as fecal leukocytes and red blood cells.

37. **What are the common infectious causes of secretory or toxigenic diarrhea?**
   - Food poisoning (toxigenic)
   - *Staphylococcus aureus*
   - *Bacillus cereus*
   - *Clostridium perfringens*
   - Enterotoxigenic *Escherichia coli*
   - *Vibrio cholerae*
   - *Giardia lamblia*
   - *Cryptosporidium* species
   - Rotavirus
   - Norwalk-like virus

38. **What are the common infectious causes of inflammatory diarrhea?**
   - *Shigella* species
   - Invasive *E. coli*
   - *Salmonella* species
   - *Campylobacter* species
   - *Clostridium difficile*
   - *Entamoeba histolytica*
   - *Yersinia enterocolitica*

39. **Why is *Salmonella enteritis* so concerning in a child who is younger than 12 months?**
   In older children with *Salmonella* gastroenteritis, secondary bacteremia and dissemination of disease rarely occur. In infants, however, 5% to 40% may have positive blood cultures for *Salmonella*, and, in 10% of these cases, *Salmonella* can cause meningitis, osteomyelitis, pericarditis, and pyelonephritis. Thus, in infants who are younger than 1 year, outpatient management of diarrhea assumes even greater significance, particularly if *Salmonella* is suspected.

40. **What is the most common cause of traveler's diarrhea?**
   Enterotoxigenic *E. coli* is clearly the most commonly identified cause. Depending on the location, however, other bacteria (such as *Campylobacter* in Southeast Asia), viruses (norovirus, rotavirus), or parasites (*Giardia, Cryptosporidium*) can be present.

41. **How can traveler's diarrhea be prevented?**
   - **Avoidance:** In high-risk areas of developing countries, avoid previously peeled raw fruits and vegetables and any foods or beverages or ice cubes prepared with tap water.
   - **Bismuth subsalicylate:** Prophylactic bismuth subsalicylate (Pepto-Bismol) has been shown to minimize diarrheal illness in up to 75% of adults. Although some authorities recommend its use in children, others argue against it because of the risk for salicylate intoxication. It can interfere with absorption of doxycycline used for malaria prevention.
   - **Anti-infective drugs:** Prophylactic use of antimicrobial agents such as trimethoprim-sulfamethoxazole, neomycin, doxycycline, and fluoroquinolones can decrease the frequency of traveler's diarrhea in children and adults. However, routine use of antibiotics is not recommended because of potential risks for allergic drug reactions, antibiotic-associated colitis, and the development of resistant organisms.
   - **Immunization:** Although potentially an ideal solution, at present it is not an alternative.

   Hill DR, Ryan ET: Management of travellers' diarrhea, *BMJ* 337:863–867, 2008.

42. **What is the most common treatment for traveler's diarrhea in children?**
   If symptoms develop, empirical therapy is indicated, and the regimen of trimethoprim-sulfamethoxazole and Imodium (for children >2 years old) is very effective. For adolescents, ciprofloxacin is an alternative.

43. **Which bacterial gastroenteritides may benefit from antimicrobial therapy?**
   See Table 7-2.

44. **List the differential diagnosis of chronic diarrhea by age group.**
   - **Newborns:** Congenital short gut, congenital lactose intolerance, malrotation with intermittent volvulus, ischemia, defective sodium-hydrogen exchange, congenital chloride diarrhea, microvillous disease
   - **Infants:** Protein sensitization, infection, parenteral diarrhea (during urinary or upper respiratory infection), immunoglobulin deficiency, diarrhea after gastroenteritis, cystic fibrosis, celiac disease, *C. difficile* infection
   - **Toddlers:** Diarrhea after gastroenteritis, food allergy, excessive ingestion of fruit juice, toddler's diarrhea, hyperthyroidism, sucrase-isomaltase deficiency, constipation and impaction with overflow, teething
   - **Older children:** Lactose intolerance, infection, inflammatory bowel disease, irritable bowel syndrome, laxative abuse

   Keating JP: Chronic diarrhea, *Pediatr Rev* 26:5–14, 2005.

   Gryboski J: The child with chronic diarrhea, *Contemp Pediatr* 10:71–97, 1993.

TABLE 7-2. BENEFITS OF ANTIMICROBIAL THERAPY IN SPECIFIC BACTERIAL GASTROENTERITIDES

Enteropathogen	Indication for or Effect of Therapy
Shigella species	Shortens duration of diarrhea
	Eliminates organisms from feces
Campylobacter jejuni	Shortens duration
	Prevents relapse
Salmonella species	Indicated for infants <12 mo
	Bacteremia
	Metastatic foci (e.g., osteomyelitis)
	Enteric fever
	Immunocompromise
Escherichia coli	
Enteropathogenic	Use primarily in infants
	Intravenous use if invasive disease
Enterotoxigenic	Most illnesses brief and self-limited
Enteroinvasive	
Yersinia enterocolitica	None for gastroenteritis alone but indicated if suspected septicemia or other localized infection
Clostridium difficile	10%-20% relapse rate

---

45. **How does osmotic diarrhea differ from secretory diarrhea?**
    See Table 7-3.

TABLE 7-3. OSMOTIC DIARRHEA VERSUS SECRETORY DIARRHEA

Stools	Osmotic Diarrhea	Secretory Diarrhea
Electrolytes	Na^+ <70 mmol/L	Na^+ >70 mmol/L
	Cl^- <25 mEq/L	Cl^- >40 mEq/L
Osmotic gap*	>135 mOsm	<50 mOsm
pH	<5.6	>6.0
Response to fasting	Improvement	None

*The osmotic gap is the osmolality of the fecal fluid minus the sum of the concentrations of the fecal electrolytes.
From Guarino A, DeMarco G: Persistent diarrhea In Walker WA, Goulet O, Kleinman RE, et al (eds): Pediatric Gastrointestinal Disease, 4th ed. Hamilton, Ontario, BC Decker, 2004, pp 180-193.

---

46. **How should children with secretory diarrhea be managed?**
    After the child is taken off feeds, a vigorous attempt must be initiated to maintain fluid and electrolyte balance. If this is successful, the child should be evaluated for proximal small bowel damage, enteric pathogens, and a baseline malabsorption workup. If

abnormalities of the mucosal integrity are suspected, a small bowel biopsy is performed; if the findings are significantly abnormal, the patient may be given parenteral alimentation and gradual refeeding. Electron microscopy may reveal congenital abnormalities of the microvillus membrane and the brush border. Hormonal causes of secretory diarrhea (e.g., a VIPoma, hypergastrinoma, or carcinoid syndrome) must be considered if initial studies are negative.

47. **What is the most common cause of bloody diarrhea in infants younger than 1 year?**
    Allergic (or nonspecific) colitis. Usually attributed to cow milk–based formula, this can occur in breastfed infants as well because of theorized transmission of maternal dietary antigens. Formula changes or maternal elimination diets are often recommended.

    Murphy MS: Management of bloody diarrhea in children in primary care, *BMJ* 336:1010–1015, 2008.

48. **What is the most common cause of antibiotic-associated colitis?**
    C. difficile. Fever, abdominal pain, and bloody diarrhea begin as early as a few days after starting antibiotics (especially clindamycin, ampicillin, and cephalosporins). Definitive diagnosis is made by sigmoidoscopy, which reveals pseudomembranous plaques or nodules (Fig. 7-4).

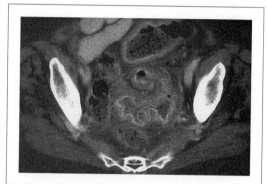

Figure 7-4. Pseudomembranous colitis. Note the multiple plaques characterizing the pseudomembranes; the plaques are characteristically yellow when viewed on endoscopy.

49. **How common is asymptomatic *C. difficile* carriage?**
    Colonization rates in infants can be up to 70%, with percentages decreasing with age. By the second year of life, the rate declines to about 6%, and above age 2 years to 3%, which is the approximate rate in adults. These high colonization rates make the interpretation of positive tests in younger infants more problematic. Toxin assays are more indicative of *C. difficile*–associated disease than culture. However, the toxin may be present without any symptoms, especially in infants, who typically do not have the toxin receptors necessary for disease.

    Bryant K, McDonald LC: *Clostridium difficile* infections in children, *Pediatr Infect Dis J* 28:145–146, 2009.

50. **What are the therapeutic alternatives for the treatment of pseudomembranous colitis?**
    If the disease is not severe, children may be treated with the withdrawal of antibiotics and supportive care. More severely ill children should be treated with oral vancomycin or metronidazole. Some clinicians have advocated cholestyramine to bind *C. difficile* toxin. A colonic clean-out with polyethylene glycol has been shown to be effective for refractory *C. difficile* infection.

51. **How helpful is eosinophilia as a diagnostic sign of parasitic disease?**
Normally, the total eosinophil count does not exceed 500/mm^3. As a screening tool for suspected parasitic disease (e.g., in symptomatic patients returning from foreign travel), it has a very poor positive-predictive value (15% to 55%). Its negative-predictive value is better (73% to 96%), particularly if sequential eosinophil counts remain normal.

   Mawhorter SD: Eosinophilia caused by parasites, *Pediatr Ann* 23:405–413, 1994.

52. **Name the three most common presenting symptoms of giardiasis.**
   - Asymptomatic carrier state
   - Chronic malabsorption with steatorrhea and failure to thrive
   - Acute gastroenteritis with diarrhea, weight loss, abdominal cramps, abdominal distention, nausea, and vomiting

53. **How reliable are the various diagnostic methods for detecting *Giardia*?**
   - Single stool examination for trophozoites or cysts: 50% to 75%
   - Three stool examinations (ideally 48 hours apart) for same: 95%
   - Single stool examination and stool enzyme-linked immunosorbent assay test for *Giardia* antigen: >95%
   - Duodenal aspirate or string test: >95%
   - Duodenal biopsy (gold standard): Closest to 100%

54. **Which patients are particularly susceptible to giardiasis?**
Those with cystic fibrosis, chronic pancreatitis, achlorhydria, agammaglobulinemia, and hypogammaglobulinemia

55. **What are the potential complications of amebiasis?**
The parasite *Entamoeba histolytica* disseminates from the intestine to the liver in up to 10% of patients and to other organs less commonly.
   - Liver abscess
   - Pericarditis
   - Cerebral abscess
   - Empyema

   Haque R, Huston CD, Hughes M, et al: Amebiasis, *N Engl J Med* 348:1565–1573, 2003.

56. **What is the triad of findings for acrodermatitis enteropathica?**
Diarrhea, **hair loss**, and **dermatitis** are the presenting signs of this rare autosomal recessive disorder. The name nicely describes the disorder: there is a classic *acral* distribution of the rash. It is usually eczematous, often with a vesiculobullous or pustular component, and it involves skin around the body orifices as well. As for *enteropathica*, serum zinc levels are extremely low as a result of impaired GI absorption. Dietary insufficiency of zinc may give an identical clinical picture. This has been found in children on long-term total parenteral nutrition without sufficient zinc and in very premature infants as a result of decreased stores and increased requirements.

57. **What features characterize "toddler's diarrhea"?**
Toddler's diarrhea, which is also known as *chronic nonspecific diarrhea*, is a clinical entity of unclear etiology that occurs in infants between 6 and 40 months of age, often following a distinct identifiable enteritis and treatment with an antibiotic. Loose, nonbloody stools (at least two per day but usually more) occur without associated symptoms of fever, pain, or growth failure. Malabsorption is not a key feature.

Multiple causes may be present: overconsumption of fruit juices, relative intestinal hypermotility, increased secretion of bile acids and sodium, and intestinal prostaglandin abnormalities. The diagnosis is one of exclusion, and toddlers should be evaluated for disaccharide intolerance, protein hypersensitivity, parasitic infestation, and inflammatory bowel disease. Treatment consists of reassurance, careful growth assessment, and psyllium bulking agents (as initial therapy). Other agents used with success have been cholestyramine and metronidazole.

58. **How does late-onset lactase deficiency vary by ethnicity?**
See Table 7-4.

TABLE 7-4. APPROXIMATE PERCENTAGE OF LOW LACTASE ACTIVITY BY ETHNIC GROUP			
United States		**Worldwide**	
White	20%	Dutch	0%
Hispanic	50%	French	32%
Black	75%	Filipino	55%
Native American	90%	Vietnamese	100%

59. **Why is *lactase deficiency* a somewhat misleading term?**
After high levels in infancy, lactase levels decline progressively; after the age of 5 years, most people have lactase levels of about 10% of those seen during infancy. Because it is statistically more common to have these lower levels, the term *deficiency* may be a misnomer. Lactose intolerance may develop if excessive lactose loads are ingested.

60. **What conditions produce secondary lactose deficiency?**
Any disorder that alters the mucosa of the proximal small intestine may result in secondary lactose intolerance. For this reason, the lactose tolerance test is commonly used as a screening test for intestinal integrity, although this has the disadvantage of concomitantly identifying all primary lactose malabsorbers. Although a combination of factors is present in many disease processes, secondary lactose intolerance can be organized into lesions of the microsurface, total surface, transit time, and site of bacterial colonization in the small bowel.
Microvillus and brush border:
■ Postenteritis
■ Bacterial overgrowth
■ Inflammatory lesions (Crohn disease)
Level of the villus:
■ Celiac disease
■ Allergic enteropathy
■ Eosinophilic gastroenteropathy
Bulk intestinal surface area:
■ Short bowel syndrome
Altered transit with early lactose entry into colon:
■ Hyperthyroidism
■ Dumping syndromes
■ Enteroenteral fistulas

61. **How is lactose intolerance diagnosed?**
The most common noninvasive method of diagnosing lactose intolerance is a breath hydrogen test. The fasted patient is fed 2 g/kg (up to 25 g) of lactose, and end-expired air is collected every 15 minutes for the next 2 to 3 hours for the purpose of measuring hydrogen concentration. Fermentation of carbohydrate by bacteria in the colon results in hydrogen expiration after lactose ingestion. A peak hydrogen level of 20 parts per million above the baseline after about 60 minutes in concert with a symptomatic response is considered a positive test. Because of the role of colonic bacteria in the mechanism of this test, it is important that the patient not have been treated with recent antibiotics.

   Direct measurement of lactase levels, as well as the other disaccharidases, can be obtained by biopsy of the duodenum or jejunum during upper endoscopy.

   Heyman MB: Lactose intolerance in infants, children and adolescents, *Pediatrics* 118: 1279–1286, 2006.

62. **What is gluten?**
After starch has been extracted from wheat flour, gluten is the residue that is left. This residue is made up of multiple proteins that are distinguished by their solubility and extraction properties. For example, the alcohol-soluble fraction of wheat gluten is wheat gliadin; it is this protein component that is primarily responsible for the mucosal injury that occurs in the small bowel in patients with celiac sprue.

63. **What classic clinical features suggest celiac disease?**
Gluten-sensitive enteropathy (celiac disease) is a relatively common cause of severe diarrhea and malabsorption in infants and children. The classic presentation of celiac disease is a 9- to 24-month-old child with failure to thrive, diarrhea, abdominal distention, muscle wasting, and hypotonia. After several months of diarrhea, growth slows; weight typically decreases before height. Often, these children become irritable and depressed and display poor intake and symptoms of carbohydrate malabsorption. Vomiting is less common. On examination, the growth defect and distention are commonly striking. There may be a generalized lack of subcutaneous fat, with wasting of the buttocks, shoulder girdle, and thighs. Edema, rickets, and clubbing may also be seen. Many patients with celiac disease, however, have a more subtle presentation rather than the classic constellation of symptoms and can present at an older age.

   DiSabatino A, Corazza GR: Coeliac disease, *Lancet* 373:1480–1493, 2009.

64. **What are possible nongastrointestinal manifestations of celiac disease?**
   ■ Dermatitis herpetiformis
   ■ Iron deficiency anemia (unresponsive to treatment with oral iron supplements)
   ■ Arthritis and arthralgia
   ■ Dental enamel hypoplasias
   ■ Chronic hepatitis
   ■ Osteopenia and osteoporosis
   ■ Pubertal delay
   ■ Short stature
   ■ Hepatitis
   ■ Arthritis

   Telega G, Bennet TR, Werlin S: Emerging new clinical patterns in the presentation of celiac disease, *Arch Pediatr Adolesc Med* 162:164–168, 2008.

   Green PHR, Cellier C: Celiac disease, *N Engl J Med* 357:1731–1743, 2007.

65. **What is the appropriate screening test for celiac disease?**
Anti–tissue transglutaminase (TTG) immunoglobulin A (IgA) and **anti–endomysial antibodies (EMA) IgA** have been demonstrated to be highly sensitive and specific for celiac disease. Because of low cost, ease of test performance, and reliability, TTG is currently recommended for initial screening of celiac disease. Antigliadin antibodies, previously the most commonly employed screening test, are not as sensitive or specific for celiac disease and are currently not recommended as first-line screening. More advanced methods of measurement of antigliadin have shown promise, however. Antibodies found in patients with celiac disease are IgA antibodies. Selective IgA deficiency is the most common primary immunodeficiency in Western countries, with a prevalence of 1.5 to 2.5 per 1,000, and is even more common in patients with celiac disease. Therefore, a quantitative IgA level should be included when measuring screening antibodies.

Guideline for the Diagnosis and Treatment of Celiac Disease in Children: Recommendations of the North American Society of Pediatric Gastroenterology, Hepatology, and Nutrition, *J Pediatr Gastroenterol Nutr* 40:1–19, 2005.

66. **How is the diagnosis of celiac disease confirmed?**
Definitive diagnosis of celiac disease requires **multiple small bowel biopsies**. In a typical sequence, the first biopsy on gluten should show villous atrophy, with increased crypt mitoses and disorganization and flattening of the columnar epithelium ("villous blunting"). This should resolve fully with repeat biopsy after a strict gluten-free diet.

67. **What common conditions are associated with an increased risk for celiac disease?**
- Type 1 diabetes
- Autoimmune thyroiditis
- Down syndrome
- Turner syndrome
- William syndrome
- Selective IgA deficiency
- First-degree relatives with celiac disease

Rodrigues AF, Jenkins HR: Investigation and management of coeliac disease, *Arch Dis Child* 93: 251–254, 2008.

68. **What is the role of stool elastase measurement?**
Measurement of fecal pancreatic elastase screens for *pancreatic insufficiency*, which can be a cause of fat malabsorption (e.g., cystic fibrosis). A decreased measurement of pancreatic elastase is associated with pancreatic insufficiency, although values can be falsely decreased when the sample is from diarrhea.

69. **How is the degree of dehydration estimated in a child?**
See Table 7-5.

70. **What three individual clinical features are the most accurate for predicting 5% dehydration?**
- Abnormal capillary refill
- Abnormal skin turgor
- Abnormal respiratory pattern

Steiner MJ, DeWalt DA, Byerley JS: Is this child dehydrated? *JAMA* 291:2746–2754, 2004.

TABLE 7-5. CLINICAL FINDINGS TO ESTIMATE THE DEGREE OF DEHYDRATION

Signs and Symptoms	Mild	Moderate	Severe
Body fluid lost (mL/kg)	<50	50-100	>100
Weight loss	<5%	5%-10%	>10%
State of shock	Impending	Compensated	Uncompensated
General appearance	Thirsty, alert, restless	Thirsty, restless, or lethargic; irritable to touch	Drowsy; limp, cold, sweaty; older may be apprehensive; infants may be comatose
Vital Signs			
Systolic blood pressure	Normal	Normal (orthostatic)	Very low or absent
Heart rate	Normal	Slight elevation (orthostatic)	Very elevated
Respiration	Normal	Deep, may be rapid	Deep and rapid (hyperpnea)
Other Examinations			
Radial pulse	Normal rate and strength	Rapid and weak	Feeble, rapid, may be impalpable
Capillary refill	<2 sec	2-3 sec	>3 sec
Skin elasticity	Retracts immediately	Retracts slowly (>3 sec)	Retracts very slowly
Anterior fontanel	Flat	Depressed	Sunken
Mucous membranes	Normal to dry	Very dry	Very dry to cracked
Tears	Present	Absent	Absent
Skin color	Pale	Gray	Mottled
Laboratory Tests			
Urine			
Volume	Decreased (<2-3 mL/kg/hr)	Oliguric (1 mL/kg/hr)	Anuric (<1 mL/kg/hr)
Osmolarity (mOsm/L)	600	800	Maximal
Specific gravity	1.010	1.25	Maximal
Blood pH	7.40-7.22	7.30-6.92	7.10-6.80

KEY POINTS: DIARRHEA AND MALABSORPTION

1. History is crucial to diagnosis and should include recent medications, ill family contacts, travel, attendance at school or day care, pets, and water sources.

2. The three keys to the assessment of dehydration are (1) capillary refill, (2) skin turgor, and (3) respiratory pattern.

3. *Salmonella* species infection is more concerning among infants who are younger than 1 year because of the increased risk for dissemination (e.g., bacteremia, meningitis).

4. Toddler's diarrhea is a common cause of chronic diarrhea in children between the ages of 6 and 40 months.

5. Celiac disease (a sensitivity to gluten) is common (up to 1% of the general population) and can present with subtle and varied symptoms.

6. Allergic or nonspecific colitis is the most common cause of bloody diarrhea in infants younger than 1 year.

71. **How accurate is blood urea nitrogen (BUN) measurement as a means of assessing dehydration in children?**
Notoriously unreliable. The BUN does not begin to rise until the glomerular filtration rate falls to about one half of normal; it then rises by about 1% each hour, and it may rise even less in a fasting child with disease. In a prospective study, Bonadio and colleagues found that 80% of patients judged to be 5% to 10% dehydrated by common physical findings may have a normal BUN.

   Bonadio WA, Hennes HH, Machi J, Madagame E: Efficacy of measuring BUN in assessing children with dehydration due to gastroenteritis, *Ann Emerg Med* 18:755–757, 1989.

72. **What is the physiologic basis for oral rehydration therapy?**
Intestinal solute transport mechanisms generate osmotic gradients by the movement of electrolytes and nutrients through the cell, and water passively follows. A coupled transport of sodium and glucose occurs at the intestinal brush border, and this is facilitated by the protein sodium glucose cotransporter 1. Oral replacement solutions are formulated with sufficient sodium, glucose, and osmolarity to maximize this cotransportation and to avoid problems of excessive sodium intake or additional osmotic diarrhea.

   King CK, Glass R, Bresee JS, Duggan C, Centers for Disease Control and Prevention: Managing acute gastroenteritis among children: oral rehydration, maintenance, and nutritional therapy, *MMWR Recomm Rep* 52:1–16, 2003.

73. **How do the various oral rehydration solutions differ in composition from other liquids that are commonly used for rehydration?**
Each solution has some advantages and disadvantages. Many home remedies are either very deficient or very excessive in electrolytes or sugar. A main problem with recommended oral rehydration solutions is their low caloric content, but the development of cereal-based and polymer-based solutions—which increase calories without increasing osmolality—is in progress. Table 7-6 lists common oral rehydration solutions.

74. **How can the World Health Organization (WHO) oral electrolyte (rehydration) solution be duplicated?**
The WHO solution is 2% glucose, 20 mEq K^+/L, 90 mEq Na^+/L, 80 mEq Cl^-/L, and 30 mEq bicarbonate/L. This solution is approximated by adding ¾ tsp of salt, 1 tsp of baking soda, 1 cup of orange juice (for KCl), and 8 tsp of sugar to 1 L of water.

TABLE 7-6. ORAL REHYDRATION SOLUTIONS

Solution	Carbohydrate (g/L)	Sodium (mEq/L)	Potassium (mEq/L)	Base (mEq/L)	Osmolality (mOsm/L)	Calories (cal/100 mL)
Diarrhea	—	50-100	25-35	25-40	250-300	—
WHO	G: 20	90	20	30	310	8
WHO/UNICEF	G: 20	75	20	25-35	245	8
Pedialyte	G: 25	45	20	30	250	10
Ricelyte	R: 30	50	25	34	210	12
Cereal-based oral rehydration solution	St: 50	60-90	20	30	315	42
Gatorade	G: 50	20	3	3	330	10
Chicken broth	0	250	5	0	450	0
Cola	F/G: 50-150	2	0.1	13	550	12-16
Apple juice	F/G/S: 100-150	3	30	0	700	15-18
Tea	0	0-1	0-1	0	0-5	0

WHO = World Health Organization; UNICEF = United Nations Children's Fund; G = glucose; R = rice syrup solids; St = starch; F = fructose; S = sucrose

75. **What are the basic principles guiding optimal treatment of children with diarrhea and mild dehydration?**
- Oral rehydration solution should be used for rehydration.
- Oral rehydration should be performed rapidly, ideally 50 to 100 mL/kg over 3 to 4 hours.
- For rapid realimentation, an age-appropriate, unrestricted diet is recommended as soon as dehydration is corrected.
- For breastfed infants, nursing should be continued.
- For formula-fed infants, diluted formula is not recommended, and special formula is usually not necessary.
- Additional oral rehydration solution should be administered for ongoing losses through diarrhea.
- No unnecessary laboratory tests or medications should be administered.

King CK, Glass R, Bresee JS, Duggan C, Centers for Disease Control and Prevention: Managing acute gastroenteritis among children: oral rehydration, maintenance, and nutritional therapy, *MMWR Recomm Rep* 52:1–16, 2003.

76. **What traditional approaches to feeding during diarrhea are no longer recommended and should be voided?**
- **Switching to lactose-free formula:** This is usually unnecessary because, for most infants, clinical trials have not shown an advantage. Certain infants with severe malnutrition and dehydration may benefit from lactose-free formula.
- **Diluted formula:** Half- or quarter-strength formula has been shown in clinical trials to be unnecessary and associated with prolonged symptoms and delays in nutritional recovery.
- **Clear liquids:** Foods high in simple sugars (e.g., carbonated soft drinks, juice drinks, gelatin desserts) should be avoided because the high osmotic load might worsen diarrhea.
- **Avoid fatty foods:** Fat may have a beneficial effect of reducing intestinal motility.
- **BRAT diet:** The bananas, rice, applesauce, and toast diet is unnecessarily restrictive and can provide suboptimal nutrition
- **Avoid food for at least 24 hours:** Early feeding decreases the intestinal permeability caused by infection, reduces illness duration, and improves nutritional outcome.

King CK, Glass R, Bresee JS, Duggan C, Centers for Disease Control and Prevention: Managing acute gastroenteritis among children: oral rehydration, maintenance, and nutritional therapy, *MMWR Recomm Rep* 52:1–16, 2003.

77. **What is the role of antiemetic agents in children with gastroenteritis?**
Guidelines have not supported the use of antiemetic medications, particularly domperidone, metoclopramide, prochlorperazine, and promethazine. Oral ondansetron, a centrally acting 5-hydroxytryptamine antagonist, has been found to be useful in decreasing the risk for persistent vomiting, lessening the need for intravenous therapy in emergency department settings and reducing the likelihood of hospitalization.

DeCamp LR, Byerley JS, Doshi N, et al: Use of antiemetic agents in acute gastroenteritis, *Arch Pediatr Adolesc Med* 162:858–865, 2008.

78. **What are nonantimicrobial drug therapies for diarrhea?**
In older children, adolescents, and adults, the following categories are used. Pediatric data are limited, and these medications are not typically approved or recommended for children younger than 3 years.
- **Antimotility agents** (loperamide [Imodium], diphenoxylate and atropine [Lomotil], tincture of opium [Paregoric]): These can cause drowsiness, ileus, and nausea and potentiate the effects of certain bacterial enteritides (e.g., *Shigella*, *Salmonella*) or accelerate the course of antibiotic-associated colitis.

- **Antisecretory drugs** (bismuth subsalicylate [Pepto-Bismol]): These involve the potential for salicylate overdose.
- **Adsorbents** (attapulgite, kaolin-pectin [Donnagel, Kaopectate]): These can cause abdominal fullness and interfere with other medications.

79. **What is the role of probiotic organisms in the treatment of antibiotic-associated diarrhea?**
   Probiotics (which are the opposite of antibiotics) are living organisms that are believed to cause health benefits by replenishing some of the more than 500 species of intestinal bacteria that antibiotics can suppress and by inhibiting the growth of more pathogenic flora. Among children receiving broad-spectrum antibiotics, about 20% to 40% are likely to experience some degree of diarrhea. *Lactobacillus GG, Bifidobacterium bifidum,* and *Streptococcus thermophilus* have been shown to limit antibiotic-associated diarrhea in children.

   Land MH, Martin MG: Probiotics: hype or helpful? *Contemp Pediatr* 25:34–42, 2008.

   Szajewska H, Ruszczynski M, Radzikowski A: Probiotics in the prevention of antibiotic-associated diarrhea in children: a meta-analysis of randomized controlled trials, *J Pediatr* 149:367–372, 2006.

FOOD ALLERGIES

80. **What are the most common food allergies in children?**
   Cow milk, eggs, and peanuts account for 75% of abnormal food challenges. Soy, wheat, fish, and shellfish are also common allergens.

   Lack G: Food allergy, *N Engl J Med* 359:1252–1260, 2008.

81. **Are food allergies in infants more or less common than generally perceived?**
   As the saying goes, "It depends on where your bread is buttered." Nearly one third of parents report that their infant has an adverse food reaction, which they equate with allergy, but the majority are nonimmunologically mediated food intolerances. In pediatric circles, a general perception is that true food allergies are relatively rare. The answer, as is custom, lies somewhere in between. A prospective study in Colorado of 489 infants followed from birth to the age of 3 years showed that 8% had allergies confirmed by food challenge. In Denmark, a prospective study of nearly 1800 infants showed a prevalence of cow milk allergy of 2.2%.

   Host A, Halken S: A prospective study of cow's milk allergy in Danish infants during the first three years of life, *Allergy* 45:587–596, 1990.

   Bock SA: Prospective appraisal of complaints of adverse reactions to foods in children during the first three years of life, *Pediatrics* 79:683–688, 1987.

82. **Do children outgrow food allergies?**
   It depends on the food. 80% of children outgrow (i.e., develop a tolerance to) certain food allergies, particularly eggs and milk, by age 10 years (often significantly earlier). Others, particularly to peanuts, are less commonly outgrown. It is estimated that only about 20% of children outgrow a peanut allergy. Food allergies that develop after 3 years of age are less likely to be outgrown.

   Kumar R: Epidemiology and risk factors for the development of food allergy, *Pediatr Ann* 37: 5552–5558, 2008.

   Sampson HA: Update on food allergy, *J Allergy Clin Immunol* 113:805–819, 2004.

83. **How are adverse food reactions characterized?**
   - **Food allergy:** Ingestion of food results in hypersensitivity reactions mediated most commonly by IgE.
   - **Food intolerance:** Ingestion of food results in symptoms not immunologically mediated, and causes may include toxic contaminants (e.g., histamine in scombroid fish poisoning), pharmacologic properties of food (e.g., tyramine in aged cheeses), digestive and absorptive limitations of host (e.g., lactase deficiency), or idiosyncratic reactions.

84. **What can be the acute manifestations of milk protein allergy in childhood?**
   - Angioedema
   - Urticaria
   - Acute vomiting and diarrhea
   - Anaphylactic shock
   - Gastrointestinal bleeding

85. **What is the most common chronic manifestation of milk protein allergy?**
   Diarrhea of variable severity. Histologic abnormalities of the small intestinal mucosa have been documented, with the most severe form seen as a flat villous lesion. Protein-losing enteropathy may result from disruption of the surface epithelium. The stools of children with primary milk protein intolerance often contain blood.

86. **What is Heiner syndrome?**
   Heiner syndrome is hematemesis and hemoptysis with failure to thrive. It is non–IgE-mediated and causes chronic pulmonary disease. It is associated with milk allergy.

87. **What likely condition does a birch-allergic child have who develops tongue swelling when eating an apple?**
   Oral allergy syndrome. In this IgE-mediated condition, allergic children develop pruritus, tingling, and swelling of the lips, palate, and tongue when ingesting certain fresh fruits and vegetables because of cross-reactivity to proteins similar to those in pollen. In this case, birch shares allergens with raw carrots, celery, and apples. Symptoms generally are limited to the mouth but occasionally can progress to anaphylaxis. Most allergens are heat labile, so this patient should be advised to stick to baked apple pie for dessert.

   Story RE: Manifestations of food allergy in infants and children, *Pediatr Ann* 37:530–535, 2008.

88. **What are the most used screening tests for food allergies?**
   - **Skin-prick testing:** Can be used in all ages, including infants; has a very high sensitivity (a <3 mm wheal excludes IgE-mediated food allergy in >95% of cases); positive test is less meaningful owing to low specificity
   - **Serum allergen-specific IgE levels:** Elevated levels correlate with increased probability of food-induced reaction; has good negative-predictive value, but positive-predictive value is much lower (many false-positive values), and screening for a wide panel of foods can result in unnecessary food avoidance; may be significant variability between laboratory tests
   - **Atopic patch testing:** Based on cutaneous, cell-mediated responses after epicutaneous application of food allergens; has a higher diagnostic efficacy for likelihood of late-phase clinical allergic reactions; not yet well standardized

   Canani RB, Ruotolo S, Discepolo V, Troncone R: The diagnosis of food allergy in children, *Curr Opin Pediatr* 20:584–589, 2008.

   Chafen JJS, Newberry SJ, Riedl MA, et al: Diagnosing and managing common food allergies, *JAMA* 303:1848–1856, 2010.

89. **Why is the DBPCFC the ultimate diagnostic test for food allergy?**
   The *double-blind, placebo-controlled food challenge*—while in need of a catchier acronym—is the gold standard for evaluating food allergies. The initial choice of food to be tested is usually based on history, skin tests, or radioallergosorbent testing. In a fasting patient without

recent antihistamine use, small quantities of the chosen food (or placebo) are given in lyophilized form (i.e., food rapidly frozen and dehydrated under high vacuum) or as capsules or liquid. The quantities are doubled every 30 to 60 minutes as the patient is observed for up to 8 hours, depending on the anticipated reaction. Observers must be capable of responding to possible anaphylaxis, which usually occurs during the first 2 hours. If no reaction has occurred, the observer should knowingly give the food being tested to ensure that a false-negative test has not occurred.

90. **Why can children who are allergic to nuts usually eat peanuts without any problem?**
Tree nuts (e.g., almonds, Brazil nuts, cashews, pecans, pistachios, or walnuts) are a relatively common cause of food allergy in adults and a less common one in children. Peanuts are a legume (like soy, green beans, and lentils) and have no cross-reactivity with members of the nut family.

Burks AW: Peanut allergy, *Lancet* 371:1538–1546, 2008.

91. **Can dietary manipulation in the first few months of life reduce the risk for atopic dermatitis and food allergies?**
Infants who are at high risk for developing allergy (at least one parent or sibling with allergic disease) may benefit from certain approaches as recommended by the American Academy of Pediatrics (AAP) Committee on Nutrition.
■ Exclusive breastfeeding for at least 4 months decreases the incidence of atopic dermatitis and cow milk allergy during the first 2 years of life
■ Use of hydrolyzed formulas may delay or prevent atopic dermatitis
■ Solid foods should not be introduced before 4 to 6 months of age because there is no evidence to support dietary intervention before this age.

Greer FR, Sicherer SH, Burks AW: Effects of early nutritional interventions on the development of atopic disease in infants and children: the role of maternal dietary restriction, breastfeeding, timing of introduction of complementary foods and hydrolyzed formulas, *Pediatrics* 121:183–191, 2008.

92. **Should highly allergic foods such as fish, eggs, and foods containing peanut protein be introduced in the diet to infants on a delayed basis to reduce the chance of allergy?**
In 2000, the AAP Committee on Nutrition recommended that in children with a high risk for allergy to dairy products, introduction should be delayed until 1 year, eggs until 2 years, and peanuts, nuts, and fish until 3 years of age. Similar restrictive guidelines have not been issued from European organizations who believe the evidence regarding the risks and benefits of the introduction of specific foods at given ages remains incomplete and inconclusive.

American Academy of Pediatrics Committee on Nutrition: Hypoallergenic infant formulas, *Pediatrics* 106:346–349, 2000.

GASTROESOPHAGEAL REFLUX AND PEPTIC ULCER DISEASE

93. **How rapidly do infants outgrow GER?**
Forty percent of healthy infants regurgitate more than once a day, and mild reflux does not represent disease. As a rule, in those infants who have more significant primary GER (about 12% of total), 25% to 50% resolve by 6 months of age, 75% to 85% by 12 months of age, and 95% to 98% by 18 months of age. GER in older children may be more widespread than appreciated. Surveys of parents of children and adolescents (3 to 17 years) revealed that symptoms of heartburn regurgitation were relatively common (2% to 8% of patients).

Campanozzi A, Boccia G, Pensabene L, et al: Prevalence and natural history of gastroesophageal reflux: pediatric prospective study, *J Pediatr* 123:779–783, 2009.

94. **When does GER become GERD (gastroesophageal reflux disease)?**
   GERD occurs when physiologic GER (a variation of normal; "happy spitters") becomes pathologic with the onset of symptoms and complications. These could include feeding refusal, poor weight gain, painful emesis, chronic respiratory problems, and others. The delineation can be imprecise, and other medical conditions can present with symptoms similar to GERD or with secondary GERD.

   Grossman AB, Liacouras CA: Gastrointestinal bleeding. In Liacouras CA, Piccoli DA, editors: *Pediatric Gastroenterology: The Requisites in Pediatrics*, Philadelphia, 2008, Mosby, pp 74–86.

95. **What are the diagnostic methods for GER?**
   The diagnosis can be made either clinically or by diagnostic testing. Clinically, reflux should be suspected in any child who demonstrates frequent, effortless vomiting or regurgitation without evidence of GI obstruction. Clinical response to medical therapy can be diagnostic.

   The upper GI barium study does not reliably indicate reflux but can assess for anatomic abnormalities, such as malrotation, which might contribute. Nuclear scintigraphy, a noninvasive test that uses radiolabeled milk ("milk scan") or a meal, can detect postprandial reflux and delay in gastric emptying but cannot distinguish between physiologic and pathologic reflux. Endoscopically, the presence of histologic esophagitis is suggestive but not diagnostic of reflux; the absence of esophagitis does not rule out reflux. The 24-hour pH probe, traditionally thought to be the most reliable test for the diagnosis of GER, only detects acid reflux and cannot detect nonacid reflux. Multichannel intraluminal impedance is a newer technology that can be performed with a pH probe to assess nonacid reflux.

   Vandenplas Y, Salvatore S, Devreker T, et al: Gastro-oesophageal reflux disease: oesophageal impedance versus pH monitoring, *Acta Paediatr* 96:956–962, 2007.

   Rosen R, Lord C, Nurko S: The sensitivity of multichannel intraluminal impedance and the pH probe in the evaluation of gastroesophageal reflux in children, *Clin Gastroenterol Hepatol* 4:167–172, 2006.

   Orenstein SR: Tests to assess symptoms of gastroesophageal reflux in infants and children, *J Pediatr Gastro Nutr* 37:S29–S32, 2003.

96. **How are the complications of GER treated?**
   Simple GER:
   - Counseling
   - Thickened feeding
   - Positional therapy
   Failure to thrive:
   - Nutritional rehabilitation
   - Nasogastric feeding
   Apnea:
   - Monitoring
   - Fundoplication, if severe
   Esophagitis:
   - Antacids
   - H_2-receptor antagonists
   - Proton pump inhibitors
   - Sucralfate
   - Prokinetic agents (bethanechol, metoclopramide)
   Recurrent aspiration:
   - Fundoplication
   - Jejunal feeding

Failure of medical and nutritional therapy:

■ Fundoplication

Orenstein SR, McGowan JD: Efficacy of conservative therapy as taught in the primary care setting for symptoms suggesting infant gastroesophageal reflux, *J Pediatr* 152:310–314, 2008.

Cezard JP: Managing gastroesophageal reflux in children, *Digestion* 69:S3–S8, 2004.

97. **An infant with known GER who periodically arches his or her back likely has what syndrome?**
    Sandifer syndrome is paroxysmal dystonic posturing with opisthotonus and unusual twisting of the head and neck (resembling torticollis) in association with GER. Typically, an esophageal hiatal hernia is also present.

98. **How effective are milk-thickening agents as a treatment for GER?**
    Milk-thickening agents do reduce the incidence of regurgitation and vomiting and result in increased weight gain. However, they do not decrease the frequency of episodes of GER and have no effect on the reflux index when pH monitoring is performed.

    Horvath A, Dziechciarz P, Szajweska H: The effect of thickened feed interventions on gastroesophageal reflux in infants: systematic review and meta-analysis of randomized, controlled trials, *Pediatrics* 122: e1268–e1277, 2008.

99. **What is the role of promotility agents in the treatment of GERD?**
    Theoretically, prokinetic agents should have an important role in GERD therapy. However, placebo-controlled studies have failed to demonstrate the effectiveness of the available promotility medications as a treatment of GERD. Cisapride is the only promotility agent that has demonstrated efficacy in GERD, but it is only available in the United States through a limited-access program because of an association with prolonged QT interval and increase in the incidence of dysrhythmias.

    Rudolph C, Mazur L, Liptak G, et al: Guidelines for evaluation and treatment of gastroesophageal reflux in infants and children: recommendations of the North American Society for Pediatric Gastroenterology, Hepatology, and Nutrition, *J Pediatr Gastroenterol* 32:S1–S31, 2001.

100. **What is the Nissen fundoplication?**
     The *Nissen fundoplication* is the most commonly performed antireflux surgical procedure. It involves wrapping a portion of the gastric fundus 360 degrees around the distal esophagus in an effort to tighten the gastroesophageal junction.

101. **Which patients are candidates for fundoplication?**
     Most infants with developmental GER do not require fundoplication. It is indicated in patients with recurrent aspiration, refractory or Barrett esophagitis, reflux-associated apnea, and reflux-associated failure to thrive that is refractory to medical therapy. Patients with severe reflux and psychomotor retardation should be evaluated for fundoplication if a feeding gastrostomy is contemplated.

102. **What are the most common complications of fundoplication?**
     Dysphagia can result if the wrap is too tight. Small bowel obstruction and paraesophageal hernia can be postsurgical complications. Gas-bloat syndrome, characterized by persistent gagging, retching, nausea, and abdominal distention, is reported. Postfundoplication dumping syndrome is also a known complication.

103. **What are the signs and symptoms of primary peptic ulcer disease in childhood?**
     Abdominal pain is the most common symptom of primary peptic ulcer disease; it is present in 90% of patients. Although the quality and character of the pain can be variable, it is usually localized to the epigastric region. Classically, ulcer pain is temporally related to

meals; however, in children, this association occurs only about half the time. Nocturnal pain occurs in about 60% of patients and is a key feature for distinguishing organic from nonorganic pain. Melena is a feature in about one third of cases. Vomiting, hematemesis, and perforation are uncommon features.

104. **What conditions are associated with secondary ulcers in children?**
   - **Systemic diseases:** Sepsis, acidosis, sickle cell anemia, cystic fibrosis, systemic lupus erythematosus, renal failure, severe hypoglycemia
   - **Traumatic injury:** Head trauma, burns, major surgery
   - **Drugs and toxins:** Corticosteroids, nonsteroidal anti-inflammatory drugs, theophylline, tolazoline, aspirin

105. **What treatments are available for peptic ulcer disease in children?**
   - **Acid-neutralizing antacids:** Effective for promoting ulcer healing; used more commonly for symptomatic pain relief because of poor compliance as a result of the large volumes (0.5 mL/kg per dose) required for therapy and potential side effects (e.g., diarrhea, constipation)
   - **H_2-receptor antagonists:** Include cimetidine, ranitidine, famotidine, and nizatidine; well-tolerated in children, with few side effects
   - **Proton pump inhibitors:** Inhibit the gastric acid pump, include lansoprazole, omeprazole, esomeprazole, and pantoprazole
   - **Sucralfate:** Chemical complex of sucrose octasulfate and aluminum hydroxide that binds to the ulcer base and acts as a barrier; adsorbs pepsin and neutralizes hydrogen ions
   - **Anticholinergics:** Decrease acid secretion; at effective doses, side effects (e.g., dry mouth, blurred vision) may be significant
   - **Antibiotics:** As treatment for *Helicobacter pylori* infection; most effective treatment remains unclear, but combination therapy with amoxicillin, proton pump inhibitor, and clarithromycin or metronidazole is currently considered first-line therapy

106. **What makes *H. pylori* such a unique bacterial pathogen?**
   It is the most common bacterial infection in humans, with 50% of the world's population estimated to be colonized. It is able to survive in an acidic environment (gastric pH of 2 or less). Colonization is chronic and may be lifelong. It is the cause of most peptic ulcer disease in adult life.

   Campbell DI, Thomas JE: *Helicobacter pylori* infection in paediatric practice, *Arch Dis Child Educ Pract Ed* 90:ep25–ep30, 2005.

107. **What is the relationship of *H. pylori* infection to antral gastritis, peptic ulcer disease, and recurrent abdominal pain in children?**
   This is an area of considerable interest, debate, and research. In adults, *H. pylori* has been associated with duodenal ulceration in more than 90% of patients and with gastric ulceration in 70% of patients. However, asymptomatic colonization complicates the picture. In asymptomatic adult volunteers, 20% to 25% of patients have *H. pylori* colonization, compared with only 4% of asymptomatic children. Studies appear to indicate that, among children, there is a strong relationship between *H. pylori* and antral gastritis (Fig. 7-5) and primary duodenal ulcer disease but a weak relationship between *H. pylori* and gastric ulcers and recurrent abdominal pain.

   Czinn SJ: *Helicobacter pylori* infection: detection, investigation, management, *J Pediatr* 146:S21–S26, 2005.

   Spee LAA, Madderom MB, Pijpers M: Association between *Helicobacter pylori* and gastrointestinal symptoms in children. *Pediatrics* 125:e651–669, 2010.

108. **What methods are available for detecting the presence of *H. pylori* in the stomach or the duodenum?**
   Noninvasive tests:
   - Stable isotope ^{13}C-urea breath test
   - Serology: Does not distinguish between past and present infection

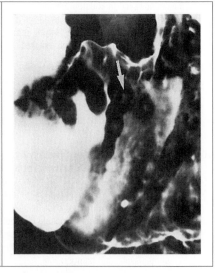

Figure 7-5. Antral gastritis. Note the thickened folds in the gastric antrum and the punctate lesions (*arrow*). (From Katz DS, Math KR, Groskin SA: Radiology Secrets. Philadelphia, Hanley & Belfus, 1998, p 106.)

- Stool antigen test

Invasive tests:
- Culture of gastric biopsy specimen
- Polymerase chain reaction testing of biopsy specimen
- Identification of histologic gastritis
- Special stains for *H. pylori*

109. **What is the basis for the ^{13}C-urea breath test for *Helicobacter*?**
    H. pylori produces urease, which can metabolize urea and produce CO_2; this is then exhaled by the patient. ^{13}C-labeled urea given orally to the patient exploits this peculiar metabolic step. If *H. pylori* is present in the proximal GI tract, labeled CO_2 is released. This is a reliable test, but it requires (nonradioactive) labeled substrate and a mass spectroscopy center for the assay.

KEY POINTS: GASTROESOPHAGEAL REFLUX AND PEPTIC ULCER DISEASE

1. More than 40% of healthy infants regurgitate effortlessly more than once per day. This does not represent significant gastroesophageal reflux.

2. Gastroesophageal reflux disease is usually a clinical diagnosis. Testing such as upper gastrointestinal testing, nuclear scintigraphy, pH and impedance monitoring, and upper endoscopy can be helpful in certain cases, but usually are not necessary.

3. By the age of 12 months, the symptoms of 95% of infants with significant reflux have resolved.

4. The most common presenting symptom of peptic ulcer disease is abdominal pain that is generally localized to the epigastric region.

5. *Helicobacter pylori* can cause gastroduodenal disease in children, including antral gastritis and primary duodenal ulcers.

GASTROINTESTINAL BLEEDING

110. What features on physical examination can help identify an unknown cause of GI bleeding?
See Table 7-7.

TABLE 7-7.	FEATURES TO IDENTIFY THE CAUSE OF GASTROINTESTINAL BLEEDING
Skin	Signs of chronic liver disease (e.g., spider angiomas, venous distention, caput medusae, jaundice)
	Signs of coagulopathy (e.g., petechiae, purpura)
	Signs of vascular dysplasias (e.g., telangiectasia, hemangiomas)
	Signs of vasculitis (e.g., palpable purpura on legs and buttocks suggests Henoch-Schönlein purpura)
	Dermatologic manifestations of inflammatory bowel disease (e.g., erythema nodosum, pyoderma gangrenosum
Head and neck	Signs of epistaxis (especially before placing a nasogastric tube, which can induce bleeding)
	Hyperpigmented spots on the lips and gums (suggests Peutz-Jeghers syndrome, which is associated with multiple intestinal polyps)
	Webbed neck (suggests Turner syndrome, which is associated with gastrointestinal vascular malformations and inflammatory bowel disease)
	Lesions on buccal mucosa (suggests trauma)
Lungs	Hemoptysis (tuberculosis, pulmonary hemosiderosis)
Cardiac	Murmur of aortic stenosis (in adults, associated with vascular malformations of the ascending colon, although this association not certain in children)
Abdomen	Splenomegaly or hepatomegaly (suggests portal hypertension and possible esophageal varices)
	Ascites (suggests chronic liver disease and possible varices)
	Palpable or tender loops of intestine (suggests inflammatory bowel disease)
Joint	Arthritis (Henoch-Schönlein purpura, IBD)
Perianal	Perianal ulcerations and skin tags (suggest inflammatory bowel disease)
	Perianal abscess (suggests IBD, chronic granulomatous disease immunodeficiency)
	Fissure (suggests constipation)
	Hemorrhoids (suggests constipation, portal hypertension)
	Rectal mass on digital examination (suggests polyp)
Growth	Failure to thrive (IBD, Hirschsprung disease)

IBD, inflammatory bowel disease.

Kamath BK, Mamula P: Gastrointestinal bleeding. In Liacouras CA, Piccoli DA, editors: *Pediatric Gastroenterology: The Requisites in Pediatrics*, Philadelphia, 2008, Mosby, pp 87–97.

111. **In patients with acute GI bleeding, how may vital signs indicate the extent of volume depletion?**
It is important to remember that, when acute bleeding occurs in children, it may take 12 to 72 hours for full equilibration of a patient's hemoglobin to occur. Vital signs are much more useful for patient management in the acute setting (Table 7-8).

TABLE 7-8. VITAL SIGNS AND BLOOD VOLUME LOSS	
Vital Signs	Blood Volume Loss
Tachycardia without orthostasis	5%-10% loss
Orthostatic changes	>10% loss
Pulse increases by 20 beats/min	
Blood pressure decreases by 10 mm Hg	
Hypotension and resting tachycardia	30% loss
Nonpalpable pulses	>40% loss

Mezoff AG, Preud'homme DL: How serious is that GI bleed? *Contemp Pediatr* 11:60–92, 1994.

112. **What is the simplest way of differentiating upper GI from lower GI bleeding?**
Nasogastric lavage. After the insertion of a soft nasogastric tube (12 Fr in small children, 14 to 16 Fr in older children), 3 to 5 mL/kg of room-temperature normal saline is instilled. If bright red blood or coffee-ground–like material is aspirated, the test is positive. A pink-tinged effluent is not a positive test because it can simply denote the dissolution of a clot and not active intestinal bleeding. By definition, upper GI bleeding occurs proximal to the ligament of Treitz. If the lavage is negative, it is unlikely that the bleeding is above this ligament, and this rules out gastric, esophageal, or nasal sources. However, bleeding from duodenal ulcers and duodenal duplications may sometimes be missed by these aspirates.

113. **How does the type of bloody stool help pinpoint the location of a GI bleed?**
   ■ **Hematochezia** (bright red blood): Normal stool spotting on toilet tissue likely suggests distal bleeding (e.g., anal fissure, juvenile colonic polyp). Mucous or diarrheal stools (especially if painful) indicate left-sided or diffuse colitis.
   ■ **Melena** (black, tarry stools): Indicates blood denatured by acid and usually implies a lesion, likely before the ligament of Treitz. However, melena can be seen in patients with Meckel diverticulum as a result of denaturation by anomalous gastric mucosa.
   ■ **Currant jelly** (dark maroon) stools usually come from the distal ileum or colon and often are associated with ischemia (e.g., intussusception).
   Because blood is a cathartic, intestinal transit time can be greatly accelerated and makes defining the site of bleeding by the magnitude and color of the blood difficult. This difficulty underscores the importance of the initial nasogastric tube insertion.

114. **What can cause false-negative and false-positive results when stool testing for blood?**
Hemoglobin and its various derivatives (e.g., oxyhemoglobin, reduced hemoglobin, methemoglobin, carboxyhemoglobin) can serve as catalysts for the oxidation of guaiac (Hemoccult) or benzidine (Hematest) when a hydrogen peroxide developer is added, thereby producing a color change. Of note, iron does not cause false-positive results.
False negatives: Ingestion of large doses of ascorbic acid; delayed transit time or bacterial overgrowth, allowing bacteria to degrade the hemoglobin to porphyrin
False positives: Recent ingestion of red meat or peroxidase-containing fruits and vegetables (e.g., broccoli, radishes, cauliflower, cantaloupes, turnips)

115. **How do the causes of *lower* GI bleeding vary by age group?**
Newborn and infant:
- *Mucosal:* Peptic ulcer disease, necrotizing enterocolitis, infectious colitis, eosinophilic or allergic colitis, Hirschsprung enterocolitis
- *Structural:* Intestinal duplication, Meckel diverticulum, intussusception

Child:
- *Mucosal:* Anal fissure, juvenile polyp, infectious colitis, inflammatory bowel disease, solitary rectal ulcer, lymphonodular hyperplasia
- *Structural:* Intestinal duplication, Meckel diverticulum, intussusception, volvulus, Dieulafoy malformation
- *Other:* Hemolytic-uremic syndrome, Henoch-Schönlein purpura, Munchausen syndrome by proxy, arteriovenous malformation, vascular malformation

Kamath BK, Mamula P: Gastrointestinal bleeding. In Liacouras CA, Piccoli DA, editors: *Pediatric Gastroenterology: The Requisites in Pediatrics*, Philadelphia, 2008, Mosby, pp 87–97.

116. **A previously asymptomatic 18-month-old child has large amounts of painless rectal bleeding (red but mixed with darker clots). What is the likely diagnosis?**
Although juvenile polyps can also cause painless rectal bleeding, the more likely diagnosis is a **Meckel diverticulum**. This outpouching occurs from the failure of the intestinal end of the omphalomesenteric duct to obliterate. Up to 2% of the population may have a Meckel diverticulum, and about half contain gastric mucosa; most are usually silent throughout life. Meckel diverticulum is twice as common in males and usually appears during the first 2 years of life as massive painless bleeding that is red or maroon in color. Tarry stools are observed in about 10% of cases. A history of previous minor episodes may be obtained. The presentation can range from shock to intussusception with obstruction, volvulus, or torsion. Meckel diverticulitis, which occurs in 10% to 20% of cases, may be indistinguishable from appendicitis.

117. **In a child with a juvenile polyp, how common are polyposis syndromes?**
Juvenile polyps are the most common type of intestinal tumor in children, usually presenting with hematochezia. Up to one third of these patients can have chronic blood loss with microcytic anemia. Juvenile polyposis is common (up to 12%) in patients with symptomatic polyps, especially with right colonic polyps, anemia, and adenomas. The importance of establishing a diagnosis of a polyposis syndrome is that some syndromes (i.e., Peutz-Jeghers [Fig. 7-6] and juvenile polyposis coli) are associated with a risk for developing adenocarcinoma as high as 30% in as few as 10 years after diagnosis.

Hoffenberg EJ, Sauaia A, Maltzman T, et al: Symptomatic colonic polyps in childhood: not so benign, *J Pediatr Gastroenterol Nutr* 28: 175–181, 1999.

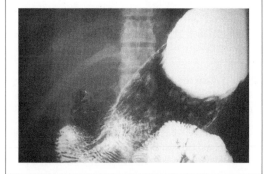

Figure 7-6. Image from a double-contrast upper gastrointestinal series reveals multiple gastric polyps in a patient with Peutz-Jeghers syndrome. (From Katz DS, Math KR, Groskin SA: Radiology Secrets. Philadelphia, Hanley & Belfus, 1998, p 139.)

118. **Worldwide, what is the most common cause of GI blood loss in children?**
Hookworm infection. Caused by the parasites *Necator americanus* and *Ancylostoma duodenale*, this infection is often asymptomatic. Progressive microscopic blood loss often leads to anemia as a result of iron deficiency.

Crompton DW: The public health importance of hookworm disease, *Parasitology* 121:S39–S50, 2000.

119. **What is a newer method for detecting the location of an obscure GI bleed that was not defined by radiographs or upper and lower endoscopy?**
Capsule endoscopy. Video capsule endoscopy is increasingly being used for detection of GI bleeding in children. The capsule camera allows for visualization of the entire small bowel, which is not attainable by upper and lower endoscopy. This method is particularly useful for detecting isolated small bowel inflammation as well as lesions that represent vascular malformations (e.g., blue rubber bleb nevus syndrome). Limitations to use include the size of the capsule, which is hard for younger children to swallow and can cause obstruction in patients with Crohn disease. An endoscopic introducer is available to place the capsule in the small bowel of patients who are not capable of swallowing it.

El-Matary W: Wireless capsule endoscopy: indications, limitations, and future challenges, *J Pediatr Gastroenterol Nutr* 46:4–12, 2008.

120. **Describe the management for massive upper GI bleeding.**
This type of hemorrhage is a life-threatening emergency, and initial therapy precedes the specific diagnostic evaluation. Management includes the following:
- Brief history and character of bleeding, previous episodes, and bleeding disorders
- Studies (complete blood cell count, liver function tests, coagulation profile, crossmatch)
- Nasogastric tube insertion
- Full history and physical examination
- Transfusion and intravascular support
- Determination of probable etiology
  Peptic ulcer disease: Diagnostic endoscopy; therapeutic endoscopy; H_2-blockers, antacids, sucralfate
  If no resolution: Surgical repair of ulcer, partial resection
  Variceal bleeding: Diagnostic endoscopy; therapeutic endoscopy; vasopressin, octreotide
  If no resolution: Sengstaken-Blakemore tube, emergency portosystemic shunt, esophageal devascularization
  Mallory-Weiss tear
  Superficial vascular anomaly: Endoscopic ablation

Chawla S, Seth D, Mahajan P et al: Upper gastrointestinal bleeding in children, *Clin Pediatr* 46: 16–21, 2007.

121. **How do the causes of upper GI bleeding vary by age group?**
- **Newborns:** Swallowed maternal blood, vitamin K deficiency, stress gastritis or ulcer, acid-peptic disease, vascular anomaly, coagulopathy, milk-protein sensitivity
- **Infants:** Stress gastritis or ulcer, acid-peptic disease, Mallory-Weiss tear, vascular anomaly, GI duplications, gastric or esophageal varices, duodenal or gastric webs, bowel obstruction
- **Children:** Mallory-Weiss tear, acid-peptic disease, varices, caustic ingestion, vasculitis, hemobilia, tumor

Gilgar MA. Upper gastrointestinal bleeding. In Walker WA, Goulet O, Kleinman RE, et al, editors: *Pediatric Gastrointestinal Disease*, ed 4, Hamilton, Ontario, 2004, BC Decker, pp 258–265.

KEY POINTS: GASTROINTESTINAL BLEEDING

1. Hemoglobin measurement is a much less reliable indicator of volume depletion than vital signs during the assessment of acute gastrointestinal bleeding.

2. Nasogastric lavage is a simple method for differentiating upper gastrointestinal bleeding from lower gastrointestinal bleeding and should always be performed in all patients suspected of having a significant gastrointestinal bleed.

3. The two most common causes of painless rectal bleeding in children are juvenile polyps and Meckel diverticulum.

122. **Why is the buffering of gastric acid important for controlling upper GI bleeding?**
    ■ Acid is ulcerogenic and can cause and propagate erosions.
    ■ Coagulation is better in a neutral or alkaline environment than in an acidic one.
    ■ Platelet plugs are disrupted by gastric pepsins, but these pepsins function less well in a neutral or alkaline environment.

    Mezoff AG, Preud'homme DL: How serious is that GI bleed? *Contemp Pediatr* 11:60–92, 1994.

123. **Name the six most common causes of massive GI bleeding in children.**
    1. Esophageal varices
    2. Meckel diverticulum
    3. Hemorrhagic gastritis
    4. Crohn disease with ileal ulcer
    5. Peptic ulcer (mainly duodenal)
    6. Arteriovenous malformation

    Treem WR: Gastrointestinal bleeding in children, *Gastrointest Endosc Clin North Am* 5:75–97, 1994.

HEPATIC AND BILIARY DISEASE

124. **What laboratory tests are commonly used to evaluate liver disease?**
    See Table 7-9.

125. **What conditions are associated with elevations of aminotransferases?**
    ■ Steatosis (fatty liver due to metabolic syndrome)
    ■ Hepatocellular inflammation (hepatitis)
    ■ Drug- or toxin-associated hepatic injury
    ■ Hypoperfusion or hypoxia
    ■ Passive congestion (right-sided congestive heart failure, Budd-Chiari syndrome, constrictive pericarditis)
    ■ Nonhepatic disorders (muscular dystrophy, celiac disease, macroenzyme of aspartate aminotransferase)

    Teitelbaum JE: Normal hepatobiliary function. In Rudolph CD, Rudolph AM, editors: *Rudolph's Pediatrics*, ed 21, New York, 2003, McGraw-Hill, pp 1479.

TABLE 7-9. LABORATORY TESTS COMMONLY USED TO EVALUATE LIVER DISEASE

Test	Clinical Significance
Alanine aminotransferase (ALT, SGPT)	Increased with damaged hepatocytes
Aspartate aminotransferase (AST, SGOT)	Less sensitive than ALT for hepatic injury
Alkaline phosphatase (AP)	Increased in cholestatic disease; also comes from bone Higher in children because of bone growth (can identify source through isoenzyme)
γ-Glutamyltransferase (GGT)	More sensitive marker for cholestasis than AP
Bilirubin	Differential diagnosis different for conjugated versus unconjugated
Albumin	Low albumin can indicate chronic impairment in hepatic synthetic function
Prealbumin	Shorter half-life; may reflect more acute synthetic capabilities
Prothrombin time (PT)	Reflects synthetic function as a result of short half-life of factors
Ammonia	Impaired removal in patients with chronic liver disease; can lead to encephalopathy

126. **What is the most frequent cause of chronically elevated aminotransferases among children and adolescents in the United States?**
   Nonalcoholic fatty liver disease associated with the metabolic syndrome. In these obese patients, hepatic steatosis (abnormal lipid deposition in hepatocytes) occurs in the absence of excess alcohol intake. The concern is that the condition could progress to nonalcoholic steatohepatitis, which adds necroinflammation and fibrosis to the original steatosis. Liver failure and portal hypertension could result.

   Sundaram SS, Zeitler P, Nadeau K: The metabolic syndrome and nonalcoholic fatty liver disease, *Curr Opin Pediatr* 21:529–535, 2009.

   Alisi A, Manco M, Vania A, et al: Pediatric nonalcoholic fatty liver disease in 2009, *J Pediatr* 155:469–474, 2009.

127. **Why is it important to determine whether an elevated bilirubin is conjugated or unconjugated?**
   Bilirubin released from erythrocytes (unconjugated) is taken up by the liver and enzymatically converted (conjugated) to a more water-soluble form. On the basis of laboratory methodology, measurements of unconjugated bilirubin are referred to as *indirect reacting* and those of conjugated bilirubin as *direct reacting*. Elevated conjugated bilirubin is associated with obstruction of the biliary tract, intrahepatic cholestasis, or poorly functioning hepatocytes. Conjugated hyperbilirubinemia always requires further evaluation.

   Harb R, Thomas DW: Conjugated hyperbilirubinemia: screening and treatment in older infants and children, *Pediatr Rev* 28:83–90, 2007.

128. **When are levels of conjugated bilirubin considered abnormal?**
>20% of total bilirubin. In significant indirect (unconjugated) hyperbilirubinemia, direct (conjugated) levels usually do not exceed 15%. The levels between 15% and 20% are thus somewhat indeterminate. Generally, direct bilirubin does not exceed more than 2 mg/dL.

129. **What are the common causes of neonatal hepatitis and neonatal cholestasis?**
See Table 7-10.

TABLE 7-10. NEONATAL CONJUGATED HYPERBILIRUBINEMIA AND NEONATAL HEPATITIS

Neonatal Hepatitis	**Metabolic**
Idiopathic	α_1-Antitrypsin deficiency
Viral	Tyrosinemia
Cytomegalovirus	Galactosemia
Herpesviruses	Cystic fibrosis
Hepatitis viruses	Bile acid synthetic disorders
Human immunodeficiency virus	Storage disorders
Enterovirus	Niemann-Pick disease
Rubella	Gaucher disease
Adenovirus	Lipidoses
Bacterial	Peroxisomal disorders
Bile Duct Obstruction	**Endocrine**
Biliary atresia	Hypothyroidism
Choledochal cyst	Panhypopituitarism
Neonatal sclerosing cholangitis	**Other Inherited Causes**
Congenital hepatic fibrosis	Alagille syndrome
Cholelithiasis	Familial intrahepatic cholestasis
Tumor or mass	Neonatal iron storage disease
	Toxic
	Parenteral nutrition
	Drugs
	Cardiovascular Disorders

Adapted from Suchy FJ: Approach to the infant with cholestasis. In Suchy FJ, Sokol RJ, Balistreri WF (eds): Liver Disease in Children, 3rd ed. New York, Cambridge University Press, 2007, pp 179-189.

---

130. **What is the likelihood of chronic hepatic disease developing after acute infections with hepatitis viruses A to G?**
   - **Hepatitis A:** 95% recover within 1 to 2 weeks of illness; chronic disease is unusual
   - **Hepatitis B:** >90% of perinatally infected infants develop chronic hepatitis B infection; 25% to 50% of children who acquire the virus between 1 and 5 years of age develop chronic infection; in older children and adults, only 6% to 10% develop chronic infection
   - **Hepatitis C:** 50% to 60% develop persistent infection
   - **Hepatitis D:** Occurs only in patients with acute or chronic hepatitis B infection; 80% develop viral persistence

■ **Hepatitis E:** Does not cause chronic hepatitis
■ **Hepatitis G:** Unknown

American Academy of Pediatrics: Hepatitis A-G. In Pickering LK, editor: *2009 Red Book, Report of the Committee on Infectious Diseases*, ed 28, Elk Grove Village, IL, 2009, American Academy of Pediatrics, pp 329–362.

131. **In addition to viral hepatitis, what are other common causes of acute and chronic hepatitis in children?**
    ■ **Metabolic and genetic disorders:** Wilson disease, α_1-antitrypsin deficiency, cystic fibrosis, steatohepatitis
    ■ **Toxic hepatitis:** Drugs, hepatotoxins, radiation
    ■ **Autoimmune:** Autoimmune hepatitis, primary sclerosing cholangitis: anti–smooth muscle antibody positive, anti–liver-kidney-microsomal antibody positive
    ■ **Anatomic**: Cholelithiasis, choledochal cyst
    ■ **Other infectious:** Cytomegalovirus, Epstein-Barr virus
    ■ **Toxic:** Ethanol, acetaminophen
    ■ **Other inherited:** Alagille syndrome, cystic fibrosis, familial intrahepatic cholestasis

132. **How is α_1-antitrypsin deficiency most likely to present in infants and children?**
    α_1-Antitrypsin deficiency is an autosomal recessive disorder that causes lung and liver disease. In the liver, injury results from intracellular accumulation of the mutant α_1-antitrypsin protein. In the lungs, the absence of functional α_1-antitrypsin leads to unchecked leukocyte elastase function, resulting in destruction of the alveolar walls and eventual emphysema. The pulmonary effects take years to evolve, so lung disease rarely is present in children. More common presenting symptoms are neonatal cholestasis, hepatomegaly, and chronic hepatitis. Although most patients do not have severe disease, this can progress to cirrhosis with liver failure.

    Perlmutter DH: Alpha-1 antitrypsin deficiency: diagnosis and treatment, *Clin Liver Dis* 8:839–859, 2004.

133. **Why is measuring the level serum level of α_1-antitrypsin not enough to diagnosis α_1-antitrypsin deficiency?**
    α_1-Antitrypsin is an acute phase reactant and might not be decreased in all cases of α_1-antitrypsin deficiency. Pi typing (short for protease inhibitor typing) by electrophoresis is necessary to make the diagnosis. MM is the normal phenotype and has the highest activity; ZZ has the lowest activity and the most common association with liver disease. PiMM is the most common Pi type, with a distribution of about 87%; PiMS represents 8%, and PiMZ 2%. The incidence of PiZZ ranges between 1 in 2000 and 1 in 5000.

    Silverman EK, Sandhaus RA: Alpha₁-antitrypsin deficiency, *N Engl J Med* 360:2749–2757, 2009.

134. **What is the metabolic defect in patients with Wilson disease?**
    Wilson disease is an autosomal recessive **defect of copper metabolism** that results in markedly increased levels of copper in many tissues, most notably the liver, basal ganglia, and cornea (Kayser-Fleischer rings). The primary defect is a mutation in the transmembrane protein ATP7B, which is key to excreting excess copper into the biliary canalicular system. The combination of markedly increased copper levels in a liver biopsy specimen, low serum ceruloplasmin, and increased urinary copper excretion strongly suggests Wilson disease.

    Ala A, Walker AP, Ashkan K, et al: Wilson's disease, *Lancet* 369:397–408, 2007.

    Panagiotataki E, Tzetis M, Manolaki N, et al: Genotype-phenotype correlations for a wide spectrum of mutations in the Wilson disease gene (ATP7B), *Am J Med Genet* 131:168–173, 2004.

135. **What are the treatments of choice for Wilson disease?**
    Copper-chelating agents. *D-Penicillamine* has traditionally been the drug of choice, but another chelator, *trientine*, has been used successfully in patients who have discontinued

penicillamine because of hypersensitivity reactions. Some advocate for trientine as an alternative agent to penicillamine due to the better safety profile. Zinc sulfate, which inhibits intestinal copper absorption, has also been used. Patients require a low copper diet for life.

136. **An infant with cholestasis, triangular facies, and a pulmonic stenosis murmur is likely to have what syndrome?**
   Alagille syndrome (arteriohepatic dysplasia). Also called *syndromic bile duct paucity*, this condition consists of a constellation of conjugated hyperbilirubinemia and cholestasis, typical triangular facies, cardiac lesions of pulmonic stenosis, peripheral pulmonic stenosis, or, occasionally, more significant lesions, butterfly vertebrae, and eye findings of posterior embryotoxon and Axenfeld anomaly or iris processes. The patient may have extreme cholestasis with pruritus and marked hypercholesterolemia. Although some patients have developmental delay, most develop appropriately. The usual mode of inheritance of Alagille syndrome is autosomal dominant.

137. **A 3-year-old child who experiences mild fluctuating jaundice in times of illness "just like his Uncle Kevin" is likely to have what condition?**
   Gilbert syndrome, which is due primarily to a decrease in hepatic glucuronyl transferase activity. Normally, bilirubin is disconjugated to glucuronic acid. In patients with Gilbert syndrome, the defective total conjugation results in the increased production of monoglucuronides in bile and mild elevation in serum unconjugated (indirect) bilirubin. The syndrome is inherited in an autosomal dominant fashion with incomplete penetrance (boys outnumber girls by 4 to 1). Frequency of this gene in the population is estimated at 2% to 6%. Elevations of bilirubin are noted during times of medical and physical stress, particularly fasting.

138. **Describe the clinical findings of portal hypertension.**
   Obstruction of portal flow is manifested by two physical signs: **splenomegaly** and **increased collateral venous circulations**. Collaterals are evident on physical examination in the anus and abdominal wall and by special studies in the esophagus. Hemorrhoids may suggest collaterals, but, in older patients, these are present in high frequency without liver disease, and thus their presence has no predictive value. Dilation of the paraumbilical veins produces a rosette around the umbilicus (the caput medusae), and the dilated superficial veins of the abdominal wall are visible. A venous hum may be present in the subxiphoid region from varices in the falciform ligament.

139. **How does autoimmune hepatitis typically present?**
   There are three typical patterns of presentation: (1) *acute hepatitis*, with nonspecific symptoms of malaise, nausea and vomiting, anorexia, jaundice, dark urine, and pale stools; (2) *insidious*, with progressive fatigue, relapsing jaundice, headache, and weight loss; and (3) despite no history of jaundice, patients present with complications of *portal hypertension* (splenomegaly, GI bleeding from varices, and weight loss). Type I autoimmune hepatitis is more common and characterized by antineutrophil antibodies and anti–smooth muscle antibodies. Type 2 AIH is characterized by anti–liver-kidney-microsomal antibodies.

140. **A patient with liver failure develops confusion. Why worry?**
   Hepatic encephalopathy can appear as either a rapid progression to coma or as mild fluctuations in mental status over an extended amount of time. A single underlying cause has not been established, but suspected toxins include ammonia, other neurotoxins, and relatively increased γ-aminobutyric acid activity. Management requires the limitation of protein intake, the use of lactulose to promote mild diarrhea, antibiotics to reduce ammonia production, intracranial pressure monitoring in advanced cases, and possible peritoneal dialysis for patients in severe coma and before liver transplantation.

KEY POINTS: HEPATIC AND BILIARY DISEASE

1. Portal hypertension manifests clinically as splenomegaly and increased collateral venous circulation.

2. Conjugated hyperbilirubinemia in any child is abnormal and deserves further investigation.

3. Extrahepatic biliary atresia is the most common pediatric indication for liver transplantation.

4. The younger the patient, the more likely it is that acute hepatitis B infection will become chronic.

141. **In children with liver failure, how should GI hemorrhage be managed?**
    - Pass a nasogastric tube to monitor upper GI hemorrhage in patients with portal hypertension
    - Administer daily vitamin K intravenously (0.2 mg/kg up to a maximum dose of 10 mg) for 3 days, and continue if response is seen
    - Use judicious administration of fresh-frozen plasma for clinical bleeding
    - Have crossmatched blood available at all times; for children with variceal bleeding, have 40 mL/kg whole blood and 0.2 U/kg platelets available
    - For gastritis or peptic ulceration, treat with an H_2-receptor antagonist or proton pump inhibitor and maintain a gastric pH level higher than 5
    - Consider the use of octreotide for a confirmed variceal bleed
    - Use endoscopic sclerotherapy or banding of varices (should be performed by an experienced gastroenterologist)

142. **What is the most common indication for pediatric liver transplantation?**
    The most common indication is **extrahepatic biliary atresia** with chronic liver failure after a Kasai hepatoportoenterostomy. Other common indications include inborn errors of metabolism (e.g., α_1-antitrypsin deficiency, hereditary tyrosinemia, Wilson disease) and idiopathic fulminant hepatic failure.

143. **Which patients are at risk for cholelithiasis?**
    See Table 7-11.

INFLAMMATORY BOWEL DISEASE

144. **What is the epidemiology of pediatric inflammatory bowel disease (IBD)?**
    The incidence of IBD in general, and Crohn disease specifically, has increased over recent decades. About 20% to 30% of all IBD cases are diagnosed before age 20 years. In the United States, the incidence of pediatric Crohn disease and ulcerative colitis are estimated at 4.5 and 2.2 cases per 100,000 children per year. It is estimated that between 50,000 and 100,000 children and adolescents in North America have IBD, and about 10,000 new cases are diagnosed annually.

Kugathasan S, Judd RH, Hoffmann RG, et al: Clinical epidemiology of inflammatory bowel disease: incidence, prevalence, and environmental influences, *Gastroenterology* 126:1504–1517, 2004.

TABLE 7-11. PATIENTS AT RISK FOR CHOLELITHIASIS

	Pigment Stone	Cholesterol Stone
Race	—	Native American
Sex	—	Female
Age	—	Adolescence
Diet	—	Obesity
Total parenteral nutrition	+++	—
Hemolytic disease (especially sickle-cell disease, thalassemia, hereditary spherocytosis)	+++	—
Cystic fibrosis	—	+++
Ileal disease	—	+++
Defects in bile salt synthesis	—	+++
Hypertriglyceridemia	—	+++
Diabetes mellitus	—	+++

+++ = increased risk

145. **How do ulcerative colitis and Crohn disease vary in intestinal distribution?**
Ulcerative colitis is limited to the superficial mucosa of the colon. It always involves the rectum and extends proximally to a variable extent. Ulcerative colitis more commonly involves the entire colon in children than in adults, who more commonly will have limited left-sided disease. Regional enteritis, or **Crohn disease**, is characterized by transmural inflammation of the bowel that may affect the entire tract from the mouth to the anus. Because of the transmural nature of the inflammation, patients can develop fistulas and abscesses more commonly with Crohn disease. The typical cobblestone appearance of Crohn disease is produced by crisscrossing ulcerations (Fig. 7-7). Crohn colitis, with no involvement of the small bowel, is more common in younger children and can be difficult to distinguish from ulcerative colitis.

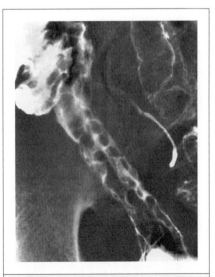

Figure 7-7. Crisscrossing ulcerations produce a cobblestone appearance in patients with Crohn disease. (From Katz DS, Math KR, Groskin SA: Radiology Secrets. Philadelphia, Hanley & Belfus, 1998, p 150.)

Bousvaros A, Antonioli DA, Colletti RB, et al: Differentiating ulcerative colitis from Crohn disease in children and young adults, *J Pediatr Gastroenterol Nutr* 44:653–674, 2007.

146. **What features differentiate ulcerative colitis from Crohn disease?**
See Table 7-12.

TABLE 7-12. FEATURES THAT DIFFERENTIATE ULCERATIVE COLITIS FROM CROHN DISEASE

	Ulcerative Colitis	Crohn Disease
Distribution	Colon only (gastritis recognized)	Entire gastrointestinal tract
		Skip lesions
	Continuous	
Clinical presentation		
Bleeding	Very common	Common
Growth failure	Uncommon	Common
Weight loss	Less common	Common
Obstruction	Uncommon	Common
Perianal disease	Rare	Common
Endoscopic findings	Continuous inflammation	Focal or segmental inflammation
	100% rectal involvement	Rectal sparing
	Erythema, edema, friability, ulceration on abnormal mucosa	Aphthous or linear ulcerations on normal-appearing mucosa
		Cobblestoning
		Abnormal terminal ileum: >50%
Histologic findings	Mucosa only	Full thickness
	No granulomas	Granulomas

Crohn's and Colitis Foundation of America: http://www.ccfa.org.

147. **What are the classic antibodies associated with IBD?**
    - Crohn disease: anti–*Saccharomyces cerevisiae* (ASCA)
    - Ulcerative colitis: Perinuclear antineutrophil cytoplasmic antibody (pANCA)

    However, as with any screening tests, the sensitivity and specificity vary greatly depending on the clinical likelihood of the condition.

    Sabery N, Bass D: Use of serologic markers as a screening tool in inflammatory bowel disease compared with elevated erythrocyte sedimentation rate and anemia, *Pediatrics* 119:193–199, 2007.

148. **What pharmacologic therapies are used in the treatment of ulcerative colitis and Crohn disease?**
    Mild disease and remission:
    - 5-Aminosalicylic acids (mesalamine, mesalazine), oral and rectal, particularly for ulcerative colitis
    - Corticosteroid enemas
    Moderate disease:
    - Metronidazole, for Crohn disease
    - Prednisone
    - Budesonide
    Refractory disease:
    - Azathioprine
    - 6-Mercaptopurine

- Cyclosporine
- Infliximab

Jacobstein D, Baldassano R: Inflammatory bowel disease. In Liacouras CA, Piccoli DA, editors: *Pediatric Gastroenterology: The Requisites in Pediatrics*, Philadelphia, 2008, Mosby, p 138.

Akobeng AK: Crohn's disease: current treatment options, *Arch Dis Child* 93:787–792, 2008.

149. **In a child who has been diagnosed with Crohn disease, what are the potential long-term complications?**
   - **Severe perianal disease** can be a debilitating complication. More prevalent in patients with Crohn disease, it may range from simple skin tags to the development of perianal abscesses or fistulas.
   - **Enteroenteral fistulas** may occur and "short circuit" the absorptive process. The thickened bowel may obstruct or perforate, thus requiring operation. The recurrence rate is high after surgery, repeated operations are often necessary, and short bowel syndrome may result. In many cases, a permanent ostomy is placed, although pouch construction and continent ileostomies have become more common.
   - **Growth retardation and delayed puberty** are seen extensively in patients with pediatric Crohn disease. The insidious onset may result in several years of linear growth failure before the correct diagnosis is made. With epiphyseal closure, linear growth is terminated, and short adult stature will be permanent.
   - **Decrease in bone mineralization** (*osteopenia*) is a more commonly recognized complication of Crohn disease, secondary to growth failure and malnutrition, disease activity, and toxic effect of corticosteroids. All patients should have a bone densitometry scan to assess for this. Treatment includes increased weight-bearing activity, correction of nutritional deficits, vitamin D and calcium supplementation, and more aggressive medical treatment of disease.
   - **Hepatic complications** of IBD include chronic active hepatitis and sclerosing cholangitis, which may require liver transplantation.
   - **Nephrolithiasis** may occur in patients with resections or steatorrhea as a result of the increased intestinal absorption of oxalate.
   - **Chronic reactive and restrictive pulmonary disease** has been noted.
   - **Arthralgias** are common, but destructive joint disease is uncommon.

KEY POINTS: INFLAMMATORY BOWEL DISEASE

1. Ulcerative colitis is limited to the superficial mucosa of the large intestine, always involves the rectum, and demonstrates no skip lesions.

2. Crohn disease can occur anywhere in the gastrointestinal tract (from the mouth to the anus) and demonstrates transmural inflammation with skip lesions; noncaseating granulomas may be found on microscopic pathology. The transmural inflammation can result in the formation of abscesses or fistulas.

3. Potential long-term complications of inflammatory bowel disease include chronic growth failure, abscesses, fistulas, nephrolithiasis, and osteopenia.

4. Surgery can be curative for ulcerative colitis, but the incidence of postoperative recurrence is high in Crohn disease.

5. Patients with inflammatory bowel disease have an increased lifetime risk for malignancy.

150. **Are children with IBD at increased risk for malignancy?**
   The risk for malignancy has not been studied systematically among pediatric populations with IBD. The risk in adults depends both on the disease and its duration. After 10 years of

ulcerative colitis, the risk rises dramatically (1% to 2% increased incidence of malignancy per year). The risk is thought to be higher in patients with pancolitis compared with those with limited left-sided disease. The carcinomas associated with ulcerative colitis are often poorly differentiated and metastasize early; they have a poorer prognosis and are more difficult to identify by radiographic and colonoscopic examinations. Most authors indicate that carcinoma of the bowel is much less common among patients with Crohn disease, although this has been disputed. The risk for lymphoma is increased in patients with Crohn disease. Immunosuppressive (e.g., 6-mercaptopurine) and biologic (e.g., infliximab) therapy may also increase the risk for neoplasia.

151. **When is surgery indicated for children with IBD?**
See Table 7-13.

TABLE 7-13. INDICATIONS FOR SURGERY FOR CHILDREN WITH IBD

Crohn Disease	Ulcerative Colitis
Perforation with abscess formation	*Urgent*:
	Hemorrhage
Obstruction with or without stenosis	Perforation
	Toxic megacolon
Uncontrolled massive bleeding	Acute fulminant colitis unresponsive to maximal medical therapy
Draining fistulas and sinuses	*Elective:*
	Chronic disease with recurrent severe exacerbations
Toxic megacolon	Continuous incapacitating disease despite adequate medical treatment
Growth failure in patients with localized areas of resectable disease	Growth retardation with pubertal delay
	Disease of >10 years' duration with evidence of epithelial dysplasia

From Hofley PM, Piccoli DA: Inflammatory bowel disease in children. Med Clin North Am 78:1293-1295, 1994.

152. **What is the postoperative prognosis for Crohn disease and ulcerative colitis?**
Patients with ulcerative colitis who undergo colectomy with ileal pouch anal anastomosis should not expect recurrence of disease. However, pouchitis, or inflammation of the ileal pouch that acts as a neorectum, is not uncommon. Alternatively, surgical resection is not curative for Crohn disease. The overall rate of clinical recurrence is estimated to be 50% 5 years after the initial resection. Medical therapy is often required after resection to decrease the risk for recurrence.

LIPID DISORDERS

153. **How are lipoproteins categorized?**
The three major lipoprotein groups are classified by their density or electrophoretic properties: **very-low-density lipoproteins** (VLDL or pre-β), **low-density lipoproteins** (LDL

or β), and **high-density lipoproteins** (HDL or α_1). In addition, chylomicrons and an intermediate-density lipoprotein (IDL or "floating β") can be found in plasma, although their quantities are typically much less, except in children with disorders of lipid metabolism.

154. **What are normal cholesterol levels for children and adolescents?**
Total cholesterol (mg/dL):
■ Acceptable: <170
■ Borderline: 170-199
■ High: >200
LDL cholesterol (mg/dL):
■ Acceptable: <110
■ Borderline: 110-129
■ High: >130

American Academy of Pediatrics: Committee on Nutrition: Cholesterol in childhood, *Pediatrics* 101:141–147, 1998.

155. **How is LDL cholesterol calculated?**

LDL cholesterol = total cholesterol − (HDL cholesterol + [total triglyceride/5])

156. **Which children should have their cholesterol measured?**
This is a controversial issue that involves both proponents and opponents of universal screening. Current recommendations, which were developed by the National Cholesterol Education Committee and the AAP, adopt a middle ground: recommended screening of all children after 2 years of age, but before 10 years, if the following are present:
■ Family history of parents or grandparents aged 55 years or younger with documented atherosclerosis, myocardial infarction, angina pectoris, peripheral vascular disease, cerebrovascular disease, or sudden cardiac death
■ History of a parent with elevated total cholesterol (>240 mg/dL)
■ Parental or family history is unobtainable, particularly for those with additional risk factors
■ Children who may be at increased risk for coronary heart disease irrespective of family history, such as those who smoke cigarettes, are overweight, obese, are diabetic, or have hypertension.
Proponents of universal screening have since argued that the guidelines are not sufficiently sensitive and may miss up to 50% of children with elevated lipids.

Daniels SR, Greer FR: AAP Committee on Nutrition: Lipid screening and cardiovascular health in childhood, *Pediatrics* 122:198–208, 2008.

O'Loughlin J, Lauzon B, Paradis G, et al: Usefulness of the American Academy of Pediatrics-recommendations for identifying youths with hypercholesterolemia, *Pediatrics* 113:1723–1727, 2004.

157. **What are the American Heart Association dietary strategies for all children older than 2 years?**
■ Balance dietary calories with physical activity to maintain normal growth
■ Engage in 60 minutes of moderate to vigorous play or physical activity daily
■ Eat vegetables and fruit daily, limit juice intake
■ Use vegetable oils and soft margarines low in saturated fat and trans fatty acids instead of butter or most other animal fats in the diet
■ Eat whole-grain breads and cereals rather than refined-grain products
■ Reduce the intake of sugar-sweetened beverages and foods
■ Use nonfat (skim) or low-fat milk and dairy products daily

- Eat more fish, especially oily fish, broiled or baked
- Reduce salt intake, including salt from processed foods

American Heart Association: Dietary recommendations for children and adolescents: a guide for practitioners, *Pediatrics* 117:544–559, 2006.

158. How are the primary genetic hyperlipidemias classified?
See Table 7-14.

TABLE 7-14. CLASSIFICATION OF PRIMARY GENETIC HYPERLIPIDEMIAS

Frederickson Type	Lipids Increased	Lipoproteins Increased	Prevalence	Clinical Findings
I	Triglyceride	Chylomicrons	Very rare	Eruptive xanthomas, pancreatitis, recurrent abdominal pain, lipemia retinalis, hepatosplenomegaly
IIa	Cholesterol	LDL	Common	Tendon xanthomas, PVD
IIb	Cholesterol, triglyceride	LDL + VLDL	Common	PVD, no xanthomas
III	Cholesterol, triglyceride	VLDL remnants (IDL)	Rare	PVD, yellow palm creases
IV	Triglyceride	VLDL	Uncommon	PVD, xanthomas, hyperglycemia
V	Triglyceride, cholesterol	VLDL + chylomicrons	Very rare	Pancreatitis, lipemia retinalis, xanthomas, hyperglycemia

IDL, intermediate-density lipoprotein; LDL, low-density lipoprotein; PVD, peripheral vascular disease; VLDL, very-low-density lipoprotein.

159. What is the most common hyperlipidemia in childhood?
Familial hypercholesterolemia, type IIA, with elevated cholesterol and LDL. This condition results from a lack of functional LDL receptors on cell membranes as a result of various mutations. When LDL cannot attach and release cholesterol to the cell, feedback suppression of hydroxymethylglutaryl coenzyme A reductase (the rate-limiting enzyme of cholesterol synthesis) does not occur, and cholesterol synthesis continues excessively. In the homozygous form of type IIa, xanthomas may appear before the age of 10 years and vascular disease before the age of 20 years. However, the homozygous form is very rare, with an incidence of 1 in 1,000,000 births. The heterozygous variety has a much higher incidence of 1 in 500, but it is less likely to produce clinical manifestations in children.

160. What are the treatment options for familial hypercholesterolemia?
- **Nonpharmacologic therapy:** Dietary restriction of cholesterol and fat; exercise and weight loss
- **Lipid-lowering resins:** Cholestyramine and the related resin, colestipol, lower plasma cholesterol by trapping bile acids in the gut, thereby causing more cholesterol to be shunted to bile acid synthesis

- **Niacin** (nicotinic acid): Reduces LDL synthesis
- **Gemfibrozil**: Enhances VLDL breakdown
- **Hydroxymethylglutaryl coenzyme A reductase inhibitors** ("statins"): Inhibitors of the rate-limiting enzyme of cholesterol synthesis
- **Cholesterol absorption inhibitors**: Newest class of agents, decrease intestinal absorption of cholesterol, have not been tested in children

Obarzanek E, Kimm SY, Barton BA, et al, DISC Collaborative Research Group: Long-term safety and efficacy of a cholesterol-lowering diet in children with elevated low-density lipoprotein cholesterol: seven year results of the Dietary Intervention Study in Children (DISC), *Pediatrics* 107:256–264, 2001.

Weigman A, Hutten BA, de Groot E, et al: Efficacy and safety of statin therapy in children with familial hypercholesterolemia: a randomized controlled trial, *JAMA* 292:331–337, 2004.

NUTRITION

161. **What are various requirements for protein, fat, and carbohydrates?**
Protein should account for 7% to 15% of caloric intake and should include a balance of the 11 essential amino acids. Protein requirements range from 0.7 to 2.5 g/kg per day. **Fats** should provide 30% to 50% of caloric intake. Although most of these calories are derived from long-chain triglycerides, sterols, medium-chain triglycerides, and fatty acids may be important in certain diets. Linoleic acid and arachidonic acid are essential for tissue membrane synthesis, and about 3% of intake must be composed of these triglycerides. The remaining 50% to 60% of calories should come from **carbohydrates**. About half of these are contributed by monosaccharides and disaccharides (e.g., sucrose, lactose) and the remainder by starches.

162. **If recommended caloric intakes are maintained, what is normal daily weight gain of young children?**
See Table 7-15.

TABLE 7-15. NORMAL DAILY WEIGHT GAIN IN YOUNG CHILDREN*

Age	Weight Gain Recommended (g)	Caloric Intake (kcal/kg/day)
0-3 mo	26-31	100-120
3-6 mo	17-18	105-115
6-9 mo	12-13	100-105
9-12 mo	9	100-105
1-3 yr	7-9	100
4-6 yr	6	90

*It should be noted that, when babies are primarily breastfed, growth during months 3-18 is less than that indicated by the table. On average, breastfed babies gain 0.65 kg less than formula-fed infants during the first year of life.
Data from Dewey KG, Heinig MJ, Nommsen LA, et al: Growth of breast-fed and formula-fed infants from 0 to 18 months: the DARLING Study. Pediatrics 89:1035-1041, 1992; and National Research Council, Food and Nutrition Board: Recommended Daily Allowances. Washington, DC, National Academy of Sciences, 1989.

163. **What are the recommended bottle feedings by age?**
See Table 7-16.

TABLE 7-16. RECOMMENDED BOTTLE FEEDINGS BY AGE		
Age	Number of Feedings	Fluid Ounces per Feeding
Birth-1 week	6-10	1-3
1 week-1 month	7-8	2-4
1-3 months	5-7	4-6
3-6 months	4-5	6-7
6-9 months	3-4	7-8

164. **Why is honey not recommended for infants during the first year of life?**
Honey has been associated with infantile botulism (so have some commercial corn syrups). *Clostridium botulinum* spores contaminate the honey and are ingested. In infants, intestinal colonization and multiplication of the organism may result in toxin production and lead to symptoms of constipation, listlessness, and weakness.

165. **How is nutritional status objectively assessed in children?**
- **Growth chart:** Anthropometric data give an estimate of the height, weight, and head circumference of a child compared with a population standard. A change in the child's percentile months may signify the presence of a nutritional problem or systemic disease.
- **Compare actual with ideal body weight** (average weight for height age): The ideal body weight is determined by plotting the child's height on the 50th percentile and recording the corresponding age. The 50th percentile weight for that age is obtained, and this ideal body weight is divided by the actual weight. The result is expressed as a percentage—the percent ideal body weight—that gives a better stratification of patients with significant malnutrition. An ideal body weight percentage of more than 120% is obese, 110% to 120% is overweight, 90% to 110% is normal, 80% to 90% is mild wasting, 70% to 80% is moderate wasting, and less than 70% is severe wasting.
- **Measurement of midarm circumference:** This provides information about the subcutaneous fat stores, and the midarm-muscle circumference (calculated from the triceps skinfold thickness) estimates the somatic protein or muscle mass.
- **Laboratory assessment:** Vitamin and mineral status can be directly assayed. Measurements of albumin (half-life, 14 to 20 days), transferrin (half-life, 8 to 10 days), and prealbumin (half-life, 2 to 3 days) can provide information about protein synthesis, but each may be affected by certain diseases. The ratio of albumin to globulin may decrease in patients with protein malnutrition.

166. **What features on examination of the scalp, eyes, and mouth suggest problems of malnutrition?**
See Table 7-17.

167. **How do marasmus and kwashiorkor differ clinically?**
- **Kwashiorkor** is edematous malnutrition as a result of low serum oncotic pressure. The low serum proteins result from a disproportionately low protein intake compared with the overall caloric intake. These children appear replete or fat, but they have dependent edema, hyperkeratosis, and atrophic hair and skin. They generally have severe anorexia, diarrhea, and frequent infections, and they may have cardiac failure.

TABLE 7-17. EFFECTS OF MALNUTRITION ON SCALP, EYES, AND MOUTH

Clinical Sign	Nutrient Deficiency
Epithelial	
Skin	
Xerosis, dry scaling	Essential fatty acids
Hyperkeratosis, plaques around hair follicles	Vitamin A
Ecchymoses, petechiae	Vitamin K
Hair	
Easily plucked, dyspigmented, lackluster	Protein calorie
Mucosal	
Mouth, lips, and tongue	B vitamins
Angular stomatitis (inflammation at corners of the mouth)	B_2 (riboflavin)
Cheilosis (reddened lips with fissures at angles)	B_2, B_6 (pyridoxine)
Glossitis (inflammation of tongue)	B_6, B_3 (niacin), B_2
Magenta tongue	B_2
Edema of tongue, tongue fissures	B_3
Spongy, bleeding gums	Vitamin C
Ocular	
Conjunctival pallor due to anemia	E (premature infants), iron, folic acid, B_{12}, copper
Bitot spots (grayish, yellow, or white foamy spots on the whites of the eyes)	A

■ **Marasmus** is severe nonedematous malnutrition caused by a mixed deficiency of both protein and calories. Serum protein and albumin levels are usually normal, but there is a marked decrease in muscle mass and adipose tissue. Signs are similar to those noted in hypothyroid children, with cold intolerance, listlessness, thin sparse hair, dry skin with decreased turgor, and hypotonia. Diarrhea, anorexia, vomiting, and recurrent infections may be noted.

168. **What are the major complications of total parenteral nutrition?**
   ■ **Mechanical:** Local or distant site thrombosis, perforation of the vasculature or heart, and accidental breakage or infiltration of the infusate into the subcutaneous, pleural, or pericardial space
   ■ **Infectious:** Particularly line-associated sepsis
   ■ **Metabolic:** Congestive heart failure and pulmonary edema from excessive infusate; hyperglycemia and hypoglycemia; electrolyte, mineral, and vitamin disorders; hyperlipidemia; metabolic acidosis; hyperammonemia; hepatic disorders (e.g., cholestasis, cholelithiasis, hepatitis)

169. **What can be done to prevent total parenteral nutrition–associated liver dysfunction?**
   ■ Limit duration of intravenous hyperalimentation
   ■ Initiate early enteral feeding
   ■ Vigilant aseptic technique and prompt treatment of suspected sepsis
   ■ Possible prophylactic administration of ursodeoxycholic acid to limit cholestasis

The factors associated with total parenteral nutrition–associated liver injury remain unclear but may involve lipid-related toxic effects of phytosterols and/or depleted levels of methionine metabolites (e.g., carnitine, cysteine, and glutathione) owing to a lack of a hepatic first-pass effect from oral feedings.

Koletzko B, Goulet O, Hunt J, et al: Guidelines on paediatric parenteral nutrition, *J Pediatr Gastroenterol Nutr* 41:S1–S87, 2005.

SURGICAL ISSUES

170. **What is the natural history of an umbilical hernia?**
Most umbilical hernias smaller than 0.5 cm spontaneously close before a patient is 2 years old. Those between 0.5 and 1.5 cm take up to 4 years to close. If the umbilical hernia is larger than 2 cm, it may still close spontaneously but may take up to 6 years or more to do so. Unlike an inguinal hernia, incarceration and strangulation are rare with an umbilical hernia.

Yazbeck S: Abdominal wall developmental defects and omphalomesenteric remnants. In Roy CC, editor: *Pediatric Clinical Gastroenterology*, ed 4, St. Louis, 1995, Mosby-Year Book, pp 134–135.

171. **Which umbilical hernias warrant surgical repair?**
Because of the high probability of self-resolution, indications for surgery are controversial. Some authorities argue that a hernia larger than 1.5 cm at the age of 2 years warrants closure as a result of its likely persistence for years. Others argue that, because the likelihood of incarceration is small for umbilical hernias, surgical closure is warranted before puberty only for persistent pain, history of incarceration, or associated psychological disturbances.

172. **When should an infant with inguinal hernia have it electively repaired?**
After the diagnosis of inguinal hernia is made, it should be repaired **as soon as possible**. In one large study of children with incarcerated hernia, 40% of patients had a known inguinal hernia before incarceration, and 80% were awaiting elective repair. Eighty percent of the children with incarceration of a hernia were infants younger than 1 year. Delay of repair should be minimized, especially in this age group. Another study found that if an infant presents with an incarcerated hernia, subsequently reduced in the emergency department, the potential for recurrent incarceration during a waiting period is increased 12-fold.

Chen LE, Zamakhshary M, Foglia RP, et al: Impact of wait time on outcome for inguinal hernia repair in infants, *Pediatr Surg Int* 25:225–232, 2009.

Stylianos S, Jacir NN, Harris BH: Incarceration of inguinal hernia in infants prior to elective repair, *J Pediatr Surg* 18:582–583, 1993.

173. **Does surgical repair of one hernia warrant intraoperative exploration for another?**
This is a controversial topic. Many surgeons opt to have pediatric patients undergo a contralateral inguinal repair because up to 10% will develop a contralateral hernia at a median of 6 months. Certain infant groups have been shown to be at higher risk for this, including those with prematurity, twin gestation, left-sided presentation, age less than 1 year, increased abdominal pressure, and female sex. Routine bilateral groin exploration in these groups has been advocated. Surveys of pediatric surgeons, however, indicate persistent widespread practice variability.

Haynes JH: Inguinal and scrotal disorders, *Surg Clin N Am* 86:371–381, 2006.

Antonoff MB, Kreykes NS, Salzman DA, et al: American Academy of Pediatrics section on surgery hernia survey revisited, *J Pediatr Surg* 40:1009–1014, 2005.

174. **How are incarcerated inguinal hernias reduced?**
Incarceration occurs most commonly during the first year of life. Because the infant will likely need to be admitted, nothing should be given to eat or drink. Reduction is most easily

accomplished if the infant is calm (preferably asleep), warm, and, if possible, in a slightly reverse Trendelenburg position. Analgesia (e.g., 0.1 mg/kg of intravenous morphine) may facilitate the relaxed state. With one hand, the examiner stabilizes the base of the hernia by the internal inguinal ring and, with the other hand, milks the sac distally to progressively force fluids and/or gas through the ring to eventually allow complete reduction. If unsuccessful, immediate surgery is indicated.

175. **Under what clinical settings should manual reduction of an inguinal hernia not be attempted?**
When the patient has clinical findings of shock, perforation, peritonitis, GI bleeding or obstruction, or evidence of gangrenous bowel (bluish discoloration of the abdominal wall).

176. **How do causes of intestinal obstruction vary by age?**
Infant and young child:
- Pyloric stenosis
- Intussusception
- Inguinal hernia
- Appendicitis
- Malrotation
- Intestinal duplication
- Intestinal atresia or stenosis
- Omphalomesenteric remnants
- Intraluminal web
- Hirschsprung disease
- Adhesions

Older child:
- Appendicitis (perforated)
- Intussusception (lead point)
- Adhesions
- Malrotation
- Inguinal hernia
- Omphalomesenteric remnants
- Inflammatory bowel disease

Caty MG, Azizhan RG: Acute surgical conditions of the abdomen, *Pediatr Ann* 23:192–194, 199–201, 1994.

177. **What is the significance of green vomiting during the first 72 hours of life?**
During the neonatal period, green vomiting should always be interpreted as a sign of potential intestinal obstruction potentially requiring surgical intervention. In one study of 45 infants with green vomiting, 20% had surgical conditions (e.g., malrotation, jejunal atresia, jejunal stenosis), 10% had nonsurgical obstruction (e.g., meconium plug, microcolon), and 70% had idiopathic vomiting that self-resolved. Plain radiographs can be frequently normal, particularly for malrotation, and thus falsely reassuring.

Williams H: Green for danger! Intestinal malrotation and volvulus, *Arch Dis Child Educ Pract Ed* 92: ep87–ep97, 2007.

Lilien LD, Srinivasan G, Pyati SP, et al: Green vomiting in the first 72 hours in normal infants, *Am J Dis Child* 140:662–664, 1986.

178. **What are the clinical findings of malrotation of the intestine?**
Malrotation of the intestine is the result of the abnormal rotation of the intestine around the superior mesenteric artery during embryologic development. Arrest of this counterclockwise rotation may occur at any degree of rotation. The lesion may display in utero volvulus, or it may be asymptomatic throughout life. Infants may display intermittent vomiting or complete

obstruction. Any infant with bilious vomiting should be considered emergent and requires careful evaluation for volvulus and other high-grade surgical obstructions. Recurrent abdominal pain, distention, or lower GI bleeding may result from intermittent volvulus. Full volvulus with arterial compromise results in intestinal necrosis, peritonitis, perforation, and an extremely high incidence of mortality. Because of the extensive nature of the lesion, postoperative short gut syndrome is present in many patients who require resection.

179. **Describe the radiographic findings associated with malrotation.**
The upper GI series will show malposition and malfixation of the ligament of Treitz. The proximal small bowel may be located in the right upper quadrant, but this is not always true. The cecum as viewed from either the upper GI series or a barium enema may be unfixed or malpositioned. In both malrotation and volvulus, the plain films may be entirely normal. There may be proximal obstruction with gastroduodenal distention. In volvulus, the barium studies may show an obstruction near the gastroduodenal junction, often with a twisted appearance.

180. **In an asymptomatic child with an incidental finding of malrotation, is surgery indicated?**
Because of the persistent possibility of acute volvulus and intestinal obstruction, surgery is always indicated when intestinal malrotation is diagnosed.

181. **In what settings should intussusception be suspected?**
Intussusception (when one portion of the bowel invaginates into the other) usually occurs before the second year of life; half of all cases occur between the ages of 3 and 9 months. Colicky pain is seen in more than 80% of cases, but it may be absent. It typically lasts 15 to 30 minutes, and the baby usually sleeps between attacks. In about two thirds of cases, there is blood in the stool (currant jelly stools). Other presenting symptoms include massive lower GI bleeding or blood streaking on the stools. The infant may appear quite toxic, dehydrated, or in shock; fever and tachycardia are common. A right lower quadrant mass may be palpable, or the area may feel surprisingly empty. Distention may accompany decreased bowel sounds.

182. **How commonly does intussusception appear with the classic findings?**
The classic triad of intussusception (colicky pain, vomiting, and passage of bloody stool) is the exception; overall, 80% of patients do not have this triad of symptoms. About 30% have blood in the stool, and this percentage may drop to about 15% if the abdominal pain was present for less than 12 hours. Palpation of a mass can suggest the diagnosis, but generally a high degree of suspicion is important.

Klein EJ, Kapoor D, Shugerman RP: The diagnosis of intussusception, *Clin Pediatr* 43:343–347, 2004.

183. **What causes intussusception?**
Intussusception is caused by one proximal segment of the bowel being invaginated and progressively drawn caudad and encased by the lumen of distal bowel. This causes obstruction and may occlude the vascular supply of the bowel segment. There is commonly a lead point on the proximal bowel that initiates the process. Lead points have included juvenile polyps, lymphoid hyperplasia, hypertrophied Peyer patches, eosinophilic granuloma of the ileum, lymphoma, lymphosarcoma, leiomyosarcoma, leukemic infiltrate, duplication cysts, ectopic pancreas, Meckel diverticulum, hematoma, Henoch-Schönlein syndrome, worms, foreign bodies, and appendicitis.

Waseem M, Rosenberg HK: Intussusception, *Pediatr Emerg Care* 24:793–800, 2008.

184. **What is the most common type of intussusception?**
Ileocolic intussusception (Fig. 7-8). It is also the most common cause of intestinal obstruction during infancy. Cecocecal and colocolic intussusceptions are less common. Gastroduodenal intussusception is rare and is usually associated with a gastric mass lesion such as a polyp or a leiomyoma. Enteroenteral intussusception is seen after surgery and in patients with Henoch-Schönlein syndrome.

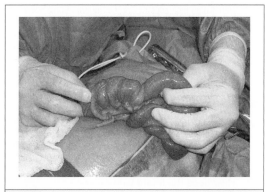

Figure 7-8. Intraoperative appearance of ileocolic intussusception through the ileocecal valve. (From Wyllie R, Hyams JS, Kay M [eds]: Pediatric Gastrointestinal and Liver Disease, 3rd ed. Philadelphia, Saunders, 2006, p 717.)

185. **How is intussusception diagnosed?**
Radiographs can demonstrate a small bowel obstruction pattern, but the sensitivity is low (45%), so this is not typically used to diagnose intussusception. Ultrasound is increasingly being used to make this diagnosis and has a role in the evaluation of reducibility, potential pathologic lead point, and exclusion of residual intussusception after enema. Traditionally, the diagnostic study of choice is a barium enema because this can be both diagnostic and therapeutic. Air enema is now considered to be better at reduction, safer, faster, and result in less radiation compared with barium enemas. In 74% of cases, air enema under fixed hydrostatic pressure will reduce the intussusception. If this is unsuccessful, surgical reduction is necessary.

Applegate KE: Intussusception in children: evidence-based diagnosis and treatment, *Pediatr Radiol* 39:S140–S143, 2009.

186. **How frequently does intussusception recur?**
Idiopathic ileocolic intussusception recurs in about 3% to 9% of all cases. Intussusceptions in older children tend to recur at a higher frequency if the causative lesion is not removed. It is important to investigate cases of recurrent intussusception for an underlying lesion.

Daneman A, Alton DJ, Lobo E, et al: Patterns of recurrence of intussusception in children: a 17-year review, *Pediatr Radiol* 28:913–919, 1998.

187. **Rotavirus vaccine and intussusception: how are they intertwined?**
Rotashield, an oral rotavirus vaccine, licensed in the United States in 1998, was suspended from use in 1999 when increased rates of intussusception were noted. A new rotavirus vaccine, RotaTeq, was introduced in 2006 and, to date, has not been shown to increase the rate of intussusception.

Haber P, Patel M, Izurieta HS, et al: Post-licensure monitoring of intussusception after RotaTeq vaccination in the United States, *Pediatrics* 121:1206–1212, 2008.

Murphy TV, Gargiullo PM, Massoudi MS, et al: Rotavirus Intussusception Investigation Team: Intussusception among infants given an oral rotavirus vaccine, *N Engl J Med* 344:564–572, 2001.

188. **Duodenal or jejunoileal atresia: which is associated with other embryonic abnormalities?**
Duodenal atresia. Duodenal atresia is caused by a persistence of the proliferative stage of gut development and a lack of secondary vacuolization and recanalization. It is associated

with a high incidence of other early embryonic abnormalities. Extraintestinal anomalies occur in two thirds of patients with this condition.

Jejunoileal atresia occurs after the establishment of continuity and patency as evidenced by distal meconium seen in these patients. The etiology is postulated to be a vascular accident, volvulus, or mechanical perforation. Jejunoileal atresias are usually not associated with any other systemic abnormality.

189. **What is the classic radiographic finding in duodenal atresia?**
The double bubble. Swallowed air distends the stomach and the proximal duodenum (Fig. 7-9).

190. **How does the infant with biliary atresia classically appear?**
In classic cases, an otherwise healthy-appearing term infant develops a recognizable jaundice by the third week of life, with increasingly dark urine and acholic stools. Usually, the child appears well, with acceptable growth. The skin color sometimes appears somewhat greenish yellow. The spleen becomes palpable after the third or fourth week, at which time the liver is usually hard and enlarged. In other cases, the jaundice is clearly present in the conjugated form during the first week of life. There is also a strong association between the polysplenia syndrome and earlier presentation of biliary atresia.

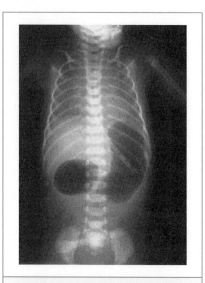

Figure 7-9. Duodenal atresia. (From Zitelli BJ, Davis HW: Atlas of Pediatric Physical Diagnosis, 5th ed. Philadelphia, Mosby, 2007, p 637.)

191. **What is the surgical procedure for biliary atresia?**
The **Kasai procedure** (hepatoportoenterostomy). The remnants of the extrahepatic biliary tree are identified, and a cholangiogram is performed to verify the diagnosis. An intestinal limb (Roux-en-Y) is attached to drain bile from the porta hepatis.

192. **When should a Kasai procedure be performed?**
As soon as possible. Earlier operation results in a dramatically improved outcome. Patients operated on when they are younger than 70 days have an increased likelihood of a successful procedure, although exceptions at both ends of this spectrum are common. Although some surgeons now suggest that infants diagnosed late in the course of disease should have a primary liver transplantation rather than a hepatoportoenterostomy because sufficient liver injury has occurred to make the Kasai procedure unlikely to be successful, there are some data to suggest that late portoenterostomy might be beneficial and result in medium-term survival with native liver in up to one third of patients.

Davenport M, Puricelli V, Farrant P, et al: The outcome of the older ($>$ or $=$100 days) infant with biliary atresia, *J Pediatr Surg* 39:575–581, 2004.

193. **Which is accompanied by more complications: high or low imperforate anus?**
High-type imperforations. The distinction is based on whether the blind end of the terminal bowel or rectum ends above (high type) or below (low type) the level of the pelvic levator musculature. The patients with high-type imperforations will have ectopic fistulas

(rectourinary, rectovaginal), urologic anomalies (hydronephrosis or double collecting system), and lumbosacral spine defects (sacral agenesis, hemivertebrae). The surgical repair in these patients is much more extensive, and future problems of incontinence, fecal impaction, and strictures are much more likely.

194. **What is the classic presentation of pyloric stenosis?**
An infant 3 to 6 weeks old has progressive nonbilious projectile vomiting leading to dehydration with hypochloremic, hypokalemic, metabolic alkalosis. On physical examination, a pyloric "olive" is palpable, and peristaltic waves are visible.

195. **How is pyloric stenosis diagnosed?**
If the classic signs and symptoms are present in association with the typical blood chemistry findings (hypochloremia, hypokalemia, metabolic alkalosis) and a mass is palpated, the diagnosis can be made on **clinical** grounds. If the diagnosis is in doubt, **ultrasound** can be used to visualize the hypertrophic pyloric musculature (Fig. 7-10). **Upper GI contrast** studies demonstrate pyloric obstruction with the characteristic "string sign" and enlarged "shoulders" bordering the elongated and obstructed pyloric channel.

196. **What is the mechanism of hyperbilirubinemia in babies with pyloric stenosis?**
Unconjugated hyperbilirubinemia has been noted in 10% to 25% of babies with pyloric stenosis. Although an enhanced enterohepatic circulation for bilirubin probably plays a role in the pathogenesis of the hyperbilirubinemia, hepatic glucuronyl transferase activity is markedly depressed in these jaundiced infants. The mechanism of diminished glucuronyl transferase activity is not known, although inhibition of the enzyme by intestinal hormones has been suggested.

197. **In a patient with suspected pyloric stenosis, why is an acidic urine very worrisome?**
As vomiting progresses in infants with pyloric stenosis, a worsening hypochloremic metabolic alkalosis develops. Multiple factors (e.g., volume depletion, elevated aldosterone levels) result in maximal renal efforts to reabsorb sodium. In the distal tubule, this is typically achieved by exchanging sodium for potassium and hydrogen. When total-body potassium levels are very low, hydrogen is preferentially exchanged, and a paradoxic aciduria develops (in the setting of an alkaline plasma). This acidic urine is an indication that intravascular volume expansion and electrolyte replenishment (especially chloride and potassium) are urgently needed.

198. **What is the connection between pyloric stenosis and erythromycin?**
In studies of infants who have received erythromycin (primarily as prophylaxis after exposure to pertussis), the incidence of pyloric stenosis is significantly increased.

Honein MA, Paulozzi LJ, Himelright IM, et al: Infantile hypertrophic pyloric stenosis after pertussis prophylaxis with erythromycin: a case review and cohort study, *Lancet* 354:2102–2105, 1999.

199. **What is the short bowel syndrome?**
The *short bowel syndrome* results from extensive resection of the small intestine. Normally, most carbohydrates, proteins, fats, and vitamins are absorbed in the jejunum and the proximal ileum. The terminal ileum is responsible for the uptake of bile acids and vitamin B_{12}. Short bowel syndrome results in failure to thrive, malabsorption, diarrhea, vitamin deficiency, bacterial contamination, and gastric hypersecretion.

200. **Why are infants with short bowel syndrome prone to renal calculi?**
Chronic intestinal malabsorption results in an increase of intraluminal fatty acids, which saponify with dietary calcium. Thus, nonabsorbable calcium oxalate does not form, excessive oxalate is absorbed, and hyperoxaluria with crystal formation results.

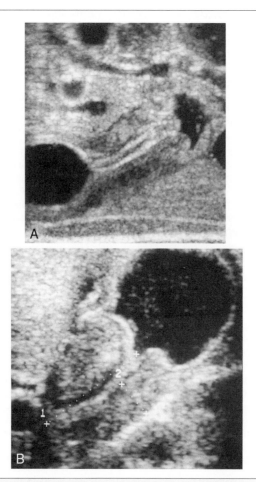

Figure 7-10. A, Ultrasound of pyloric stenosis. Note the elongated and curved pyloric channel with parallel walls and the thickened muscle with a "shoulder" projecting into the antrum. **B**, Longitudinal sonograph of the pylorus in a patient with pyloric stenosis. 1, canal length = 1.7 cm; 2, muscle wall thickness = 0.6 cm. (From Glick PL, Pearl RH, Irish MS, Caty MG: Pediatric Surgery Secrets. Philadelphia, Hanley & Belfus, 2001, p 203.)

201. **In extensive small bowel resection, how much is "too much"?**
Infants who retain 20 cm of small bowel as measured from the ligament of Treitz can survive if the ileocecal valve is intact. If the ileocecal valve has been removed, the infant usually requires a minimum of 40 cm of bowel to survive. The importance of the ileocecal valve appears to relate to its ability to retard transit time and minimize bacterial contamination of the small intestine.

202. **What conditions may mimic appendicitis?**
   - Gastroenteritis
   - Ruptured ovarian follicle and ovarian torsion
   - Mesenteric adenitis
   - Inflammatory bowel disease
   - Constipation
   - Henoch-Schönlein purpura

- Pelvic inflammatory disease
- Primary peritonitis
- Pyelonephritis
- Perforated peptic ulcer
- Right lower lobe pneumonia
- Pancreatitis

Caty MG, Azizhan RG: Acute surgical conditions of the abdomen, *Pediatr Ann* 23:192–194, 199–201, 1994.

KEY POINTS: SURGICAL ISSUES

1. Bilious (dark green) emesis in a newborn is a true gastrointestinal emergency; it is a sign of potential obstruction.

2. Malrotation is diagnosed on the basis of the malposition or malfixation of the ligament of Treitz, as seen on an upper gastrointestinal series. Malrotation can lead to acute volvulus and should always be repaired.

3. The classic triad of intussusception consists of the following: (1) colicky abdominal pain, (2) vomiting, and (3) bloody stools with mucous. However, it occurs in fewer than 20% of patients.

4. In patients younger than 2 years, intussusception is the most common abdominal emergency.

5. Pyloric stenosis typically appears with progressive, nonbilious, projectile vomiting and a hypochloremic, hypokalemic metabolic alkalosis in an infant between the ages of 3 and 6 weeks.

6. The classic picture of appendicitis is anorexia followed by pain followed by nausea and vomiting, with subsequent localization of findings to the right lower quadrant. However, there is a large degree of variability, particularly in younger patients.

203. **Appendicitis in children: clinical, laboratory, or radiologic diagnosis?**
The diagnosis of appendicitis has traditionally been a clinical one. The classic picture in children is a period of **anorexia followed by pain, nausea, and vomiting**. Abdominal pain begins periumbilically and then shifts after 4 to 6 hours to the right lower quadrant. Fever is low grade. Peritoneal signs are detected on examination. In unequivocal cases, experienced surgeons would argue that no laboratory tests are needed.

Laboratory studies have limited value in equivocal cases. White blood cell count of more than 18,000/mm^3 or a marked left shift is unusual in uncomplicated cases and suggests perforation or another diagnosis. A urinalysis with many white blood cells suggests a urinary tract infection as the primary pathology.

Limited computed tomography (CT) scanning with rectal contrast is a powerful tool for diagnosis with sensitivities and specificities between 98% and 100% in children. Three percent diatrizoate meglumine saline solution is instilled into the colon in a slow controlled drip; oral and intravenous contrast are not needed. Diagnosis is based on the visualization of an abnormal appendix or pericecal inflammation or abscess with or without the presence of an appendicolith. This type of imaging can supplement or supplant abdominal ultrasound studies; plain abdominal films are of limited value.

Acheson J, Banerjee J: Management of suspected appendicitis in children, *Arch Dis Child Educ pract ED* 95:9–13, 2010.

Garcia Pena BM, Cook EF, Mandl KD: Selective imaging strategies to diagnose pediatric appendicitis, *Pediatrics* 113:24–28, 2004.

Kwok MY, Kim MK, Gorelick MH: Evidence-based approach to the diagnosis of appendicitis in children, *Pediatr Emerg Care* 20:690–698, 2004.

204. **How specific is the diagnosis of appendicitis if an appendicolith is noted on radiograph?**

Although an appendicolith (or fecalith) on radiographic studies (plain film or CT scan) is significantly associated with appendicitis, it is not sufficiently specific to be the sole basis for the diagnosis. On CT scanning, these can be noted in 65% of patients with appendicitis and in up to 15% of patients without appendicitis. The positive-predictive value of finding an appendicolith is about 75%; in its absence, the negative-predictive value is only 26%.

Lowe LH, Penney MW, Scheker LE, et al: Appendicolith revealed on CT in children with suspected appendicitis: How specific is it in the diagnosis of appendicitis? *AJR Am J Roentgenol* 175:981–984, 2000.

205. **Should a digital rectal examination be performed on all children with possible appendicitis?**

Tradition says yes, but reviews of studies of the practice indicate that in children it can be emotionally and physically traumatic and associated with a high false-positive interpretation. It may be most helpful in equivocal cases involving pelvic or retrocecal appendicitis (about one third of cases), suspected abscess formation, or for attempted palpation of adnexal or cervical tissues when vaginal examination is not indicated. Thus, many clinicians now view it as "investigatory" rather than "routine" and only when results will change management.

Brewster GS, Herbert ME: Medical myth: a digital rectal examination should be performed on all individuals with possible appendicitis, *West J Med* 173:207–208, 2000.

206. **In children taken to surgery for suspected appendicitis, how often is perforation of the appendix present?**

It depends to a large extent on the age of the child (and, of course, on the skill of the clinician). Unfortunately, as a result of the variable location of the appendix, the clinical presentation of pain in appendicitis is often very different from the classic case. The younger the child, the more difficult the diagnosis. In infants younger than 1 year, nearly 100% of patients who come to surgery have a perforation. Fortunately, appendicitis is rare in this age group because the appendiceal opening at the cecum is much larger than the tip, and obstruction is unusual. In children younger than 2 years, 70% to 80% are perforated; in those 5 years and younger, 50% are perforated. Particularly in younger children, a high index of suspicion is necessary, and rapid diagnosis is critical. If the onset of symptoms can be pinpointed (usually anorexia related to a meal), 10% of patients will have perforation during the first 24 hours, but more than 50% will perforate by 48 hours.

207. **Should children with acute abdominal pain be given analgesia before a diagnosis?**

A controversial question because a long-held fear has been that treating the pain may mask the symptoms, change the physical findings, and potentially delay the diagnosis of a possible surgical problem. However, there is a growing evidence that the use of opiate analgesia in patients, including children, with acute abdominal pain does not result in increased mortality or morbidity.

Bailey B, Bergeron S, Gravel J, et al: Efficacy and impact of intravenous morphine before surgical consultation in children with right lower quadrant pain suggestive of appendicitis: a randomized controlled trial, *J Pediatr* 50:371–378, 2007.

Ranji SR, Goldman LE, Simel DL, et al: Do opiates affect the clinical evaluation of patients with acute abdominal pain? *JAMA* 296:1764–1774, 2006.

ACKNOWLEDGMENT

The editors gratefully acknowledge contributions by Drs. Douglas Jacobstein, Peter Mamula, Jonathan E. Markowitz, and David A. Piccoli that were retained from previous editions of *Pediatric Secrets*.

CHAPTER 8

GENETICS

Kwame Anyane-Yeboa, MD

CLINICAL ISSUES

1. **What genetically inherited disease has the highest known mutation rate per gamete per generation?**

   Neurofibromatosis. The estimated mutation rate for this disorder is 1.3×10^{-4} per haploid genome. The clinical features are café-au-lait spots and axillary freckling in childhood followed by the development of neurofibromas in later years. There is about a 10% risk for malignancy with this condition, and mental deficiency is common.

   National Neurofibromatosis Foundation: http://www.nf.org.

   NF, Inc.: http://www.nfinc.org.

2. **Which disorders with ethnic and racial predilections most commonly warrant maternal screening for carrier status?**

   See Table 8-1.

TABLE 8-1. MATERNAL SCREENING ACCORDING TO ETHNIC AND RACIAL PREDILECTIONS		
Disorder	**Ethnic or Racial Group**	**Screening Test**
Tay-Sachs disease	Ashkenazi Jewish, French, French Canadian	Decreased serum hexosaminidase A concentration, DNA studies
Familial dysautonomia	Ashkenazi Jewish	DNA
Gaucher disease	Ashkenazi Jewish	DNA
Canavan disease	Ashkenazi Jewish	DNA
Bloom syndrome	Ashkenazi Jewish	DNA
Fanconi anemia	Ashkenazi Jewish	DNA
Niemann-Pick disease (type A)	Ashkenazi Jewish	DNA
Mucolipidosis IV	Ashkenazi Jewish	DNA
Cystic fibrosis	Pan ethnic	DNA
Sickle cell anemia	Black, African, Mediterranean, Arab, Indian, Pakistani	Presence of sickling in hemolysate followed by confirmatory hemoglobin electrophoresis

3. **Why are mitochondrial disorders transmitted from generation to generation by the mother and not the father?**

   Mitochondrial DNA abnormalities (e.g., many cases of ragged red fiber myopathies) are passed on from the mother because mitochondria are present in the cytoplasm of the egg and not the sperm. Transmission to males or females is equally likely; however, expression is variable because mosaicism with normal and abnormal mitochondria in varying proportions is very common.

Johns DR: Mitochondrial DNA and disease, *N Engl J Med* 333:638–644, 1995.

4. **Which syndromes are associated with advanced paternal age?**
Advanced paternal age is well documented to be associated with **new dominant mutations.** The assumption is that the increased mutation rate is the result of the accumulation of new mutations from many cell divisions. The more cell divisions, the more likely an error (mutation) will occur. The mutation rate in fathers who are older than 50 years is five times higher than the mutation rate in fathers who are younger than 20 years. Autosomal dominant new mutations have been mapped and identified, including **achondroplasia, Apert syndrome**, and **Marfan syndrome**.

5. **What is the most common genetic lethal disease?**
Cystic fibrosis (CF). A genetic lethal disease is one that interferes with a person's ability to reproduce as a result of early death (before childbearing age) or impaired sexual function. CF is the most common autosomal recessive disorder in whites, occurring in 1 in 1600 infants (1 of every 20 individuals is a carrier for this condition). CF is characterized by widespread dysfunction of exocrine glands, chronic pulmonary disease, pancreatic insufficiency, and intestinal obstructions. Males are azoospermic. The median survival is about 29 years.

Cystic Fibrosis Foundation: http://www.cff.org.

6. **Assuming that the husband is healthy and that no one in the wife's family has CF, what is the risk that a couple will have a child with CF if the husband's brother has the disease?**
See Fig. 8-1.

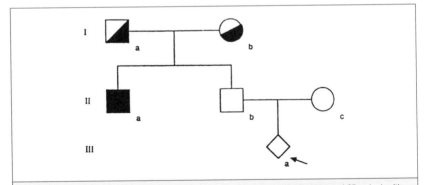

Figure 8-1. Risk for cystic fibrosis (CF) in offspring of a mother with no family history of CF and a healthy father whose brother has CF. (1) Because IIa is affected with CF, both his parents must be carriers. (2) The chance of IIb being a carrier is two out of three because we know that he is not affected by CF. (3) The risk of IIc being a carrier is 1 in 20 (the population risk). (4) The chance of IIIa being affected is calculated as follows: father's carrier risk × mother's carrier risk × chance that both will pass on their recessive CF gene to their child = $2/3 \times 1/20 \times 1/4 = 1/120$.

7. **What are the "fat baby" syndromes?**
   - **Prader-Willi** (obesity, hypotonia, small hands and feet)
   - **Beckwith-Wiedemann** (macrosomia, omphalocele, macroglossia, ear creases)
   - **Sotos** (macrosomia, macrocephaly, large hands and feet)

- **Weaver** (macrosomia, accelerated skeletal maturation, camptodactyly)
- **Bardet-Biedl** (obesity, retinal pigmentation, polydactyly)
- **Infants of diabetic mothers**

8. **What is the "H_3O" of Prader-Willi syndrome?**
   Hyperphagia, hypotonia, hypopigmentation, and **obesity**. About 70% of Prader-Willi patients will have a deletion of an imprinted gene *SNPRN* on the long arm of paternally derived chromosome 15; in about 20% of these patients, both copies of the chromosome are maternally derived. The phenomenon in which a child inherits two complete or partial copies of the same chromosome from only one parent is referred to as *uniparental disomy*. The maternal uniparental disomy for chromosome 15 results in Prader-Willi syndrome, just as does a deletion of the paternal copy of the chromosome.

9. **What syndrome is associated with unprovoked outbursts of laughter?**
   Angelman syndrome. In 1965, Harry Angelman described a syndrome in three "puppet children," as he called them. Other characteristics include severe mental retardation, lack of speech, unsteady gait, microcephaly, and seizures. Facial features include maxillary hypoplasia, large mouth (often with protruding tongue), and prognathism (large chin).

10. **What is the genetic basis of Angelman syndrome?**
    About 70% of cases are due to deletions of an imprinted gene, *UBE3A* (E6-associated protein ubiquitin-protein ligase gene), which resides on the long arm of the maternally derived chromosome 15. About 25% of cases are due to *UBE3A* mutations, and a small percentage of cases are due to paternal disomy of chromosome 15. (Both copies of chromosome 15 are derived from the father.)

11. **A child with supravalvular aortic stenosis, small and abnormally shaped primary teeth, low muscle tone with joint laxity, and elevated calcium noted on testing is likely to have what syndrome?**
    Williams syndrome, also known as Williams-Beuren syndrome. The genetic abnormalities are microdeletions on chromosome 7 in an area that codes for the gene elastin. The loss of this gene is thought to contribute to the cardiac and musculoskeletal features found in Williams syndrome. Other characteristic features include frequent ear infections, hyperacusis (sensitivity to loud noises), failure to thrive at a younger age, and personality traits of a strong social orientation ("cocktail party personality") combined with anxiety problems.

    Prober BR: Williams-Beuren syndrome, *N Engl J Med* 362:239-252, 2010.

    Waxler JL, Levine K, Pober BR: Williams syndrome: a multidisciplinary approach to care, *Pediatr Ann* 38:456–463, 2009.

12. **What is the likely diagnosis in a 15-month-old boy with microcephaly, an upturned nose, syndactyly of the second and third toes, and developmental delay?**
    Smith-Lemli-Opitz syndrome. This is an autosomal recessive disease caused by a *defect in cholesterol metabolism*. A deficiency of the enzyme 7-dehydrocholesterol (7-DHC) due to mutations on the *DHCR7* gene on chromosome 11 prevents the conversion of 7-DHC to cholesterol. Low cholesterol results and treatment has included cholesterol supplementation. Prognosis is discouraging, with most children having moderate to severe mental retardation.

13. **Name the two most common forms of dwarfism that are recognizable at birth.**
    - **Thanatophoric dwarfism:** This is the most common, but it is a *lethal* chondrodysplasia that is characterized by flattened, U-shaped vertebral bodies; telephone receiver–shaped femurs; macrocephaly; and redundant skinfolds that cause a puglike appearance. *Thanatophoric* means death loving (an apt description). The incidence is 1 in 6400 births.

■ **Achondroplasia:** This is the most common viable skeletal dysplasia, occurring in 1 in 26,000 live births. Its features are small stature, macrocephaly, depressed nasal bridge, lordosis, and a trident hand.

14. **What chromosomal abnormality is found in cri-du-chat syndrome?**
This syndrome is the result of a deletion of material from the short arm of chromosome 5 (i.e., 5p−), which causes many problems, including growth retardation, microcephaly, and severe mental retardation. Patients have a characteristic catlike cry during infancy, from which the syndrome derives its name. In 85% of cases, the deletion is a de novo event. In 15%, it is due to malsegregation from a balanced parental translocation.

    http://www.geneclinics.org.

15. **Why are patients with Marfan syndrome at risk for sudden cardiac death?**
A mutation in the fibrillin gene located on chromosome 15 in patients with Marfan syndrome results in abnormal cross-linking of collagen and elastin. Degeneration of elastic elements in the aortic root leads to dilation, which can acute dissect or rupture. Marfan syndrome is autosomal dominant. Tall individuals with suggestive features (thin habitus, hypermobile joints, long digits, pectus excavatum or carinatum, kyphoscoliosis) require consultation with a geneticist.

16. **What syndrome is associated with CATCH22?**
This acronym has been used to describe the salient features of **DiGeorge/velocardiofacial syndrome**:
   ■ **C**ongenital heart disease
   ■ **A**bnormal face
   ■ **T**hymic aplasia or hypoplasia
   ■ **C**left palate
   ■ **H**ypocalcemia
   ■ **22:** Microdeletion of chromosome 22q11
   The cardiovascular lesions frequently encountered are tetralogy of Fallot, truncus arteriosus, interrupted aortic arch, right-sided aortic arch, and double-outlet right ventricle. Any infant with any of these cardiovascular lesions should be screened for DiGeorge/velocardiofacial syndrome.

    Kobrynski LJ, Sullivan KE: Velocardiofacial syndrome, DiGeorge syndrome: the chromosome 22q11.2 deletion syndromes, *Lancet* 370:1443–1452, 2007.

17. **List the syndromes and malformations associated with congenital limb hemihypertrophy.**
   ■ Beckwith-Wiedemann syndrome
   ■ Conradi-Hünermann syndrome
   ■ Klippel-Trenaunay-Weber syndrome
   ■ Proteus syndrome
   ■ Neurofibromatosis
   ■ Hypomelanosis of Ito
   ■ CHILD syndrome (**c**ongenital **h**emidysplasia, **i**chthyosiform erythroderma, **l**imb **d**efects)

18. **For what condition are these patients with isolated limb hypertrophy at risk?**
Embryonal cell tumors, including Wilms tumor, adrenal tumors, and hepatoblastoma. The risk in patients with isolated hemihypertrophy is about 6%; in patients with Beckwith-Wiedemann syndrome, it is 7.5%. Surveillance with abdominal ultrasound and α-fetoprotein measurements every 3 months is recommended until the child is at least **5** years old. In patients with Beckwith-Wiedemann syndrome, facial appearance is also affected (Fig. 8-2).

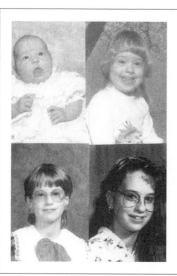

Figure 8-2. Facial shape in Beckwith-Wiedemann syndrome, illustrated from birth to adolescence in a single person. In infancy and early childhood, the face is round with prominent cheeks and relative narrowing of the forehead. Note that by adolescence the trend is toward normalization. (From Allanson JE: Pitfalls of genetic diagnosis in the adolescent: the changing face. Adolesc Med State Art Rev 13:257-268, 2002.)

19. **What are the most common microchromosome deletion syndromes?**
    - DiGeorge/velocardiofacial syndrome (DGS/VCF)
    - Prader-Willi syndrome (PWS)
    - Angelman syndrome (AS)
    - William syndrome (WS)
    - Alagille syndrome
    - Rubinstein-Taybi syndrome (RTS)
    - Wilms tumor/aniridia/ambiguous genitalia/mental retardation syndrome (WAGR)
    - Miller-Dieker syndrome
    - Smith-Magenis syndrome

    Ensenauer RE, Michels VV, Reinke SS: Genetic testing: practical, ethical, and counseling considerations, *Mayo Clin Proc* 80:63–73, 2005.

20. **After Down syndrome, what is the next most common autosomal trisomy in live-born children?**
    Trisomy 18. Occurring in about 1 in 3000 children, this diagnosis should be suspected in newborns with intrauterine growth retardation, microcephaly, prominent occiput, micrognathia, and an overlapping of fingers. The prognosis is poor, with very high mortality and morbidity.

    http://www.trisomy.org.

    http://www.trisomy18.org.

21. **What are the reasons that a condition might be genetically determined but the family history would be negative?**
    - Autosomal recessive inheritance
    - X-linked recessive inheritance
    - Genetic heterogeneity (e.g., retinitis pigmentosa may be transmitted as autosomal recessive or dominant or X-linked recessive)
    - Spontaneous mutation
    - Nonpenetrance
    - Expressivity (i.e., variable expression)

- Extramarital paternity
- Phenocopy (i.e., an environmentally determined copy of a genetic disorder)

Juberg RC: ...but the family history was negative, *J Pediatr* 91:693–694, 1977.

22. **What online resources are available for a pediatrician who suspects a child has a genetic syndrome or would like additional information about a patient already diagnosed with a genetic problem?**
Two sites are particularly superb.
Online Mendelian Inheritance in Man (OMIM; http://www.ncbi.nlm.nih.gov/omim/): This site is a comprehensive compendium of human genes and genetic phenotypes. It is now edited primarily under the auspices of Johns Hopkins University School of Medicine.
GeneTests (http://www.ncbi.nih.gov/sites/GeneTests/): This site provides a wealth of genetic information, including peer-reviewed articles (*GeneReviews*) with disease descriptions, including diagnosis and management information. It is sponsored by the University of Washington at Seattle.

DOWN SYNDROME

23. **What are the common physical characteristics of children with Down syndrome?**
- Upslanted palpebral fissures with epicanthal folds
- Small, low-set ears with overfolded upper helices
- Short neck with excess skinfolds in newborns
- Prominent tongue
- Flattened occiput
- Exaggerated gap between first and second toe
- Hypotonia

National Down Syndrome Society: http://www.ndss.org.

24. **Are Brushfield spots pathognomonic for Down syndrome?**
No. Brushfield spots are speckled areas that occur in the periphery of the iris. They are seen in about 75% of patients with Down syndrome but also in up to 7% of normal newborns.

25. **What is the chance that a newborn with a simian crease has Down syndrome?**
A single transverse palmar crease is present in 5% of normal newborns. Bilateral palmar creases are found in 1%. These features are twice as common in males as they are in females. However, about 45% of newborn infants with Down syndrome have a single transverse crease. Because Down syndrome occurs in 1 in 800 live births, the chance that a newborn with a simian crease has Down syndrome is only 1 in 60.

26. **Why is an extensive cardiac evaluation recommended for newborns with Down syndrome?**
About 40% to 50% have congenital heart disease, but most infants are asymptomatic during the newborn period. Defects include atrioventricular canal (most common, 60%), ventriculoseptal defect, and patent ductus arteriosus.

Down Syndrome: *Health Issues*. http://www.ds-health.com.

27. **What proportion of infants with Down syndrome have congenital hypothyroidism?**
About 2% (1 in 50), compared with 0.025% (1 in 4000) for all newborns. This emphasizes the importance of the state-mandated newborn thyroid screen.

28. **What other conditions of increased risk should not be overlooked during early infancy?**
   - **Gastrointestinal malformations,** including duodenal atresia and tracheoesophageal fistula
   - **Cryptorchidism**
   - **Lens opacities and cataracts**
   - **Strabismus**
   - **Hearing loss,** both sensorineural and conductive

KEY POINTS: INCREASED RISKS FOR PATIENTS WITH DOWN SYNDROME DURING THE NEWBORN PERIOD AND EARLY INFANCY

1. Congenital heart disease: Atrioventricular canal defects, ventriculoseptal defects

2. Gastrointestinal malformations: duodenal atresia, tracheoesophageal atresia

3. Congenital hypothyroidism

4. Lens opacities and cataracts

5. Hearing loss

6. Cryptorchidism

29. **What is the expected intelligence quotient (IQ) of a child with Down syndrome?**
   The IQ range is generally 25 to 50, with a mean reported IQ of 54; occasionally, the IQ may be higher. Intelligence deteriorates during adulthood, with clinical and pathologic findings consistent with advanced Alzheimer disease. By age 40 years, the mean IQ is 24.

30. **Down syndrome is a risk factor for what malignancy?**
   Leukemia. Its frequency in these individuals is 50-fold higher for younger children (0 to 4 years old) and 10-fold higher for individuals 5 to 29 years old, for a 20-fold increase in lifetime risk. Before leukemia becomes apparent, children with Down syndrome are at increased risk for other unusual white blood cell problems, including transient myeloproliferative disorder (a disorder of marked leukocytosis, blast cells, thrombocytopenia, and hepatosplenomegaly, which spontaneously resolves) and a leukemoid reaction (markedly elevated white blood cell count with myeloblasts without splenomegaly, which also spontaneously resolves).

   Olney HJ, Gozzetti A, Rowley JD: Chromosomal abnormalities in childhood hematologic malignant disease. In Nathan DG, Orkin SD, Ginsburg D, Look AT, editors: *Nathan and Oski's Hematology of Infancy and Childhood*, ed 6. Philadelphia, 2003, WB Saunders, pp 1120–1121.

31. **What is the genetic basis for Down syndrome?**
   The syndrome can be caused by trisomy of all or part of chromosome 21:
   - Full trisomy 21: 94%
   - Mosaic trisomy 21: 2.4%
   - Translocation: 3.3%

32. **What chromosomal abnormalities are related to maternal age?**
All trisomies and some sex chromosomal abnormalities (except 45,X and 47,XYY).

33. **How does the risk for having an infant with Down syndrome change with advancing maternal age?**
See Table 8-2. Most cases of Down syndrome involve nondisjunction at meiosis I in the mother. This may be related to the lengthy stage of meiotic arrest between oocyte development in the fetus until ovulation, which may occur as much as 40 years later.

TABLE 8-2. APPROXIMATE RISK FOR DOWN SYNDROME BY MATERNAL AGE	
Maternal Age (yr)	Approximate Risk for Down Syndrome
30	1:1,000
35	1:365
40	1:100
45	1:50

34. **What percentage of all babies with Down syndrome are born to women over the age of 35?**
Only 20%. Although their individual risk is higher, women in this age bracket account for only 5% of all pregnancies in the United States.

Haddow JE, Palomaki GE, Knight GJ, et al: Prenatal screening for Down syndrome with use of maternal serum markers, *N Engl J Med* 327:588–593, 1992.

35. **Does advanced paternal age increase the risk for having a child with trisomy 21?**
There does not appear to be an increased risk for Down syndrome associated with paternal age until after age 55 years. Some studies have noted an increased risk for having children with Down syndrome after this age, although others have not. The reports are controversial, and the statistical analysis needed to perform such a study is cumbersome. It is known that about 10% of all trisomy 21 cases derive the extra chromosome 21 from the father.

36. **Which is technically correct: Down's syndrome or Down syndrome?**
In 1866, John Langdon Down, physician at the Earlswood Asylum in Surrey, England, described the phenotype of a syndrome that now bears his name. However, it was not until 1959 that it was determined that this disorder is caused by an extra chromosome 21. The correct designation is *Down syndrome.*

DYSMORPHOLOGY

37. **How common are major and minor malformations in newborns?**
Major malformations are unusual morphologic features that cause medical, cosmetic, or developmental consequences to the patient. **Minor anomalies** are features that do not cause medical or cosmetic problems. About 14% of newborn babies have a minor anomaly, whereas only 2% to 3% have a major malformation.

38. **What is the clinical significance of a minor malformation?**

The recognition of minor malformations in a newborn may serve as an indicator of altered morphogenesis or as a valuable clue to the diagnosis of a specific disorder. The presence of several minor malformations is unusual and often indicates a serious problem in morphogenesis. For example, when three or more minor malformations are discovered in a child, there is a more than 90% risk for a major malformation also being present. The most common minor malformations involve the face, ears, hands, and feet. Almost any minor defect may occasionally be found as an unusual familial trait.

39. **What is LEOPARD syndrome?**

This autosomal dominant condition is also known as *multiple lentigines* syndrome.
- **L**entigines
- **E**lectrocardiogram abnormalities
- **O**cular hypertelorism
- **P**ulmonic stenosis
- **A**bnormal genitalia
- **R**etarded growth
- **D**eafness

40. **Describe the most common anomaly associations.**

An *association* is a nonrandom occurrence of multiple anomalies without a known sequence initiator or causal relationship but with such a frequency that the malformations have a statistical connection.
- **CHARGE:** **C**oloboma of the eye, **h**eart defects, **a**tresia of the choanae, **r**etardation (mental and growth), **g**enital anomalies (in males), and **e**ar anomalies
- **MURCS:** **M**üllerian duct aplasia, **r**enal aplasia, and **c**ervicothoracic **s**omite dysplasia
- **VATER:** **V**ertebral, **a**nal, **t**racheoesophageal, and **r**enal or **r**adial anomalies
- **VACTERL:** VATER anomalies plus **c**ardiac and **l**imb anomalies

41. **What is the underlying genetic mechanism for CHARGE syndrome?**

It is an autosomal dominant condition, and almost all cases are due to de novo mutations in the *CHD7* gene. Rare familial cases have been reported. *CHD7* (chromodomain helicase DNA-binding protein 7) is the only gene currently known to be mutated in CHARGE syndrome. In 70% of CHARGE syndrome patients, a mutation can be identified in this gene.

42. **What is the proper way to test for low-set ears?**

This designation is made when the upper portion of the ear (helix) meets the head at a level below a horizontal line drawn from the lateral aspect of the palpebral fissure. The best way to measure is to align a straight edge between the two inner canthi and determine whether the ears lie completely below this plane (Fig. 8-3). In normal individuals, about 10% of the ear is above this plane.

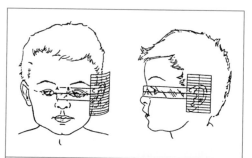

Figure 8-3. How to test for low-set ears. (From Feingold M, Bossert WH: Normal values for selected physical parameters: an aid to syndrome delineation. In Bergsma D [ed]: The National Foundation—March of Dimes Birth Defects Series 10:9, 1974.)

43. **What is the most common genetic mutation in infants with prelingual hearing loss?**

    GJB2 (gap junction β-2) gene. In patients with congenital nonsyndromic deafness, about 75% are due to mutations, and this is the most common. The *GJB2* gene encodes the protein connexin 26, which is critical for gap junctions between cochlear cells. Prelingual hearing loss is hearing loss detected before speech development. All congenital hearing loss is prelingual, with a prevalence of 1 in 500 newborn infants. Connexin mutations are usually autosomal recessive. Another mutation classified as 167delT is found exclusively in the Ashkenazi Jewish population.

    Smith RJ, Robin NH: Genetic testing for deafness—GJB2 and SLC26A4 as causes of deafness, *J Commun Disord* 35:367–377, 2002.

44. **What is the inheritance pattern of cleft lip and palate?**

    Most cases of cleft lip and palate are inherited in a polygenic or multifactorial pattern. The male-to-female ratio is 3:2, and the incidence in the general population is about 1 in 1000. Recurrence risk after one affected child is 3% to 4%; after two affected children, it is 8% to 9%.

45. **How can hypertelorism be rapidly assessed?**

    If an imaginary third eye would fit between the eyes, hypertelorism is possible. Precise measurement involves measuring the distance between the center of each eye's pupil. This is a difficult measurement in newborns and uncooperative patients because of eye movement. In practice, the best way to determine hypotelorism or hypertelorism is to measure the inner and outer canthal distances and to then plot these measurements on standardized tables of norms.

46. **Which syndromes are associated with iris colobomas?**

    Colobomas of the iris (Fig. 8-4) are the result of abnormal ocular development and embryogenesis. They are frequently associated with chromosomal syndromes (most commonly trisomy 13, 4p−, 13q−) and triploidy. In addition, they may be commonly found in patients with the CHARGE association, Goltz syndrome, and Rieger syndrome. Whenever iris colobomas are noted, chromosome analysis is recommended. The special case of complete absence of the iris (aniridia) is associated with the development of Wilms tumor and may be caused by an interstitial deletion of the short arm of chromosome 11.

    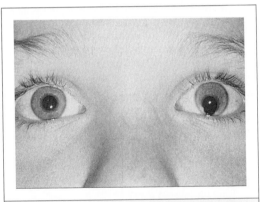

    Figure 8-4. Left iris coloboma. (From Zitelli BJ, Davis HW: Atlas of Pediatric Physical Diagnosis, 4th ed. St. Louis, Mosby, 2002, p 674.)

GENETIC PRINCIPLES

47. **What is the risk for having a child with a recessive disorder when the parents are first or second cousins?**

    First cousins may share more than one deleterious recessive gene. They have ⅛ of their genes in common, and their progeny are homozygous at 1/16 of their gene loci.

Second cousins have only $1/32$ of their genes in common. The risk that consanguineous parents will produce a child with a severe or lethal abnormality is 6% for first-cousin marriages and 1% for second-cousin marriages.

48. **Identify the common symbols used in the construction of a pedigree chart.**
See Fig. 8-5.

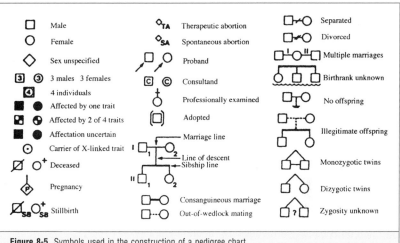

□	Male	♂TA	Therapeutic abortion	□—O	Separated	
O	Female	♂SA	Spontaneous abortion	□—O	Divorced	
◇	Sex unspecified		Proband	□—O—□	Multiple marriages	
③ ③	3 males 3 females	C ©	Consultand		Birthrank unknown	
④	4 individuals		Professionally examined	□—O	No offspring	
■ ●	Affected by one trait					
■ ●	Affected by 2 of 4 traits	[□]	Adopted	□┄┄O	Illegitimate offspring	
■ ●	Affectation uncertain		Marriage line			
⊙	Carrier of X-linked trait		Line of descent			
Ø O⁺	Deceased		Sibship line		Monozygotic twins	
◈	Pregnancy				Dizygotic twins	
	Stillbirth	□—O	Consanguineous marriage		Zygosity unknown	
		□┄O	Out-of-wedlock mating			

Figure 8-5. Symbols used in the construction of a pedigree chart.

49. **How can the same genotype lead to different phenotypes?**
In parental imprinting (an area of the regulation of gene expression that is incompletely understood), the expression of an identical gene is dependent on whether the gene is inherited from the mother or the father. For example, in patients with Huntington disease, the clinical manifestations occur much earlier if the gene is inherited from the father rather than the mother. Modification of the genes by methylation of the DNA during development has been hypothesized as one explanation of the variability.

50. **What is FISH?**
Fluorescence *in situ* hybridization (FISH) is a molecular cytogenetic technique that is used to identify abnormalities of chromosome number or structure using a single-stranded DNA probe (for a known piece of DNA or chromosome segment). The probe is labeled with a fluorescent tag and targeted to a single-strand DNA that has been denatured in place on a microscope slide. The use of fluorescent microscopy enables the detection of more than one probe, each of which is labeled with a different color. An example of the use of FISH is for the rapid prenatal diagnosis of trisomies with the use of amniotic fluid or chorionic villi testing using interphase cells from cultured specimens and probes for the most common chromosomal abnormalities (13, 18, 21, X, and Y). Although interphase FISH for prenatal diagnosis has low false-positive and false-negative rates, it is considered investigational and is used only in conjunction with standard cytogenetic analysis.

51. **What is currently the best method for detecting microchromosome deletions and duplications?**
Microarray-based comparative genomic hybridization (aCGH) is currently the best method of detecting DNA copy number variations (CNVs). This test scans the whole genome for variations in DNA copy numbers. Standard chromosome analysis can detect chromosomal

imbalances that are at least 5Mb in size, whereas aCGH is able to detect cryptic changes (deletions and duplications) that are not visible on standard chromosome analysis. It has become the method of choice for infants and children with multiple congenital anomalies and/or developmental delays. Five percent of such children have visible abnormalities on routine chromosome analysis, but an additional 10% to 15% will have an abnormality when screened with aCGH. It will eventually replace the current FISH analysis for detection of conditions such as DiGeorge syndrome and Williams syndrome. It is important to note that not all CNVs are deleterious; some are polymorphisms that are frequently carried by one parent. Parental studies are thus important in interpreting aCGH results when the results are not clear.

Shaffer LG, Bejjani BA: Using microarray-based molecular cytogenic methods to identify chromosome abnormalities, *Pediatr Ann* 38:440–447, 2009.

Veltman JA: Genomic microarrays in clinical diagnosis, *Curr Opin Pediatr* 18:598–603, 2006.

SEX-CHROMOSOME ABNORMALITIES

52. **What did Lyon hypothesize?**
The *Lyon hypothesis* is that, in any cell, only one X chromosome will be functional. Any other X chromosomes present in that cell will be condensed, late replicating, and inactive (called the *Barr body*). The inactive X may be either paternal or maternal in origin, but all descendants of a particular cell will have the same inactive parentally derived chromosome.

53. **Is it possible to get identical twins of different sexes?**
Yes. If anaphase lag (loss) of a Y chromosome occurs at the time of cell separation into twin embryos, a female fetus with karyotype 45,X (Turner syndrome) and a normal male fetus (46,XY) result.

54. **What are the features of the four most common sex-chromosome abnormalities?**
See Table 8-3.

55. **Of the four most common types of sex-chromosome abnormalities, which is identifiable at birth?**
Only infants with Turner syndrome have physical features that are easily identifiable at birth.
Loscalzo ML: Turner syndrome, *Pediatr Rev* 29:219–227, 2008.

KEY POINTS: TURNER SYNDROME

1. Majority: 45,X

2. Newborn period: Only sign may be lymphedema of feet and/or hands

3. Adolescence: Primary amenorrhea due to ovarian dysplasia

4. Short stature often prompts initial workup

5. Normal mental development

6. Classic features: Webbed neck with low hairline, broad chest with wide-spaced nipples

7. Increased risk for congenital heart disease: Coarctation of the aorta

TABLE 8-3. MOST COMMON SEX CHROMOSOME DISORDERS

	47,XXY (Klinefelter)	47,XYY	47,XXX	45,X (Turner)
Frequency of live births	1 in 2000	1 in 2000	1 in 2000	1 in 8000
Maternal age association	+	–	+	–
Phenotype	Tall, eunuchoid habitus, underdeveloped secondary sexual characteristics, gynecomastia	Tall, severe acne, indistinguishable from normal males	Tall, indistinguishable from normal females	Short stature, webbed neck, shield chest, pedal edema at birth, coarctation of the aorta
IQ and behavior problems	80-100; behavioral problems	90-110; behavioral problems; aggressive behavior	90-110; behavioral problems	Mildly deficient to normal intelligence; spatial-perceptual difficulties
Reproductive function	Extremely rare	Common	Common	Extremely rare
Gonad	Hypoplastic testes; Leydig cell hyperplasia, Sertoli cell hypoplasia, seminiferous tubule dysgenesis, few spermatogenic precursors	Normal-size testes, normal testicular histology	Normal-size ovaries, normal ovarian histology	Streak ovaries with deficient follicles

From Donnenfeld AE, Dunn LK: Common chromosome disorders detected prenatally. Postgrad Obstet Gynecol 6:5, 1986.

56. **What are the similarities between Noonan syndrome and Turner syndrome?**
    - Dorsal hand and pedal edema
    - Low posterior hairline
    - Web neck (pterygium colli)
    - Congenital elbow flexion (cubitus valgus)
    - Broad chest with wide-spaced nipples
    - Narrow, hyperconvex nails
    - Prominent ears
    - Short fourth metacarpal and/or metatarsal

57. **Describe the differences between Noonan syndrome and Turner syndrome.**
    See Table 8-4.

TABLE 8-4. DIFFERENCES BETWEEN TURNER SYNDROME AND NOONAN SYNDROME	
Turner Syndrome	**Noonan Syndrome**
Affects females only	Affects both males and females
Chromosome disorder	Normal chromosomes
(45,X)	Autosomal dominant disorder
Near-normal intelligence	Mental deficiency
Coarctation of aorta is the most common cardiac defect	Pulmonary stenosis is the most common cardiac defect
Amenorrhea and sterility due to ovarian dysgenesis	Normal menstrual cycle in females

58. **What is the most common inherited form of mental retardation?**
    Fragile X syndrome. It affects an estimated 1 in 1000 males and 1 in 2000 females. About 2% to 6% of male subjects and 2% to 4% of female subjects with unexplained mental retardation will carry the full fragile X mutation.

    FRAXA Research Foundation: http://www.fraxa.org.

    National Fragile X Foundation: http://www.fragilex.org.

59. **What is the nature of the mutation in fragile X syndrome?**
    Expansion of trinucleotide repeat sequences. When the lymphocytes of an affected male are grown in a folate-deficient medium and the chromosomes examined, a substantial fraction of X chromosomes demonstrate a break near the distal end of the long arm. This site—the fragile X mental retardation-1 gene (*FMR1*)—was identified and sequenced in 1991. At the center of the gene is a repeating trinucleotide sequence (CGG) that, in normal individuals, repeats 6 to 45 times. However, in carriers, the sequence expands to 50 to 200 copies (called a premutation). In fully affected individuals, it expands to 200 to 600 copies.

    Visootsak J, Warren ST, Anido A, et al: Fragile X syndrome: an update and review for the primary pediatrician, *Clin Pediatr* 44:37–381, 2005.

60. **What are the associated medical problems of fragile X syndrome in males?**
Flat feet (80%), macroorchidism (80% after puberty), mitral valve prolapse (50% to 80% in adulthood), recurrent otitis media (60%), strabismus (30%), refractive errors (20%), seizures (15%), and scoliosis (>20%).

Lachiewicz AM, Dawson DV, Spiridigliozzi GA: Physical characteristics of young boys with fragile X syndrome: reasons for difficulties in making a diagnosis in young males, *Am J Med Genet* 92:229–236, 2000.

61. **What is the outcome for girls with fragile X?**
Heterozygous females who carry the fragile X chromosome have more behavioral and developmental problems (including attention deficit hyperactivity disorder), cognitive difficulties (50% with an IQ in the mentally retarded or borderline range), and physical differences (prominent ears, long and narrow face). Cytogenetic testing is recommended for all sisters of fragile X males.

Hagerman RJ, Berry-Kravis E, et al: Advances in the treatment of fragile X syndrome, *Pediatrics* 123:378–390, 2009.

KEY POINTS: FRAGILE X SYNDROME

1. Most common cause of inherited mental retardation

2. Prepubertal: Elongated face, flattened nasal bridge, protruding ears

3. Pubertal: Macro-orchidism

4. Heterozygous females: 50% with IQ in the borderline or mentally retarded range

5. First recognized trinucleotide repeat disorder

TERATOLOGY

62. **Which drugs are known to be teratogenic?**
Most teratogenic drugs exert a deleterious effect in a minority of exposed fetuses. Exact malformation rates are unavailable because of the inability to perform a statistical evaluation on a randomized, controlled population. Known teratogens are summarized in Table 8-5.

63. **Describe the characteristic features of the fetal hydantoin syndrome.**
Craniofacial: Broad nasal bridge, wide fontanel, low-set hairline, broad alveolar ridge, metopic ridging, short neck, ocular hypertelorism, microcephaly, cleft lip and palate, abnormal or low-set ears, epicanthal folds, ptosis of eyelids, coloboma, and coarse scalp hair
Limbs: Small or absent nails, hypoplasia of distal phalanges, altered palmar crease, digital thumb, and dislocated hip
About 10% of infants whose mothers took phenytoin (Dilantin) during pregnancy have a major malformation; 30% have minor abnormalities.

64. **Does cocaine cause fetal malformations?**
Yes. Several malformations are associated with maternal cocaine use. All are believed to be due to a disruption in normal organ growth and development as a result of vascular

TABLE 8-5. KNOWN TERATOGENS

Drug	Major Teratogenic Effect
Thalidomide	Limb defects
Lithium	Ebstein tricuspid valve anomaly
Aminopterin	Craniofacial and limb anomalies
Methotrexate	Craniofacial and limb anomalies
Phenytoin	Facial dysmorphism, dysplastic nails
Trimethadione	Craniofacial dysmorphism, growth retardation
Valproic acid	Neural tube defects
Diethylstilbestrol	Müllerian anomalies, clear cell adenocarcinoma
Androgens	Virilization
Tetracycline	Teeth and bone maldevelopment
Streptomycin	Ototoxicity
Warfarin	Nasal hypoplasia, bone maldevelopment
Penicillamine	Cutis laxa
Accutane (retinoic acid)	Craniofacial and cardiac anomalies

insufficiency. Intestinal atresias due to mesenteric artery vasoconstriction or thrombosis and urinary tract anomalies, including urethral obstruction, hydronephrosis, and hypospadias, are most commonly reported. Limb reduction defects, which are often described as transverse terminal defects of the forearm or amputation of the digits of the hands and feet, have also been identified.

65. **What amount of alcohol is safe to ingest during pregnancy?**
This is unknown. The full dysmorphologic manifestations of fetal alcohol syndrome are associated with heavy intake. However, most infants will not display the full syndrome. For infants born to women with lesser degrees of alcohol intake during pregnancy and who demonstrate more subtle abnormalities (e.g., cognitive and behavioral problems), it is more difficult to ascribe risk because of confounding variables (e.g., maternal illness, pregnancy weight gain, other drug use [especially marijuana]). Furthermore, for reasons that are unclear, it appears that infants who are prenatally exposed to similar amounts of alcohol are likely to have different consequences. Because current data do not support the concept that any amount of alcohol is safe during pregnancy, the American Academy of Pediatrics recommends abstinence from alcohol for women who are pregnant or who are planning to become pregnant.

Koren G, Caprara D, Chan D, et al: Is it all right to drink a little during pregnancy? *Can Fam Phys* 50:1643–1644, 2004.

Committee on Substance Abuse and Committee on Children with Disabilities: Fetal alcohol syndrome and fetal alcohol effects, *Pediatrics* 91:1004–1006, 1993.

66. **What are the frequent facial features of the fetal alcohol syndrome?**
   - **Skull:** Microcephaly, midface hypoplasia
   - **Eyes:** Short palpebral fissures, epicanthal folds, ptosis, strabismus
   - **Mouth:** Hypoplastic philtrum, thin upper lip, prominent lateral palatine ridges, retrognathia in infancy, micrognathia or relative prognathia in adolescence
   - **Nose:** Flat nasal bridge, short and upturned nose (Fig. 8-6)

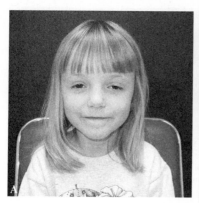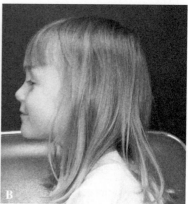

Figure 8-6. Patient with fetal alcohol syndrome. **A**, Note bilateral ptosis, short palpebral fissures, smooth philtrum, and thin upper lip. **B**, Short palpebral fissures are sometimes more noticeable in profile. Head circumference is second percentile. (From Seaver LH: Adverse environmental exposures in pregnancy: teratology in adolescent medicine practice. Adolesc Med State Art Rev 13:269-291, 2002.)

Hoyme HE, May PA, Kalberg WO, et al: A practical clinical approach to diagnosis of fetal alcohol spectrum disorders: clarification of the 1996 Institute of Medicine criteria, *Pediatrics* 115:39–47, 2005.

KEY POINTS: FETAL ALCOHOL SYNDROME

1. Growth deficiencies: Prenatal and postnatal

2. Microcephaly with neurodevelopmental abnormalities

3. Short palpebral fissures

4. Smooth philtrum

5. Thin upper lip

67. **What happens to children with fetal alcohol syndrome when they grow up?**
    A follow-up study of 61 adolescents and adults revealed that relative short stature and microcephaly persisted, but facial anomalies became more subtle. Academic functioning, particularly in arithmetic, was delayed to the early grade-school level. Intermediate or significant maladaptive behavior was present in 100% of patients. Severely unstable family environments were common.

    Streissguth AP, Aase JM, Clarren SK, et al: Fetal alcohol syndrome in adolescents and adults, *JAMA* 265:1961–1967, 1991.

    National Organization on Fetal Alcohol Syndrome: http://www.nofas.org.

ACKNOWLEDGMENT

The editors gratefully acknowledge contributions by Drs. Elain H. Zackai, JoAnn Bergoffen, Alan E. Donnenfeld, and Jeffrey E. Ming that were retained from the first three editions of *Pediatric Secrets*.

CHAPTER 9

HEMATOLOGY

Steven E. McKenzie, MD, PhD

BONE MARROW FAILURE

1. **What are the types of bone marrow failure?**

   Bone marrow failure manifests as pancytopenia or, at times, cytopenia of a single cell type. It can be acquired (acquired aplastic anemia) or inherited/genetic (e.g., Fanconi anemia, Kostmann syndrome, Diamond-Blackfan anemia, amegakaryocytic thrombocytopenia, thrombocytopenia-absent radius).

   > Alter BP: Bone marrow failure syndromes in children, *Pediatr Clin North Am* 49:973–988, 2002.

2. **What are the causes of acquired aplastic anemia?**

   After careful exclusion of the known causes listed below, more than 80% of cases remain classified as idiopathic. A variety of associated conditions include the following:

   Radiation

   Drugs and chemicals
   - Regular: Cytotoxic, benzene
   - Idiosyncratic: Chloramphenicol, anti-inflammatory drugs, antiepileptics, gold

   Viruses
   - Epstein-Barr virus
   - Hepatitis (primarily B)
   - Parvovirus (in immunocompromised hosts)
   - Human immunodeficiency virus (HIV)

   Immune diseases
   - Eosinophilic fasciitis
   - Hypogammaglobulinemia

   Thymoma

   Pregnancy

   Paroxysmal nocturnal hemoglobinuria

   Preleukemia

   > Shimamura A, Guinana EC: Acquired aplastic anemia. In Nathan DG, Orkin SD, Ginsburg D, Look AT, editors: *Nathan and Oski's Hematology of Infancy and Childhood*, ed 6, Philadelphia, 2003, WB Saunders, p 257.

3. **What is the definition of severe aplastic anemia?**

   Severe disease includes a hypocellular bone marrow biopsy (<30% of the normal hematopoietic cell density for age) and decreases in at least two of three peripheral blood counts: neutrophil count less than 500 cells/mm^3, platelet count less than 20,000 cells/mm^3, or reticulocyte count less than 1% after correction for the hematocrit. Categorization has important prognostic and therapeutic implications.

4. **What are the treatments and prognosis for children with aplastic anemia?**

   In the absence of definitive treatment, less than 20% of children with severe acquired aplastic anemia survive more than 2 years. When bone marrow transplantation is performed using a human leukocyte antigen (HLA)-identical sibling donor, the 2-year survival rate exceeds 85%.

The usual approach to the newly diagnosed child with severe acquired aplastic anemia is to perform bone marrow transplantation if there is an HLA-identical sibling to serve as the donor.

About 80% of children with severe aplastic anemia do not have a sibling donor for bone marrow transplantation. These children receive medical therapy, usually the combination of antithymocyte, cyclosporine, and hematopoietic growth factors, such as granulocyte-macrophage colony-stimulating factor or granulocyte colony-stimulating factor (G-CSF). Two-year response and survival rates for combination medical therapy now exceed 80% in children.

Locasciulli A: Acquired aplastic anemia in children: incidence, prognosis and treatment options, *Paediatr Drugs* 4:761–766, 2002.

Trigg ME: Hematopoietic stem cells, *Pediatrics* 113:S1051–S1057, 2004.

5. **What is the probable diagnosis of a 6-year-old child with pancytopenia, short stature, abnormal thumbs, and areas of hyperpigmentation?**
   Fanconi anemia, or constitutional aplastic anemia, is a genetic disorder in which numerous physical abnormalities are often present at birth, and aplastic anemia occurs at about the age of 5 years. The more common physical abnormalities include hyperpigmentation, anomalies of the thumb and radius, small size, microcephaly, and renal anomalies (e.g., absent, duplicated, or pelvic horseshoe kidneys). Patients with Fanconi anemia are also susceptible to leukemia and epithelial carcinomas.

6. **How is the diagnosis of Fanconi anemia made?**
   Chromosomal breakage analysis can be used to make the diagnosis, and molecular diagnosis can confirm the diagnosis and be used to test relatives. In studies of peripheral blood lymphocytes, a high percentage of patients with Fanconi anemia have chromosomal breaks, gaps, or rearrangements. Many genes causing the Fanconi anemia syndrome have now been identified, and molecular diagnosis has assumed increasing importance as studies linking genotype and phenotypes such as aplastic anemia and leukemia can be analyzed.

Tischkowitz M, Dokal I: Fanconi anaemia and leukemia—clinical and molecular aspects, *Br J Haematol* 126:176–191, 2004.

7. **What is transient erythroblastopenia of childhood (TEC) and Diamond-Blackfan anemia?**
   Both are disorders of red blood cell (RBC) production that occur during early childhood. Both disorders are characterized by a low hemoglobin level and an inappropriately low reticulocyte count. The bone marrow of patients with these conditions may be indistinguishable, showing reduced or absent erythroid activity in both cases.

8. **Why is distinguishing between the two conditions extremely important?**
   TEC is a self-limited disorder, whereas Diamond-Blackfan syndrome usually requires lifelong treatment.

9. **How are the two conditions diagnosed?**
   Although there is an overlap in the age of presentation, Diamond-Blackfan syndrome commonly causes anemia during the first 6 months of life, whereas TEC occurs more frequently after the age of 1 year. The RBCs in patients with Diamond-Blackfan syndrome have fetal characteristics that are useful for distinguishing this disorder from TEC, including increased mean cell volume, elevated level of hemoglobin F, and presence of i antigen. The level of adenine deaminase may be elevated in patients with Diamond-Blackfan syndrome but normal in children with TEC. Twenty-five percent of white patients with Diamond-Blackfan anemia have been found to have mutations in the gene for ribosomal protein S19, and molecular diagnosis for these mutations is helpful when positive. Recently, additional gene mutations have been identified in Diamond-Blackfan anemia. These also affect ribosomal proteins. In total, about three fourths of Diamond-Blackfan patients can be identified by mutational analysis.

Drpatchinskaia N, Gustavsson P, Andersson B, et al: The gene encoding ribosomal protein S19 is mutated in Diamond-Blackfan anaemia, *Nat Genet* 21:169–175, 1999.

Willig TN, Niemeyer CM, Leblanc T, et al: Identification of new prognosis factors from the clinical and epidemiologic analysis of a registry of 229 Diamond-Blackfan anemia patients. DBA group of Societe d'Hematologie et d'Immunologie Pediatrique (SHIP), Gesellshaft fur Padiatrische Onkologie und Hamatologie (GPOH), and the European Society for Pediatric Hematology and Immunology (ESPHI), *Pediatric Res* 46:553–561, 1999.

10. **What is Kostmann syndrome?**

Kostmann syndrome is severe congenital neutropenia. At birth or shortly thereafter, very severe neutropenia (absolute neutrophil count of 0 to 200/mm^3) is noted, often at the time of significant bacterial infection (e.g., deep skin abscess, pneumonia, sepsis). Even with antibiotic treatment, there is a high mortality rate during infancy unless G-CSF therapy is used to elevate the neutrophil count. Some recipients of G-CSF have survived the infection risk but have developed myelodysplastic syndrome or acute myeloid leukemia. Therefore, individualized judgment and monitoring are essential in G-CSF treatment of severe congenital neutropenia. An alternative treatment is bone marrow transplantation from an HLA-identical sibling donor.

CLINICAL ISSUES

11. **What is the hemoglobin value below which children are considered to be anemic (lower limit of normal)?**
    - Newborn (full term): 13.0 g/dL
    - 3 months: 9.5 g/dL
    - 1–3 years: 11.0 g/dL
    - 4–8 years: 11.5 g/dL
    - 8–12 years: 11.5 g/dL
    - 12–16 years: 12.0 g/dL

Dallman P, Siimes MA: Percentile curves for hemoglobin and red-cell volume in infancy and childhood, *J Pediatr* 94:26–31, 1979.

12. **In patients with severe chronic anemia, how rapidly can transfusions be given?**

When anemia is chronic, there has been cardiovascular adaptation and a relatively normal blood volume. Excessively rapid transfusions can lead to congestive heart failure. For patients with a hemoglobin level of less than 5 g/dL who exhibit no signs of cardiac failure, a safe regimen is to transfuse packed red blood cells at a rate of 1 to 2 mL/kg per hour by continuous infusion until the desired target is reached. In most patients, 3 mL/kg will raise the hematocrit level by 1%. Judicious use of a diuretic like furosemide (or automated erythrocytapheresis, in larger children) can be considered.

Jayabose S, Tugal O, Ruddy R, et al: Transfusion therapy for severe anemia, *Am J Pediatr Hematol Oncol* 15:324–327, 1993.

13. **When does the physiologic anemia of infancy occur?**

Physiologic anemia occurs at 8 to 12 weeks in full-term infants and at 6 to 8 weeks in premature infants. Full-term infants may exhibit hemoglobin levels as low as 9 g/dL at this time, and very premature infants may have levels as low as 7 g/dL.

14. **Why does the physiologic anemia of infancy occur?**

The mechanisms responsible for physiologic anemia are not completely understood. RBC survival time is decreased in both premature and full-term infants. Furthermore, the ability to increase erythropoietin production in response to ongoing tissue hypoxia is somewhat blunted, although the response to exogenous erythropoietin is normal.

15. **In what settings of shortened RBC survival can the reticulocyte count be normal or decreased?**

As a rule, the reticulocyte count is elevated in conditions of shortened RBC survival (e.g., hemoglobinopathies, membrane disorders, immune hemolysis) and decreased in anemias that are characterized by impaired RBC production (e.g., iron deficiency, aplastic anemia). The reticulocyte count may be unexpectedly low in a setting of shortened RBC survival in the following conditions:

■ Aplastic or hypoplastic crisis is occurring at the same time, as is seen in patients with human parvovirus B19 infection.

■ An autoantibody in immune-mediated hemolysis reacting with antigens that are present on reticulocytes leads to increased clearance of these cells.

■ In patients in chronic states of hemolysis, the marrow may become unresponsive as a result of micronutrient deficiency (e.g., iron, folate) or because of a reduction in erythropoietin production, as is seen in patients with chronic renal failure.

16. **How does the pathophysiology of anemia differ in chronic and acute infection?**

Chronic infection and other inflammatory states impair the release of iron from reticuloendothelial cells, thereby decreasing the amount of this necessary ingredient that are available for RBC production. The lack of mobilizable iron may be the result of the action of proinflammatory cytokines (e.g., interleuking-1, tumor necrosis factor-α). Giving additional iron under these circumstances further increases reticuloendothelial iron stores and does little to help the anemia.

Acute infection may cause anemia through a variety of mechanisms, including bone marrow suppression, shortened RBC life span, RBC fragmentation, and immune-mediated RBC destruction.

17. **Describe the differential diagnosis for children with splenomegaly and anemia.**

Key question: Is the anemia the cause of the splenomegaly, or is the splenomegaly the cause of the anemia?

Anemia causing splenomegaly

■ Membrane disorders
■ Hemoglobinopathies
■ Enzyme abnormalities
■ Immune hemolytic anemia

Splenomegaly causing anemia

■ Cirrhotic liver disease
■ Cavernous transformation of portal vessels
■ Storage diseases
■ Persistent viral infections

18. **A 14-month-old child presents symptoms including marked cyanosis, lethargy, and normal oxygen saturation by pulse oximetry after drinking from a neighbor's well. What is the likely diagnosis?**

Methemoglobinemia should always be considered when a patient presents symptoms of cyanosis without demonstrable respiratory or cardiac disease. Methemoglobin is produced by the oxidation of ferrous iron in hemoglobin into ferric iron. Methemoglobin cannot transport oxygen. Normally, it constitutes less than 2% of circulating hemoglobin. Oxidant toxins (e.g., antimalarial drugs, nitrates in food or well water) can dramatically increase the concentration. Patients with cyanosis as a result of methemoglobinemia can have normal oxygen saturation as measured by pulse oximetry because the oximeter operates by measuring only hemoglobin that is available for saturation.

19. **How can the diagnosis of methemoglobinemia be made at the bedside?**
In patients with methemoglobinemia, the inability of the RBC to maintain hemoglobin iron in the ferrous (Fe^{2+}) state leads to a loss of oxygen-carrying capacity. When a drop of blood from a patient with methemoglobinemia is placed on a piece of filter paper, it generally has a brownish color. When the filter paper is waved in the air, the color of the blood remains brown because the hemoglobin is unable to bind oxygen. By contrast, blood from a normal individual turns from brown to red when the filter paper is waved in the air.

20. **What is the treatment for methemoglobinemia?**
In an acute situation in which levels of methemoglobin are higher than 30%, treatment consists of 1 to 2 mg/kg of 1% methylene blue administered intravenously over 5 minutes and repeated in 1 hour if levels have not fallen to normal. Failure to respond to therapy should raise the possibility of glucose-6-phosphate-dehydrogenase (G6PD) deficiency, which prevents the conversion of methylene blue to the metabolite that is active in the treatment of methemoglobinemia. In these cases, hyperbaric oxygen therapy or exchange transfusion may be necessary.

21. **Why are infants at greater risk for the development of methemoglobinemia?**
   ■ Antioxidant defense mechanisms (e.g., soluble cytochrome b_5 and NADH-dependent cytochrome b_5 reductase) are 40% lower in infants than teenagers.
   ■ Infants' intestinal pH is relatively alkaline compared with older children's. If nitrates are ingested (e.g., from fertilizer-contaminated well water), this higher pH more readily allows bacterial conversion of nitrate to nitrite, which is a potent oxidant.
   ■ Infants are more susceptible to various oxidant exposures: nitrate reductase from foods such as undercooked spinach, menadione (vitamin K_3) for the prevention of neonatal hemorrhage, over-the-counter teething preparations with benzocaine, and metoclopramide for gastroesophageal reflux.

   Bunn HF: Human hemoglobins: normal and abnormal. In Nathan DG, Orkin SH, editors: *Nathan and Oski's Hematology of Infancy and Childhood*, ed 5, Philadelphia, 1998, WB Saunders, pp 729–751.

22. **What are the indications for the use of leukoreduced red blood cells?**
When packed RBCs are prepared from whole blood and then filtered, most of the remaining white cells are removed from the product. Because febrile transfusion reactions are usually the result of leukocytes, filtered products should be used for patients who have experienced such reactions to previous blood transfusions. Filtered RBCs are also effective for reducing the transmission of cytomegalovirus in at-risk individuals. In addition, the use of filtered blood components reduces the risk of HLA alloimmunization, which is desirable for patients who have undergone repeated transfusions and for those who may need stem cell or solid organ transplantation. Currently, many RBC products are leukoreduced at the time of collection (i.e., prestorage). Other products can be leukoreduced at the time of administration.

COAGULATION DISORDERS

23. **What features on history or physical examination help pinpoint the cause of a bleeding problem?**
   ■ **Platelet problems:** Although there can be considerable overlap, in general, platelet problems (platelet dysfunction or von Willebrand disease) result in petechiae, especially

on dependent parts of the body and mucosal surfaces. Additional manifestations of platelet disorders include epistaxis, hematuria, menorrhagia, and gastrointestinal hemorrhages.

- **Coagulation factor deficiencies or platelet problems:** Ecchymoses are suspicious for coagulation factor deficiencies or platelet problems when they occur in unusual areas (particularly not limited to the extremities), are out of proportion with the extent of described trauma, or are present in different stages of healing. Child abuse must also be considered with these features. Delayed bleeding from old wounds and extensive and deep tissue hemorrhage (particularly into joint spaces or intramuscular after immunizations) are also suggestive of coagulation protein disorders. Severe epistaxis (requiring an emergency department visit), bilateral bleeding, and a family history of similar bleeding problems suggest an underlying bleeding disorder.
- **Disseminated intravascular coagulation (DIC):** Bleeding from multiple sites in an ill patient is worrisome for DIC. If a patient has tolerated tonsillectomy and/or adenoidectomy or extraction of multiple wisdom teeth without major hemorrhage, a significant inherited bleeding disorder is unlikely.

Sharathkumar AA, Pipe SW: Bleeding disorders, *Pediatr Rev* 29:121–129, 2008.

24. **What do the activated partial thromboplastin time (aPTT) and the prothrombin time (PT) measure in the basic clotting cascade?**
    See Fig. 9-1.

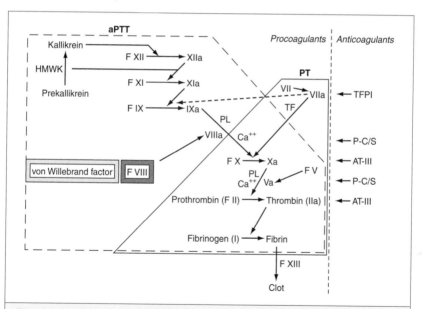

Figure 9-1. Simplified pathways of blood coagulation. The area inside the *dotted line* is the intrinsic pathway measured by the activated partial thromboplastin time (aPTT). The area inside the *solid line* is the extrinsic pathway, measured by the prothrombin time (PT). The area encompassed by both lines is the common pathway. AT-III, antithrombin III; F, factor; HMWK, high-molecular-weight kininogen; P-C/S, protein C/S; PL, phospholipid; TFPI, tissue factor pathway inhibitor. (Adapted from Montgomery RR, Scott JP: Hemostasis. In Behrman RE, Kliegman RM, Jenson HB [eds]: Nelson Textbook of Pediatrics, 16th ed. Philadelphia, WB Saunders, 2000.)

25. **What are the possible causes of a prolonged aPTT and PT?**
    See Table 9-1.

TABLE 9-1. COMMON CAUSES OF PROLONGED PROTHROMBIN TIME (PT) AND ACTIVATED PARTIAL THROMBOPLASTIN TIME (aPTT)		
Scenario	Common and Important Causes	Comments
Prolonged PT	Vitamin K deficiency Liver disease Warfarin Factor VII deficiency Disseminated intravascular coagulation (DIC)	Isolated PT elevation is sensitive marker early in DIC development
Prolonged aPTT	Von Willebrand disease Hemophilia (factor VIII, IX, or XI deficiency) Heparin Antiphospholipid antibodies (associated with minor infections or, rarely, autoimmune or thromboembolic disease)	Rare deficiencies of factor XII, congenital abnormalities of the receptor for vitamin B_{12}-intrinsic factor complex Gastric mucosal defects that interfere with the secretion of intrinsic factor or phosphokinase may also elevate aPTT but are not clinically significant Half of children with prolonged aPTT do not have a bleeding disorder
Prolonged PT and aPTT	Heparin Warfarin Liver disease DIC	Fibrinogen measurement can help distinguish among liver disease and DIC (decrease in fibrinogen) and vitamin K (no decrease in fibrinogen)

From Savage W, Takemoto C: Bleeding and bruising. Contemp Pediatr 26:66, 2009.

26. **What is the INR?**
    The *international normalized ratio (INR)* results from a calculation in which an individual patient PT test value is divided by the laboratory's pooled normal plasma standard PT, then raised to an exponent applicable to each individual PT-initiating reagent available. Its utility is in monitoring coumarin use, in that the reported value has clinical utility regardless of which laboratory performed the PT test. The INR for individuals with normal coagulation proteins not receiving coumarin therapy is 1.0 ($\pm$ about 0.1 to 0.2, based on the laboratory's upper and lower range). For those receiving coumarin therapy, the desired INR varies with the condition being treated but is often 2.0 to 3.0.

27. **What are the inheritance patterns of common bleeding and clotting disorders?**
- **Von Willebrand disease:** This is the most common coagulopathy, and it is autosomal dominant in most cases.
- **Factor VIII deficiency** (hemophilia A) and **factor IX deficiency** (hemophilia B): These conditions are inherited in an X-linked pattern so that females are carriers and males are affected. Inquiry about affected maternal male first cousins or uncles is appropriate. In general, heterozygotes for clotting factor deficiencies are not clinically affected.
- **Factor V Leiden, protein C,** and **antithrombin III**: These are not sex-linked disorders; heterozygosity for factor V mutation is present in 3% to 6% of white children, and evidence indicates that some of these heterozygous individuals may have problems related to hypercoagulation (e.g., venous thrombosis).

Journeycake JM, Buchanan GR: Coagulation disorders, *Pediatr Rev* 24:83–91, 2003.

28. **Why is the lack of a family history of bleeding problems only moderate evidence against the likelihood of hemophilia A in a patient?**
The abnormal factor VIII gene responsible for hemophilia A exhibits marked heterogeneity, and up to one third of cases (either the immediate-carrier mother or the son) may have developed a spontaneous mutation. Molecular diagnosis of the most common mutation in severe factor VIII deficiency—a gene inversion in the distal portion of the gene in the affected male, the mother, and maternal relatives—may help the physician with understanding the family history.

29. **Which is most common: von Willebrand disease, factor VIII deficiency, or factor IX deficiency?**
Von Willebrand disease. Frequency is estimated to be between 1 in 100 to 1 in 1000. Factor VIII deficiency (hemophilia A) is more common (1 in 5000) than factor IX deficiency (hemophilia B), affecting 80% to 85% of all patients with clinically diagnosed factor deficiency.

30. **What are the clinical classifications for hemophilia A and B?**
- **Severe:** <1% factor VIII or IX activity; spontaneous bleeding common; bleeding often involves joints, soft tissue, brain (intracranial hemorrhages in neonates), postcircumcision; most common type (50% to 70% of cases)
- **Moderate:** 1% to 5% factor VIII or IX activity; bleeding after minor trauma, but not usually spontaneous; may involve joints and soft tissue, but less commonly central nervous system (CNS) or postcircumcision; least common type (10% of cases)
- **Mild:** 6% to 30% factor VIII or IX activity; bleeding only after major trauma or surgery; joint and soft tissue involvement, but uncommon after circumcision; more common than moderate type (30% to 40% of cases)

National Hemophilia Foundation: http://www.hemophilia.org.

Sharathkumar AA, Pipe SW: Bleeding disorders, *Pediatr Rev* 29:121–129, 2008.

31. **What are the primary measures for achieving hemostasis in individuals with bleeding disorders?**
Never forget anatomic or surgical technical causes and corrections for hemorrhage. As a result, primary measures are local measures ("push on it, put a stitch or staple in it"), supplemented occasionally with licensed topical prothrombotics. Replacement of the deficient blood components is also important, but pharmacologic measures such as desmopressin acetate (DDAVP, which increase von Willebrand factor [vWF]), antifibrinolytics such as epsilon aminocaproic acid (which stabilize clots), and topical hemostatic preparations such as fibrin glue can be useful.

32. **How are the doses of replacement factor calculated for a hemophiliac patient with or without life-threatening hemorrhage?**

It is important to note that recombinant factor replacement products are widely available, and many are produced in ways that never use any human or animal protein during production. While reducing or eliminating the risk of blood-borne infection, many recombinant factor replacement products will have a unique pharmacokinetic profile. Therefore, it is the practice at many hemophilia treatment centers to perform a yield and survival study of the levels of factor over time in the bloodstream of individual patients with the specific product they use before any major surgery.

For moderate (1% to 5% of normal factor levels) to severe (<1% of normal) hemophilia, recombinant factor VIII or factor IX concentrates are the treatments of choice. Each unit of factor VIII or factor IX is equivalent to the activity of 1 mL of normal plasma. With the recombinant products, a dose of 1 unit/kg should increase the factor VIII level by 1.5% to 2% and the factor IX level by 1%. If there is an antibody inhibitor of the replacement factor, correction will not be achieved. Under these circumstances, alternate therapies are needed, such as porcine factor VIII, factor VIII inhibitor bypassing activity complexes, or recombinant factor VIIa.

For minor hemorrhages (e.g., knee and elbow bleeds), factor levels should be increased to 20% to 30% of normal.

For major bleeding episodes (e.g., hip bleeds, intracranial hemorrhage, bleeding around the airway), factor levels should be raised to 70% to 100% and repeat dosing strongly considered under close medical supervision.

Kelly KM, Butler RB, Farace L, et al: Superior *in vivo* response of recombinant factor VIII concentrate in children with hemophilia A, *J Pediatr* 130:537–540, 1997.

Lee C: Recombinant clotting factors in the treatment of hemophilia, *Thromb Haemost* 82: 516–524, 1999.

KEY POINTS: HEMOPHILIA

1. Hemophilia A: Factor VIII abnormalities (75% to 85% of total cases)

2. Family history is not always positive; up to one third of cases of factor VIII deficiency are caused by a spontaneous mutation.

3. Hemophilia B: Factor IX abnormalities

4. Severity based on factor levels: Severe (<1%), moderate (1% to 5%), mild (5% to 25%)

5. Common initial presentation: Bleeding after circumcision

33. **In patients with severe hemophilia, can prophylaxis with factor replacement prevent severe hemorrhage?**

In a study of boys with severe hemophilia A given regular recombinant factor VIII infusions up to 6 years of age, prophylaxis prevented joint damage and decreased the frequency of joint and other hemorrhages. Prophylaxis works. However, the cost was nearly $300,000 annually. How to reconcile the benefits and costs of effective expensive therapies remains a challenge for the health care system.

Manco-Johnson MJ, Abshire TC, Shapiro AD, et al: Prophylaxis versus episodic treatment to prevent joint disease in boys with severe hemophilia, *N Engl J Med* 357:535–544, 2007.

Roosendaal G, Lafeber F: Prophylactic treatment for prevention of joint disease in hemophilia—cost versus benefit, *N Engl J Med* 357:603–605, 2007.

34. **What are the half-lives of exogenously administered factors VIII and IX?**
The half-lives for the *first* doses of factors VIII and IX are 6 to 8 hours and 4 to 6 hours, respectively. With *subsequent* doses, factor VIII has a half-life of 8 to 12 hours, whereas factor IX has a half-life of 18 to 24 hours. Thus, for serious bleeding, the second dose of factor VIII should be given 6 to 8 hours after the first, whereas the second dose of factor IX should be given 4 to 6 hours after the first. Subsequent doses are usually given every 12 hours for factor VIII replacement and every 24 hours for factor IX replacement, but the measurement of actual factor levels may be necessary to guide therapy in life-threatening situations.

   Gill JC: Transfusion principles for congenital coagulation disorders. In Hoffman R, Benz EJ, Shattil SJ, et al, editors: *Hematology: Basic Principles and Practice*, ed 3. New York, 2000, Churchill Livingstone, pp 2282–2290.

35. **Can someone with isolated factor XII deficiency causing an elevated aPTT undergo surgery?**
The aPTT test requires functional factor XII in the test tube to activate factor XI, and, in patients with factor XII deficiency, the aPTT is prolonged. However, because there is an alternative for activation of factor XI in the body through the FVII/TF (extrinsic pathway) that leads to the generation of thrombin, the risk for perioperative bleeding with isolated factor XII deficiency is considered to be that of the average patient. It is prudent to know the personal and family bleeding histories in an individual with a prolonged aPTT; to rule out factor XI, IX, VIII, and vWF deficiencies; and to rule out the presence of an inhibitor of coagulation before the diagnosis of isolated factor XII deficiency can be made.

36. **What can cause an elevation of the PT when other coagulation testing is normal?**
Factor VII deficiency. PT measures the function of the common pathway factors (including X, V, II, and fibrinogen) as well as the extrinsic pathway (tissue factor and factor VII). The aPTT measures the common pathway plus the function of the intrinsic pathway (including factors XII, XI, IX, and VIII). Isolated factor VII deficiency selectively elevates the PT. Other causes of elevated PT (e.g., liver disease, vitamin K deficiency, warfarin toxicity) are not selective for lowering factor VII activity.

37. **Who gets hemophilia C?**
More commonly called factor XI deficiency, this is an uncommon type of hemophilia (<5% of total hemophilia patients). Unlike the X-linked nature of hemophilias A and B, it is an autosomal recessive disease that occurs most frequently in Ashkenazi Jews.

   Asadai R, et al: Factor XI deficiency in Ashkanazi Jews in Israel, *N Engl J Med* 325:153–158, 1991.

38. **Why is factor IX deficiency also called "Christmas disease"?**
In 1952, investigators in England noted that, when blood from one group of hemophiliacs was added to the blood of another group of hemophiliacs, the clotting time was shortened. This provided the basis for the discovery of plasma substances in addition to what was then called "antihemophilic globulin" (and now called factor VIII), which is responsible for normal clotting. The name was derived because the first patient examined in detail with the unusual clotting deficiency (later designated as factor IX) was a boy named Christmas. The publication of the landmark article in fact occurred during the last week of December in 1952.

   Biggs R, Douglas AS, Macfarlane RG, et al: Christmas disease: a condition previously mistaken for haemophilia, *BMJ* 262:1378–1382, 1952.

39. **What is vWF?**

Synthesized in megakaryocytes and endothelial cells, vWF is a large multimeric protein that binds to collagen at points of endothelial injury. It serves as a bridge between damaged endothelium and adhering platelets, and it facilitates platelet attachment. It also serves as a carrier protein for factor VIII in circulation; it minimizes the clearance of factor VIII from plasma and accelerates its cellular synthesis.

40. **What are the coagulation abnormalities in von Willebrand disease?**

Von Willebrand disease is actually a group of disorders caused by qualitative or quantitative abnormalities in vWF. Coagulation abnormalities in children with severe disease can include a prolonged bleeding time, prolonged partial thromboplastin time, decreased factor VIII coagulant activity, decreased factor VIII antigen, and decreased ability of patient plasma to induce aggregation of normal platelets in the presence of ristocetin (the so-called ristocetin cofactor activity).

41. **What are the common variants of von Willebrand disease?**

See Table 9-2.

TABLE 9-2. COMMON VARIANTS OF VON WILLEBRAND DISEASE

	Type I	Type IIA	Type IIB	Type IIN
Frequency	65%-80%	10%-12%	3%-5%	1%-3%
Genetic transmission	Autosomal dominant	Autosomal dominant	Autosomal dominant	Autosomal dominant
Ristocetin cofactor activity	Low	Low	Low	Normal
Low-dose ristocetin-induced platelet aggregation	Normal	Normal	Increased	Normal
Multimeric electrophoretic pattern	Normal mix (various sizes)	Large, intermediate forms absent	Large multimers absent	Multimers normal
Response to desmopressin	Good	Poor	Decreases platelets	Raises low factor VIII

Data from Montgomery RR, Gill JC, Scott JP, et al: Hemophilia and von Willebrand disease. In Nathan DG, Orkin SD, Ginsburg D, Look AT (eds): Hematology of Infancy and Childhood, 6th ed. Philadelphia, WB Saunders, 2003, p 1561.

42. **What are initial diagnostic tests for suspected von Willebrand disease?**
   - Quantification of vWF antigen
   - Measurement of vWF function (either ristocetin-based platelet aggregation test, known as *ristocetin cofactor assay*) or vWF collagen-binding assay
   - Factor VIII clotting activity

   Screening tests for bleeding disorders (such as aPTT and bleeding time) can be normal in mild disease. Bleeding times are becoming less commonly used in pediatrics. Stress, pregnancy, or medications (e.g., oral contraceptives) can cause daily variation in a patient. The platelet function analyzer (PFA-100) is a recent coagulation screening device that detects most forms of von Willebrand disease; its use in routine clinical practice is evolving.

Robertson J, Lillicrap D, James PD: von Willebrand disease, *Pediatr Clin N Am* 55:377–392, 2008.

Favaloro EJ: The utility of the PFA-100 in the identification of von Willebrand disease: a concise review, *Semin Thromb Hemost* 32:537–545, 2006.

43. **What does the ristocetin cofactor assay measure?**
    vWF activity. vWF will bind to the glycoprotein IB receptor on platelets in the presence of the antibiotic ristocetin. A patient's plasma is serially diluted and mixed with platelets. The presence of vWF allows for platelet agglutination, which can then be quantified on the basis of the dilutions.

44. **How is von Willebrand disease treated?**
    Treatment depends on the variant of vWD disease that is identified:
    - If protein is normal but diminished in quantity, DDAVP is given to stimulate endogenous release. DDAVP is now available for intravenous use and for intranasal use (Stimate). It is important to test vWD patients for the safety and efficacy of either form of DDAVP before clinical use. It is also important to note that the form of intranasal DDAVP used for vWF therapy is different from that used for enuresis management.
    - If protein is abnormal but bleeding is mild, desmopressin may also be of value.
    - If protein is abnormal but bleeding is severe, licensed vWF concentrates may be administered. In 2009 in the United States, a plasma-derived but highly purified product (Humate P) provides both vWF and factor VIII in a useful way because the ristocetin cofactor activity is quantitated for each vial, allowing more precise use.

45. **How does DDAVP work in the treatment of von Willebrand disease?**
    DDAVP is a synthetic analog of the vasopressin, the antidiuretic hormone. Within 1 to 2 hours of its administration (either intravenous, subcutaneous, or intranasal), plasma vWF levels increase by twofold to eightfold. DDAVP appears to act by causing the release of vWF from endothelial cells. Factor VIII levels also increase in part owing to increased stabilization of the vWF factor VIII complex by DDAVP, which lessens proteolytic degradation.

Robertson J, Lillicrap D, James PD: von Willebrand disease, *Pediatr Clin N Am* 55:377–392, 2008.

46. **Should children awaiting surgery undergo routine preoperative screening for potential abnormal bleeding?**
    This is controversial. A study from Philadelphia of 1600 pediatric patients scheduled for tonsillectomy who had a PT, aPTT, and bleeding time found only 2% with abnormal results, of which most were an isolated elevated aPTT. Of these patients, most had antiphospholipid antibody, which was transient. A recent study of patients referred for isolated aPTT found that in the absence of symptoms and a negative family history, the diagnosis of a bleeding disorder was unlikely. Others argue that screening should be used despite the small yield to avoid missing an undiagnosed bleeding disorder.

Shah MD, O'Riordan MA, Alexander SW: Evaluation of prolonged aPTT values in the pediatric population, *Clin Pediatr* 45:347–353, 2006.

Burk CD, Miller L, Handler SD, et al: Preoperative history and coagulation screening in children undergoing tonsillectomy, *Pediatrics* 89:691, 1992.

47. **In an adolescent with menorrhagia, how likely is a bleeding disorder?**
    Up to 20% may have a bleeding disorder, particularly vWD. The American College of Obstetrics and Gynecology recommends screening for any patient under age 18 with menorrhagia.

Kulp JL, Mwangi CN, Loveless M: Screening for coagulation disorders in adolescents with abnormal uterine bleeding, *J Pediatr Adolesc Gynecol* 21:27, 2008.

48. **What is the role of vitamin K in coagulation?**
Vitamin K is essential for the γ-carboxylation of both procoagulants (including factors II, VII, IX, and X) and anticoagulants (proteins C and S). γ-Carboxylation occurs in the liver and converts the proteins to their functional forms. Vitamin K is obtained in three ways: (1) as dietary fat-soluble K_1 (phytonadione) from leafy vegetables and fruits; (2) as K_2 (menaquinone) from synthesis by intestinal bacteria; and (3) as water-soluble K_3 (menadione) from commercial synthesis.

49. **In what settings outside the newborn period can vitamin K abnormalities contribute to a bleeding diathesis?**
- Malabsorptive intestinal disorders (e.g., cystic fibrosis, Crohn disease, celiac disease, short bowel syndrome)
- Prolonged antibiotic therapy (this diminishes intestinal bacteria)
- Prolonged hyperalimentation without supplementation
- Malnutrition
- Chronic hepatic disorders (hepatitis, α_1-antitrypsin deficiency) that can diminish both the absorption of fat-soluble vitamin K (as a result of diminished bile salt production) and the use of vitamin K in factor conversion
- Drugs that can disrupt vitamin K include phenobarbital, phenytoin, rifampin, and warfarin

50. **What is the best test for distinguishing coagulation disturbances resulting from hepatic disease, DIC, and vitamin K deficiency?**
Factors II, V, VII, IX, and X are made in the liver, and all these factors (except factor V) are vitamin K dependent. Therefore, the measurement of factor V is a useful test to distinguish liver disease from vitamin K deficiency because this factor is reduced in the former and normal in the latter disorder. Factor VIII is reduced in patients with DIC because of the consumptive process, but this factor is normal or increased in patients with liver disease and vitamin K deficiency. Therefore, the factor VIII level is a good test to distinguish DIC from the other two disorders (Table 9-3).

TABLE 9-3. COAGULATION ABNORMALITIES IN LIVER DISEASE, VITAMIN K DEFICIENCY, AND DISSEMINATED INTRAVASCULAR COAGULATION

	Factor V	Factor VII	Factor VIII
Liver disease	Low	Low	Normal or increased
Vitamin K deficiency	Normal	Low	Normal
Disseminated intravascular coagulation	Low	Low	Low

51. **What is DIC?**
DIC is an acquired syndrome that is precipitated by a variety of diseases and characterized by diffuse fibrin deposition in the microvasculature, consumption of coagulation factors, and endogenous generation of thrombin and plasmin. The process is uncontrolled, and the result can be significant microthrombus formation with ischemic injury to multiple organ systems.

52. **What tests are valuable for the diagnosis of suspected DIC?**
See Table 9-4.

TABLE 9-4. TESTS FOR DIAGNOSIS OF DISSEMINATED INTRAVASCULAR COAGULATION	
Test	**Usual Results**
Prothrombin time; activated partial thromboplastin time	Prolonged
Fibrinogen	<100 mg/dL*
Platelet count	Low
D-Dimer	>2 μg/mL
Factors II, V, and VIII	Usually low*

*These results may be normal, however, especially in patients with mild disseminated intravascular coagulation because synthesis increases with accelerated consumption.

Data from Nathan DG, Orkin SH, Ginsburg D, Look AT (eds): Nathan and Oski's Hematology of Infancy and Childhood, 6th ed. Philadelphia, WB Saunders, 2003, p 1524.

53. **What is the treatment of choice for DIC?**
DIC occurs most commonly in the context of bacterial sepsis and hypotension. The best treatment is reversal of the underlying cause through treatment of the infection and appropriate fluid and pressor management. If bleeding is severe or if hemorrhage is occurring in a life-threatening location, platelets and fresh-frozen plasma should be given to make up for the loss of these elements, which is occurring from consumption. Heparin has not been proved to be effective for increasing survival in patients with sepsis and DIC. The replenishment of depleted antithrombin III levels with antithrombin III concentrate may decrease the risk for new thromboses.

54. **What are the common hereditary disorders that predispose a child to thrombosis?**
- **Factor V Leiden:** This is an abnormal factor V protein that is resistant to the normal antithrombotic effect of activated protein C.
- **Protein C deficiency:** Protein C inactivates factors V and VIII and stimulates fibrinolysis.
- **Protein S deficiency:** Protein S serves as a cofactor for the activity of protein C.
- **Antithrombin III deficiency:** Antithrombin III is involved in the inhibition of thrombin, factor X, and, to a lesser extent, factor IX.
- **Prothrombin variation** (gene position 20210 AT).
- **Hyperhomocysteinemia** is often the result of a mutation of the *MTHFR* gene. Those with predisposition to hyperhomocystenemia due to thermolabile *MTHFR* variants benefit from folate supplementation, sometimes with vitamins B_6 and B_{12} in addition.
- **Antiphospholipid antibodies.** These are passed from mother to infant prenatally. They can also be acquired, often in adolescence in the presence of systemic autoimmune diseases such as systemic lupus erythematosus.

Goldberg NA, Bernard TJ: Venous thromboembolism in children, *Pediatr Clin N Am* 55:305–322, 2008.

Beck MJ, Berman B: Review of thrombophilic states, *Clin Pediatr* 44:193–199, 2005.

55. **What are common acquired causes of thrombosis in childhood and adolescence?**
In infancy and childhood, these are usually catheter-related, often in the setting of prolonged parenteral nutrition or cancer therapy, or related to significant dehydration. In adolescence, use of oral contraceptives and cigarette smoking may contribute. Occasionally, thoracic outlet syndrome and upper vessel thrombi may result from extensive exercise such as weight lifting.

56. **What are low-molecular-weight heparin (LMWH) and pentasaccharide?**
   LMWH is the sulfated oligosaccharide heparin, derived from natural sources such as beef lung and pig intestine, that has been subjected to heparinase treatment to reduce the average molecular weight. Dosing and bioavailability become more standardized, with less frequent or no monitoring of the anti–factor Xa activity, depending on clinical circumstances. LMWH still works by binding antithrombin to enhance its anti–factor IIa and anti–factor Xa activities. Pentasaccharide is a synthetic five-sugar agent that binds antithrombin and primarily inhibits factor Xa. It has a longer half-life and reduced monitoring advantages over heparin, but currently no antidote is available clinically.

57. **What are the direct thrombin inhibitors?**
   There are two classes of direct thrombin inhibitors, anticoagulant drugs that block the enzymatic activity of thrombin without binding to antithrombin. The first class includes natural or synthetic derivatives of leech hirudin, usually cleared renally. The second class includes synthetic small molecule drugs such as brand argatroban, usually cleared hepatically. Use in children remains under investigation.

HEMATOLOGY LABORATORY

58. **Of the seven RBC parameters given by a Coulter counter, which are measured and which are calculated?**
   The Coulter counter, which is the most commonly used automated electronic cell counter, uses the impedance principle. A precise volume of blood passes through a narrow aperture and impedes an electrically charged field, and each "blip" is counted as a cell. The larger the RBC, the greater the electric displacement. In a separate chamber, the same volume is hemolyzed and colorimetrically analyzed to determine the hemoglobin concentration.
   Measured values:
   - RBC count
   - Mean corpuscular volume (MCV)
   - Hemoglobin (Hb)

   Calculated values:
   - Mean corpuscular hemoglobin (MCH, measured in pg/cell) = $(10 \times [Hb/RBC])$
   - Mean corpuscular hemoglobin concentration (MCHC, measured in g/dL) = $(100 \times [Hb/Hct])$
   - Hematocrit (Hct, given as a percentage) = $(RBC \times [MCV/10])$
   - RBC distribution width (RDW) = coefficient of variation in RBC size

59. **How does the MCV help provide a quick screen of the possible causes of anemia?**
   - **Microcytic:** Iron deficiency, thalassemias, sideroblastic anemia
   - **Normocytic:** Autoimmune hemolytic anemia, hemoglobinopathies, enzyme deficiencies, membrane disorders, anemia of chronic inflammation
   - **Macrocytic:** Disorders of B_{12} and folic acid metabolism, bone marrow failure

60. **What is a quick rule of thumb for approximating MCV?**
   $70 + $ (age in years). This number (in mm^3) approximates the lower limit of MCV in children younger than 8 years old, below which microcytosis is present. From 8 to 12 years, the lower limit for normal MCV is 77 mm^3, and from 12 to 18 years, it is 78 mm^3.

61. **In addition to an elevated reticulocyte count, what laboratory studies suggest increased destruction (rather than decreased production) of RBCs as a cause of anemia?**
   - **Increased serum erythrocyte lactate dehydrogenase:** More commonly seen in patients with hemolytic diseases, it can be greatly elevated in patients with ineffective erythropoiesis (e.g., megaloblastic anemia).

- **Decreased serum haptoglobin:** When RBCs lyse, serum haptoglobin binds the released hemoglobin and is excreted. However, up to 2% of the population has congenitally absent haptoglobin.
- **Hyperbilirubinemia (indirect):** This is usually increased with RBC lysis. However, it may also be elevated in patients with ineffective erythropoiesis (e.g., megaloblastic anemia). Additionally, 2% of the population has Gilbert disease. In these patients, acute infection can cause a transient elevation of bilirubin as a result of liver enzymatic dysfunction rather than hemolysis.

62. **What is the difference between the direct and indirect Coombs tests?**
Coombs serum is rabbit antihuman immunoglobulin.
- **Direct test:** Coombs serum is added directly to a patient's washed RBCs. The occurrence of agglutination means that the patient's RBCs have been sensitized *in vivo* by the antibody. Direct Coombs testing is vital for diagnosing autoimmune hemolytic anemias.
- **Indirect test:** This involves incubating a patient's serum with RBCs of a known type and adding Coombs serum. If *in vitro* sensitization occurs, agglutination will result, which indicates that antibodies are present against the known blood type. Indirect testing is key for blood crossmatching.

63. **How is the corrected reticulocyte count calculated?**
Because the reticulocyte count is expressed as a percentage of total RBCs, it must be corrected according to the extent of anemia with the following formula: reticulocyte % $\times$ (patient Hct/ normal Hct) = corrected reticulocyte count. For example, a very anemic 10-year-old patient with a hematocrit level of 7% (in contrast with an expected normal hematocrit of 36%) and a reticulocyte count of 5% has a corrected reticulocyte count of 1.0%: 5% $\times$ (7%/36%) = 1%. This is not appropriately elevated, as might be seen in patients with severe iron deficiency. The key concept is the appropriateness of the reticulocyte response to anemia. The corrected "retic count" should be elevated if the bone marrow is working properly and has all the right nutrients for making RBCs, including iron, folate, and vitamin B_{12}.

64. **What is the significance of targeting on an RBC smear?**
RBC targets on a peripheral smear are caused by excessive membrane relative to the amount of hemoglobin. Therefore, target cells are found when the membrane is increased (e.g., in patients with liver disease) or when the intracellular hemoglobin is diminished (e.g., in patients with iron deficiency or thalassemia trait). Target cells may also be found in patients with certain hemoglobinopathies (e.g., hemoglobins C and SC). In these instances, the target cells are caused by aggregation of the abnormal hemoglobin.

65. **In what conditions are Howell-Jolly bodies found?**
Howell-Jolly bodies are nuclear remnants that are found in the RBCs of patients with reduced or absent splenic function and in patients with megaloblastic anemias. They are occasionally present in the RBCs of premature infants. Howell-Jolly bodies are dense, dark, and perfectly round, and their characteristic appearance makes them easily distinguishable from other RBC inclusions and from platelets overlying red cells.

66. **What is the cause of Heinz bodies?**
Heinz bodies represent precipitated denatured hemoglobin in the RBC. Heinz bodies occur when the hemoglobin is intrinsically unstable (e.g., as in hemoglobin Koln) or when the enzymes that normally protect hemoglobin from oxidative denaturation are abnormal or deficient (e.g., as in G6PD deficiency). These inclusions are not visible with a routine Wright-Giemsa stain but can be seen readily with methyl violet or brilliant cresyl blue stains.

67. **What makes an "atypical lymphocyte" atypical?**
Atypical lymphocytes (Fig. 9-2) are young lymphocytes (not lymphoblasts) that are characterized by an irregular plasma membrane with a large nucleus. Cytoplasm is typically basophilic. On a blood smear, where an atypical lymphocyte abuts an RBC, the shape of the lymphocyte will deform around it. Atypical lymphocytes are seen in a variety of illnesses, most commonly infectious mononucleosis.

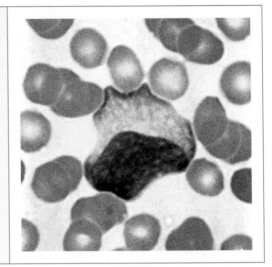

Figure 9-2. Atypical lymphocyte. Note the deformation of the lymphocyte by the adjacent red cells. (From Zitelli BJ, Davis HW: Atlas of Pediatric Physical Diagnosis, 5th ed. Philadelphia, Mosby, 2007, p 421.)

HEMOLYTIC ANEMIA

68. **What clinical features are suspicious for hemolytic anemia?**
   - Discolored urine (dark, brown, red)
   - Jaundice
   - Pallor
   - Tachycardia
   - Splenic and/or liver enlargement
   - If very severe, hypovolemic shock or congestive heart failure

69. **What two types of RBC forms are commonly seen on the peripheral smear in patients with hemolytic anemia?**
   - **Spherocytes or microspherocytes:** These forms can be seen in any hemolytic anemia that results from a loss of RBC membrane surface area (e.g., Coombs-positive hemolytic anemia, DIC, or hereditary spherocytosis).
   - **Schistocytes:** These various forms of fragmented RBCs can be seen in patients with microangiopathic hemolytic anemia, which is a form of intravascular hemolysis caused by mechanical disruption (e.g., prosthetic heart valves, hemolytic-uremic syndrome, cavernous hemangioma).

70. **Name the two most common inherited disorders of RBC membranes.**
Hereditary spherocytosis is characterized by hemolysis (anemia, reticulocytosis, jaundice, splenomegaly), spherocytosis, and, in most cases, a family history of hemolytic anemia. The diagnosis can be made by establishing the presence of the clinical findings and by the

finding of increased osmotic fragility of the RBCs. Hereditary spherocytosis is inherited as an autosomal dominant disorder about 75% of the time.

Hereditary elliptocytosis is characterized by variable hemolysis, with a predominance of elliptocytes on the blood smear. It is usually inherited in an autosomal dominant pattern.

71. **Which disorder is most commonly associated with an elevated MCHC?**
Hereditary spherocytosis. The hyperchromic appearance of spherocytes and microspherocytes is the result of the loss of surface membrane, an excess of hemoglobin, and mild cellular dehydration. In other hemolytic anemias that are associated with spherocytosis, the percentage of spherocytes is usually insufficient to raise the MCHC.

72. **What is the osmotic fragility test?**
This is a test to confirm the diagnosis of hereditary spherocytosis. A normal red blood cell is discoid in shape as a result of its relative excess of surface area per cell volume from the redundancy of its cell membrane. In increasingly hypotonic solutions, more and more RBCs will swell and burst at a standard rate. In spherocytosis, because there is less surface area to cell volume, more cells burst compared with normal in these hypotonic solutions, particularly after incubating at 37°C for 24 hours. This tendency toward earlier lysis makes them osmotically fragile (Fig. 9-3).

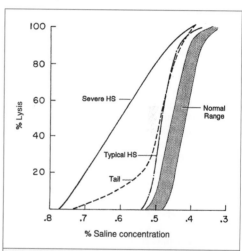

Figure 9-3. Osmotic fragility curves in hereditary spherocytosis. (From Nathan DG, Orkin SH, Ginsburg D, Look AT [eds]: Nathan and Oski's Hematology of Infancy and Childhood, 6th ed. Philadelphia, WB Saunders, 2003, p 610.)

Shah S, Vega R: Hereditary spherocytosis, *Pediatr Rev* 25:166–171, 2004.

73. **What is the difference between alloimmune and autoimmune hemolytic anemia?**
- **Alloimmune hemolytic anemia:** Antibodies responsible for hemolysis are directed against another's RBCs.
- **Autoimmune hemolytic anemia:** Antibodies are directed against the host's RBCs.

74. **In which settings do alloimmune and autoimmune hemolytic anemia most commonly appear?**
Isoimmune: RBC antigen incompatibility between mother and fetus transfusion of incompatible blood
Autoimmune: *Primary:* Autoimmune hemolytic anemia (AIHA)
- Secondary infections (e.g., *Mycoplasma pneumoniae*, Epstein-Barr virus, varicella, viral hepatitis)
- Drugs (e.g., antimalarials, penicillin, tetracycline)
- Systemic autoimmune disorders (e.g., systemic lupus erythematosus, dermatomyositis)

75. **How does the cause of AIHA vary by age?**
AIHA in children younger than 10 years is more likely to be primary. In children older than 10 years, AIHA is more likely to be secondary to an underlying disease.

76. **What is the most important test to establish the diagnosis of AIHA?**
The **Coombs test**. The diagnosis of AIHA requires the presence of autoantibodies that bind to erythrocytes. However, in about 10% of patients with AIHA, the Coombs test is negative. Thus, patients should be treated for AIHA if the disease is strongly suspected, even if the direct Coombs test is negative.

77. **What are the differences between autoimmune hemolytic anemias caused by "warm" and "cold" erythrocyte autoantibodies?**
   - **Warm** (usually immunoglobulin G [IgG] antibodies with maximal activity at 37°C): These are most commonly directed against the Rh antigens and generally do not require complement for in vivo hemolysis. Hemolysis is predominantly extravascular—consumption occurs primarily in the spleen. Warm antibody-mediated hemolytic anemia is more likely to be associated with underlying disease (especially systemic lupus erythematosus in females) and to become chronic. Splenectomy and immunosuppression (e.g., with steroids) are often effective therapies.
   - **Cold** (IgM antibodies with maximal activity between 0° and 30°C): These are most commonly directed against I or i antigen. Hemolysis is most commonly intravascular, through complement activation. Extravascular hemolysis that does occur primarily involves hepatic consumption. Cold antibody-mediated hemolytic anemia is more commonly associated with acute infection (e.g., *Mycoplasma pneumoniae*, cytomegalovirus). Patients are less likely to develop chronic hemolysis, and therapy (e.g., splenectomy, immunosuppression) is often ineffective.

78. **An 8-year-old black male developed jaundice and very dark urine 24 to 48 hours after beginning nitrofurantoin for a urinary tract infection. What is the likely diagnosis?**
G6PD deficiency is the most common hemolytic anemia caused by an RBC enzymatic defect. The enzyme G6PD is a key component of the pentose phosphate pathway, which ordinarily generates sufficient nicotinamide adenine dinucleotide phosphate hydrogen to maintain glutathione in a reduced state (and to make it available for combating oxidant stresses). The deficiency is inherited in an X-linked recessive fashion. In patients who are deficient (most commonly those of African, Mediterranean, or Asian ancestry), oxidant stresses (particularly certain drugs) can result in hemolysis.

79. **In a patient with G6PD deficiency, why is the initial diagnosis often difficult in the acute setting?**
The amount of G6PD enzymatic activity depends on the age of the RBC. Older RBCs have the least, and reticulocytes have the most. In an acute hemolytic episode, the older cells are destroyed first; younger ones may remain, and reticulocytes may increase. If erythrocytic G6PD levels are measured at this point, the result may be misleadingly near or above the normal range. If clinical suspicions remain, repeating the test when the reticulocyte count is reduced will give a more accurate measurement.

80. **What is favism?**
Favism refers to the clinical syndrome of acute hemolytic anemia from the ingestion of fava beans as an oxidative challenge in patients with G6PD deficiency. This is particularly common in portions of the Mediterranean and Asia, where fava beans are a dietary staple.

IRON DEFICIENCY ANEMIA

81. **At what age do exclusively breastfed infants become at risk for iron deficiency?**
Healthy term infants who are exclusively breastfed are at risk for iron deficiency after they are 6 months old. The age of risk for exclusively breastfed premature infants can be more complicated, particularly for the smaller and sicker infants, and recommendations vary. The lower iron stores of premature infants are more rapidly depleted compared with term babies.

Leung AK, Chan KW: Iron deficiency anemia, *Adv Pediatr* 48:385–408, 2001.

82. **Why are infants who begin consuming cow milk at an early age susceptible to iron deficiency anemia?**
Lower bioavailability. Although breast milk and cow milk contain about the same amount of iron (0.5 to 1.0 mg/L), nonheme iron is absorbed at 50% efficiency from breast milk but at only 10% from cow milk. In addition, cow milk may cause microscopic gastrointestinal bleeding in younger infants as a result of mucosal injury, possibly from sensitivity to bovine albumin. In older infants, cow milk may interfere with iron absorption from other sources.

Fuchs G, DeWier M, Hutchinson S, et al: Gastrointestinal blood loss in older infants: impact of cow milk versus formula, *J Pediatr Gastroenterol Nutr* 16:4–9, 1993.

Sullivan P: Cow's milk-induced intestinal bleeding in infancy, *Arch Dis Child* 68:240–245, 1993.

83. **For which pediatric groups should screening for iron deficiency anemia be considered?**
   - Low birthweight
   - Consumption of whole cow milk before the age of 7 months
   - Use of formula not fortified with iron
   - Low socioeconomic status
   - Exclusive breastfeeding (without solid or formula supplementation) beyond the age of 6 months
   - Perinatal blood loss
   - Teenage females (if menstruation is heavy or if pregnant)

Oski F: Iron deficiency in infancy and childhood, *N Engl J Med* 329:190–193, 1993.

84. **How common is anemia in teenage athletes?**
Significant anemia is uncommon. However, iron deficiency without anemia may be found in about half of adolescent female athletes and in up to one eighth of male athletes, particularly long-distance runners. However, an adverse effect of this iron deficiency on athletic performance in the absence of anemia has never been conclusively demonstrated. On the other hand, iron depletion (with or without anemia) may be associated with lassitude, decreased concentration ability, and mood swings.

Ballin A, Berar M, Rubinstein U, et al: Iron state in female adolescents, *Am J Dis Child* 146:803–805, 1992.

Rowland TW: Iron deficiency in the young athlete, *Pediatr Clin North Am* 37:1153–1162, 1990.

85. **As iron becomes depleted from the body, what is the progression at which laboratory tests change?**
The left end of the line for each test indicates the point at which the result deviates from its baseline. As shown in Fig. 9-4, in general, the depletion of marrow, liver, and spleen reserves (as represented by ferritin) occurs first. This is followed by a decrease in transport iron (as represented by transferrin saturation) and finally a fall in hemoglobin and MCV. The figure illustrates that the absence of anemia does not exclude the possibility of iron deficiency and that iron depletion is relatively advanced before anemia develops. Tests of soluble transferrin receptor have become of interest in patients with iron deficiency anemia because the elevated levels are very sensitive indicators.

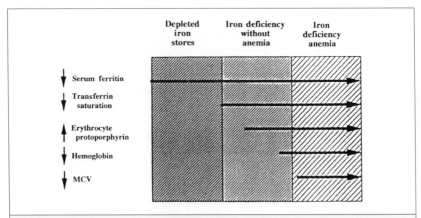

Figure 9-4. Progression of laboratory test changes with iron depletion. (From Dallman PR, Yip R, Oski FA: Iron deficiency and related nutritional anemias. In Nathan DG, Oski FA [eds]: Hematology of Infancy and Childhood, 4th ed. Philadelphia, WB Saunders, 1993, p 427.)

86. **How might the reticulocyte hemoglobin content be helpful for the diagnosis of iron deficiency?**
Because the reticulocyte is the most recently produced RBC in circulation, the earliest sign of iron deficiency may be a fall in the concentration of hemoglobin in reticulocytes. This number can be calculated from automated counting equipment and may be a reliable and inexpensive alternative to ferritin. Studies have indicated that patients with a concentration of at least 25 pg per cell have a very low likelihood of iron deficiency.

Mateos ME, Dela-Cruz J, López-Laso E, et al: Reticulocyte haemoglobin content for the diagnosis of iron deficiency, *J Pediatr Hematol Oncol* 30:539–542, 2008.

87. **Why are tests for iron stores more difficult to interpret during acute inflammatory states?**
The ferritin level, which is used to monitor body iron stores, is exquisitely sensitive to inflammation, increasing even with mild upper respiratory infections. Elevations of ferritin may persist for some time. By contrast, serum iron, transferrin level, and percent transferrin saturation may decrease with infection or inflammation. Free erythrocyte protoporphyrin should not be affected by acute inflammation but may increase in chronic inflammatory states.

88. **What is the role of hepcidin in iron metabolism?**
Hepcidin is part of the system of iron regulatory proteins about which our understanding has increased explosively. The iron regulatory system controls intestinal iron absorption, blood transport, tissue deposition, and mobilization of stores for utilization. Hepcidin is synthesized in the liver and participates in the orchestration of uptake and utilization.

Collard KJ: Iron homeostasis in the neonate, *Pediatrics* 123:1208–1216, 2009.

89. **What are the causes of microcytic anemia in children?**
- **More common:** Iron deficiency (from nutritional insufficiency and/or blood loss), thalassemia (α and β; major, minor, or trait)
- **Less common:** Lead toxicity, hemoglobinopathy (with or without thalassemia), chronic inflammation, copper deficiency, sideroblastic anemia

90. **Why is the red cell distribution width (RDW) helpful for diagnosing microcytic anemia?**

The RDW is a quantification of anisocytosis (variation in RBC size). It is derived from the RBC size histogram that is measured by automated cell counters, and it is reported as a percentage. In children, normal values range from about 11.5% to 14.5% but can vary among instruments. Statistically, it is the coefficient of variation of RBC volume distribution.

91. **How is the RDW useful for distinguishing causes of microcytic anemia?**

When elevated in a patient with microcytosis, it suggests that iron deficiency is a more likely cause of anemia than the thalassemia trait. Children with the thalassemia trait tend to have values that overlap with normal RDW values. The combination of an RDW above the normal range with a free erythrocyte protoporphyrin level of more than 35 μg/dL is more sensitive and specific for iron deficiency anemia.

Jain S, Kamat D: Evaluation of microcytic anemia, *Clin Pediatr* 48:7–13, 2009.

92. **What is the Mentzer index?**

MCV/RBC. This is one of the formulas that is used to distinguish the hypochromic, microcytic anemias of the thalassemia trait from iron deficiency. As a general rule, iron deficiency causes alterations in RBCs that tend to be variable, whereas thalassemia generally results in more uniformly smaller cells. In patients with the β-thalassemia trait, the Mentzer index is usually less than 13; in patients with iron deficiency, it is usually greater than 13.

93. **In a child with suspected iron deficiency anemia, is a therapeutic trial with iron an acceptable diagnostic approach?**

Yes. If an infant or child is otherwise well, a therapeutic trial of 4 to 6 mg/kg per day of elemental iron can substitute for additional diagnostic testing (e.g., ferritin, transferrin saturation, free erythrocyte protoporphyrin) because dietary iron deficiency is the most likely cause of microcytic anemia. If the child is iron deficient, is compliant with therapy, and does not have ongoing undetected blood loss, the hemoglobin should rise by more than 1 g/dL in about 2 weeks. If the hemoglobin does rise, therapy should be continued for an additional 2 months to replenish iron stores.

94. **After iron therapy is initiated, how early can a response be detected?**

2 to 5 days: Increase in reticulocyte count

7 to 10 days: Increase in hemoglobin level

For patients with mild iron deficiency anemia, the hemoglobin level should be checked after several weeks of therapy. For patients with more severe anemia, it may be useful to check the hemoglobin and reticulocyte levels after several days to make certain that the hemoglobin has not declined to dangerous levels and that the reticulocyte response is beginning.

95. **What foods affect the bioavailability of nonheme iron?**

It is decreased by phosphates, tannates, polyphenols, and oxalates found in cereal, eggs, milk, cheese, tea, and complex carbohydrates. It is increased by fructose, citrate, and especially ascorbic acid found in red kidney beans, cauliflower, and bananas. In children with iron deficiency, the administration of replacement iron with a vitamin C–fortified fruit juice 30 minutes before a meal makes physiologic sense.

96. **What are the options for use of parenteral iron therapy?**

When oral iron therapy has failed or cannot be used, there are several formulations of iron for intravenous use with generally good tolerance. These include formulations such as iron sucrose and sodium ferric gluconate. Usually, repletion of iron stores requires multiple treatments over time. Care must be exercised in administration to avoid untoward side effects. Monitoring is required to ensure that anemia is reversed and that iron stores are restored.

KEY POINTS: IRON DEFICIENCY ANEMIA

1. The introduction of whole cow milk before the age of 1 year increases risk as a result of occult gastrointestinal bleeding.

2. Red blood cell distribution width is increased because deficiency results in uneven red blood cell size (anisocytosis).

3. Low levels of ferritin indicate diminished tissue iron stores.

4. This condition impairs cognitive development in infants.

5. Absence of anemia does not exclude the possibility of iron deficiency. Iron depletion is relatively advanced before anemia develops.

97. **What are the differences between pica, geophagia, and pagophagia?**
    All are clinical markers that suggest the diagnosis of iron deficiency. *Pica* is a more general term that indicates a hunger for material that is not normally consumed as food. *Geophagia* refers to the consumption of dirt or clay, and *pagophagia* refers to the excessive consumption of ice. These are distinguished from *cissa,* which is the physiologic craving during pregnancy for unusual food items or combinations.

98. **What is the derivation of the term *pica*?**
    The condition comes from the Latin term for the magpie, *Pica hudsonia.* This bird is believed to eat almost anything, hence the term pica for the tendency to eat non-nutritional substances.

    Borgna-Pignatti C, Marsella M: Iron deficiency in infancy and childhood, *Pediatr Ann* 37:332–333, 2008.

99. **Discuss the relationship between iron deficiency and development in infants and toddlers.**
    Multiple studies have shown an association between iron deficiency in infants between 9 and 24 months old and lower motor and cognitive scores and increased behavioral problems compared with nonanemic controls. Some longer-term studies suggest that the developmental impairments may be long lasting. Debate remains about whether this relationship is causal and, if so, whether the correction of anemia leads to a reversal of the problems.

    Buchanan GR: The tragedy of iron deficiency during infancy and childhood, *J Pediatr* 135: 413–415, 1999.

100. **Why are iron-deficient children at increased risk for lead poisoning?**
     - Pica associated with iron deficiency increases the likelihood of ingestion of lead-contaminated items.
     - Gastrointestinal absorption of lead may be increased in patients who consume less iron-containing nutrients.

     Watson WS, Morrison J, Bethel MI, et al: Food iron and lead absorption in humans, *Am J Clin Nutr* 44:248–256, 1986.

101. **How does lead cause microcytic anemia?**
     - As a divalent metal, lead interferes with iron absorption and iron utilization in heme pathways (microcytosis is thought to be due to iron deficiency)
     - Lead can directly inhibit the enzymes involved in heme synthesis

     Richardson W: Microcytic anemia, *Pediatr Rev* 28:5–13, 2007.

MEGALOBLASTIC ANEMIA

102. **What is megaloblastic anemia?**
Megaloblastic anemia is a macrocytic anemia that is characterized by large RBC precursors (megaloblasts) in the bone marrow and that is usually caused by nutritional deficiencies of either folic acid (folate) or vitamin B_{12} (cobalamin).

103. **Is megaloblastic anemia the most common cause of macrocytic anemia?**
No. Macrocytic anemia can be found in conditions associated with a high reticulocyte count (e.g., hemolytic anemia, hemorrhage), bone marrow failure (e.g., Fanconi's anemia, aplastic anemia, Diamond-Blackfan anemia), liver disease, Down syndrome, and hypothyroidism.

104. **What findings on a complete blood count are suggestive of megaloblastic anemia?**
   - **RBCs:** Elevated MCH and mean cell volume (often 106 fl or more), with normal MCHC; marked variability in cell size (anisocytosis) and shape (poikilocytosis)
   - **Neutrophils:** Hypersegmentation (>5% of neutrophils with five lobes or a single neutrophil with six lobes)
   - **Platelets:** Usually normal; thrombocytopenia in more severe anemia

105. **What are the causes of vitamin B_{12} (cobalamin) deficiency in children?**
Decreased intake
   - May occur in vegetarians who consume no animal products
   - Seen in exclusively breastfed infants of vitamin B_{12}–deficient mothers
   - General malnutrition

Decreased absorption
   - Ileal mucosal abnormalities (e.g., Crohn disease)
   - Surgical resection of terminal ileum
   - Competition for cobalamin in bacterial overgrowth syndromes or infection with the fish tapeworm *Diphyllobothrium latum*
   - Congenital abnormalities of the receptor for vitamin B_{12}–intrinsic factor complex
   - Gastric mucosal defects that interfere with the secretion of intrinsic factor

106. **What are the best dietary sources of folate and vitamin B_{12}?**
   - **Folate:** Folate-rich foods include liver, kidney, and yeast. Good sources also include green vegetables (particularly spinach) and nuts. Moderate sources include fruits, bread, cereals, fish, eggs, and cheese. Pasteurization or boiling destroys folate.
   - **Vitamin B_{12}:** Humans do not manufacture B_{12}; bacteria and fungi do. Animals require it, whereas plants do not. Consequently, our major dietary source of vitamin B_{12} is the consumption of animal tissue, milk, or eggs. Fish, which live on bacterial diets, are also a good dietary source. Of note is that B_{12} is required for normal folate metabolism.

107. **What is pernicious anemia?**
Pernicious anemia is a megaloblastic anemia that is caused by a lack of intrinsic factor. Intrinsic factor is a glycoprotein that is released from the gastric parietal cells and binds to vitamin B_{12} to form a complex that is ultimately absorbed in the terminal ileum.

108. **A 10-month-old child who was exclusively fed goat milk is likely to develop what type of anemia?**
Megaloblastic anemia as a result of folic acid deficiency. Goat milk contains very little folic acid compared with cow milk. Infants who are consuming large amounts of goat milk—especially if they are not receiving significant supplemental solid foods—are susceptible to this type of anemia. In addition, the diagnosis can be complicated by the higher risk for coexistent iron deficiency anemia in this age group.

PLATELET DISORDERS

109. **How can a platelet count be estimated from a peripheral smear?**
As a rule, each platelet that is visible on a high-power microscopic field (100× objective) represents 15,000 to 20,000 platelets/mm^3. If platelet clumps are observed, the count is usually higher than 100,000/mm^3.

110. **How much does a platelet transfusion raise the platelet count?**
In general, 0.1 to 0.2 U/kg of transfused platelets should raise the platelet count by 40,000/mm^3 (or 1.0 U/m^2 should raise the count by 10,000/mm^3). In normal patients, platelet survival time is 7 to 10 days, but this is often considerably shorter in thrombocytopenic patients as a result of a variety of causes.

111. **What are the main pathophysiologic processes that can result in thrombocytopenia?**
- Peripheral destruction
- Consumptive coagulopathy
- Splenic sequestration
- Bone marrow failure

112. **A previously healthy 3-year-old child develops mucosal petechiae, multiple ecchymoses, and a platelet count of 20,000/mm^3 2 weeks after a bout of chickenpox. What is the most likely diagnosis?**
Acute idiopathic (immune) thrombocytopenic purpura (ITP). ITP is one of the most common bleeding disorders of childhood, and the presentation of symptoms occurs after infection in about 50% of cases.

113. **What microscopic features would suggest a diagnosis other than ITP in a patient with a platelet count of 20,000?**
- Platelet clumps (*in vitro* phenomenon caused by EDTA that results in artifactually low platelet count)
- Leukemic blasts
- RBC fragments (suggest a microangiopathic etiology such as hemolytic-uremic syndrome or Kasabach-Merritt syndrome)
- Large platelets (seen in inherited platelet disorders such as Bernard Soulier syndrome, MYH9 syndromes, DiGeorge syndrome)
- Atypical lymphocytes (thrombocytopenia rarely occurs as part of infectious mononucleosis)
- Uniformly small platelets (a feature of Wiskott-Aldrich syndrome)

    Thachil J, Hall GW: Is this immune thrombocytopenic purpura? *Arch Dis Child* 93:76–81, 2008.

    Drachman JG: Inherited thrombocytopenia: when a low platelet count does not mean ITP, *Blood* 103:390–398, 2004.

114. **What is the natural history of acute childhood ITP?**
With or without medical treatment, 50% to 60% of patients with acute ITP will have normal platelet counts within 1 to 3 months of diagnosis, and 75% are well after 6 months. By 1 year, only 10% of children with ITP remain thrombocytopenic, and some of the children with chronic ITP still improve as long as 5 to 10 years after diagnosis. About 5% of patients have recurrent ITP. Because of this predominantly benign natural course of ITP, careful consideration is necessary before instituting treatment that is hazardous or irreversible.

115. **In a toddler with suspected ITP, what is the significance of a palpable spleen on examination?**
Although patients with ITP may rarely have a palpable spleen tip, the presence of splenomegaly in a patient with thrombocytopenia warrants more aggressive evaluation for an associated problem (e.g., collagen vascular disease, hypersplenism).

116. **In patients with suspected ITP, should a bone marrow evaluation be done?**
This is a topic of much debate. A major concern is that, without a bone marrow aspiration, the diagnosis of leukemia may be delayed or the course of illness worsened by treatment (typically corticosteroids) that is begun for presumed ITP. However, it is rare that patients with leukemia present with symptoms of isolated thrombocytopenia. Local custom will likely prevail regarding the need for bone marrow examination in the setting of classic acute ITP, but generally it is not necessary for children with newly diagnosed ITP whose initial management involves either observation, intravenous immunoglobulin (IVIG), or anti-D. Heightened consideration should be given if the following are present: (1) other cell lines are involved; (2) history and physical examination have atypical features (e.g., weight loss, protracted fever, bone or joint pain, hepatosplenomegaly); and (3) steroid therapy is to be used.

Blanchette V, Bolton-Maggs P: Childhood immune thrombocytopenic purpura: diagnosis and management, *Pediatr Clin N Am* 55:393–420, 2008.

117. **When should medical treatment be given for acute ITP without active bleeding?**
Because the long-term prognosis of ITP does not appear to be influenced by medical treatment, the management of a newly diagnosed child with ITP and no serious bleeding remains controversial. The principal concern is susceptibility to intracranial bleeding, which occurs in less than 1% of affected patients (but can have a 30% to 50% mortality rate), almost always when the platelet count is less than 10,000/mm³. Local custom will prevail, but some authorities will treat medically when the platelet count is less than 10,000/mm³ and/or there is active mucous membrane hemorrhage; this minimizes the chance of intracranial catastrophe and avoids the excessive limitations of physical activity that might otherwise be imposed on a child with ITP.

118. **How do treatments for ITP compare?**
   - **IVIG:** 0.8 to 1.0 g/kg per day, raises the platelet count in about 85% of patients. The response usually occurs within 48 hours and persists for 3 to 4 weeks. Up to 75% of patients will have some degree of limited adverse reaction (e.g., nausea, vomiting, headaches, fever). IVIG is more expensive than steroids.
   - **Corticosteroids:** Corticosteroids are similarly effective, but oral steroids take about twice as long (4 days) to raise the platelet count significantly. The steroid effect may be multifactorial because signs of hemorrhage tend to decrease before the increase in platelets occurs. This may include microvascular endothelial stability. Side effects of long-term frequent steroid use are multiple.
   - **Anti-D immunoglobulin:** Anti-D immunoglobulin (immunoglobulin with antibody Rho [D]) should be given intravenously to individuals with adequate hemoglobin count, (Rh)D-positive RBCs, and intact splenic function. It is given more rapidly than IVIG, with a slightly smaller proportion of responders.
   - **Splenectomy**: When done laparoscopically, splenectomy successfully restores the platelet count to safe (>50 K/μL) or normal (>150 K/μL) levels in three fourths to four fifths of severe patients who fail drug therapy. Preoperative immunization against encapsulated bacteria is necessary to minimize the risk for postsplenectomy sepsis; many advocate oral antibiotic prophylaxis as well postoperatively.
   - **Anti-CD20 (rituximab)**: In refractory severe cases, antibody therapy directed at B-lymphocyte CD20 has achieved some partial and complete responses that are sustained.

119. **Is there a role for stimulating platelet production in ITP therapy?**
In chronic, severe, refractory ITP, use of agonists of the thrombopoietin receptor have shown efficacy in raising platelet counts to safe levels. The effect lasts only during the time period while the drug is being administered.

120. **Which children with ITP are candidates for splenectomy?**
Splenectomy improves the platelet count in up to 90% of patients. Because spontaneous remission is common in acute ITP, splenectomy is usually limited to bleeding that is life threatening and unresponsive to medical therapies. Patients with ITP lasting more than 1 year with continued bleeding, severe thrombocytopenia, or unacceptable restrictions may be reasonable candidates for splenectomy.

121. **What evaluations should be considered in a patient with persistent refractory thrombocytopenia?**
    - Antinuclear antibody, double-stranded DNA, C3, C4, p-ANCA, c-ANCA (to rule out systemic lupus erythematosus and other collagen vascular diseases)
    - Quantitative immunoglobulin levels, pneumococcal titers (to rule out common variable immune deficiency)
    - Evaluation for *Helicobacter pylori* (stool antigen test or urea breath test)
    - Bone marrow aspiration or biopsy (to evaluate for possible myelodysplastic syndrome or marrow failure)
    - Viral studies (including polymerase chain reaction for HIV, hepatitis C, Epstein-Barr virus, cytomegalovirus, parvovirus, and human herpesviruses 6 and 8)

    Kalpatthi R, Bussel JB: Diagnosis, pathophysiology and management of children with refractory immune thrombocytopenic purpura, *Curr Opin Pediatr* 20:8–16, 2008.

122. **What is the association between ITP and *Helicobacter pylori*?**
H. pylori, in addition to being a gastrointestinal troublemaker, has been implicated in autoimmune diseases including ITP. Noncontrolled studies have suggested a possible benefit for refractory ITP with increasing platelet counts on the eradication of *H. pylori*. One possible mechanism is the cross-reactivity between surface proteins of *H. pylori* and platelet-associated antigens.

    Bisogno G, Errigo G, Rossetti F, et al: The role of Helicobacter pylori in children with chronic idiopathic thrombocytopenic purpura, *J Pediatr Hematol Oncol* 30:53–57, 2008.

123. **What is neonatal alloimmune thrombocytopenia and how is it diagnosed and treated?**
When a fetus expresses platelet antigens inherited from the father that the mother lacks, some mothers, especially those with "permissive" HLA types, form IgG antibodies that cross the placenta and cause moderate to severe thrombocytopenia in the fetus. Infants of mothers with first pregnancies can be affected, and there is a high recurrence risk. Both mother and father should have the common platelet alloantigens typed for incompatibility, and the mother should be tested for IgG antiplatelet antibodies recognizing that difference. In second and subsequent pregnancies at risk, especially for intracranial hemorrhage, maternal IVIG has been demonstrated to be of benefit. Infants should receive washed maternal platelets, antigen-matched platelets, or in exceptionally dire circumstances, untyped platelets. Under investigation is whether prenatal platelet typing is of benefit in prevention of the substantial proportion of cases in first pregnancies.

    Bussel JB, Sola-Visner M: Current approaches to the evaluation and management of the fetus and neonate with immune thrombocytopenia, *Semin Perinatol* 33:35–42, 2009.

124. **In what conditions of children is thrombocytosis most commonly seen?**
- Acute infections (e.g., upper and lower respiratory tract infections)
- Chronic infections (e.g., tuberculosis)
- Iron deficiency anemia
- Hemolytic anemia
- Medications (e.g., vinca alkaloids, epinephrine, corticosteroids)
- Inflammatory disease (e.g., Kawasaki disease)
- Malignancy (e.g., chronic myelogenous or megakaryocytic leukemia)

Schafer AI: Thrombocytosis, *N Engl J Med* 350:1211–1219, 2004.

Yohannan MD, Higgy KE, al-Mashhadani SA, Santhosh-Kumar CR: Thrombocytosis: etiologic analysis of 663 patients, *Clin Pediatr* 33:340–343, 1994.

125. **What level of thrombocytosis requires treatment?**
A high platelet count in most children does not appear to be a cause of significant morbidity because it is often transient. In some centers, aspirin in doses of 81 mg daily are administered when the platelet count exceeds $1.5 \times 10^6/mm^3$. The early introduction of aspirin therapy may be more important if the patient has other problems that might contribute to hyperviscosity, such as a high white blood cell count or hemoglobin level.

Denton A, Davis P: Extreme thrombocytosis in admissions to paediatric intensive care: no requirement for treatment, *Arch Dis Child* 92:515–516, 2007.

SICKLE CELL DISEASE

126. **What is the mutation that results in sickle cell disease?**
On the β chain, valine is substituted for glutamic acid at position 6 on chromosome 11. Only a single nucleotide substitution ensues (GTG for GAG), but the result is sickle hemoglobin (HbS), which polymerizes on deoxygenation, makes the RBC more rigid, and causes structural damage to the RBC membrane. This change leads to hemolytic anemia and contributes to vaso-occlusion. The α chain is normal.

NHLBI Comprehensive Sickle Cell Center: http://www.sicklecell-info.org.

Sickle Cell Disease Association of America: http://www.sicklecelldisease.org.

127. **Why is sickle cell disease often asymptomatic during the first months of life?**
During the neonatal period, the presence of large amounts of fetal hemoglobin reduces the rate of polymerization of HbS and the sickling of RBCs that contain this abnormal hemoglobin. As the amount of fetal hemoglobin decreases after age 3 to 6 months, patients with sickle cell disease are increasingly likely to experience their first clinical manifestations.

128. **What are the various genotypes that can occur in sickle cell disease?**
Genotypes depend on which two genes make up the β chain component. In general, severity varies from with SS > Sβ^{0-} thalassemia > SC > Sβ^+ thalassemia > S-hereditary persistence of fetal hemoglobin (HPFH). Hemoglobin concentrations increase from an average of 6 to 8 g/dL with Hb-SS to 11 to 14 g/dL for Hb-HPFH, which contribute to the variation in clinical severity. Only Sβ^+-thalassemia has any hemoglobin A on electrophoresis (5% to 30%).

Driscoll MC: Sickle cell disease, *Pediatr Rev* 28:259–267, 2007.

129. **What are the two major pathophysiologic mechanisms in sickle cell anemia that cause the morbidities associated with the disease?**
- **Hemolysis:** Sickled RBCs undergo both intravascular and extravascular hemolysis, which leads to anemia, reticulocytosis, jaundice, gallstones, and occasional aplastic crisis.

It now appears that chronic hemolysis affects the use and bioavailability of nitric oxide, a potent vasoactive agent. Long-term hemolysis has been associated with pulmonary hypertension and right-sided heart failure.

- **Vaso-occlusion:** Intermittent and chronic vaso-occlusion result in both acute exacerbations (e.g., painful crisis, stroke) and chronic disease manifestations (e.g., retinopathy, renal disease). The adhesion of sickled erythrocytes to inflamed vascular endothelium is a principal pathologic component. Activation of leukocytes and platelets, as well as components of the coagulation protein cascade, is also prominent.

130. **A 6-month-old black male has painful swelling of both hands. What is the most likely diagnosis?**
Hand-foot syndrome, or **dactylitis**. This common early manifestation of sickling disorders in infants and young children is characterized by painful swelling of the hands, feet, and proximal fingers and toes caused by symmetrical infarction in the metacarpals, metatarsals, and phalanges (Fig. 9-5). A lack of systemic signs, the presence of symmetrical involvement, and young patient age help distinguish hand-foot syndrome from the much less common osteomyelitis, which may also complicate sickle cell disease.

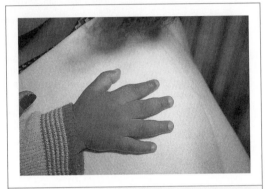

Figure 9-5. Swelling of the fingers from dactylitis. (From Lissauer T, Clayden G: Illustrated Textbook of Pediatrics. London, Mosby, 1997, p 238.)

131. **When does functional asplenia occur in children with sickle cell disease?**
It may begin as early as 5 or 6 months of age, and it may precede the presence of Howell-Jolly bodies in the peripheral smear. By 6 years of age, 90% have functional asplenia with a small, atrophied spleen. Clinical experience indicates that the period of increased risk for serious bacterial infection parallels the development of functional asplenia. Consequently, in addition to routine vaccinations, antibiotic prophylaxis with penicillin is recommended beginning at 2 months of age. Loss of splenic function usually occurs later in patients with HbSC or HbS β-thalassemia.

Claster S, Vichinsky EP: Managing sickle cell disease, *BMJ* 327:1151–1155, 2003.

132. **What are the three main categories of crises in patients with sickle cell disease?**
- **Aplastic crisis:** Hemoglobin may fall as much as 10% to 15% per day without reticulocytosis
- **Vaso-occlusive crisis:** Includes painful crises (most common), acute chest syndrome, acute central nervous system events (stroke), and priapism
- **Acute splenic sequestration:** May occur rapidly, with profound hypotension and cardiac decompensation

Dover GJ, Platt OS: Sickle cell disease. In Nathan DG, Orkin SH, Ginsburg D, Look AT (eds): *Nathan and Oski's Hematology of Infancy and Childhood*, ed 6, Philadelphia, 2003, WB Saunders, pp 802–811.

133. **What is the most common cause of death in children with sickle cell disease?**
Infection. Splenic dysfunction causes increased susceptibility to meningitis and sepsis (particularly pneumococcal).

134. **How should a child with a vaso-occlusive (painful) crisis be managed?**
For outpatients with an acute painful crisis, ibuprofen or acetaminophen and codeine are reasonable choices. Patients with intensely painful crises require day unit or inpatient hospitalization for opioid (including morphine and meperidine) analgesics, ideally given intravenously. Patient-controlled analgesia offers the dual benefit of a constant infusion and intermittent boluses of an analgesic. Other supplementary agents, including nonsteroidal analgesics (e.g., ketorolac), vasodilators and membrane active agents (e.g., cetiedil citrate), and high-dose methylprednisone, are under study. For severe crises, blood transfusions to reduce the percentage of sickle cells to less than 30% may be beneficial.

Jacob E, Miaskowski C, Savedra M, et al: Management of vaso-occlusive pain in children with sickle cell disease, *J Pediatr Hematol Oncol* 25:307–311, 2003.

Melzer-Lange MD, Walsh-Kelly CM, Lea G, et al: Patient-controlled analgesia for sickle cell pain crisis in a pediatric emergency department, *Pediatr Emerg Care* 20:2–4, 2004.

135. **How should children with sequestration crisis be managed?**
Acute sequestration crisis represents a true emergency in sickle cell disease and is the second leading cause of death in young children with sickle cell disease. The clinical problem is primarily one of hypovolemic shock as a result of the pooling of blood in the acutely enlarged spleen. The hemoglobin level may drop to as low as 1 to 2 g/dL. The major therapeutic effort should be directed toward volume replacement with whatever fluid is handy. In most instances, normal saline or colloid solutions will be adequate until properly cross-matched blood is available. Acute sequestration crisis is one of the few instances for patients with sickle cell disease in which transfusion with whole blood is appropriate because the problem is one of hypovolemia and anemia rather than anemia alone. If whole blood is not available, packed RBCs alone or packed RBCs plus plasma may be an alternative therapy.

136. **What is the "acute chest syndrome" in sickle cell patients?**
Acute chest syndrome refers to the constellation of findings (e.g., fever, cough, chest pain, pulmonary infiltrates) that can resemble pneumonia or pulmonary infarction. The exact mechanism is unknown, and the cause is likely multifactorial. Various infections (e.g., viral, chlamydial, mycoplasmal) may initiate respiratory inflammation, which ultimately causes localized hypoxia; increased pulmonary sickling may then result. Rib and other bone infarcts can also occur, and hypoventilation may result from chest splinting. Pulmonary fat embolism has been seen to occur, particularly in the setting of a preceding bony painful crisis (e.g., the thigh).

Gladwin MT, Vichinsky E: Pulmonary complications of sickle cell disease, *N Engl J Med* 359: 2254–2265, 2008.

137. **How should the acute chest syndrome in sickle cell patients be treated?**
- **Aggressively** because rapid progression to respiratory failure is possible
- **Optimization of ventilation** is vital, including supplemental oxygen, analgesics adequate to minimize splinting, incentive spirometry, and other possible measures (e.g., bronchodilators, nitrous oxide).
- **Judicious hydration:** Overly vigorous hydration can lead to pulmonary edema.
- **Antibiotics:** These should typically be given to cover *Chlamydia* species, *Mycoplasma* species, and *Streptococcus pneumoniae*.

■ **Blood transfusion,** including erythrocytapheresis (automated RBC exchange transfusion), has been shown to improve the status of patients with acute chest syndrome; this should be considered for patients with severe or worsening disease.

Graham LM: Sickle cell disease: pulmonary management options, *Pediatr Pulmonol* 26:S191–S193, 2004.

138. **How often is priapism a problem in children with sickle cell disease?**
Priapism is an unwanted, painful erection that is usually unrelated to sexual activity. It is an underappreciated morbidity in adolescents with sickle cell disease, usually occurring at least once by the age of 20 years and typically by the age of 12 years. Most patients are unaware of the term and the consequences; early intervention may prevent irreversible penile fibrosis and impotence.

Maples BL, Hagemann TM: Treatment of priapism in pediatric patients with sickle cell disease, *Am J Health Sys Pharm* 61:355–363, 2004.

KEY POINTS: SICKLE CELL DISEASE

1. A genetic mutation leads to an abnormal β-globin chain.

2. Eight percent of African Americans have the sickle cell trait.

3. Crises include vaso-occlusive, sequestration, and aplastic.

4. The risk for serious bacterial infection is increased among these patients as a result of functional asplenia.

5. Dactylitis (painful hand and foot swelling) is often the earliest manifestation.

139. **What are the approaches to the prevention of stroke in children with sickle cell disease?**
Children should undergo transcranial Doppler ultrasound measurements of intracranial arterial blood flow velocity. Confirmed abnormal values portend a risk for stroke that is minimized by regular RBC transfusion to keep the HbS percentage reduced (often <30% initially, later <50%).

Armstrong-Wells J, Grimes B, Sidney S, et al: Utilization of TCD screening for primary stroke prevention in children with sickle cell disease, *Neurology* 72:1316–1321, 2009.

Adams RJ: Big strokes in small persons, *Arch Neurol* 64:1567–1574, 2007.

140. **What are the long-term morbidities associated with sickle cell disease?**
■ Stroke
■ Pulmonary arterial hypertension
■ Chronic lung disease
■ Renal insufficiency
■ Congestive heart failure
■ Retinal damage
■ Leg ulcers
■ Osteonecrosis of femoral and/or humeral heads
■ Poor growth
■ Cholelithiasis

141. **What is the primary mechanism by which hydroxyurea is beneficial for sickle cell disease?**
Hydroxyurea is a cytotoxic drug that had been used primarily to treat chronic myelogenous leukemia and polycythemia vera. However, its use was shown to increase hemoglobin F (HbF) totals. Increased concentrations of HbF (particularly >20%) is associated with fewer vaso-occlusive painful events, transfusions, and hospitalizations. Long-term benefits are unclear.

Platt OS: Hydroxyurea for the treatment of sickle cell anemia, *N Engl J Med* 358:1362–1369, 2008.

Strouse JJ, Lanzkron S, Beach MC, et al: Hydroxyurea for sickle cell disease: a systematic review for efficacy and toxicity in children, *Pediatrics* 122:1332–1342, 2008.

142. **How common is the sickle cell trait in the United States?**
Heterozygosity for the sickle gene occurs in about 8% of blacks in the United States, 3% of Hispanics in the eastern United States, and a much smaller percentage of individuals of Italian, Greek, Arabic, and Veddah Indian heritage. Of note is that 2% of blacks in the United States have the hemoglobin C trait.

143. **Does sickle cell trait have any significant morbidity?**
Under normal physiologic conditions, no. RBCs in individuals with sickle cell trait contain only 30% to 40% sickle hemoglobin, which is insufficient to cause sickling. However, in hypoxic settings, sickling may occur. Portions of the kidney may have physiologically low oxygen concentrations that can interfere with function and lead to an inability to concentrate urine (hyposthenuria) and hematuria (usually microscopic and asymptomatic). At high altitudes (e.g., when mountain climbing or in an unpressurized aircraft), splenic infarction is possible.

144. **What is the second most common worldwide hemoglobin variant?**
Hemoglobin E. This variant is particularly high in the southeast Asian population (especially those of Laotian, Thai, and Cambodian heritage). Heterozygotes are asymptomatic; homozygotes can have a mild microcytic anemia. The most common abnormal findings on a peripheral smear are microcytosis and target cells.

THALASSEMIA

145. **What are the thalassemias?**
The thalassemias are a heterogeneous group of disorders of hereditary anemia due to diminished or absent normal globin chain production. Normally, four α-globin genes and two β-globin genes are expressed to make the tetrameric globin protein, which then combines with a heme moiety to make the predominant hemoglobin that is found in RBCs, HbA (subunits $\alpha_2 \beta_2$). Depending on the number of genes that are deleted, the production of polypeptide chains is diminished. In patients with α-thalassemia, α-globin production is lowered; in patients with β-thalassemia, β-globin production is lowered. When one class of polypeptide chains is diminished, this leads to a relative excess of the other chain. The result is ineffective erythropoiesis, precipitation of unstable hemoglobins, and hemolysis as a result of intramedullary RBC destruction.

Cooley's Anemia Foundation: http://www.thalassemia.org.

146. **Where was β-thalassemia first described?**
Despite its incidence being highest in the Mediterranean region, β-thalassemia was first described by a hematologist, Dr. Denton Cooley, in 1925 in Detroit. Why Detroit and not Europe for the first recognition? Speculation is that the condition was thought to be malaria, endemic to that region and with similar clinical features of hemolysis, anemia, and splenomegaly.

Weatherall DJ, Clegg JB: Historical perspectives: the many and diverse routes to our current understanding of the thalassemias. In Weatherall DJ, Clegg JB, editors: *The Thalassemia Syndromes*, ed 4, Oxford, 2001, Blackwell Science, p 3–62.

147. **What accounts for the variability in the clinical expression of the thalassemias?**
Clinical heterogeneity results from variability in the number of gene deletions (particularly in α-thalassemia). As a rule, the greater the number of deletions, the more severe the symptoms. A large number of point mutations have been identified in various populations; this can contribute to the phenotypic diversity. In addition, the inheritance of other thalassemia genes (e.g., δ-thalassemia) or the persistence of fetal hemoglobin can modify the clinical course.

148. **How is the diagnosis of thalassemia made in most clinical laboratories?**
Homozygous β-thalassemia is detected by the absence (β^0) or reduction (β^+) of the amount of HbA ($\alpha_2 \beta_2$) relative to HbF ($\alpha_2 \gamma_2$ or fetal hemoglobin) on hemoglobin electrophoresis. The carrier state for β-thalassemia is characterized by a low mean cell volume and, in most instances, an increased level of HbA_2 ($\alpha_2 \delta_2$) or HbF. The levels of these two hemoglobins are most accurately measured by column chromatography. Estimation or quantitation from electrophoretic patterns is frequently misleading.

The α-thalassemia trait remains a diagnosis of exclusion (low mean cell volume in the absence of an identifiable cause) in the clinical laboratory, although the enumeration of missing α genes for the most common deletions in specific ethnic populations is accomplished by molecular techniques. Newer polymerase chain reaction–based DNA tests for the common variants have become very useful.

149. **Describe the clinical features of the α-thalassemia syndromes.**
When all four α-globin genes are missing or nonfunctional, this results in severe intrauterine anemia and hydrops fetalis. Extraordinary therapy such as **in utero** transfusion may result in survival. Absence of three functional α-globin genes results in HbH disease, which is a chronic moderate to severe anemia with jaundice and splenomegaly that may necessitate RBC transfusion therapy. Absence of two α-globin genes is associated with mild microcytic anemia. Absence of one α-globin gene is clinically silent (Table 9-5).

TABLE 9-5.   CLINICAL FEATURES OF α-THALASSEMIA

Syndrome	Usual Genotype	α Gene Number	Clinical Features
Normal	αα/αα	4	Normal
Silent carrier	α-/αα	3	Normal
α-Thalassemia trait	α-/α-	2	Mild microcytic anemia
HbH disease	- -/αα	1	Moderate microcytic anemia Splenomegaly Jaundice

150. **What are the clinical features of the β-thalassemia syndromes?**
   ■ **Thalassemia minor:** Minimal or no anemia (hemoglobin 9 to 12 g/dL); microcytosis; elevated RBC count

- **Thalassemia intermedia:** Microcytic anemia with hemoglobin usually higher than 7 g/dL; growth failure; hepatosplenomegaly; hyperbilirubinemia; thalassemic facies (i.e., frontal bossing, mandibular malocclusion, prominent malar eminences due to extramedullary hematopoiesis) develop between the ages of 2 and 5 years
- **Thalassemia major** (Cooley anemia): Severe anemia (hemoglobin 1 to 6 g/dL) usually during the first year of life; hepatosplenomegaly; growth failure

Rund D, Rachmilewitz E: β-Thalassemia, *N Engl J Med* 353:1135–1146, 2005.

151. **How can coexistent iron deficiency increase the difficulty of diagnosing β-thalassemia?**
The β-thalassemia trait is usually diagnosed by hemoglobin electrophoresis, with quantitative hemoglobins revealing elevated HbA_2 and/or HbF levels. Iron deficiency can cause a lowering of HbA_2, thereby masking the diagnosis. With iron replacement, the hemoglobin A_2 will rise to the expected elevated levels seen in patients with the β-thalassemia trait.

KEY POINTS: THALASSEMIA

1. Normal hemoglobin (HbA): Tetramer of two α and two β chains

2. Associated with quantitative reduction in globin synthesis

3. Homozygous β-thalassemia is most severe form with pallor, jaundice, hepatosplenomegaly, growth retardation

4. Expansion of facial bones resulting from extramedullary hematopoiesis

5. Severity of α-thalassemia depends on number of genes deleted (1 to 4)

6. α-Thalassemia: More common among people of Southeast Asian ethnicity

7. β-Thalassemia: More common in people of Mediterranean ethnicity

152. **What are the adverse effects of chronic transfusional iron overload in children with thalassemia?**
- **Cardiac:** Congestive heart failure, dysrhythmias, and, less frequently, pericarditis
- **Endocrine:** Delays in growth and sexual development, hypoparathyroidism, hypothyroidism; diabetes as a result of iron overload is irreversible, even with intensive chelation
- **Hepatic:** Progressive liver fibrosis and cirrhosis

153. **What are the two most common diseases that are associated with transfusion-related iron overload?**
Thalassemia major and sickle cell disease.

154. **How do you reduce iron accumulation in children who require repeated transfusions?**
- **Chelation therapy:** Subcutaneous or intravenous deferoxamine has been the standard therapy for transfusional overload. Oral iron chelators are now available and in routine clinical use worldwide.
- **Splenectomy:** This is used primarily in patients with thalassemia (and a small subgroup of sickle cell patients) who have hypersplenism, which results in the premature destruction of RBCs and increased transfusion requirements.

- **Diet:** Drinking tea with meals reduces dietary iron absorption and may be most helpful in patients with diseases such as thalassemia intermedia, in which the bulk of excessive iron is dietary in origin.
- **Erythrocytapheresis:** Automated erythrocytapheresis rather than repeated simple transfusions may markedly reduce transfusional iron loading in patients with sickle cell disease.

Kwiatkowski JL: Oral iron chelators, *Pediatr Clin N Am* 55:461–482, 2008.

ACKNOWLEDGMENT

The editors gratefully acknowledge contributions by Dr. Anne F. Reilly that were retained from the third edition of *Pediatric Secrets*.

CHAPTER 10

IMMUNOLOGY

Georg A. Holländer, MD, and Anders Fasth, MD, PhD

CLINICAL ISSUES

1. **What are the immunoglobulin G (IgG) subclasses?**
   IgG can be classified according to structural, chemical, and biologic differences into four subclasses: IgG1, IgG2, IgG3, and IgG4. The relative contributions of each to total IgG are 70%, 20%, 7%, and 3%, respectively. In response to protein antigens, IgG1 and IgG3 subclasses predominate, whereas IgG2 and IgG4 are typically noted with polysaccharide antigens.

2. **What is an IgG subclass deficiency?**
   A disproportionately low level of one subclass with normal levels of total IgG. In the mid-1970s, reports began to appear describing children with recurrent infections (primarily sinopulmonary) who had selective subclass deficiencies. Most common was IgG2 deficiency, but multiple other combinations have since been described.

3. **Why is there controversy about the diagnostic significance of subclass deficiencies?**
   - IgG values have a very wide and age-dependent range.
   - Methodologic variability among laboratories is widespread.
   - Specific antibody responses may be more important than absolute subclass quantities.
   - Coexistent immunologic problems (e.g., IgA deficiency) may be present.
   - Subclass deficiencies can be the presenting abnormality in more serious immunologic disorders (e.g., ataxia-telangiectasia, common variable immunodeficiency, chronic mucocutaneous candidiasis, adenosine deaminase deficiency).
   - Some younger patients with subclass deficiencies have immunoglobulin levels that return to normal with maturation.

   Shackelford PG: IgG subclasses: importance in pediatric practice, *Pediatr Rev* 14:291–296, 1993.

4. **What are the immunologic risks for asplenic patients?**
   Overwhelming bacterial infections have been noted in children and adults with anatomic or functional asplenia. The incidence of mortality from septicemia is increased 50-fold in individuals after the traumatic loss of splenic function. The risk for bacteremia is higher in younger (versus older) children and may be greater during the first few years after splenectomy. *Streptococcus pneumoniae*, *Haemophilus influenzae* type B, and *Neisseria meningitidis* are the most frequent pathogens observed in asplenic children.

5. **What is the significance of a leukemoid reaction?**
   A *leukemoid reaction* usually refers to a white blood cell count of greater than 50,000/mm^3 and an accompanying shift to the left (i.e., the differential count shows an increase in immature cells). Causes include bacterial sepsis, tuberculosis, congenital syphilis, congenital or acquired toxoplasmosis, and erythroblastosis fetalis. Infants with Down syndrome may also have a leukemoid reaction that is often confused with acute leukemia during the first year of life.

6. **Name the three most common causes of eosinophilia in children in the United States.**
   Eosinophilia, which is usually defined as more than 10% eosinophils or an absolute eosinophil count of 1000/mm^3 or greater, is most commonly seen in three atopic conditions: **atopic dermatitis**, **allergic rhinitis**, and **asthma**.

7. **What conditions are associated with extreme elevations of eosinophils in children?**
   - Visceral larval migrans (toxocariasis)
   - Other parasitic disease (trichinosis, hookworm, ascariasis, strongyloidiasis)
   - Eosinophilic leukemia
   - Hodgkin disease
   - Drug hypersensitivity
   - Idiopathic hypereosinophilic syndrome

8. **What is the first immune disorder to involve a congenital defect in programmed cell death (apoptosis)?**
   Autoimmune lymphoproliferative syndrome (also known as *Canale-Smith syndrome*). Patients display a nonmalignant, noninfectious lymphoproliferation with splenomegaly, chronic lymphadenopathy, and, often, hepatomegaly. Lymphocytes persist that normally would die. Diagnosis rests on increases in α/β T-cell antigen receptor positive, CD4$^-$, CD8$^-$ (i.e., double-negative) T cells, and defective in vitro Fas-mediated lymphocyte apoptosis.

9. **What is the preferred vaccination strategy for recipients of solid organ transplants?**
   To induce early vaccine-specific immunologic memory, vaccinations are best delivered before transplantation and as early as possible in the course of the medical illness for which a solid organ transplantation (SOT) is needed. Live vaccines should not be given 1 month before SOT or while receiving immunosuppressive therapy. When necessary, an accelerated primary vaccine schedule can be attempted. Patients receiving SOT are usually immunosuppressed and hence compromised in their response to vaccine and other antigens. The immunologic response to routine vaccination (primary vaccines, booster injections) is best when patients have been without immunosuppression for at least 6 months. Vaccinations are commonly not recommended in the first 6 months after SOT because of a lack of a sufficient immune response and the risk for graft rejection or dysfunction.

   Campbell AL, Herold BC: Immunization of pediatric solid-organ transplantation, *Pediatr Transplant* 9:652–661, 2005.

10. **What are the most prominent effects of glucocorticoids on the immune system?**
    Glucocorticoids have **immunosuppressive, anti-inflammatory**, and **anti-allergic** effects. They inhibit leukocyte traffic and access to sites of inflammation, induce apoptosis of lymphocytes, and interfere with the effector functions of leukocytes, endothelial cells, and fibroblasts through suppression of mediators of inflammation. Specifically, glucocorticoids increase the number of circulating neutrophils but decrease: (1) monocyte-macrophages owing to a decrease in myelopoiesis and release from the bone marrow, (2) T cells owing to redistribution, and (3) basophils and eosinophils. The synthesis of proinflammatory cytokines and prostaglandins and the cell surface expression of major histocompatibility (MHC) class II molecules and Fc receptors is decreased in monocyte-macrophages exposed to glucocorticoids. In T cells, production and action are diminished. Endothelial cells decrease their vessel permeability and the expression of adhesion molecules. The production of inflammatory mediators (e.g., interleukin-1 [IL-1], prostaglandins) is reduced in response to glucocorticoids.

DEVELOPMENTAL PHYSIOLOGY

11. **How do immunoglobulin levels change during the first years of life?**
    - IgG levels in a full-term baby are equal or higher (5% to 10%) than maternal levels as a result of active placental transport. With an IgG half-life of 21 days, this transported maternal IgG reaches a nadir after 3 to 5 months. As the infant begins to make IgG, the level begins to rise slowly; it is 60% of adult level at 1 year of age, and it achieves the adult level by 6 to 10 years of age.
    - IgM concentrations are normally very low at birth, and 75% of normal adult concentrations are usually achieved by about 1 year of age.
    - IgA is the last immunoglobulin produced and approaches 20% of adult value by 1 year; however, full adult levels are not reached until adolescence. Because delays in the production of IgA are not unusual, the diagnosis of IgA deficiency is difficult to make with certainty in a child who is younger than 2 years.
    - IgD and IgE, both of which are present in low concentrations in the newborn, reach 10% to 40% of adult concentrations by 1 year of age.

12. **Which are the characteristics of immunoglobulin transport across the placenta?**
    IgG is the only isotype that is transferred across the placenta. All IgG subclasses cross the placenta, and their relative concentrations in the cord serum are comparable with those of the maternal serum. Transfer of IgG can first be detected as early as 8 weeks of gestation, and levels rise steadily between 18 and 22 weeks. By 30 weeks, the serum concentrations of IgG are about 50% of those observed in neonates born at term. IgG concentrations comparable with those of the mother are achieved by 34 weeks of gestation, and values at term can be higher by about 10% compared with maternal serum levels as a result of the active transport across the placenta.

13. **How does the complement system of the neonate compare with that of an adult?**
    The alternative and the classic complement pathway activity is moderately (50% lysis of target cells through the alternative pathway [AP_{50}]: 50% to 65% of adult values) to slightly (the quantity of dilution of serum required to lyase 50% of red blood cells in a standard hemolytic complement assay [CH_{50}]: 55% to 90% of adult values) diminished in the term neonate. In preterm neonates, these activities may be further decreased. Most notably, the serum concentrations for factors C8 and C9 are about 20% of those seen in adults.

14. **What determines immunoglobulin levels during infancy?**
    Immunoglobulin serum concentrations are determined by the amount of maternal IgG transported across the placenta, by catabolism of maternal IgG, and by the rate of synthesis of the infant's own IgM, IgG, and IgA. The development of specific antibodies is dependent on antigen exposure, antigen presentation, and the availability of T-cell help and T-cell maturation. Newborns readily produce antibodies against (vaccine) proteins, whereas polysaccharides fail to induce an adequate response during the first 2 years of life.

15. **Why are antibodies not produced by the fetus in appreciable quantities?**
    - The fetus is in a sterile environment and is not exposed to foreign antigens.
    - The active transport of maternal IgG across the placenta may suppress fetal antibody synthesis.
    - Fetal and neonatal monocyte-macrophages may not process foreign antigens normally.

16. **What is the role of the thymus?**
    The thymus is the primary lymphoid organ for the production and generation of T cells bearing the α/β T-cell antigen receptor. The thymus is responsible for the central selection of the T-cell repertoire, which allows for the establishment of tolerance toward self-antigens and responsiveness to nonself (i.e., foreign) antigens.

17. **At what age does thymic function cease?**
At birth, the thymus is at two thirds of its mature weight, and it reaches its peak mass at about 10 years of age. Subsequently, thymic size declines, but substantial function (as measured by the output of new T cells) persists into very late adulthood (70 to 80 years of age).

Douek DC, McFarland RD, Keiser PH, et al: Changes in thymic function with age and during the treatment of HIV infection, *Nature* 396:690–695, 1998.

18. **What are the advantages of breast milk for the immune systems of infants?**
Several studies have reported that human milk enhances the development of the immune system, especially with regard to measuring antibody formation. For example, antibody levels in response to immunization with conjugate *H. influenzae* type B vaccine are significantly higher in breastfed babies than in formula-fed babies; this suggests that breastfeeding enhances the active immune response during the first year of life.

Pabst HF, Spady DW: Effect of breast-feeding on antibody response to conjugate vaccine, *Lancet* 336:269–270, 1990.

19. **How does neutrophil function in the neonate compare with that of adults?**
There is a diminished neutrophil storage in the neonate, and the cells display a reduced adhesion and migration capacity in response to chemotactic stimuli. By contrast, the efficiency for the ingestion and killing of bacteria is normal for these cells. Under suboptimal conditions, however, these effector functions may be diminished, and neutrophils from sick and stressed neonates can display a decreased microbicidal activity.

NEUTROPENIA

20. **How is neutropenia defined?**
Neutropenia is arbitrarily defined as an absolute neutrophil count (ANC) of less than 1500/mm³. The ANC is determined by multiplying the percentage of bands and neutrophils by the total white blood cell count. An ANC of less than 500/mm³ is severe neutropenia. Agranulocytosis is defined as ANC of less than 100/mm³. As a rule, the lower the ANC, the greater the risk for infectious complications.

KEY POINTS: INFECTIONS IN IMMUNODEFICIENCIES

1. Increased frequency

2. Increased and prolonged severity

3. Unusual organisms (frequently opportunistic microorganisms)

4. Unexpected or severe complications of infection

5. Repeated infections without a symptom-free interval

21. **How do children with neutrophil disorders present?**
Neutrophil disorders include those that affect quantity (e.g., various neutropenias) and those that affect function (e.g., chemotaxis, phagocytosis, bactericidal activity). These defects should be considered part of the differential diagnosis in patients with delayed separation of the umbilical cord, recurrent infections with bacteria or fungi of low virulence (but minimal problems with recurrent viral or protozoal infections), poor wound healing, and specific locales of infection (e.g., recurrent furunculosis, perirectal abscesses, gingivitis).

22. **What is the most common cause of transient neutropenia in children?**
    Viral infections, including influenza, adenovirus, Coxsackie virus, respiratory syncytial virus, hepatitis A and B, measles, rubella, Epstein-Barr virus, cytomegalovirus, and varicella. The neutropenia usually develops during the first 2 days of illness and may persist for up to a week. Multiple factors likely contribute to the neutropenia, including a redistribution of neutrophils (increased margination rather than circulation), sequestration in reticuloendothelial tissue, increased use in injured tissues, and marrow suppression. In general, otherwise healthy children with transient neutropenia as a result of viral infections are at low risk for serious infectious complications.

23. **Excluding intrinsic defects in myeloid stem cells, what conditions are associated with neutropenia in children?**
    - **Infection:** Viral marrow suppression, bacterial sepsis-endotoxin suppression
    - **Bone marrow infiltration:** Leukemia, myelofibrosis
    - **Drugs**
    - **Immunologic factors:** Neonatal alloimmune (secondary to maternal IgG directed against fetal neutrophils) and autoimmune (e.g., autoimmune neutropenia of childhood, systemic lupus erythematosus, Evans syndrome)
    - **Metabolic factors:** Hyperglycinemia, isovaleric acidemia, propionic acidemia, methylmalonic acidemia, glycogen storage disease type IB
    - **Nutritional deficiencies:** Anorexia nervosa, marasmus, B_{12}/folate deficiency, copper deficiency
    - **Sequestration:** Hypersplenism

    Segel GB, Halterman S: Neutropenia in pediatric practice, *Pediatr Rev* 29:12–23, 2008.

24. **Which drugs are frequently associated with neutropenia?**
    Many drugs can cause neutropenia, and this is frequently the result of either a dose-dependent bone marrow suppression or a hapten-induced generation of antineutrophil antibodies. Neutropenia is also relatively frequently observed in patients treated with phenothiazine, sulfonamides, semisynthetic penicillins, nonsteroidal anti-inflammatory agents, and antithyroid medications. Within days after stopping the drug, immature neutrophils usually reappear in the peripheral blood.

25. **Which is the most common form of chronic childhood neutropenia?**
    Autoimmune neutropenia of infancy (ANI). This disorder displays a 3:2 female predominance and is caused by a chronic depletion of mature neutrophils. About 90% of all cases are detected within the first 14 months of life. The median duration of neutropenia is 20 months, and 95% of patients with this condition have fully recovered by the time they are 4 years old. The ANC of infants with ANI is usually below 500/mm^3, and the bone marrow displays normal cellularity despite an arrest at late stages of metamyelocytes or at the band stage. Antineutrophil antibodies are occasionally detected, but their presence is not necessary for the diagnosis of ANI.

26. **Which primary immune deficiencies that affect lymphocytes are typically associated with neutropenia?**
    - **X-linked agammaglobulinemia:** One third of patients will have neutropenia at some point during the course of their disease.
    - **Hyper-IgM syndrome:** This is typically associated with cyclic or persistent neutropenia.
    - Several **T-cell defects** as well as the rare **natural killer (NK)-cell deficiencies** can be associated with neutropenia.

27. **Which hematologic disorder is frequently observed in neonates delivered from mothers with severe pregnancy-induced hypertension?**
    About half of all neonates born to women with severe pregnancy-induced hypertension display **neutropenia**. Because the neutrophils are only transiently depressed, an increased risk for infection is not observed.

PRIMARY IMMUNODEFICIENCIES

28. **How common are primary immunodeficiencies?**
    - Primary immune deficiencies: 1:10,000 (excluding asymptomatic IgA deficiency)
    - B-cell defects: 65%
    - Combined cellular and antibody deficiencies: 15% (severe combined immunodeficiency: 1 in 100,000 newborns)
    - Phagocytic disorders: 10%
    - T-cell–restricted deficiencies: 5%
    - Complement component disorders: 5%

    In a survey study of 10,000 American households, the calculated prevalence of a diagnosed immunodeficiency was 1 in 2000 in children, 1 in 1200 in people of all ages, and 1 in 600 households.

    Boyle JM, Buckley RH: Population prevalence of diagnosed primary immunodeficiency diseases in the United States, *J Clin Immunol* 27:497–502, 2007.

    Immune deficiency foundation: http://www.primaryimmune.org.

    International Patient Organization for Primary Immunodeficiencies: http://www.ipopi.org.

    The Jeffrey Modell Foundation: http://www.jmfworld.org.

29. **What are the typical clinical findings of the various primary immunodeficiencies?**
    See Table 10-1.

30. **What are the typical features of transient hypogammaglobulinemia of infancy (THI)?**
    THI is characterized by diminished concentrations of one or more classes of immunoglobulin. This deficiency is most commonly understood as an age-related delay in the acquisition of the ability to produce normal immunoglobulin isotype concentrations, and it can be also understood as a rare physiologic event. The frequency of THI has been estimated to be lower than 1 in 1000, and it represents less than 5% of all of the diagnoses of primary immunodeficiencies. Typically, no consistent immunologic defects are observed among individuals with THI. None of the infections noted in these patients are usually life-threatening. In sharp contrast with patients with X-linked agammaglobulinemia, children with THI respond to immunizations with tetanus and diphtheria toxoids; they also have isohemagglutinin titers and a normal number of T and B cells.

31. **Why are male children more likely to suffer from a primary immunodeficiency?**
    Several primary immunodeficiency disorders are linked to the X-chromosome: agammaglobulinemia, hyper-IgM syndrome, severe combined immunodeficiency (the common cytokine receptor δ-chain deficiency), lymphoproliferative syndrome, Wiskott-Aldrich syndrome, one form of chronic granulomatous disease, and properidine deficiency. This fact accounts for the observation that the male-to-female ratio is 4:1 among patients with a primary immunodeficiency who are younger than 16 years.

32. **Which is the most common type of primary immunodeficiency?**
    Selective IgA deficiency is the most common primary immunodeficiency. The prevalence of selective IgA deficiency has been calculated to range from 1 in 220 to 1 in 3000, depending on the population studied. However, most IgA-deficient subjects remain healthy, which has been attributed to a compensatory increase of IgM in bodily secretions. A minority of these patients demonstrate normal levels of secretory IgA and normal numbers of IgA-bearing mucosal plasma cells. Although IgA represents less than 15% of total immunoglobulin, it is predominant on mucosal surfaces. Therefore, most patients with symptoms have recurrent diseases involving mucosal surfaces, including otitis media, sinopulmonary infections, and chronic diarrhea. Systemic infections are rare.

TABLE 10-1. CLINICAL FINDINGS OF PRIMARY IMMUNODEFICIENCIES

	Predominant B-Cell Deficiency	Predominant T-Cell Deficiency	Phagocytic Defects	Complement Defects
Age at onset	After maternal antibodies have disappeared (usually >6 mo)	Early infancy	Early infancy	Any age
Type of infection	Gram-positive or gram-negative (encapsulated) bacteria; *Mycoplasma*; *Giardia*; *Cryptosporidium*; *Campylobacter*; enteroviruses	Viruses, particularly CMV-1 and CBV; systemic BCG after vaccination; fungal; *Pneumocystis carinii*	Gram-positive or gram-negative bacteria; catalase-positive organisms in CGD, especially *Aspergillus*	*Streptococcus*; *Neisseria*
Clinical findings	Recurrent respiratory tract infections; diarrhea; malabsorption; ileitis; colitis; cholangitis; arthritis; dermatomyositis; meningoencephalitis	Poor growth and failure to thrive; oral candidiasis; skin rashes; sparse hair; opportunistic infections; graft-versus-host disease; bony abnormalities; hepatosplenomegaly	Poor wound healing; skin diseases (e.g., seborrheic dermatitis, impetigo, abscess); cellulitis without pus; suppurative adenitis; periodontitis; liver abscess; Crohn disease; osteomyelitis; bladder outlet obstruction	Rheumatoid disorders; angioedema; increased susceptibility to infection

BCG, bacille Calmette-Guérin; CBV, Coxsackie B virus; CGD, chronic granulomatous disease; CMV-1, cytomegalovirus type 1.

33. **What are the diagnostic criteria for IgA deficiency?**
Serum concentrations of IgA lower than 0.05 g/L are diagnostic and almost invariably associated with a concomitant lack of secretory IgA. Serum levels for IgM are normal, and concentrations for IgG (particularly IgG1 and IgG3) may be increased in one third of all IgA-deficient patients.

34. **What is the association of autoimmune disorders and IgA deficiency?**
Autoimmune disorders have been described in up to 40% of patients with selective IgA deficiency. These include systemic lupus erythematosus, rheumatoid arthritis, thyroiditis, celiac disease, pernicious anemia, Addison disease, idiopathic thrombocytopenic purpura, and autoimmune hemolytic anemia.

35. **What are the allergies associated with IgA deficiency?**
There is a strong association between IgA deficiency and allergic disorders. The most common diseases are allergic conjunctivitis, rhinitis, urticaria, atopic eczema, food allergies, and asthma.

   National Institute of Allergy and Immunology: http://www.niaid.nih.gov.

36. **Why is immunoglobulin therapy not used as a treatment for selective IgA deficiency?**
Unless a patient has a concurrent IgG subclass deficiency (even in this setting, therapy is controversial), γ-globulin therapy is not indicated and is in fact relatively contraindicated because of the following:
   - The short half-life of IgA makes frequent replacement therapy impractical.
   - γ-Globulin preparations have insufficient IgA quantities to restore mucosal surfaces.
   - Patients can develop anti-IgA antibodies with the potential for hypersensitivity complications, including anaphylaxis.

   http://www.jmfworld.org.

37. **In an infant with panhypogammaglobulinemia, how can the quantitation of B and T lymphocytes in peripheral blood help distinguish the diagnostic possibilities?**
   - Normal numbers of T lymphocytes, no detectable B lymphocytes: X-linked agammaglobulinemia (Bruton disease)
   - Normal numbers of T and B lymphocytes: Transient hypogammaglobulinemia of infancy, common variable immunodeficiency
   - Decreased numbers of T lymphocytes, normal or decreased numbers of B lymphocytes: Severe combined immunodeficiency
   - Decreased CD4 lymphocytes: Human immunodeficiency virus (HIV) infection

38. **What are the criteria for the diagnosis of X-linked (Bruton) agammaglobulinemia (XLA)?**
   - Onset of recurrent bacterial infections before 5 years of age
   - Serum immunoglobulin values for IgG, IgM, and IgA well below 2 standard deviations of the normal for age
   - Absent isohemagglutinins
   - Poor to absent response to vaccines
   - Less than 2% peripheral B cells (CD19)

39. **What are the typical clinical manifestations of XLA?**
Newborns with XLA have normal serum levels of IgG at birth and few—if any—symptoms. Typically, symptoms begin at the age of 4 to 12 months, although as many as 20% of

patients with XLA present with clinical symptoms as late as 3 to 5 years of age. Infections are the most common clinical manifestation and frequently occur as a result of encapsulated bacteria, *Staphylococcus aureus; Salmonella, Campylobacter,* and *Mycoplasma* species; and *Giardia lamblia.* Infections may be localized to the respiratory tract (e.g., otitis media, sinusitis, pneumonia), the skin (e.g., pyoderma), or the gastrointestinal tract (e.g., diarrhea), or they may spread hematogenously (e.g., sepsis, meningitis, septic arthritis).

KEY POINTS: WARNING SIGNS OF IMMUNODEFICIENCY ✔

1. Eight or more new ear infections within 1 year

2. Two or more serious sinus infections within 1 year

3. Two or more months on antibiotics with little effect

4. Two or more severe pneumonia infections within 1 year

5. Failure of an infant to gain weight and grow normally

6. Recurrent deep skin or organ abscesses

7. Persistent thrush in mouth or elsewhere on skin after 1 year of age

8. Need for intravenous antibiotics to clear infections

9. Two or more deep-seated infections such as meningitis, osteomyelitis, cellulitis, or sepsis

10. A family history of primary immunodeficiency

40. **How frequently is the mother *not* the carrier of the disease in XLA?**
    About one third of all XLA cases are thought to be caused by new mutations.

41. **Which are the typical immunologic laboratory findings in patients with the complete form of XLA?**
    Low to absent concentrations of all immunoglobulin isotypes; absent or low B cells; lack of germinal centers in lymph nodes; absence of tonsils; a complete or almost complete block at the developmental pre–B-cell stage; normal T-cell and NK-cell numbers and functions.

42. **What are the typical laboratory findings of common variable immunodeficiency (CVID)?**
    Laboratory evaluations in patients with CVID typically demonstrate low IgG levels and low to absent IgA and IgM serum concentrations. Similarly, specific antibodies to previously encountered pathogens and to vaccines and isohemagglutinins are low to absent. A large proportion of patients with CVID exhibit a depressed switch from IgM to IgG. Although lymphocyte subsets are normal in most patients with CVID, standard T-cell function tests (e.g., *in vitro* proliferation in response to mitogens, nominal antigens, and allogeneic cells) are subnormal in about half of all patients.

43. **What are the clinical features of CVID?**
    Although symptoms can occur at any time of life, the first peak is ages 5 to 10 years and later as a young adult between 20 and 30 years. The most frequent clinical presentation involves recurrent bacterial infections of the sinopulmonary system caused by encapsulated bacteria. Other manifestations include involvement of the gastrointestinal tract (e.g., infections with *G. lamblia* and *Campylobacter jejuni,* chronic malabsorption, nodular lymphoid

hyperplasia, gastric atrophy with achlorhydria); and autoimmune disorders (e.g., rheumatoid arthritis, autoimmune hemolytic anemia, pernicious anemia, neutropenia, thrombocytopenia, chronic active hepatitis, vitiligo, parotitis).

Glocker E, Ehl S, Grimbacher B: Common variable immunodeficiency in children, *Curr Opin Pediatr* 19:685–692, 2007.

44. **Which is the treatment of choice for CVID?**
The treatment of CVID may include lifelong periodic intravenous (or subcutaneous) immunoglobulin replacement, immunosuppressive therapy, antibiotics, and physiotherapy for chest disease. The effect of a higher dose of immunoglobulin to maintain trough levels of IgG at low-normal levels may be beneficial with regard to a decrease in the incidence of infections and the frequency of hospitalization. If SCID is attributable to the lack of adenosine deaminase, gene therapy may be a safe and effective treatment.

45. **What is the underlying disorder in an 8-year-old girl with atypical eczema, pneumatoceles, and bouts of severe furunculosis?**
Hyper-IgE syndrome is the most likely diagnosis. This disease is clinically characterized by the following:
- Recurrent infections (almost invariably caused by *S. aureus*) of the skin, lungs (causing frequently persistent pneumatoceles), ears, sinuses, eyes, joints, and viscera
- Atypical eczema with lichenified skin
- Coarse facial features, especially the nose
- Osteopenia of unknown cause
- Delayed tooth exfoliation (i.e., prolonged retention of primary teeth)

The laboratory evaluation of the hyper-IgE syndrome reveals massively elevated IgE levels associated with IgG subclass and specific antibody deficiencies; variable dysfunctions of neutrophils; and an imbalance of cytokine production as a result of a T_H2 predominance (IL-4, IL-5).

Grimbacher B, Holland SM, Gallin JI, et al: Hyper-IgE syndrome with recurrent infections—an autosomal dominant multisystem disorder, *N Engl J Med* 340:697–702, 1999.

46. **What is the molecular cause of the autosomal dominant form of the hyper-IgE syndrome?**
Lymphocytes in patients with hyper-IgE syndrome have a diminished response to the cytokine IL-6. In an analysis of the intracellular signaling molecules involved in the response to IL-6, missense mutations, and single-codon in-frame deletions in the gene that encodes the signal transducer and activator of transcription 3 (STAT3) were found to be the predominant (and at present only defined) molecular cause of the hyper-IgE syndrome.

Holland SM, DeLeo FR, Elloumi HZ, et al: STAT3 mutations in the hyper-IgE syndrome, *N Engl J Med* 357:1608–1619, 2007.

47. **Which is the medical treatment of choice for the hyper-IgE syndrome?**
Continuous antimicrobial therapy is usually necessary to control the deep-seated infections. No specific immunotherapeutic regimen has been successful; in particular, intravenous substitution of immunoglobulins and interferon are of no proven benefit for patients with this disorder.

48. **What are the proven indications for intravenous immunoglobulin therapy?**
The first five listed below have U.S. Food and Drug Administration approval, but a growing list of other conditions appear to have clinical benefit from immunoglobulin therapy:
- Humoral and combined primary immune deficiencies with low to absent levels of IgM and/ or IgG (XLA, CVID, hyper-IgM syndrome, severe combined immune deficiency [SCID], Wiskott-Aldrich syndrome, ataxia telangiectasia, antibody deficiencies with normal serum

immunoglobulins, selected cases of symptomatic IgG subclass deficiencies despite antibiotic treatment)
- Kawasaki disease
- B-cell chronic lymphocytic leukemia
- HIV
- Idiopathic thrombocytopenic purpura
- Guillain-Barré syndrome (acute inflammatory demyelinating polyradiculopathy)
- Chronic inflammatory demyelinating polyradiculoneuropathy
- Graves ophthalmopathy
- Cytomegalovirus-induced pneumonia in solid organ transplant recipients
- Toxic epidermal necrolysis

Orange JS, Hossny EM, Weiler CR, et al: Use of intravenous immunoglobulin in human disease, *J Allergy Clin Immunol* 117:S525–S553, 2006.

49. **What are the pharmacologic characteristics of intravenous immunoglobulin (IVIG)?**
After the infusion, 100% of the IgG stays in the intravascular compartment. Over the course of the next 3 to 4 days, IgG equilibrates with the extra cellular space, with 85% of the infused IgG still situated in the circulation. By the end of the first week, half of the IgG given has left the circulation, and by 4 weeks after the infusion, the serum levels have returned to baseline. However, these data apply to healthy individuals with a regular catabolism, and they have to be adjusted for both patients with a higher metabolic rate and for individuals transfused with increased IgG concentrations.

50. **What are the adverse reactions to IVIG?**
The common, infusion rate-related adverse events are chills, headache, fatigue and malaise, nausea and vomiting, myalgia, arthralgia, and back pain. Less frequent are abdominal and chest pains, tachycardia, dyspnea, and changes in blood pressure. Serious but rare side effects include aseptic meningitis, thrombosis, disseminated intravascular coagulation, renal and pulmonary insufficiency, and anaphylaxis in complete IgA-deficient individuals due to IgE antibodies specific for IgA. Subcutaneous therapy can reduce the occurrence of systemic adverse events in selected patients.

Orange JS, Hossny EM, Weiler CR, et al: Use of intravenous immunoglobulin in human disease, *J Allergy Clin Immunol* 117:S525–S553, 2006.

51. **Which viral infections can result in hypogammaglobulinemia in the immunocompetent individual?**
Epstein-Barr virus, HIV, and congenital rubella. Single cases of hypogammaglobulinemia have also been described among children infected with cytomegalovirus and parvovirus B19.

52. **What is the classic triad of Wiskott-Aldrich syndrome?**
Thrombocytopenia with small platelets volume, eczema, and immunodeficiency. This syndrome is an X-linked disorder, and the initial manifestations are often present at birth and consist of petechiae, bruises, and bloody diarrhea as a result of thrombocytopenia. The eczema is similar in presentation to classical atopic eczema (antecubital and popliteal fossa). Infections are common and include (in decreasing frequency): otitis media, pneumonia, sinusitis, sepsis, and meningitis. The severity of immunodeficiency may vary but usually affects both T- and B-cell functions. It is important to note that this immunodeficiency is progressive and associated with a high risk for developing cancer; a teenager with this condition has a 10% to 20% statistical risk for developing a lymphoid neoplasm. Only about one third of patients with Wiskott-Aldrich syndrome present with the classic triad.

Puck J, Candotti F: Lessons from the Wiskott-Aldrich syndrome, *N Engl J Med* 355:1759–1761, 2006.

53. **What is the likely diagnosis of a patient presenting with a progressive ataxia and recurrent bacterial sinopulmonary infections?**
Ataxia-telangiectasia. In patients with ataxia-telangiectasia, primarily progressive cerebella ataxia develops during infancy and is typically associated with other neurologic symptoms (e.g., the loss or decrease of deep tendon reflexes, choreoathetosis, apraxia of eye movements). The signs of telangiectasia occur usually after the onset of ataxia, generally between 2 and 8 years of age. The telangiectasias are primarily at the bulbar conjunctivae. Recurrent infections (as a consequence of a humoral and cellular immunodeficiency) are observed in 80% of patients with ataxia-telangiectasia and are typically localized to the middle ear and the upper airways.

KEY POINTS: SUSPECT IMMUNODEFICIENCY IN INFANTS WITH THESE CONDITIONS

1. Failure to thrive

2. Persistent cough

3. Persistent candidiasis

4. Absolute lymphocyte count $<2000/mm^3$

54. **Which laboratory tests support the diagnosis of ataxia-telangiectasia?**
Although the diagnosis of ataxia-telangiectasia chiefly relies on the clinical presentation, several laboratory findings support the diagnosis. The peripheral blood count usually reveals lymphopenia and eosinophilia. There is often a reduction of IgA (70% of all cases), IgG2/IgG4, and IgE; a poor antipolysaccharide response; and an increased frequency of autoantibodies, including antibodies to IgA and IgG. T-cell immunity is abnormal in about 60% of patients.

55. **What is the single most important laboratory test if SCID is suspected?**
A full blood count to document **lymphopenia** ($2000/mm^3$) is the single most important laboratory test during the initial evaluation of a patient for suspected SCID. However, a minority of patients with SCID (about 20%) may have a normal absolute lymphocyte count.

56. **What are the most common forms of SCID?**
   - X-linked form: 50%
   - Janus-associated kinase 3 deficiency: 10%
   - IL-7 receptor deficiency: 10%
   - Adenosine deaminase deficiency: 8%

57. **What are the typical clinical features of SCID?**
   - Recurrent bacterial infections (typically pneumonia, otitis media, and sepsis)
   - Persistent viral infections (respiratory syncytial virus, enterovirus, parainfluenza, cytomegalovirus)
   - Opportunistic infections (*Pneumocystis carinii, Pneumocystis jiroveci* fungi)
   - Failure to thrive
   - Diarrhea (enterovirus, rotavirus)
   - May include skin rash (due to maternal-fetal engraftment with graft-versus-host disease)

   http://www.scid.net.

58. **What disease did the "bubble boy" have?**
Adenosine deaminase (ADA) deficiency. In this form of SCID, the lack of ADA results in abnormalities of B- and T-cell function and increased susceptibility to infection. The bubble served as a means of minimizing contagion but also promoted social isolation. Although bone marrow transplantation has been curative as a treatment of this condition, ADA deficiency is the first disease to be treated by gene therapy (i.e., insertion of functional ADA genes into the patient's autologous cells and followed by infusion).

Aiuti A, Cattaneo F, Galimberti S, et al: Gene therapy for immunodeficiency due to adenosine deaminase deficiency, *N Engl J Med* 360:447–458, 2009.

59. **What are the clinical phenotypes of adenosine deaminase deficiency?**
- **Neonatal or infantile onset** (80% to 90%): Clinically and immunologically virtually indistinguishable from all forms of classic SCID; lymphopenia with absent humoral and cellular immune functions; failure to thrive; severe infections with fungal, viral, and opportunistic pathogens. Half of these patients have skeletal abnormalities at the costochondral junction (flared ribs).
- **Delayed onset** (15% to 20%): Recurrent infections, particularly sinopulmonary infections and septicemia, with a frequent failure to generate specific antibodies. Increased IgE levels, IgG subclass deficiencies, and autoimmunity (hypoparathyroidism, type 1 diabetes, hemolytic anemia, and idiopathic thrombocytopenia) provide evidence of immune dysregulation.

Shovlin CL, Simmonds HA, Fairbanks LD, et al: Adult onset immunodeficiency caused by inherited adenosine deaminase deficiency, *J Immunol* 153:2331–2339, 1994.

60. **Describe the molecular defect of chronic granulomatous disease (CGD).**
CGD is characterized by a profound defect in the oxygen metabolic burst in myeloid cells following the phagocytosis of microbes. The molecular mechanisms responsible for this disease are heterogenous because any defect of the four subunits that constitute the nicotinamide adenine dinucleotide phosphate hydrogen-oxidase can cause CGD. As a consequence, superoxide, oxygen radicals, and peroxide production are lacking, and patients with CGD cannot kill catalase-positive pathogenic bacteria and fungi (e.g., *S. aureus; Nocardia, Serratia,* and *Aspergillus* species).

61. **Which laboratory tests are used for the diagnosis of CGD?**
Patients suspected to have CGD can be diagnosed as a result of their failure to generate reactive oxygen species during the respiratory burst or, alternatively, as a result of their inability to kill catalase-positive bacteria (*S. aureus, Escherichia coli*) in vitro with their phagocytes. The screening tests for the production of superoxide are the slide nitroblue tetrazolium reduction test and the flow cytometric 2′,7′-dichlorofluorescein test.

62. **What types of infections are commonly seen in children with CGD?**
Superficial staphylococcal skin infections, particularly around the nose, eyes, and anus, are common. Severe adenitis, recurrent pneumonia, indolent osteomyelitis, and chronic diarrhea are frequent. A male child with a liver abscess should be considered to have chronic granulomatous disease until it is proved otherwise.

63. **What are the cornerstones of CGD treatment?**
- Prevention of infections through immunization and prophylactic antibiotic and anti-*Aspergillus* treatment; avoidance of certain sources of pathogens
- Use of prophylactic recombinant human interferon-γ (the use is questioned by some clinicians)
- Early and aggressive use of parenteral antibiotics
- Surgical treatment of recalcitrant infections

Marciano BE, Wesley R, De Carlo ES, et al: Long-term interferon-gamma therapy for patients with chronic granulomatous disease, *Clin Infect Dis* 39:692–699, 2004.

64. **Which disorder has to be considered in a newborn patient with delayed separation of the umbilical cord?**
Patients with **leukocyte adhesion deficiency type 1** (LAD1) suffer from a profound impairment of leukocyte mobilization into extravascular sites. The hallmark of this disorder is the complete absence of neutrophils at the site of infection and inflammation (e.g., wound healing).

65. **What are the typical features of patients with LAD1?**
LAD1 is clinically divided into a severe and a moderate phenotype. Characteristic pathologic findings in LAD1-patients are *persistent neutrophil leukocytosis*, the *lack of neutrophils at sites of infection* (resulting in necrotic areas without pus), the *severe depletion of lymphocytes* in lymphoid tissues, and the impaired healing of traumatic or surgical wounds.
- **Severe disease** (residual CD18 cell surface expression on leukocytes, <0.5% of normal): delayed separation of the umbilical cord (which occurs normally on average by 10 days of life, range 3 to 45 days), omphalitis, and persistent leukocytosis in the newborn period. In children after infancy, features include severe sinusitis, destructive periodontitis, and recurrent infections, mostly with *S. aureus* and gram-negative enteric bacteria, but commonly also with fungi. Children with the severe form of LAD1 usually die from infections before 2 years of age.
- **Moderate disease** (>1% of normal CD18 expression): normal timing of the umbilical cord separation, usually live beyond childhood, and their infections are fewer and less severe.

66. **An infant with hypocalcemic tetany, a loud cardiac murmur, and dysmorphic facies probably has what syndrome?**
DiGeorge or **22q11.2 deletion syndrome**. The clinical pattern results from microdeletions of the long arm of chromosome 22q11 with maldevelopment of the third and fourth pharyngeal pouches during embryogenesis. This results in a spectrum of malformations and clinical findings, including the following:
- Cardiac defects: Aortic arch and conotruncal anomalies, especially truncus arteriosus
- Parathyroid absence or hypoplasia with abnormal calcium homeostasis
- Abnormal facies, including round and broad low-set ears with folded helix, short philtrum, hypertelorism, notched ear pinna, hooped eyelids, malar flatness, micrognathia, and down-slanting palpebral fissures
- Mild mental retardation (intelligence quotient of about 70)
- Language and speech problems
- Behavior disorder
- Thymic hypoplasia: Degree of thymic maldevelopment is variable and usually results in diminished numbers of T cells; clinically significant immunologic abnormalities often absent

67. **Which diagnosis needs to be considered in a 3-month-old infant with type 1 diabetes, severe diarrhea, and eczema?**
IPEX (**i**mmunodysregulation, **p**olyendocrinopathy, **e**nteropathy, **X**-linked). IPEX is caused by a deficiency in the fork-head DNA-binding protein FOXP3, which is required for regulatory T cells to maintain peripheral immunological tolerance. Most patients have eosinophilia and increased IgE and IgA serum concentrations but usually a normal T and B cellularity. Severe diarrhea and failure to thrive secondary to severe enteropathy are frequently the earliest presenting symptoms with other autoimmune features occurring including type 1 diabetes mellitus, hypothyroidism, and hemolytic anemia.

68. **Which primary immune deficiencies are defined by the occurrence of autoimmunity?**
- **Autoimmune polyglandular syndrome-1 (APS-1):** Also known as the APECED syndrome (**a**utoimmune **p**oly**e**ndocrinopathy, **c**andidiasis, **e**ctodermal **d**ysplasia). Autosomal recessive disorder characterized by chronic mucocutaneous candidiasis (≤5 years of age), hypoparathyroidism (<10 years of age), and Addison disease (<15 years of age).

- **Autoimmune lymphoproliferative syndrome (ALPS):** Autoimmune manifestations occur in up to 70% of patients and typically include autoimmune hemolytic anemia, idiopathic thrombocytopenia, and autoimmune neutropenia. ALPS is caused by different gene defects that result in a failure to undergo programmed cell death (apoptosis).
- **IPEX**

69. **Which two primary immunodeficiencies are mitochondriopathies?**
Even though mitochondria are primarily perceived as energy producers alone, they also host one of the major pathways of apoptosis. Two nuclear genes code for proteins of the intermembrane space of the mitochondria that when mutated produce immunodeficiency due to defective apoptosis.

- **Reticular dysgenesis:** A rare autosomal recessive form of SCID associated with severe neutropenia and sensorineural deafness is caused by mutation in the adenylate kinase 2 (*AK2*) gene
- **Kostmann disease:** A severe congenital neutropenia caused by mutations in *HAX1*, a gene product required for the prevention of apoptosis in myeloid, lymphoid, and neuronal cells

Lagresle-Peyrou C, Six EM, Picard C, et al: Human adenylate kinase 2 deficiency causes a profound haematopoietic defect associated with sensorineural deafness, *Nat Genet* 41:106 –111, 2009.

Klein C, Grudzien M, Appaswamy G, et al: HAX1 deficiency causes autosomal recessive severe congenital neutropenia (Kostmann disease), *Nat Genet* 39:86–92, 2009.

70. **What are the two main phenotypes associated with complement component deficiencies?**
Generally, deficiencies of the *early* complement components (C1, C2, C3, and C4; factor I and factor H) are associated with autoimmune diseases (glomerulonephritis, systemic lupus erythematosus, dermatomyositis, scleroderma, and vasculitis) or with a predisposition to infections with encapsulated organisms. Deficiencies of the *terminal* components (C5, C6, C7, C8, and possibly C9) are associated with recurrent neisserial diseases.

71. **Which are the genetic complement deficiencies?**
Genetic deficiencies have been described for all complement components (including the regulatory inhibitors). C4 and C2 deficiencies are the most frequent. Complement deficiencies are common in countries in Southern Africa, the Northern African Coast, and the Eastern Mediterranean.

72. **Which potential life-threatening disorder of the complement system is associated with nonpruritic swelling and occasional recurrent abdominal pain?**
Hereditary C1 inhibitor deficiency. Angioedema of any part of the body—including the airway and the intestine—can occur as a consequence of failure to inactivate the complement and kinin systems. The condition has also been called hereditary angioneurotic edema. Infections, oral contraceptives, pregnancy, minor trauma, stress, and other variables have been noted to precipitate this autosomal dominant disease. Diagnosis is confirmed by direct assay of the inhibitor level. Clinical presentations include the following:

- **Recurrent facial and extremity swelling:** Acute, circumscribed edema that is not painful, red, or pruritic, thereby clearly distinguished from urticaria; usually self-resolves in 72 hours
- **Abdominal pain:** Recurrent and often severe, colicky pain as a result of interstitial wall edema with vomiting and/or diarrhea; may be misdiagnosed as an acute abdomen
- **Hoarseness, stridor:** A true emergency because death by asphyxiation may occur as a result of laryngeal edema; epinephrine, hydrocortisone, and antihistamines are often of only limited benefit; and tracheostomy is needed if there is progression of symptoms

Zuraw BL: Hereditary angioedema, *N Engl J Med* 359:1027–1036, 2008.

LABORATORY ISSUES

73. **Which are the initial screening tests for a suspected immunodeficiency?**
The basic screening tests should include **complete blood count** (including hemoglobin, morphology, and absolute cellularity); **quantification of immunoglobulin levels** (IgM, IgG, IgE, and IgA); **antibody responses to previous antigen exposures** (e.g., vaccines, pathogen-defined infections); **determination of isohemagglutinin titers**; assessment of the classic complement pathway by determining the **CH_{50}**; and **workup of infections**, including determination of C-reactive protein, blood cultures, and appropriate radiography. The choice of the laboratory tests is generally dependent on the clinical findings and the immunodeficiency suspected, and the results have to be compared with age-matched controls. It is important to note that there is no justification for a blanket screening; tests should only be ordered if their results will affect either the diagnosis or management of the patient.

74. **Which laboratory tests allow for a broad evaluation of the humoral immune system?**
Serum immunoglobulin levels, quantitative: IgM, IgG, IgA, and IgE. A combined IgG, IgA, and IgM level of less than 400 mg/dL suggests immunoglobulin deficiency; more than 5000 IU/mL for IgE suggests hyper-IgE syndrome.

IgG subclasses: These immunoglobulins should generally be measured primarily in patients more than 6 years old, in certain circumstances (e.g., in patients with selective IgA deficiency and normal to low IgG concentrations but demonstrated functional antibody deficiency), and in patients with recurrent sinopulmonary infections.
- Specific antibody titers: In response to documented infections and vaccinations
- Isohemagglutinin titer (anti-A, anti-B): 1:4 or less after the age of 1 year suggests specific IgM deficiency
- Tetanus, diphtheria (IgG1)
- Pneumococcal polysaccharide antigens (IgG2)
- Viral respiratory agents (IgG3)

Determination of B-cell numbers: In the peripheral blood with the use of flow cytometry (CD19, CD20)

B-cell proliferation and immunoglobulin production: With the use of in vitro assays

75. **Which diagnostic tests allow for the specific evaluation of T-cell functions?**
- **Total lymphocyte count:** Although most T-cell immunodeficiencies are not associated with a decreased lymphocyte count, a total count of less than 1500/mm^3 suggests a deficiency.
- **T-cell subpopulations:** Total T cells with less than 60% mononuclear cells, helper (CD4) cells less than 200/μL, or CD4/CD8 less than 1.0 suggest T-cell deficiency.
- **Delayed-type hypersensitivity skin testing**
- **Proliferative responses** to mitogens, antigens, and allogeneic cells
- **Acquisition of activation markers** on T cells (using flow cytometry)
- **Cytotoxic assay**
- **Cytokine synthesis**
- **Adenosine deaminase** and **purine nucleoside phosphorylase** determination in red blood cells
- **Molecular biologic studies** (including karyotyping and fluorescent in situ hybridizations)
- **Histology** of thymic and lymph-node biopsies

76. **What is the value of skin testing for the diagnosis of T-cell deficiencies?**
Skin tests for the assessment of delayed-type hypersensitivity are difficult to evaluate. A positive test is useful for eliminating the diagnosis of severe T-cell deficiency, whereas a negative test may reflect a T-cell defect, or it may result from the lack of an anamnestic response to the antigens used. Seventy-five percent of normal children between the ages of 12 and 36 months will respond to *Candida* skin testing at 1:10 dilution, and, by 18 months,

about 90% of normal children will respond to one of a panel of recall antigens (tetanus toxoid, trichophyton, and *Candida*); the younger the child, the less likely the reactivity. The cell-mediated reaction may be obscured by a humoral (Arthus) reaction as a result of previous priming.

77. **What is the importance of the CD4/CD8 ratio?**
The CD4/CD8 ratio is an index of helper to suppressor and cytotoxic cells and may be significantly altered in patients with a variety of immunodeficiencies. In normal individuals, the ratio ranges from 1.4:1.0 to 1.8:1.0. In patients with viral infections (particularly HIV), the ratio can be reduced; in patients with bacterial infections, it can be increased.

78. **Which laboratory tests appropriately evaluate the phagocytic system?**
Absolute granulocyte count
Antineutrophil antibodies (however, antineutrophil antibodies are found in only one half of the cases of autoimmune neutropenia of infancy)
Bone marrow biopsy (to differentiate increased consumption from decreased production)
Specific *in vitro* and *in vivo* assays:
- *Determination of chemotaxis*: in vivo (skin wounds) or in vitro (Boyden chambers): Measurements are not routinely used for diagnostic purposes
- *Quantification of neutrophil adherence*: Measurement of cell surface expression of leukocyte function antigen-1 (CD11/CD18) by flow cytometry; adherence to inert surfaces such as nylon, wool, or plastic
- *Determination of the respiratory burst*: (1) Nitroblue tetrazolium test (NBT) measures the ability of phagocytic cells to ingest and reduce a yellow dye to an intercellular blue crystal; (2) Dihydrorhodamine (DHR)—in activated granulocytes reactive oxygen intermediates reduce DHR 123 to rhodamine 123, which results in an increase in fluorescence that can be quantified by flow cytometry
- *Enzyme assays* (myeloperoxidase, glucose-6-phosphate dehydrogenase, glutathione peroxidase, NADPH-oxidase)
- *Test treatment with rHu granulocyte colony-stimulating factor*. Autoimmune forms of neutropenia in small children respond to minor doses (1 mcg/kg) within a couple of days, whereas congenital forms require larger doses with responses after 2 to 3 weeks of treatment
- *Mutational analysis*

79. **How is the classic complement cascade evaluated?**
The primary screening test is the CH_{50}. This test assesses the ability of an individual's serum (in varying dilutions) to lyse sheep red blood cells after those cells are sensitized with rabbit IgM antisheep antibody. The CH_{50} is an arbitrary unit that indicates the quantity of complement necessary for 50% lysis of the red blood cells in a standardized setting. Test results are usually expressed as a derived reciprocal of the test dilution needed for 50% lysis. The test is relatively insensitive because major reductions in individual complement components are necessary before the CH_{50} is altered. Therefore, determination **C3** and **C4 levels** are often included in the initial screening of a child with a suspected complement deficiency.

CHAPTER 11

INFECTIOUS DISEASES

Mark F. Ditmar, MD

ANTI-INFECTIVE THERAPY

1. **What are the differences among classes of penicillins?**
   - **Penicillins** (penicillins G [intravenous] and V [oral]): Penicillin G is the drug of choice for *Treponema pallidum* infection (syphilis) and is useful for the treatment of certain other infections (e.g., group A streptococcal pharyngitis and some anaerobic infections).
   - **Aminopenicillins** (ampicillin and amoxicillin): The spectrum is similar to that of penicillin but includes additional activity against aerobic gram-negative bacteria.
   - **Penicillinase-resistant penicillins** (methicillin, oxacillin, nafcillin, and dicloxacillin): These have excellent activity against sensitive strains of *Staphylococcus aureus*.
   - **Antipseudomonal penicillins** (piperacillin and ticarcillin): These have an expanded gram-negative spectrum and can be used to treat susceptible strains of *Pseudomonas aeruginosa*.

   The spectrum of certain penicillins can be increased by the addition of a β-lactamase inhibitor. β-Lactamases are a common basis for penicillin resistance in some bacteria (e.g., methicillin-sensitive *S. aureus*) but not in other species (e.g., *Streptococcus pneumoniae*). Available combinations include amoxicillin-clavulanate, ampicillin-sulbactam, piperacillin-tazobactam, and ticarcillin-clavulanate.

2. **In patients for whom the history lists "penicillin allergy," how commonly is a true allergy present on testing?**
   ≤20%. In patients reporting a penicillin allergy, skin tests and radioallergosorbent tests are frequently negative. Because nonpruritic maculopapular rashes occur frequently in patients taking oral ampicillin (3% to 7%), these are unlikely to be immunoglobulin E (IgE) mediated and are not contraindications to future penicillin use. A rash that develops in the second week of the initial exposure of an antibiotic and is pruritic is more likely to be allergic.

   Pichichero ME, Pichichero DM: Diagnosis of penicillin, amoxicillin, and cephalosporin allergy: reliability of examination assessed by skin and oral challenge, *J Pediatr* 132:137–143, 1998.

3. **How can the emergence of antibiotic-resistant pathogens be minimized?**
   - Appropriate hand hygiene, contact isolation, and environmental decontamination to reduce the transmission of resistant organisms to other patients
   - Use of the most potent, narrowest spectrum antibiotic possible for an appropriate length of time
   - Minimization of the empirical use of broad-spectrum antibiotics
   - Avoidance of antibiotic treatment of illnesses that are likely viral
   - Awareness of local antibiotic resistance patterns

4. **How much has community-associated methicillin-resistant *S. aureus* (CA-MRSA) increased in the United States?**
   MRSA was first reported in the United States in 1968. CA-MRSA has been defined as MRSA infections diagnosed by the primary care provider or if isolated within 24 to 72 hours after

admission. Initially, cases were most commonly seen in patients residing in long-term care facilities and those recently hospitalized. However, during the 1990s, cases began to increase of children with CA-MRSA infections without any risk factors. These infections have now achieved epidemic proportions. Depending on the locale in the United States, up to 75% of all staphylococcal isolates in hospitalized patients with staphylococcal infections are CA-MRSA.

5. **What has been the most important antibiotic-susceptibility difference between hospital-acquired and community-associated MRSA?**
Differences in clindamycin susceptibility. Previously, most hospital-acquired MRSAs were not susceptible to clindamycin, whereas most CA-MRSAs were. This resistance is thought to be conferred by the a bacterial ribosome modification that allows resistance to macrolides, lincosamides, and streptogramin B (the MLS_B phenotype). There is, however, increasing resistance to clindamycin in the CA-MRSA isolates.

6. **Why is the *D-test* done?**
The *D-test* is done with MRSA isolates that are susceptible to clindamycin and resistant to erythromycin to evaluate whether that isolate might have the MLS_B resistance not constitutively expressed (i.e., always produced) but *inducible by exposure to macrolides*. If patients with this type of MRSA are begun on clindamycin, they may have a higher likelihood of recrudescence. The test involves placing antibiotic disks for erythromycin and clindamycin in close proximity on the agar plate. A flattening of the clindamycin zone of bacterial growth adjacent to the erythromycin disk produces a "D" appearance and indicates the MRSA isolate has inducible MLS_B resistance.

7. **Is mupirocin useful in the eradication of *S. aureus* in colonized children?**
Colonization of the nasal mucosa or skin is common in children. About 15% to 40% of healthy children are carriers of methicillin-sensitive *S. aureus* (MSSA). MRSA nasal carriage ranges from 1% to 24% in various studies involving day care, emergency room visits, or hospitalized children. The use of mupirocin applied twice daily for 1 to 21 days was shown in some adult studies to significantly but variably decrease colonization and recurrent invasive disease. However, eradication is difficult, recolonization is common, and protracted use of mupirocin leads to increased rates of MRSA resistance. Thus, mupirocin is not recommended for routine use in children to decrease colonization in children.

Fergie J, Purcell K: The epidemic of methicillin-resistant *Staphylococcus aureus* colonization and infection in children: effects on the community, health systems, and physician practices, *Pediatr Ann* 36:404–412, 2007.

8. **Which antibiotic is associated with the "red man syndrome"?**
The red man syndrome is a frequent occurrence with the rapid infusion of **vancomycin** and is characterized by flushing of the neck, face, and thorax. The histamine release underlying this reaction is directly caused by vancomycin. It is not mediated by IgE and therefore does not represent a true hypersensitivity reaction. Generally, the reaction can be avoided by slowing the rate of drug infusion. Administration of an H_1-receptor antagonist (e.g., diphenhydramine) before vancomycin is given is also effective for preventing this reaction.

9. **How should infections with vancomycin-resistant enterococci be managed?**
Resistance to vancomycin has been observed in both *Enterococcus faecium* and *Enterococcus faecalis*. Many patients have succumbed to bacteremia or other invasive infections with vancomycin-resistant enterococci (VRE). Most of these infections are acquired nosocomially, which reflects the fact that the organism can survive on inanimate surfaces (including medical equipment) for weeks. Basic tenets of anti-infective therapy apply: foreign bodies should be removed, infected fluid collections should be drained, and patients should

be placed on contact isolation to prevent spread. The combination streptogramin agent quinupristin-dalfopristin (Synercid) and the oxazolidinone antibiotic linezolid (Zyvox) have shown effectiveness and safety in limited data. Of note is that quinupristin-dalfopristin has activity against *E. faecium* but not *E. faecalis*.

10. **Is vancomycin still effective against all staphylococci?**
Within a few years of the emergence of VRE, isolates of *S. aureus* with reduced susceptibility and resistance to vancomycin were reported. In some of these isolates, acquisition of resistance genes from VRE has been demonstrated. Fortunately, these isolates have retained susceptibility to a variety of other antibiotics. Appropriate use of vancomycin is key to prevent overuse and to limit the likelihood of further emergence of vancomycin resistance.

11. **In what situations may treatment with vancomycin be considered appropriate?**
   - Serious infections (e.g., meningitis) attributable to β-lactam–resistant gram-positive organisms
   - Infections attributable to gram-positive microorganisms in patients with serious allergies to β-lactam antibiotics
   - Antimicrobial-associated colitis (e.g., *Clostridium difficile*) that fails to respond to metronidazole or that is life threatening
   - Prophylaxis, as recommended by the American Heart Association, for endocarditis in certain high-risk patients
   - Prophylaxis for certain procedures (e.g., implantation of prosthetic materials or devices) at institutions with high rates of MRSA

   American Academy of Pediatrics: Antimicrobial agents and related therapy. In Pickering LK, editor: *2009 Red Book: Report of the Committee on Infectious Diseases*, ed 28, Elk Grove Park, IL, 2009, American Academy of Pediatrics, pp 742–743.

12. **Are fluoroquinolones safe to use in children?**
Members of the fluoroquinolone class of antibiotics act against bacterial DNA gyrase and topoisomerase II, two enzymes that are required for bacterial DNA replication. No member of the class is approved by the U.S. Food and Drug Administration (FDA) for use in patients younger than 18 years. Part of the basis for this recommendation is the occurrence of arthropathy in immature beagle dogs treated with ciprofloxacin or other quinolones. However, there is growing anecdotal experience with the use of these antibiotics in adolescents and children, primarily those with cystic fibrosis in whom endogenous *P. aeruginosa* strains may display high-level resistance to other antibiotic classes (e.g., antipseudomonal penicillins, carbapenems, aminoglycosides). FDA-approved pediatric indications for ciprofloxacin include postexposure treatment for inhalation anthrax and for complicated urinary tract infection. They may also be considered when parenteral therapy is not feasible and the infection is caused by multidrug-resistant organisms for which there are no other effective oral agents available.

   Murray TS, Baltimore RS: Pediatric uses of fluoroquinolone antibiotics, *Pediatr Ann* 36:336–342, 2007.

13. **What are the differences among first-, second-, third-, and fourth-generation cephalosporins?**
First-generation cephalosporins (e.g., cefazolin, cephalexin, cefadroxil)
   - Alternative drugs for patients allergic to penicillins, although there is a 5% to 10% risk for cross-reactivity
   - Prophylaxis for orthopedic and cardiovascular surgery
   - Better *S. aureus* coverage (MSSA) compared with second- and third-generation cephalosporins
   - Lack of efficacy against *Haemophilus influenzae*

Second-generation cephalosporins (e.g., cefaclor, cefuroxime, cefprozil, cefpodoxime)
- Increased spectrum of activity, including many gram-negative organisms
- Prophylaxis for intra-abdominal and pelvic surgery (e.g., cefoxitin)
- Improved compliance with oral medications (most with twice-daily dosing)
- Poor penetration into the cerebrospinal fluid (CSF)
- No antipseudomonal activity

Third-generation cephalosporins (e.g., ceftriaxone, cefotaxime, cefixime, cefdinir, ceftazidime)
- Broadest spectrum, including excellent activity against gram-negative bacteria
- Generally less activity against gram-positive organisms than earlier generations
- Very high blood and CSF levels achievable in relation to minimal inhibitory concentration for bacterial strains
- Wide therapeutic index with generally minimal toxicity (similar to previous generations)
- Some offer single-daily dosing
- Ceftazidime: the first cephalosporin with antipseudomonal coverage
- More expensive

Fourth-generation cephalosporins (e.g., cefepime)
- Spectrum similar to third-generation agents, with the addition of antipseudomonal activity

Harrison CJ, Bratcher D: Cephalosporins: a review, *Pediatr Rev* 29:264–272, 2008.

14. **Can cephalosporins be safely given to patients who are allergic to penicillin?**

Previous estimates of cross-sensitivity to cephalosporins among penicillin-allergic patients were thought to be 8% to 18%, but these rates have been criticized as inaccurate and excessive. Side-chain–specific antibodies appear to be key in the immune response to cephalosporins. The incidence of allergic cross-reactivity varies with the chemical side-chain similarity of the cephalosporin to penicillin or amoxicillin. For first-generation cephalosporins, the attributable increased risk is thought to be only 0.4%. For certain second- and third-generation cephalosporins (e.g., cefuroxime, cefpodoxime, and cefdinir), the risk is thought to be close to zero. No evidence supports an increase of anaphylaxis with cephalosporins among penicillin-allergic patients. American Academy of Pediatrics guidelines do endorse the use of selected second-generation and third-generation cephalosporins for penicillin-allergic patients as long as the penicillin reaction is not severe.

Pichichero ME: A review of the evidence supporting the American Academy of Pediatrics recommendation for prescribing cephalosporin antibiotics for penicillin-allergic patients, *Pediatrics* 115:1048–1057, 2005.

15. **Why is chicken soup so helpful for upper respiratory infections (URIs)?**

The benefits of chicken soup have been of lore for hundreds of years, beginning in the 12th century, when physician and philosopher Maimonides extolled its virtue. The precise mechanisms of its anecdotal therapeutic benefits remain elusive. One study at the University of Nebraska found that the nonparticulate component of chicken soup *in vitro* inhibited neutrophil migration in a concentration-dependent manner. This anti-inflammatory effect may be one mechanism by which chicken soup mitigates the symptoms of URIs.

Rennard BO, Ertl RF, Gossman GL, et al: Chicken soup inhibits neutrophil chemotaxis in vitro, *Chest* 118:1150–1157, 2000.

16. **Is there any physiologic basis to the adage "starve a fever, feed a cold"?**

Some studies indicate that anorexia increases the number of T_H2 cells, which are key in fighting bacterial infections. This would serve as a potentially useful behavioral adaptation, particularly in preantibiotic times. Eating, on the other hand, promotes T_H1 cells by gastrointestinal stimulation of vagal and neurohormonal factors. The T_H1 cells are essential components of the antiviral immune reaction, which might include rhinoviruses and others involved in the common cold.

Bazar KA, Yun AJ, Lee PY: "Starve a fever and feed a cold": feeding and anorexia may be adaptive behavioral modulators of autonomic and T helper balance, *Med Hypotheses* 64:1080–1084, 2005.

CLINICAL ISSUES

17. **Name the three stages of pertussis infection (whooping cough).**
    1. **Catarrhal** (1 to 2 weeks): Low-grade fever, upper respiratory infection symptoms
    2. **Paroxysmal** (2 to 4 weeks): Severe cough occurring in paroxysms, onset of inspiratory "whoop"
    3. **Convalescent** (1 to 2 weeks): Resolution of symptoms

18. **What is the most common cause of death in children with whooping cough?**
    Ninety percent of deaths are attributable to **pneumonia**, which most often develops as a secondary bacterial infection. These cases can be easily missed during the paroxysmal phase, when respiratory symptoms are so prominent and usually attributed solely to pertussis. A new spiking fever should prompt a careful search for an evolving pneumonia.

19. **Is erythromycin of value in pertussis infection?**
    If used during the first 14 days of illness or before the paroxysmal stage, erythromycin can decrease the severity of symptoms during the paroxysmal stage. If the diagnosis is established later in the course, erythromycin should still be administered to eliminate the nasopharyngeal carriage of *Bordetella pertussis* and limit the spread of disease. Evidence suggests that treatment with azithromycin or clarithromycin for 5 to 7 days is also effective for eradicating carriage and preventing transmission.

20. **Do antibiotics prevent the development of pneumonia after a URI?**
    More than 90% of URIs are caused by viruses, and children younger than 5 years (especially those in day care environments) can experience six to eight URI episodes per year. Multiple studies have shown that antibiotic treatment of URIs does not shorten their course or prevent the development of pneumonia.

    Gadomski AM: Potential interventions for preventing pneumonia among young children: lack of effect of antibiotic treatment for upper respiratory infections, *Pediatr Infect Dis J* 12:115–120, 1993.

21. **Sternal edema is classically the sign of what infection?**
    Mumps.

22. **How does Hatchcock sign help distinguish swelling as a result of mumps from swelling caused by adenitis?**
    Upward pressure applied to the angle of the mandible produces tenderness with mumps (Hatchcock sign); this maneuver produces no tenderness with adenitis. Another way to distinguish it is to have the patient sip on lemon juice or suck a lemon wedge. Stimulation of salivation will cause pain in mumps with enlargement of the parotid gland, but no change is noted in patients with adenitis.

23. **Summarize the distinguishing features of staphylococcal scalded skin syndrome, staphylococcal toxic shock syndrome, and streptococcal toxic shock syndrome.**
    See Table 11-1.

TABLE 11-1. DISTINGUISHING FEATURES OF STAPHYLOCOCCAL SCALDED SKIN SYNDROME, STAPHYLOCOCCAL TOXIC SHOCK SYNDROME, AND STREPTOCOCCAL TOXIC SHOCK SYNDROME

Clinical Features	Staphylococcal Scalded Skin Syndrome	Staphylococcal Toxic Shock Syndrome	Group A Streptococcal Toxic Shock-like Syndrome
Organism	*Staphylococcus aureus* Usually phage group 11, type 71	*Staphylococcus aureus* Usually phage group 1, type 29	Group A streptococci Usually type 1, 3, or 18 Exotoxin A production
Site of infection	Usually focal Mucocutaneous border: nose, mouth, diaper area Sometimes inapparent	Mucous membranes Infected wound or furuncle Sometimes inapparent	Blood, abscess, pneumonia, empyema, cellulitis, necrotizing fasciitis Sometimes inapparent
Skin rash	Tender erythroderma: face, neck, generalized Bullae, no petechiae	Tender erythroderma: trunk, hands, feet Edema of hands, feet	Erythroderma: trunk, extremities
Desquamation	Early, first 1-2 days, generalized, feet	Late, 7-10 days, mostly hands and feet Hyperemia of oral and vaginal mucosa	Late, 7-10 days, mostly hands Hyperemia of oral and vaginal mucosa
Mucous membranes	Normal	Hypertrophy of tongue papillae	Hypertrophy of tongue papillae
Conjunctivae	Normal	Markedly injected	Injected
Course	Insidious, 4-7 days Benign, <1% mortality	Fulminant, shock with secondary multiorgan failure, 10% mortality	Fulminant, shock with early primary multiorgan failure, 30%-50% mortality

Adapted from Bass JW: Treatment of skin and skin structure infections. Pediatr Infect Dis J 11:152-155, 1992.

24. **What percentage of cases of staphylococcal toxic shock syndrome are nonmenstrual?**
    During the past two decades, the epidemiology of toxic shock syndrome has changed, reflecting changes in tampon composition and a decrease in absorbency. More than 50% of reported cases are now nonmenstrual. The syndrome occurs in the setting of focal staphylococcal colonization or focal infections, including empyema, osteomyelitis, soft tissue abscess, surgical infections, and burns.

25. **In the setting of clinical signs and symptoms of encephalitis, what electroencephalogram pattern is suggestive of herpes simplex virus (HSV) disease?**
    Periodic lateralized epileptiform discharges. These may be seen in other, rarer forms of encephalitis, such as Epstein-Barr virus (EBV) encephalitis, Creutzfeldt-Jakob disease, and subacute sclerosing panencephalitis.

26. **Can acyclovir be used to prevent or treat oral HSV infections?**
    In immunocompetent hosts, oral acyclovir offers significant therapeutic benefit in primary HSV gingivostomatitis but has limited efficacy for the treatment of recurrent herpes labialis. Topical acyclovir has not shown consistent benefit in either of these settings. Prophylaxis with oral acyclovir can reduce the number of recurrences in adults with herpes labialis, but it has not been well-studied in children.

27. **How quickly do central lines become colonized?**
    The timing and rate of central line colonization depend on a number of factors. Manipulation of the catheter (e.g., for blood drawing, medication administration, or flushing) and poor handwashing by health care providers are probably the most important factors that increase the risk for colonization. In general, the likelihood of colonization increases with the length of time that the catheter has been in place. Colonization rates have been reported to be less than 10% for catheters less than 3 days old, about 15% for catheters 3 to 7 days old, and about 20% for catheters in place for more than 7 days.

28. **What is the proper medical term for oral thrush?**
    Acute pseudomembranous candidiasis. Quite a mouthful. Although thrush is sometimes confused with residual formula in the mouth in infants, formula is more easily removed with a tongue blade. When thrush is scraped, small bleeding points often occur on the underlying mucosa.

29. **What is the most common specific etiology diagnosed in patients with systemic febrile illness after international travel?**
    Malaria, both in children and adults. Next in frequency are dengue fever, typhoid fever, rickettsioses, and leptospirosis. Malaria should be considered in the differential diagnosis in anyone with fever who has travelled to an endemic area in the previous year. More than half of the world's population lives in areas where malaria is endemic.

    Wilson ME, Weld LH, Boggild A, et al: Fever in returned travellers: results from the GeoSentinel surveillance network, *Clin Infect Dis* 44:1560–1568, 2007.

    Freedman DO, Weld LH, Kozarsky PE, et al: Spectrum of disease and relation to place of exposure among ill returned travellers, *N Engl J Med* 354:119–130, 2006.

30. **What is the classic triad of malaria?**
    Spiking fevers, anemia, and splenomegaly. Malaria is caused by species of *Plasmodium* (transmitted by the *Anopheles* mosquito), which infect red blood cells (RBCs); certain species

can have a dormant liver stage. The classic malarial fever involves a periodicity (typically 48 to 72 hours) associated with the rupture of RBCs. Chills, headache, abdominal pain, and myalgias are also common symptoms.

Cavagnaro CS, Brady K, Siegel C: Fever after international travel, *Clin Pediatr Emerg Med* 9:250–257, 2008.

31. **How is malaria diagnosed?**
 Thick and thin blood smears. Thick smears are made by applying the blood film twice to a slide (and incorporating more RBCs). Giemsa stain is applied to both with an attempt to identify parasites in the cells. The thick smear is better for determining the presence of parasites, and the thin smear for species identification. A determination of parasite density (a rough gauge to severity of infection) can be made. Therapy depends on the species identified. If smears are negative and clinical suspicion remains strong, repeat smears should be obtained in multiple times (every 12 to 24 hours) over a 3-day period.

32. **Which illness is associated with the term "breakbone fever"?**
 Dengue fever. The term refers to the classic presentation of fever, severe headache, retro-orbital pain, fatigue, and severe myalgias or arthralgias. Most cases are less severe. The illness is caused by an arbovirus, transmitted by mosquitoes, which is endemic in tropical areas worldwide, including the Caribbean and Central and South America. Leukopenia, thrombocytopenia, and mild elevations of hepatic transaminases are common. Children, more commonly than adults, may develop *dengue hemorrhagic fever*, which encompasses fever, epistaxis, mucosal bleeding, and platelet counts lower than 100,000/μL. This may progress to *dengue shock syndrome* with significant mortality.

33. **What causes leptospirosis?**
 Spirochetes of the genus *Leptospira*. These are typically acquired from animal contact, or water or soil contaminated by the urine of dogs, rats, or livestock in the course of recreation or work. Animals may remain asymptomatic shedders for years, and the organisms can remain viable after shedding for weeks to months. Acquisition of illness is more common after heavy rainfalls or flooding. The incubation period can be up to 1 month. In 90% of cases, the disease is self-limited.

American Academy of Pediatrics: Leptospirosis. In Pickering LK, editor: *2009 Red Book: Report of the Committee on Infectious Diseases*, ed 28, Elk Grove Park, IL, 2009, American Academy of Pediatrics, pp 427–428.

34. **What are the phases of leptospirosis?**
 - **Septicemic phase:** Initially—nonspecific symptoms of fever, chills, headache, transient rash. A conjunctivitis without purulent discharge occurs in about one third of cases. Eighty percent of cases feature severe myalgias of the calves and lumbar area. Symptoms may last up to 1 week and improve for 1 to 4 days, when the second phase occurs.
 - **Immune-mediated:** Fever returns, accompanied by potentially more severe findings, including aseptic meningitis and Weil syndrome (jaundice, nonoliguric renal failure, hemorrhage due to thrombocytopenia). Severe pulmonary hemorrhages with hemoptysis may develop. The protein manifestations are due to the pathophysiology as a generalized vasculitis.

35. **How is the diagnosis of leptospirosis made?**
 Although the spirochete can be cultured from blood or CSF, the organism is difficult to grow and can take up to 4 months. Diagnosis more commonly is made by acute and convalescent serology.

36. **Which organisms are particularly dangerous to clinical microbiology laboratory workers?**

    The laboratory should be alerted when highly transmissible bacterial agents are suspected in specimens that have been submitted for culture. These bacteria include *Francisella tularensis* (the causative agent of tularemia), *Bacillus anthracis* (anthrax), and *Coxiella burnetii* (Q fever). In addition, the laboratory may process fungal cultures that contain molds and dimorphic fungi (e.g., *Histoplasma*, *Blastomyces*) in a biosafety cabinet to prevent exposure to spores.

CONGENITAL INFECTIONS

37. **Which congenital infections cause cerebral calcifications?**

    Cerebral calcifications are most frequently observed in **congenital *Toxoplasma*** and **cytomegalovirus (CMV)** infections. They are seen occasionally in patients with congenital HSV infection and rarely in patients with congenital rubella infection.

38. **What are the late sequelae of congenital infections?**

    The late sequelae of chronic intrauterine infections are relatively common and may occur in infants who are asymptomatic at birth. Most sequelae present symptoms later in childhood rather than infancy.

    ■ CMV: Hearing loss,* minimal to severe brain dysfunction* (motor, learning, language, and behavioral disorders)
    ■ Rubella: Hearing loss,* minimal to severe brain dysfunction* (motor, learning, language, and behavioral disorders), autism,* juvenile diabetes, thyroid dysfunction, precocious puberty, progressive degenerative brain disorder*
    ■ Toxoplasmosis: Chorioretinitis,* minimal to severe brain dysfunction,* hearing loss, precocious puberty
    ■ Neonatal herpes: Recurrent eye and skin infection, minimal to severe brain dysfunction
    ■ Hepatitis B virus: Chronic subclinical hepatitis, rarely fulminant hepatitis

    Plotkin SA, Alpert G: A practical guide to the diagnosis of congenital infections in the newborn infant, *Pediatr Clin North Am* 33:465–479, 1986.

39. **What is the most common congenital infection?**

    Congenital CMV infection, which in some large screening studies occurs in up to 1.3% of newborns. However, 90% to 95% of infected neonates are asymptomatic. Some infants who are asymptomatic at birth later develop hearing loss.

40. **How is CMV transmitted from mother to infant?**

    CMV can be transmitted by the transplacental route or through contact with cervical secretions or breast milk. On occasion, transmission may occur by contact with saliva or urine.

41. **Should congenital CMV be treated?**

    Treatment is recommended for infants with life- or vision-threatening disease, such as severe retinitis, interstitial pneumonitis, hepatitis, or thrombocytopenia. Ganciclovir is approved for use in children.

42. **How do complications vary between newborns with CMV infection who are symptomatic and those who are asymptomatic at birth?**

    See Table 11-2.

---

*Seen with infections that are subclinical during early infancy.

TABLE 11-2. **COMPLICATIONS IN SYMPTOMATIC VERSUS ASYMPTOMATIC NEWBORNS WITH CYTOMEGALOVIRUS**

Complication	Symptomatic Occurrence (%)	Asymptomatic Occurrence (%)
Death	6	0
Microcephaly	38	2
Sensorineural hearing loss	58	7
Bilateral hearing loss	37	3
Moderate to profound hearing loss (60-90 dB)	27	2
Chorioretinitis	20	3
Intelligence quotient of <70	55	4
Seizures	23	1
Paresis, paralysis	13	0

Adapted from Remington JS, Klein JO: Infections of the Fetus and Newborn Infant, 5th ed. Philadelphia, W.B. Saunders, 2001, p 408.

43. **What is the risk to the fetus if the mother is infected with parvovirus B19 during pregnancy?**
    The risk of fetal loss is 2% to 10% and is greatest when maternal infection occurs during the first half of pregnancy. Fetal loss occurs as a consequence of hydrops, which develops as a result of parvovirus-induced anemia. An elevated maternal serum α-fetoprotein level may be a marker for an adverse outcome. The signs of parvovirus infection in adults are not very distinctive but may include fever, a maculopapular or lacelike rash, and joint pain.

44. **What are the consequences of primary varicella infection during the first trimester?**
    The congenital varicella syndrome consists of a constellation of features:
    ■ Limb atrophy, usually associated with a cicatricial (scarring) lesion
    ■ Neurologic and sensory defects
    ■ Eye abnormalities (chorioretinitis, cataracts, microphthalmia, Horner syndrome)
    ■ Cortical atrophy and mental retardation
        This syndrome usually follows maternal infection during the first trimester, although it may be seen after infection up to 20 weeks into gestation. The largest prospective study reported to date found four cases of fetal varicella syndrome in 141 pregnancies, yielding an incidence of less than 3%.

45. **When should varicella zoster immunoglobulin (VZIG) be given to a newborn?**
    VZIG should be given as soon as possible to a newborn whose mother developed varicella from 5 days before to 2 days after delivery. During this period of high risk, the fetus is exposed to high circulating titers of the virus without the benefit of maternal antibody synthesis. Premature neonates exposed to varicella during the neonatal period are also candidates for VZIG:
    ■ If the infant is 28 weeks' gestation or older and the mother has no history of chickenpox or positive varicella serology
    ■ If the infant is less than 28 weeks' gestation or weighs 1000 g or less, regardless of maternal history, because little maternal antibody crosses the placenta before the third trimester of pregnancy

46. **Do urogenital mycoplasmas have a role in neonatal disease?**
Ureaplasma urealyticum has been associated with low birthweight and bronchopulmonary dysplasia. This organism has been recovered from neonates with respiratory distress, pneumonia, and meningitis, but a causative role in these diseases has not been proved. Several reports of apparent *Mycoplasma hominis* meningitis and eye infection have been published.

47. **If a mother is culture positive for *U. urealyticum* or *M. hominis*, what is the likelihood of transmission to the newborn infant?**
Vertical transmission occurs in up to 60% of exposed newborns. Risk for transmission is higher in preterm and low-birthweight infants and correlates with the prolonged rupture of membranes and maternal fever. Infants delivered by cesarean section over intact membranes have a very low rate of colonization compared with infants delivered vaginally.

48. **What are the features of congenital rubella syndrome?**
The most characteristic features of congenital rubella syndrome are congenital heart disease, cataracts, microphthalmia, corneal opacities, glaucoma, and radiolucent bone lesions. The features of congenital rubella syndrome can be divided into three broad categories:
- **Transient:** Low birthweight, hepatosplenomegaly, thrombocytopenia, hepatitis, pneumonitis, and radiolucent bone lesions
- **Permanent:** Deafness, cataracts, and congenital heart lesions (patent ductus arteriosus > pulmonary artery stenosis > aortic stenosis > ventricular septal defects)
- **Developmental:** Psychomotor delay, behavioral disorders, and endocrine dysfunction

49. **Should all pregnant women be screened for HSV infection during pregnancy?**
Existing data indicate that antepartum cultures of the maternal genital tract fail to predict viral shedding at the time of delivery. As a consequence, routine antepartum cultures are not recommended.

50. **What are risk factors for the development of neonatal HSV disease?**
Among infants born vaginally to mothers with primary herpes genitalis, 30% to 50% will develop HSV disease. Only 3% to 5% of infants born to mothers with active recurrent disease become infected. Distinguishing between primary and recurrent herpes infections by history and clinical examination is often difficult. Low birthweight is an independent risk factor. Fetal scalp monitoring may result in direct inoculation of the virus into the baby's scalp.

Many experts advocate cesarean birth for women who are in labor at term and have visual evidence of active genital HSV lesions, especially if membranes have been ruptured for less than 4 to 6 hours. If membranes have been ruptured for longer periods of time, operative delivery is less effective for reducing the risk for neonatal infection.

Corey L, Wald A: Maternal and neonatal herpes simplex virus infections, *N Engl J Med* 361: 1376–1385, 2009.

51. **What are the three forms of neonatal HSV disease?**
Occurring with about equal frequency, the three patterns of neonatal HSV disease are as follows:
- Mucocutaneous disease (localized to the skin, eye, or mouth)
- Encephalitis
- Disseminated disease (± central nervous system [CNS] involvement) with a picture that resembles bacterial sepsis
It is important to note that only one third of infants with either localized encephalitis or disseminated disease will have visible skin lesions.

52. **In which newborns or infants should HSV infection be suspected?**
In full-term infants younger than 4 weeks and premature infants (<32 weeks' gestation) younger than 8 weeks, HSV infection should be considered in the following cases:
   - History of third-trimester HSV lesions in the mother
   - Skin lesions suspicious for HSV on the infant (may be single or grouped vesicles, pustules, bullae, or denuded skin)
   - Ill-appearing infant with findings of poor feeding, irritability, lethargy, vomiting, and hypothermia
   - Seizure associated with the current illness
   - Abnormal liver function tests (alanine aminotransferase or aspartate aminotransferase >100 U/L)
   - CSF pleocytosis (bloody, uninterruptible CSF must be considered case by case)

   Baker MD, Avner JR: The febrile infant: what's new? *Clin Pediatr Emerg Med* 9:213–220, 2008.

53. **How should the neonate with suspected HSV disease be treated?**
Intravenous acyclovir is the preferred drug and is administered pending definitive diagnosis. For mucocutaneous disease, treatment is continued for 14 days. For encephalitis and disseminated disease, treatment is continued for 21 days. Acyclovir has been shown to be superior to vidarabine, another antiviral agent evaluated for treatment for neonatal HSV infection.

54. **In which groups of women is prenatal hepatitis B surface antigen (HBsAg) screening recommended?**
In the past, women were screened for HBsAg if they fell into a high-risk group based on ethnic origin, immunization status, or history of exposure to blood products, intravenous drugs, or a high-risk partner. However, historic information reveals only a portion of HBsAg carriers were captured using these screening criteria, and thus it is recommended that all pregnant women be screened for HBsAg.

55. **What is the relationship between age of acquisition of hepatitis B virus and the likelihood of chronic hepatitis B infection?**
Chronic hepatitis B virus infection with persistence of HBsAg occurs in as many as 90% of infants who are infected by perinatal transmission, in an average of 30% of children who are 1 to 5 years old when infected, and in 2% to 6% of older children, adolescents, and adults who become infected.

   Liaw Y-F, Chu C-M: Hepatitis B virus infection, *Lancet* 373:582–592, 2009.

56. **How should infants born to mothers with hepatitis A infection be managed?**
Neonates born to mothers with active hepatitis A infection are unlikely to contract the virus, and efficacy of postnatal prophylaxis with hepatitis A immunoglobulin has not been proved. Some experts recommend immunoglobulin if the mother's symptoms begin within 2 weeks before or 1 week after delivery, but this is controversial.

   American Academy of Pediatrics: Hepatitis A. In Pickering LK, editor: *2009 Red Book: Report of the Committee on Infectious Diseases*, ed 28, Elk Grove Park, IL, 2009, American Academy of Pediatrics, p 336.

57. **How should infants born to mothers with hepatitis B infection be managed?**
For infants born to women who are HBsAg positive, hepatitis B immunoglobulin (0.5 mL intramuscularly) and the first dose of hepatitis B vaccine should be administered within 12 hours of delivery to reduce the risk for infection. Although breast milk is capable of transmitting the hepatitis B virus, the risk for transmission in HBsAg-positive mothers whose infants have received timely hepatitis B immunoglobulin and hepatitis B vaccine is not increased by breastfeeding.

58. **How should infants born to mothers with hepatitis C infection be managed?**
The risk for vertical transmission of hepatitis C virus is about 5%, and no preventive therapy exists. Nucleic amplification testing can be done at 1 to 2 months of age, if desired, to assess for neonatal infection. Antibody testing cannot be done until after 18 months because that is the expected duration of the presence of passive maternal antibody in infants. Mothers with hepatitis C infection should be advised that transmission of hepatitis C by breastfeeding has not been documented. Accordingly, maternal hepatitis C infection is not a contraindication to breastfeeding, although mothers with cracked or bleeding nipples should consider abstaining.

Maheshwari A, Ray S, Thuluvath PJ: Acute hepatitis C, *Lancet* 372:321–332, 2008.

American Academy of Pediatrics: Hepatitis C. In Pickering LK, editor: *2009 Red Book: Report of the Committee on Infectious Diseases*, ed 28, Elk Grove Park, IL, 2009, American Academy of Pediatrics, p 360.

59. **How do the clinical features of early and late congenital syphilis differ?**
The manifestations of congenital syphilis are protean and may be divided into early and late findings. Early manifestations occur during the first 2 years of life; late manifestations occur after 2 years of age (Table 11-3).

60. **Describe the appearance of Hutchinson teeth.**
The permanent central incisors are typically **peg shaped** or **notched.**

TABLE 11-3. EARLY AND LATE MANIFESTATIONS OF CONGENITAL SYPHILIS

Early Congenital Syphilis (310 Patients)		Late Congenital Syphilis (271 Patients)	
Hepatomegaly	32%	Pseudoparalysis of Parrot	87%
Skeletal abnormalities	29%	Short maxilla	84%
Splenomegaly	18%	High palatal arch	76%
Birthweight <2500 g	16%	Hutchinson triad	75%
Pneumonia	16%	Saddle nose	73%
Severe anemia, hydrops, edema	16%	Mulberry molars	65%
Skin lesions	15%	Hutchinson teeth	63%
Hyperbilirubinemia	13%	Higoumenakia sign	39%
Snuffles, nasal discharge	9%	Relative protuberance of mandible	26%
Painful limbs	7%	Interstitial keratitis	9%
Cerebrospinal fluid abnormalities	7%	Rhagades	7%
Pancreatitis	5%	Saber shin	4%
Nephritis	4%	Eighth nerve deafness	3%
Failure to thrive	3%	Scaphoid scapulae	0.7%
Testicular mass	0.3%	Clutton joint	0.3%
Chorioretinitis	0.3%		
Hypoglobulinemia	0.3%		

Adapted from Sanchez PJ, Gutman LT: Syphilis. In Feigin RD, Cherry JE, Demmler GJ, Kaplan SL (eds): Pediatric Infectious Diseases, 5th ed. Philadelphia, W.B. Saunders, 2004, pp 1730-1732.

61. **How is the diagnosis of congenital syphilis made?**
    - Pregnant women and infants should be screened for possible infection with a nontreponemal test for *Treponema pallidum*. Such tests include the rapid plasma reagin card test and the Venereal Disease Reference Laboratory (VDRL) slide test.
    - If blood from the mother or infant yields a positive nontreponemal serologic test, a specific treponemal test should be performed on the infant's blood. Examples include the fluorescent treponemal antibody absorption test and the microhemagglutination test for *T. pallidum*.
    - Evaluation of infants with suspected congenital syphilis should also include a complete blood count, analysis of the CSF (including a CSF VDRL), and long-bone radiographs (unless the diagnosis has been otherwise established).

62. **What are the pitfalls of rapid plasma reagin and VDRL testing?**
    - Cord blood specimens from the infant can produce false-positive results; therefore, serum from the infant is preferred.
    - A mother who has been treated adequately for syphilis during pregnancy can still passively transfer antibodies to the neonate, which results in a positive titer in the infant in the absence of infection. In this circumstance, the infant's titer is usually less than the mother's and reverts to negative over several months.

63. **What is the leading cause of preventable blindness worldwide?**
    Trachoma. Rarely seen in the United States, trachoma is an infection caused by certain serotypes of *Chlamydia trachomatis*. If untreated, a chronic follicular keratoconjunctivitis results in neovascularization and extensive scarring of the cornea. In children, the acute disease is generally mild and self-limited, whereas the chronic, scarring disease occurs more commonly in adults. Prevalence is more common in socioeconomically disadvantaged areas with crowding and inadequate water supplies. The World Health Organization estimates that about 6 million people are blind as a result of an untreated infection.

    Chandran L, Boykan R: Chlamydial infections in children and adolescents, *Pediatr Rev* 30:243–249, 2009.

64. **If a pregnant woman is found to have *C. trachomatis* in her birth canal, what is the most appropriate course of action?**
    A pregnant woman with a known chlamydial infection should be treated with oral erythromycin or azithromycin to reduce the risk for neonatal chlamydial pneumonia and conjunctivitis. Untreated mothers may transmit *Chlamydia* to babies born vaginally about 50% of the time. Simultaneous treatment of the male partners with doxycycline or azithromycin should also be undertaken.

65. **Should newborns of mothers with untreated chlamydial infection receive prophylactic antibiotic therapy?**
    Although these infants are at increased risk for infection, the efficacy of prophylactic antibiotics is not known, and treatment is not indicated. Infants should be followed carefully for signs of conjunctivitis or pneumonia and treatment initiated if indicated. If close follow-up cannot be ensured, some pediatric infectious disease experts would advise preemptive therapy.

    American Academy of Pediatrics: *Chlamydia trachomatis*. In Pickering LK, editor: *2009 Red Book: Report of the Committee on Infectious Diseases*, ed 28, Elk Grove Park, IL, 2009, American Academy of Pediatrics, p 257.

66. **What is the risk to a fetus after primary maternal *Toxoplasma* infection?**
    The risk depends on the time during pregnancy that the mother becomes infected. Assuming that the mother is untreated, first-trimester infection is associated with a fetal infection rate of about 25%, second-trimester infection with a rate of more than 50%, and third-trimester infection with a rate of roughly 65%. The severity of clinical disease in

congenitally infected infants is inversely related to gestational age at the time of primary maternal infection.

67. **What is the typical presentation of congenital toxoplasmosis?**
At birth, 70% to 90% are asymptomatic. As with other congenital infections, the symptomatic neonatal presentations are varied, ranging from severe disease with fever, hepatosplenomegaly, chorioretinitis, and/or neurologic features (e.g., seizures, hydrocephalus, microcephaly) in about 10% of infected infants. Among asymptomatic infants, intracranial calcifications are often present, and long-term risks include impaired vision, learning disabilities, mental retardation, and seizures.

68. **How can a woman minimize the chance of acquiring a *Toxoplasma* infection during pregnancy?**
Measures relate to personal hygiene, food preparation, and exposure to cats.
■ Prepare meat by cooking it to more than 65.5°C (150°F), smoking it, or curing it in brine.
■ Wash fruits and vegetables before consumption.
■ Wash hands and kitchen surfaces thoroughly after contact with raw meat and unwashed fruits or vegetables, and wash thoroughly after gardening.
■ Avoid changing cat litter boxes, or wear gloves while changing the litter and wash hands thoroughly afterward. Changing the litter every 1 to 2 days will also reduce risk.
■ Avoid untreated water in developing countries.

THE FEBRILE CHILD

69. **Fever in children: is it friend or foe?**
In certain situations, fever is beneficial, and in others, it is detrimental. Gonococci and some treponemes are killed at temperatures of 40°C (104°F) and higher, and benefits from fever therapy have been reported in cases of gonococcal urethritis and neurosyphilis. In addition, fever appears to hamper the growth of some types of pneumococci and some viruses. Fever is also associated with a decrease in the amount of free serum iron, which is an essential nutrient for many pathogenic bacteria. Modest fever can accelerate a variety of immunologic responses, including phagocytosis, leukocyte chemotaxis, lymphocyte transformation, and interferon production.

On the other hand, other data indicate that high fever can impair the immune response. In addition, although the metabolic effects of fever are well tolerated by most children, in some situations, these effects can be dangerous. Examples include patients at risk for cardiac or respiratory failure and those with neurologic disease or with septic shock. Fever can precipitate febrile seizures in the susceptible population, which are children between 6 months and about 5 years of age. Especially in smaller children, fever can contribute to dehydration, increased sleepiness, and discomfort.

70. **At what temperature does a child have fever?**
This is a simple question without a simple answer. Because body temperatures vary among individuals and age groups and vary over the course of the day in a given individual (lowest around 4:00 to 5:00 am and highest in late afternoon and early evening), a precise cutoff point is difficult to determine. In children between the ages of 2 and 6 years, diurnal variation can range up to 0.9°C (1.6°F). Infants tend to have a higher baseline temperature pattern, with 50% having daily rectal temperatures higher than 37.8°C (100.0°F); after the age of 2 years, this elevated baseline falls. In addition, activity and exercise (within 30 minutes), feeding or meals (within 1 hour), and hot foods (within 1 hour) can cause body temperature elevations. Most authorities agree that, for a child younger than 3 months, a rectal temperature higher than 38°C (100.4°F) constitutes fever. In infants between the ages of

3 and 24 months (who tend to have a higher baseline), a temperature of 38.3°C (101°F) or higher likely constitutes fever. In those older than 2 years, as the baseline falls, fever more commonly is defined as a rectal temperature higher than 38°C (100.4°F).

71. **Where did the popular notion that a normal temperature is 98.6°F originate?**
The temperature 98.6°F was established as the mean healthy temperature in 1868 after more than 1 million temperatures from 25,000 patients were analyzed. Ironically, these were axillary temperatures, and the waters of what constitutes normal have been muddied since.

Mackowiak PA, Wasserman SS, Levine MM: A critical appraisal of 98.6°F, the upper limit of the normal body temperature, and other legacies of Carl Reinhold August Wunderlich, *JAMA* 268:1578–1580, 1992.

72. **How does temperature vary among different body sites?**
There can be significant variability in the relationship between different sites, and conversions should be done with caution. As a general guideline:
- Rectal: Standard
- Oral: 0.5° to 0.6°C (1°F) lower
- Axillary: 0.8° to 1.0°C (1.5° to 2.0°F) lower
- Tympanic: 0.5° to 0.6°C (1°F) lower

73. **How accurate is parental palpation for fever in infants?**
It is common for parents to report a subjective fever by palpation without measuring a temperature by thermometry. Palpation by parents has a sensitivity and specificity of about 80% in children older than 3 months. In infants younger than 3 months, the positive-predictive value of a parent reporting a palpable fever is about 60%, with a negative-predictive value of 90%. For these younger infants, for whom identification of fever carries potentially greater clinical repercussions, parents seem to overestimate the presence of a fever, but they are more accurate when a child is afebrile.

Katz-Sidlow RJ, Rowberry JP, Ho M: Fever determination in young infants: prevalence and accuracy of parental palpation, *Pediatr Emerg Care* 25:12–14, 2009.

Zomorrodi A, Attia MW: Fever: parental concerns, *Clin Pediatr Emerg Med* 9:238–243, 2008.

74. **How should the temperature of young infants be taken?**
In infants who are younger than 3 months (when fever can be more significant clinically), a rectal temperature is the preferred method. Tympanic recordings are much less sensitive in this age group because the narrow, tortuous external canal can collapse, thereby resulting in readings obtained from the cooler canal rather than the warmer tympanic membrane. Cutaneous infrared thermometry has reduced diagnostic accuracy in this age group. Axillary temperatures often underestimate fever. The oral route is usually not used until a child is 5 to 6 years old.

Hausfater P, Zhao Y, Defrenne S, et al: Cutaneous infrared thermometry for detecting febrile patients, *Emerg Infect Dis* 14:1255–1258, 2008.

El-Radhi AS, Barry A: Thermometry in paediatric practice, *Arch Dis Child* 91:351–356, 2006.

75. **Can excessive bundling raise an infant's temperature?**
Prospective studies have found mixed results. One study of newborns in a warm environment of 80°F found that rectal temperatures in bundled infants could be elevated to more than 38°C, which is the "febrile range." Another study of infants 3 months old and younger found that, in room temperatures of 22.2° to 23.8°C (72° to 75°F), the bundling of infants for

up to 65 minutes did not produce any rectal temperatures higher than 38°C. A clinical method that may help to distinguish disease-related fevers from possible environmental overheating is the "abdomen-toe" temperature differential. A foot as warm as the abdomen suggests an overly warm environment, whereas a foot that is cooler suggests fever with peripheral vasoconstriction.

Grover C, Berkowitz CD, Lewis RJ, et al: The effects of bundling on infant temperature, *Pediatrics* 94:669–673, 1994.

Cheng TL, Partridge JC: Effect of bundling and high environmental temperatures on neonatal body temperature, *Pediatrics* 92:238–240, 1993.

76. **Does teething cause fever?**
Long a doctrine of grandmothers, the suggested association between teething and temperature elevation may have some basis in fact. In one study of 46 healthy infants with rectal temperatures recorded for 20 days before the eruption of the first tooth, nearly half had a new temperature elevation of more than 37.5°C on the day of the eruption. Other studies have shown some statistical association with slight temperature increase. In any event, significantly elevated fever should not be ascribed simply to teething. Listen to the grandmothers, but verify.

Macknin ML, Piedmonte M, Jacobs J, Skibinski C: Symptoms associated with infant teething: a prospective study, *Pediatrics* 105:747–752, 2000.

Jaber L, Cohen IJ, Mor A: Fever associated with teething, *Arch Dis Child* 67:233–234, 1992.

77. **What is occult bacteremia?**
Occult bacteremia refers to the finding of bacteria in the blood of patients, usually between the ages of 3 and 36 months, who are febrile without a clinically apparent focus of infection. This term should be distinguished from *septicemia*, which refers to the growth of bacteria in the blood of a child with the clinical picture of toxicity and shock.

78. **How has the pneumococcal vaccine affected the incidence of occult bacteremia?**
In trials done after the introduction of the Hib vaccine (1990) but before the introduction of the pneumococcal conjugate vaccine (2000), bacteremia rates for pneumococcus ranged from 1.6% to 3.1% in highly febrile (≥39.0°C), non–toxic-appearing children from ages 2 to 36 months. Since the introduction of the vaccine, bacteremia rates for *S. pneumoniae* have fallen to less than 1%. Children who are incompletely immunized are at higher risk compared with the fully immunized. In the post–pneumococcal conjugate vaccine era, rates of false-positive results (contaminants) now exceed true-positive rates.

Wilkinson M, Bulloch B, Smith M: Prevalence of occult bacteremia in children ages 3 to 36 months presenting to the emergency department in the postpneumococcal conjugate vaccine era, *Acad Emerg Med* 16:220–225, 2009.

Waddle E, Jhaveri R: Outcomes of febrile children without localizing signs after pneumococcal conjugate vaccine, *Arch Dis Child* 94:144–147, 2009.

79. **What is meant by "serotype replacement"?**
This is an increase in infections caused by serotypes not included in a vaccine. In the case of the conjugate pneumococcal vaccine, 7 vaccine serotypes and 2 cross-reactive serotypes composed the vaccine and accounted for about 80% of invasive pneumococcal disease. Pneumococci have more than 90 serotypes, and since the introduction of the vaccine,

there has been a rise of infections caused by nonvaccine serotypes (particularly 19A). The overall incidence of invasive disease still remains well below the prevaccine level. A 13-valent conjugate vaccine, which adds serotype 19A, was licensed in 2010. This is expected to further modify serotype replacement patterns.

Muñoz-Almagro C, Jordan I, Gene A, et al: Emergence of invasive pneumococcal disease caused by nonvaccine serotypes in the era of the 7-valent conjugate vaccine, *Clin Infect Dis* 46: 183–185, 2008.

CDC. Licensure of a 13-valent pneumococcal conjugate vaccine (PCV13) and recommendations for use among children, 2010, *JAMA* 303:2026–2028, 2010.

80. **What are the Yale Observation Scales?**

    This set of six items of observation and physical signs was designed at Yale to assist in detecting serious illness in febrile children who were younger than 24 months old. Normal (1 point), moderate impairment (3 points), and severe impairment (5 points) scores are given for quality of cry, reaction to parental stimulation, state of alertness, color, hydration, and response to social overtures. Scores of 10 or less correlate with a low likelihood of serious illness, primarily in infants older than 2 months.

    McCarthy PL, Sharpe MR, Spiesel SZ, et al: Observation scales to identify serious illness in febrile children, *Pediatrics* 70:802–809, 1982.

81. **What is the proper way to evaluate and manage febrile illness in infants who are younger than 60 days?**

    This remains a contentious issue even in the era of the conjugate pneumococcal vaccine. On average, up to 10% of febrile infants who are younger than 2 months have serious bacterial infections (bacteremia, meningitis, osteomyelitis, septic arthritis, urinary tract infection, or pneumonia). The incidence of bacterial meningitis, however, is thought to be declining, in part owing to lower rates in older infants because of vaccinations. Additionally, a well physical appearance does not rule out the presence of bacterial disease because up to 65% of febrile infants with serious bacterial infection may appear well on initial examination. In the past, combinations of clinical and laboratory criteria were developed to identify patients who might be at "low risk" for serious bacterial infection and might be managed as outpatients. These were not found to be reliable in infants younger than 1 month. In general, patients younger than 1 month with fever ($\geq$38.0°C) warrant aggressive evaluation, including blood, urine, and CSF cultures, because of higher rates of bacteremia (including pathogens from the neonatal period such as group B streptococci) and greater difficulty in global assessment of wellness. For infants between 1 and 2 months for whom development may vary (e.g., ability to socially smile, quality of reaction to parental stimulation), the approach can be more varied (including possible omission of lumbar puncture [LP]), particularly if diagnostic testing meets low-risk criteria and reliable follow-up is ensured. One laboratory approach to the outpatient management of the febrile infant (29 to 60 days; temperature $\geq$38°C) is one from the Children's Hospital of Philadelphia. Patients are categorized as "low risk" and followed as outpatients without antibiotic therapy if the following criteria are met:

    ■ Well-appearing infant
    ■ No evidence of focal infection on physical examination
    ■ Total peripheral blood white blood cell (WBC) count 5000 to 15,000/mm^3
    ■ CSF WBC count less than 8/mm^3 and gram negative (if done)
    ■ Urinalysis: less than 10 WBCs per high-power field and 3 or less bacteria per high-power field on spun specimen
    ■ No pulmonary infiltrate on chest radiograph, if performed

    Baker MD, Avner JR: The febrile infant: what's new? *Clin Pediatr Emerg Med* 9:213–220, 2008.

82. **How should older infants and toddlers (3 to 36 months old) with fever and no apparent source be managed?**
The widespread use of vaccines for *H. influenzae* type b and *S. pneumoniae* has dramatically reduced invasive bacterial disease. Previously, much of the evaluation that centered on febrile children in this age group dealt with identifying possible occult bacteremia with the intent of using empiric antibiotic treatment to lessen the chance of dissemination to focal complications (particularly meningitis). However, rates of bacteremia and meningitis have fallen dramatically. The most common cause of serious bacterial infection in children with fever without a source is an occult urinary tract infection. Most pediatric infectious disease experts no longer recommend a complete blood count and/or blood culture or any laboratory tests (other than urinalysis and urine culture in certain settings) in the evaluation of a well-appearing febrile infant older than 90 days who has received Hib and pneumococcal vaccines because of the low risk for bacteremia and meningitis.

Avner JR, Baker MD: Occult bacteremia in the post pneumococcal conjugate vaccine era: does the blood culture stop here? *Acad Emerg Med* 16:258–260, 2009.

Mahajan P, Stanley R: Fever in the toddler-aged child: old concerns replaced with new ones, *Clin Pediatr Emerg Med* 9:221–227, 2008.

83. **When is a chest radiograph indicated for a febrile young infant?**
Although some clinicians believe that chest radiographs should be performed for all febrile infants who are younger than 2 to 3 months, others reserve this study for infants who have respiratory symptoms or signs, including cough, tachypnea, irregular breathing, retractions, rales, wheezing, or decreased breath sounds. In a study of infants younger than 8 weeks who were admitted with fever, 31% of patients with respiratory manifestations had an abnormal chest radiograph, compared with only 1% of asymptomatic infants. That study was done in the pre–pneumococcal vaccine era. Leukocytosis (>20,000/mL) in febrile (>39°C) patients younger than 5 years increases the likelihood of an "occult pneumonia." In most cases, it is not possible to differentiate viral from bacterial pneumonias radiologically.

Murphy CG, van de Pol AC, Harper MB, et al: Clinical predictors of occult pneumonia in the febrile child, *Acad Emerg Med* 14:243–249, 2007.

Crain EF, Bulas D, Bijur PE, Goldman HS: Is a chest radiograph necessary in the evaluation of every febrile infant less than 8 weeks of age? *Pediatrics* 88:821–824, 1991.

84. **How long should one wait before a blood culture is designated negative?**
Bacterial growth is evident in most cultures of infected blood within 48 hours or earlier. With the use of continuous monitoring techniques, a study at Children's Hospital of Philadelphia of 200 cultures from central venous catheters found that the median time for a positive blood culture was 14 hours. In addition, 99.2% of cultures with gram-negative bacteria were positive by 36 hours, and 97% of cultures with gram-positive bacteria were positive by 36 hours. A study from Australia of neonatal blood cultures found that the median time for positivity for group B streptococcus was 9 hours, that for *Escherichia coli* was 11 hours, and that for coagulase-negative staphylococci was 29 hours.

Although 36 to 48 hours is generally sufficient time to isolate common bacteria present in the bloodstream, fastidious organisms may take longer to grow. Therefore, when one suspects anaerobes, fungi, or other organisms with special growth requirements, a longer time should be allowed before concluding that a culture is negative.

Shah SS, Downes KJ, et al: How long does it take to "rule out" bacteremia in children with central venous catheters? *Pediatrics* 121:135–141, 2008.

Jardine L, Davies MW, Faoagali J: Incubation time required for neonatal blood cultures to become positive, *J Paediatr Child Health* 42:797–802, 2006.

85. **How should a child with fever and petechiae be evaluated?**
In these patients, the most significant concern is serious systemic bacterial infection, particularly meningococcemia. When prospectively evaluated in one large study from Boston Children's Hospital, the incidence of bacteremia or clinical sepsis in patients with petechiae and fever was low (<2%), and no well-appearing children had meningococcemia when evaluated. Another study found that five physical findings, if any were present, increased the likelihood of invasive disease: ill appearance, nuchal rigidity, purpuric skin hemorrhages, universal distribution, and skin hemorrhages larger than 2 mm. Important features of the evaluation are as follows:
- **History:** Elicit information about exposures, travel, animal contacts, and immunizations.
- **Physical examination:** Assess vital signs, general appearance, signs of toxicity, evidence of nuchal rigidity, presence of purpura, and distribution of petechiae (patients with systemic bacterial infection rarely have petechiae confined to the head and neck).
- **Laboratory:** Obtain blood culture, complete blood count with differential, and prothrombin and partial thromboplastin times; consider the examination of cerebrospinal fluid.

Nielsen HE, Anderson EA, Anderson J, et al: Diagnostic assessment of hemorrhagic rash and fever, *Arch Dis Child* 85:160–165, 2001.

Mandl KD, Stack AM, Fleisher GR: Incidence of bacteremia in infants and children with fever and petechiae, *J Pediatr* 131:398–404, 1997.

86. **When is a fever considered a fever of unknown origin (FUO)?**
FUO is defined as the presence of daily (or nearly daily) fever (temperature of >38.3°C [101°F]) in a single illness in a patient for whom a careful history, thorough physical examination, and preliminary laboratory data after 1 week fail to reveal the probable cause. Definitions of duration in children vary but range from 14 to 21 days.

87. **What is the eventual etiology of fever in children with FUO?**
The differential diagnosis is extremely broad. The three major categories for pediatric patients are infections, collagen-vascular diseases (e.g., vasculitis, rheumatoid arthritis), and neoplasms. A large number of cases have no identifiable cause, and the fever resolves without explanation. The largest category is *infections*. As a general rule, in children younger than 6 years, the most common causes involve respiratory or genitourinary tract infections, localized infections (abscess, osteomyelitis), juvenile rheumatoid arthritis, and, infrequently, leukemia. Adolescents, on the other hand, are more likely to have tuberculosis, inflammatory bowel disease, another autoimmune process, or, infrequently, lymphoma.

Edwards KM, Halasa NB: Fever of unknown origin (FUO) and recurrent fever. In Bergelson JM, Shah SS, Zaoutis TE, editors: *Pediatric Infectious Diseases: The Requisites in Pediatrics*, Philadelphia, 2008, Mosby Elsevier, pp 266–273.

88. **How should a child with FUO be evaluated?**
FUO is more likely to be an unusual presentation of a common disorder than a common presentation of a rare disorder. A complete and detailed history is key, with particular attention to possible exposures, including animals, unpasteurized milk (*Yersinia* or *Campylobacter*), uncooked poultry, ticks, pica, or dirt ingestion (possible *Toxocara* or *Toxoplasma*), rabbits (*Tularemia*), mosquitoes, stagnant water, and reptiles (*Salmonella*). Travel history is also important. After performing a thorough physical examination, one should avoid indiscriminately ordering a large battery of tests. Initial tests include a complete blood count, screen for inflammation (C-reactive protein or erythrocyte sedimentation rate), tests of renal function, liver enzymes, uric acid, LDH, urinalysis, urine and blood cultures, tuberculin skin test and chest radiograph. Laboratory studies should subsequently be directed as much as possible toward the most likely diagnostic possibilities.

Tolan RW Jr: Fever of unknown origin: a diagnostic approach to this vexing problem, *Clin Pediatr* 49:207–213, 2010.

89. **What is PFAPA?**

    PFAPA is the acronym for the syndrome of **p**eriodic **f**ever, **a**phthous stomatitis, **p**haryngitis, and cervical **a**denitis, a clinical syndrome of unclear etiology that is responsive to very short courses of corticosteroids for individual episodes and is perhaps the most common cause of regular, recurrent fevers in children.

    Feder HM, Salazar JC: A clinical review of 105 patients with PFAPA (a periodic fever syndrome), *Acta Paediatr* 99:178–184, 2010.

90. **In addition to PFAPA, which syndromes are associated with periodic fevers?**

    Predictable periodic fever is a cardinal feature of a small number of *autoinflammatory disorders*, which are thought to be due to primary dysregulation of the innate immune system and may involve mutated proteins. Many are hereditary and have ethnic predilections. Many present during childhood. Periodic fever is uncommon in infectious diseases and malignancies. The most common periodic fever syndromes are summarized in Table 11-4.

TABLE 11-4. CHARACTERISTICS OF PFAPA VERSUS OTHER SELECTED FEVER SYNDROMES			
	PFAPA	**Familial Mediterranean Fever**	**Hyper-IgD Syndrome (HIDS)**	**TNF-Receptor-Associated Periodic Syndrome (TRAPS)**
Age at onset	Childhood	<10 yr (80%)	Childhood	Variable
Length of fever episode	4 days	2 days	4-6 days	1-3 wk
Interval between fever episodes	2-8 wk	Irregular	Irregular	Irregular
Associated symptoms and signs	Aphthous stomatitis, pharyngitis, adenitis	Painful pleuritis, peritonitis, oligoarthritis, foot and ankle rash	Abdominal pain, cervical adenopathy, splenomegaly	Abdominal pain, pleuritis, rash, myalgias, orbital edema
Inheritance	Random	Autosomal recessive	Autosomal recessive	Autosomal dominant

IgD, immunoglobulin D; PFAPA, syndrome of periodic fever, aphthous stomatitis, pharyngitis, and cervical adenitis; TNF, tumor necrosis factor.
Data from Goldsmith DP: Periodic fever syndromes. Pediatr Rev 30: e34-e41, 2009.

HUMAN IMMUNODEFICIENCY VIRUS INFECTION

91. **When did human immunodeficiency virus (HIV) testing begin on blood that was intended for transfusion?**
Spring of 1985. Patients at greatest risk for acquired immunodeficiency syndrome (AIDS) from a transfusion are those who received their transfusions from 1978 to the spring of 1985.

92. **How common is the maternal-to-infant transmission of HIV?**
Virtually all infants born to HIV-1–seropositive mothers will acquire antibody to the virus transplacentally. About 25% (range, 13% to 39%) of these infants will ultimately develop active HIV infection. In nonbreastfeeding populations, about 30% of maternal-to-infant HIV transmission occurs *in utero*, and the remainder occurs intrapartum. Vertical transmission of HIV-2 is less common, occurring in 0% to 4% of cases.

DeCock KM, Fowler MG, Mercier E, et al: Mother-to-child transmission of HIV-1: timing and implications for prevention, *Lancet Infect Dis* 11:726–732, 2006.

Abrams EJ, Weedon J, Bertolli J, et al, New York City Pediatric Surveillance of Disease Consortium, Centers for Disease Control and Prevention: Aging cohort of perinatally human immunodeficiency virus-infected children in New York City. New York City Pediatric Surveillance of Disease Consortium, *Pediatr Infect Dis J* 20:511–517, 2001.

93. **What drugs have been proved effective for reducing the maternal-to-infant transmission of HIV?**
In a landmark study published in 1994, treatment with zidovudine (AZT) administered antepartum and intrapartum to the mother and postnatally to the infant reduced transmission by about two thirds. In another study conducted in Africa, treatment with nevirapine administered intrapartum to the mother (200 mg at the onset of labor) and postnatally to the infant (2 mg/kg at 72 hours of life or time of discharge) resulted in a 47% decrease in the rate of transmission. However, this regimen of nevirapine appears to result in high rates of nevirapine resistance.

Currently, interventions to prevent transmission target the late intrauterine and intrapartum periods when the highest likelihood of transmission occurs. HIV-infected pregnant women in the United States are treated the same as nonpregnant adults, generally with combination antiretroviral therapy. Treatment with AZT alone is reserved for the rare pregnant woman with a normal CD4 count and a low or undetectable viral load who otherwise would not require therapy. All HIV-exposed newborn infants should receive AZT at 2 mg/kg/dose orally every 6 hours for the first 6 weeks of life. Among infants born to mothers with high viral loads and multidrug-resistant strains, treatment with additional agents is advisable. Elective caesarean delivery is also recommended for women with high HIV loads.

Committee on Pediatric AIDS: HIV testing and prophylaxis to prevent mother-to-child transmission in the United States, *Pediatrics* 122:1127–1134, 2008.

Jackson JB, Musoke P, Fleming T, et al: Intrapartum and neonatal single dose nevirapine compared with zidovudine for prevention of mother to child transmission of HIV-1 in Kampala, Uganda: 18-month follow-up of the HIVNET 012 randomised trial, *Lancet* 354:795–802, 1999.

Connor EM, Sperling RS, Gelber RS, et al: Reduction of maternal-infant transmission of human immunodeficiency virus type 1 with zidovudine treatment, *N Engl J Med* 331:1173–1180, 1994.

94. **What are the risk factors for perinatal transmission of HIV?**
- AZT monotherapy during pregnancy (compared with combination antiretroviral therapy)
- High maternal viral load
- Rupture of membranes more than 4 hours before delivery

- Fetal instrumentation with scalp electrodes and forceps
- Vaginal delivery (especially with high maternal viral loads)
- Episiotomies and vaginal tears
- Prematurity and low birthweight (possible impaired fetal or placental membranes)
- Concurrent maternal HSV-2 infection (increased shedding of HIV in genital secretions)
- Breastfeeding

Paintsil E, Andiman WA: Update on successes and challenges regarding mother-to-child transmission of HIV, *Curr Opin Pediatr* 21:95, 2009.

95. Should HIV-infected women breastfeed?

No and yes. HIV has been shown to be present in breast milk and also to be transmissible by breastfeeding. Worldwide, up to one third to one half of maternal-to-child transmission of HIV may occur through breastfeeding. This risk is increased when the infection is acquired after birth. Thus, in developed countries where alternative means of nutrition (i.e., formula) are readily available, breastfeeding is not recommended. In developing countries where breastfeeding may be protective against other causes of significant morbidity and mortality (e.g., diarrheal and respiratory illnesses) and alternative means of nutrition are less reliably available, recommendations remain a dilemma. The World Health Organization recommends exclusive breastfeeding when replacement feeding is not acceptable, feasible, affordable, or safe. Exclusive breastfeeding appears to have lower rates of transmission than mixed (e.g., formula and solid foods) breastfeeding. It remains unclear what is the optimal duration of breastfeeding to balance its protective effect and yet to minimize HIV transmission. Also unclear is whether maternal antiretroviral treatment during lactation will reduce the risk for HIV-1 transmission during breastfeeding.

Kuhn L, Reitz C, Abrams EJ: Breastfeeding and AIDS in the developing world, *Curr Opin Pediatr* 21: 83–93, 2009.

Coovadia HM, Rollins NC, Bland RM, et al: Mother-to-child transmission of HIV-1 infection during exclusive breastfeeding in the first 6 months of life: an intervention cohort study, *Lancet* 369:1107–1116, 2007.

96. How is a newborn infant whose mother is infected with HIV confirmed to also be infected?

Because maternal antibody may persist in the infant well into the second year of life, enzyme-linked immunosorbent assay testing and Western blot testing are unreliable until about 18 months of age. The diagnosis of HIV infection in the newborn therefore usually relies on the direct detection of the virus or viral components in the infant's blood or body fluids. The gold standard for diagnostic testing of infants and children younger than 18 months is HIV-1 NAAT, which can directly detect HIV-1 DNA or RNA.

Infants born to HIV-infected women, who have not taken antiretroviral therapy, should be tested by HIV-1 NAAT during the first few days of life to determine whether *in utero* acquisition has occurred. If a mother has been taking antiretroviral therapy since the second trimester, has a virus load undetectable the week before delivery, and has received 3 hours of zidovudine intravenously before delivery, the risk for *in utero* transmission is low. An HIV-1 NAAT should be done at 14 days of life. If negative, the test is repeated at 4 weeks. (If negative again, a *presumptive* diagnosis of disease exclusion is made.) A negative HIV-1 NAAT at 8 weeks also *presumptively* indicates disease exclusion. For those who are presumptively negative, a repeat HIV-1 NAAT at 4 months, if negative, is thought to *definitively* exclude HIV-1 infection. Any time a positive result is obtained, testing should be repeated on a second blood sample as soon as possible. The diagnosis of HIV infection is established if two separate samples are found to be positive by polymerase chain reaction. For children with negative testing, many experts recommend HIV-1 antibody assay testing at 12 to 18 months to confirm the absence of HIV infection.

Havens PL, Mofenson LM: Evaluation and management of the infant exposed to HIV-1 in the United States, *Pediatrics* 123:175–187, 2009.

Schutzbank WS, Steele RW: Management of the child born to an HIV-positive mother, *Clin Pediatr* 48:467–471, 2009.

97. **Can cord blood be used for newborn testing for HIV-1?**
    No. Cord blood has an unacceptably high rate of false-positive test results owing to possible contamination from maternal blood.

    Havens PL, Mofenson LM: Evaluation and management of the infant exposed to HIV-1 in the United States, *Pediatrics* 123:175–187, 2009.

98. **What are the earliest and most common manifestations of congenital HIV infection?**
    - Most infants with congenital HIV infection are asymptomatic at birth, although occasional patients have diffuse lymphadenopathy and hepatosplenomegaly.
    - Older infants with HIV infection commonly present symptoms of failure to thrive, mucocutaneous candidiasis (especially after 1 year), hepatosplenomegaly, interstitial pneumonitis, or a combination of these features.
    - Toddlers and older children with HIV infection may have generalized lymphadenopathy, recurrent bacterial infections, recurrent or chronic parotitis, or progressive encephalopathy and loss of developmental milestones.

    Simpkins EP, Siberry GK, Hutton N: Thinking about HIV infection, *Pediatr Rev* 30:337–348, 2009.

99. **When should *Pneumocystis* prophylaxis begin and end for an HIV-exposed infant?**
    Historically, the peak incidence of *Pneumocystis* pneumonia in HIV-infected infants occurred at the age of 3 months (range, 4 weeks to 6 months). Given that vertical transmission of HIV cannot be definitely excluded until the patient is at least 4 months old, *Pneumocystis* prophylaxis should be initiated at the age of 4 to 6 weeks and continued until the infant is at least 4 months old. If the HIV status of the child is indeterminate or confirmed positive, *Pneumocystis jiroveci* pneumonia prophylaxis should be continued until the child is 12 months old, at which time reassessment is done (based on CD4 T-lymphocyte counts).

100. **Among patients younger than 13 years of age with HIV infection, how does the CD4 count influence classification?**
    According to the 1994 revised Pediatric HIV Classification System, for children 12 months of age and younger, three categories are used (Table 11-5).

TABLE 11-5. CLASSIFICATION OF HUMAN IMMUNODEFICIENCY VIRUS

Category	Age-Specific CD4 T-Lymphocyte Count and Percentage of Total Lymphocytes		
	<12 mo	1-5 yr	6-12 yr
Category 1 (no immunosuppression)	≥1500 μL	≥1000 μL	≥500 μL
	≥25%	≥25%	≥25%
Category 2 (moderate suppression)	750-1499 μL	500-999 μL	200-499 μL
	15%-24%	15%-24%	15%-24%
Category 3 (severe suppression)	<750 μL	<500 μL	<200 μL
	<15%	<15%	<15%

American Academy of Pediatrics: Human immunodeficiency virus. In Pickering LK, editor: *2009 Red Book: Report of the Committee on Infectious Diseases*, ed 28, Elk Grove Park, IL, 2009, American Academy of Pediatrics, p 384.

101. **What is the significance of the "viral load"?**
   Viral load refers to a quantification of HIV viral RNA as measured by various assays. It is a measure of the degree of infection and can range from 40 to 50 copies/mL to 20 to 50 million copies/mL. Higher levels are associated with increased likelihoods of rapid disease progression and poorer long-term prognosis. Viral loads are used as an ongoing measure of efficacy of treatment with the goal to achieve an undetectable level for as long as possible.

102. **What are the major classes of antiretroviral agents (ARTs) used to treat HIV?**
   - **Nucleoside reverse transcriptase inhibitors** (NRTIs) competitively inhibit the HIV reverse transcriptase (which converts HIV RNA into DNA) and terminate the elongation of viral DNA. They require intracellular phosphorylation for activation. NRTIs have little or no effect on chronically infected cells because their site of action is before the incorporation of viral DNA into host DNA. This class of drugs includes zidovudine, lamivudine, stavudine, zalcitabine, didanosine (ddI), and abacavir.
   - **Nonnucleoside reverse transcriptase inhibitors** (NNRTIs) also inhibit the HIV reverse transcriptase, although they do so at a different site than do the NRTIs. They bind directly to the active site of HIV reverse transcriptase and do not require activation. This class of drugs includes efavirenz and nevirapine.
   - **Protease inhibitors** (PIs) inhibit the HIV protease, which cuts HIV polyprotein precursors before viral budding. This class of drugs includes amprenavir, nelfinavir, ritonavir, indinavir, saquinavir, and lopinavir.
   - Other types of agents include **fusion inhibitors, nucleotide reverse transcriptase inhibitors, integrase inhibitors,** and **entry inhibitors.**

   Guidelines for treatment of HIV-infected children and adolescents are regularly updated and available at http://www.aidsinfo.nih.gov/Guidelines. Generally, triple- or four-drug therapy (so-called highly active antiretroviral therapy, or HAART, regimens) is often recommended, including at least one PI or NNRTI.

   Patel K, Hernán MA, Williams PL, et al: Long-term effectiveness of highly active antiretroviral therapy on the survival of children and adolescents with HIV infection: a 10-year follow-up study, *Clin Infect Dis* 46:507–515, 2008.

103. **What are the common bone marrow toxicities associated with antiretroviral therapy?**
   - Anemia occurs in up to 9% of children receiving AZT (compared with 4% to 5% of those on other regimens). Neutropenia occurs in 6% to 27% of children receiving antiretroviral therapy, particularly those taking AZT and ddI.
   - Thrombocytopenia occurs in 30% of untreated children with HIV infection and is more commonly an initial presentation of HIV infection than a complication of antiretroviral therapy. In initial trials, severe thrombocytopenia was seen in 2% of children receiving either ddI and AZT or lamivudine and AZT.
   - Lipodystrophy occurs in children treated with protease inhibitors.

104. **How common is the transmission of HIV from infected children to household contacts?**
   Extremely rare. Only a handful of reports clearly implicate an infected sibling as the source of HIV infection. Nevertheless, children with HIV infection should be instructed regarding good hygiene and appropriate behavior, and their families should be counseled about HIV and its transmission.

105. **Should a classroom teacher be told that a child is HIV positive?**
There is no absolute requirement to inform a classroom teacher, a school principal, or any other school official about a child's HIV status. It is not necessary for anyone except the child's physician to be aware of the diagnosis. Nevertheless, in certain circumstances, it may be advisable for a family to communicate with a teacher or a principal.

> American Academy of Pediatrics: School health. In Pickering LK, editor: *2009 Red Book: Report of the Committee on Infectious Diseases*, ed 28, Elk Grove Park, IL, 2009, American Academy of Pediatrics, p 146.

KEY POINTS: HUMAN IMMUNODEFICIENCY VIRUS INFECTION

1. Interventions to prevent maternal HIV transmission target the late intrauterine and intrapartum periods when the highest likelihood of transmission occurs.

2. Most infants with congenital HIV infection are asymptomatic at birth.

3. The gold standard for diagnostic testing of infants and children younger than 18 months is HIV-1 nucleic acid amplification testing (NAAT), which can directly detect HIV-1 DNA or RNA.

4. Viral loads are used as an ongoing measure of treatment efficacy.

5. Triple- or four-drug therapy (so-called highly active antiretroviral therapy, or HAART, regimens) is often recommended for HIV-infected children.

6. Risk factors for increased HIV transmission after a needlestick injury include a high viral inoculum, large volume of blood, and deep puncture wound.

106. **What are the risk factors for HIV transmission after a needlestick injury?**
- High viral inoculum (patient with advanced disease)
- Large volume of blood (from a large-diameter needle)
- Deep puncture wound

Overall, the risk for transmission from needles contaminated with the blood of an HIV-infected patient is roughly 0.3%. Risk from a puncture wound found in the community is thought to be lower. There are no known transmissions from accidental nonoccupational (community) needlesticks. These risk factors were identified in a case-control study that involved 33 health care workers and 665 controls.

> American Academy of Pediatrics: Human immunodeficiency virus infection. In Pickering LK, editor: *2009 Red Book: Report of the Committee on Infectious Diseases*, ed 28, Elk Grove Park, IL, 2009, American Academy of Pediatrics, pp 399–400.

> Cardo DM, Culver DH, Ciesielski CA, et al: A case-control study of HIV seroconversion in health care workers after percutaneous exposure. Centers for Disease Control and Prevention Needlestick Surveillance Group, *N Engl J Med* 337:1485–1490, 1997.

107. **When should postexposure prophylaxis be given after a needlestick injury?**
Data from health care workers suggest that prophylaxis is most effective when given within 1 to 2 hours of exposure, and data from animal studies suggest that prophylaxis is not effective if it is initiated more than 24 to 72 hours after exposure. It is recommended that postexposure prophylaxis be continued for 4 weeks. With exposure to known HIV-infected

blood, postexposure prophylaxis has been shown to reduce the transmission of HIV in health care workers by about 81%. Guidelines for extent of therapy (up to three drugs) have been developed depending on percutaneous injuries that are either less severe (solid needle or superficial injury) or more severe (large-bore hollow needle, deep puncture, visible blood on device, or needle used in patient's artery or vein). The severity of HIV disease in the patient also factors in the type of treatment. A National Clinicians' Post-Exposure Prophylaxis Hotline is available at 888-448-4911.

U.S. Public Health Service: Updated U.S. Public Health Service guidelines for the management of occupational exposures to HIV and recommendations for postexposure prophylaxis, *MMWR Recomm Rep* 54:1–17, 2005.

IMMUNIZATIONS

108. **Why are the buttocks a poor location for intramuscular injections in infants?**
The gluteus maximus is not a good choice for injections because of the following:
- The gluteus muscles are incompletely developed in some infants.
- There is a potential for injury to the sciatic nerve or the superior gluteal artery if the injection is misdirected.
- Some vaccinations may be less effective if they are injected into fat (e.g., vaccines for rabies, influenza, and hepatitis B).

If injections into the buttocks are given to older children, the proper site is the gluteus medius in the upper outer quadrant rather than the gluteus maximus, which is more medial.

Zuckerman JN: The importance of injecting vaccines into muscle, *BMJ* 321:1237–1238, 2000.

109. **When administering an intramuscular vaccination, is aspiration necessary before injection?**
Traditionally, the plunger has been withdrawn to verify that the needle tip is not in a vein. However, when vaccinations are given as recommended in the anterior-lateral thigh in an infant or in the deltoid in toddlers older than 18 months, aspiration before injection is *not* required because no large blood vessels are located at those preferred sites. Additionally, the process of aspiration before injection is more painful and takes longer to administer.

Ipp M: Vaccine-related pain: randomized controlled trial of two injection techniques, *Arch Dis Child* 92:1105, 2007.

American Academy of Pediatrics: Acute immunization. In Pickering LK, editor: *2009 Red Book: Report of the Committee on Infectious Diseases*, ed 28, Elk Grove Park, IL, 2009, American Academy of Pediatrics, p 20.

110. **Do shorter or longer needles result in more local reactions when immunizations are given to infants?**
When compared, longer needles (25 mm) result in fewer local reactions following vaccination compared with shorter needles (16 mm). Although it would seem intuitive that a shorter needle would result in less trauma and less reaction, the longer needles are more likely to reach the muscle for deposition of the vaccine. Injection into subcutaneous tissue where blood vessels are fewer may allow more time for vaccine components to linger and create more local inflammation.

Diggle L, Deeks JJ, Pollard AJ: Effect of needle size on immunogenicity and reactogenicity of vaccines in infants: randomized, controlled trial, *BMJ* 333:571, 2006.

111. **Is there any risk associated with administering multiple vaccines simultaneously?**
Most vaccines can be administered simultaneously at separate sites without concern about effectiveness because the immune response to one vaccine generally does not interfere

with immune responses to others. The immune system is capable of recognizing hundreds of thousands of antigens. However, some exceptions exist. For example, the simultaneous administration of cholera vaccine and yellow fever vaccine is associated with interference.

112. **Should premature babies receive immunization on the basis of postconception age or chronologic age?**
In most cases, premature babies should be immunized in accordance with postnatal chronologic age. If a premature infant is still in the hospital at 2 months of age, the vaccines routinely scheduled for that age should be administered, including diphtheria, tetanus, acellular pertussis, *H. influenzae* type B, heptavalent pneumococcal, and inactivated poliovirus vaccines.

Among premature infants who weigh less than 2 kg at birth, seroconversion rates to hepatitis B vaccine are relatively low when immunization is initiated shortly after birth. Accordingly, in these infants, if the mother is HBsAg negative, immunization should be delayed until just before hospital discharge or until 30 days of age.

Saari TN, American Academy of Pediatrics Committee on Infectious Diseases: Immunization of preterm and low birth weight infants. American Academy of Pediatrics Committee on Infectious Diseases, *Pediatrics* 112:193–198, 2003.

113. **Which vaccines are egg-embryo–based vaccines?**
Of the immunizations that are commonly administered to children, **measles-mumps-rubella** (MMR) vaccine preparations are grown in chick embryo fibroblast culture. Recent studies indicate that children with egg allergy are at low risk for anaphylaxis to MMR and do not require skin testing before the administration of this vaccine.

Influenza vaccine contains egg protein and on rare occasions induces immediate hypersensitivity reactions, including anaphylaxis. In children who have a history of severe anaphylactic reactions to eggs and who are scheduled to receive influenza vaccine, skin testing is recommended. However, in most cases, these children should not receive the influenza vaccine and should instead be prescribed chemoprophylaxis as necessary.

The vaccine for **yellow fever** is prepared in eggs and contains egg protein.

114. **What is the difference between whole-cell and acellular pertussis vaccines?**
Whole-cell pertussis vaccines consist of whole bacteria that have been inactivated and are nonviable. These vaccines contain lipo-oligosaccharide and other cell wall components that result in a high incidence of adverse effects.

Acellular pertussis vaccines contain one or more *B. pertussis* proteins that serve as immunogens. All acellular pertussis vaccines contain at least detoxified pertussis toxin, and most contain other antigens as well, including filamentous hemagglutinin, fimbrial proteins, and pertactin. The acellular vaccines are associated with a much lower incidence of side effects and thus are preferred for all doses in the United States.

115. **What are the absolute contraindications to pertussis immunization?**
The adverse events after pertussis immunization that represent absolute contraindications to further administration of pertussis vaccine include the following:
- Immediate anaphylactic reaction
- Encephalopathy within 7 days of vaccination

The adverse events that represent precautions for further administration of pertussis vaccine include the following:
- A seizure (with or without fever) within 3 days of immunization
- Persistent, severe, inconsolable screaming or crying for 3 hours or longer within 2 days of immunization
- Collapse or shocklike state within 2 days of vaccination

■ Body temperature of 40.5°C or higher (≥104.8°F), unexplained by another cause, within 2 days of immunization

When a contraindication to pertussis immunization exists, diphtheria-tetanus vaccine should be administered instead.

American Academy of Pediatrics: Pertussis. In Pickering LK, editor: *2009 Red Book: Report of the Committee on Infectious Diseases*, ed 28, Elk Grove Park, IL, 2009, American Academy of Pediatrics, p 514.

116. **How long does protection against pertussis last after immunization?**
Vaccine-induced immunity to pertussis is relatively short lived. On the basis of studies of patients who have been immunized with a whole-cell pertussis vaccine and exposed to a sibling with pertussis, protection against infection is about 80% during the first 3 years after immunization, dropping to 50% at 4 to 7 years and to near 0% at 11 years. Teenagers and adults thus become susceptible to pertussis and serve as vectors for infants, for whom morbidity and mortality are much higher. Because of the slow, steady resurgence of pertussis in the past two decades and the availability of an acellular pertussis Vaccines combined with diphtheria and tetanus toxoid (Tdap), the Advisory Committee on Immunization Practices of the Centers for Disease Control and Prevention has recommended that all adolescents >11 should receive a booster dose.

Halperin SA: The control of pertussis—2007 and beyond, *N Engl J Med* 356:110–113, 2007.

117. **Which vaccines offer protection against cervical cancer?**
Vaccination for **human papillomavirus (HPV).** The first vaccine against HPV (Gardasil) was approved in 2006. It is a quadrivalent vaccine (HPV4) that prevents disease cause by HPV types 6, 11, 16, and 18. A bivalent vaccine (HPV2, Cervarix) was approved in 2009. HPV types 16 and 18 have been causally linked with cervical, vulvar, and vaginal cancers with the peak incidence occurring among the 40- to 49-year-old age group.

Jenson HB: Human papillomavirus vaccine: a paradigm shift for pediatricians, *Curr Opin Pediatr* 21:112–121, 2009.

118. **How effective is the pneumococcal conjugate vaccine?**
The heptavalent pneumococcal conjugate vaccine is highly effective against invasive pneumococcal disease, reducing rates by up to 98% for vaccine-associated serotypes in children fully vaccinated during the first 2 years of life. The greatest decline in invasive disease has been in the number of children experiencing bacteremia without a focus. This vaccine has a modest effect on pneumococcal otitis media, preventing about 35% of culture-confirmed cases in young children. A concern has been the possible shift of pneumococcal serotypes causing invasive disease to those not covered by the vaccine, particularly serotype 19a.

Alter SJ: Pneumococcal infections, *Pediatr Rev* 30:155–164, 2009.

119. **What is the "grandparent effect" of vaccination?**
The rate of invasive pneumococcal disease has declined in people older than 65 years since the introduction of the conjugate pneumococcal in 2000. Meningitis rates have declined by 54%. Decreased nasopharyngeal carriage among vaccinated infants has likely reduced transmission to older individuals caring for them. This type of "herd effect" in elderly people is referred to as the *grandparent effect*.

Hsu HE, Shutt KA, Moore MR, et al: Effect of pneumococcal conjugate vaccine on pneumococcal meningitis, *N Engl J Med* 360:244–256, 2009.

Millar EV, Watt JP, Bronsdon MA, et al: Indirect effect of 7-valent pneumococcal conjugate vaccine on pneumococcal colonization among unvaccinated household members, *Clin Infect Dis* 47:989–996, 2008.

120. **What serogroup capable of causing meningococcal infections is lacking in licensed vaccines in the United States?**

Serogroup B isolates account for about one third of cases of meningococcal disease, but serogroup B polysaccharide is absent from these vaccines. Two quadrivalent meningococcal vaccines containing capsular polysaccharide from serogroups A, C, Y, and W135 are available in the United States, including a plain polysaccharide vaccine that is approved for use in children at least 2 years old and a polysaccharide diphtheria toxoid conjugate vaccine that is licensed for use in individuals 11 to 55 years old. A study in infants with the a new tetravalent vaccine using a nontoxic mutant of diphtheria toxoid as the carrier protein has demonstrated good immunogenicity and may become part of the vaccination schedule for infants in the future.

All 11- to 12-year-olds should be vaccinated with the conjugate vaccine routinely. In addition, unvaccinated college freshmen living in dormitories should be offered either the plain polysaccharide vaccine or the conjugate vaccine. Vaccination is considered advisable for children at least 2 years old who are in high-risk groups, including those with functional or anatomic asplenia or complement deficiency.

A meningococcal vaccine is given to all military recruits in the United States and should be considered for individuals traveling to areas of epidemic or hyperendemic disease. In addition, the current vaccines may be useful as an adjunct to chemoprophylaxis for the control of outbreaks caused by a vaccine serogroup.

Snape MD, Perrett KP, Ford KJ, et al: Immunogenicity of a tetravalent meningococcal glycoconjugate vaccine in infants: a randomized controlled trial, *JAMA* 299:173–184, 2008.

Bilukha OO, Rosentein N: Prevention and control of meningococcal disease: recommendations of the Advisory Committee on Immunization Practices, *MMWR* 54:1–21, 2005.

121. **How effective is the varicella vaccine if given after exposure to the illness?**

The varicella vaccine is highly effective (95% for the prevention of any disease, 100% for the prevention of moderate to severe disease) when used within 36 hours of exposure in an environment involving close contact. The reason for the high efficacy is that naturally acquired varicella-zoster virus usually takes 5 to 7 days to propagate in the respiratory tract before primary viremia and dissemination occur, whereas vaccine virus may elicit humeral and cellular immunity in significantly less time.

Watson B, Seward J, Yang A, et al: Postexposure effectiveness of varicella vaccine, *Pediatrics* 105: 84–88, 2000.

122. **Why is a varicella booster now recommended?**

The varicella vaccine was introduced in 1996, and by 2005, 88% of eligible children had been vaccinated in large part because most states had made varicella immunization mandatory for school entrance. Compared with the prevaccine era, cases declined by 71% to 84%. However, breakthrough disease was reported with increasing frequency in vaccinated children because a single dose of the vaccine was found to be only 85% effective. Data also indicated waning protection from a single dose over 5 years. In 2007, the recommendations by the Advisory Committee on Immunization Practices were for the first dose of a varicella-containing vaccine at 12 to 15 months of age and a second dose at 4 to 6 years.

Asch-Goodkin J: Varicella vaccines: time for a second dose, *Contemp Pediatr* 24:9S–10S, 2007.

123. **Of the vaccines included in the routine schedule, which ones contain live viruses?**

MMR and **varicella**. Oral polio vaccine is a live attenuated virus vaccine, but it is no longer recommended for routine use. Other live virus vaccines include cold-adapted, live-attenuated influenza, rotavirus, and yellow fever virus vaccines.

KEY POINTS: IMMUNIZATIONS

1. Premature babies should be immunized in accordance with postnatal chronologic age.

2. Without a booster after age 5 years, protection against pertussis infection is about 80% during the first 3 years after immunization, dropping to 50% at 4 to 7 years and to near zero at 11 years.

3. Live vaccines: measles-mumps-rubella, varicella, cold-adapted, live-attenuated influenza, rotavirus, yellow fever virus, oral polio.

4. Vaccination for human papillomavirus offers protection against cervical cancer.

5. When administering an intramuscular vaccination, aspiration is not necessary before injection.

124. **What are the indications for palivizumab?**
    Palivizumab is a humanized mouse monoclonal antibody that is directed against a respiratory syncytial virus (RSV) protein and that is approved for the prevention of RSV disease in selected children. It is typically administered intramuscularly monthly beginning in November for an additional 2 to 4 months. According to the American Academy of Pediatrics, recommendations for the consideration of palivizumab administration include the following:
    - Infants and children younger than 2 years with chronic lung disease who are requiring medical therapy
    - Infants born before 32 weeks' gestation within 6 months of the expected RSV season
    - Infants and children younger than 2 years with congenital heart disease requiring medical therapy
    - Certain infants with neuromuscular disease or congenital abnormalities of the airways that compromise handling of respiratory secretions

    American Academy of Pediatrics: Respiratory syncytial virus. In Pickering LK, editor: *2009 Red Book: Report of the Committee on Infectious Diseases*, ed 28, Elk Grove Park, IL, 2009, American Academy of Pediatrics, pp 563–567.

125. **What are the recommendations regarding the administration of live-virus vaccines to patients receiving corticosteroid therapy?**
    Children receiving corticosteroid treatment can become immunosuppressed. Although some uncertainty exists, there is adequate experience to make recommendations about the administration of live-virus vaccines to previously healthy children receiving steroid treatment. In general, live-virus vaccines should not be administered to children who have received prednisone or its equivalent in a dose of 2 mg/kg day or greater (or $\geq$20 mg per day for individuals whose weight is >10 kg) for more than 14 days. Treatment for shorter periods, with lower doses, or with topical preparations or local injections should not contraindicate the use of these vaccines.

    American Academy of Pediatrics: Immunization in special clinical circumstances. In Pickering LK, editor: *2009 Red Book: Report of the Committee on Infectious Diseases*, ed 28, Elk Grove Park, IL, 2009, American Academy of Pediatrics, pp 78–79.

126. **What is thimerosal?**
    Thimerosal is a mercury-containing preservative that has been used as an additive to vaccines for decades because of its effectiveness for preventing contamination, especially in open, multidose containers. In an effort to reduce exposure to mercury, vaccine manufacturers, the FDA, the American Academy of Pediatrics, and other groups

have worked to remove thimerosal from vaccines that contain this compound. By the end of 2001, all vaccines in the routine schedule for children and adolescents were free or virtually free of thimerosal with the exception of the some inactivated influenza vaccines.

American Academy of Pediatrics: Active immunization. In Pickering LK, editor: *2006 Red Book: Report of the Committee on Infectious Diseases*, ed 27, Elk Grove Park, IL, 2006, American Academy of Pediatrics, p 48.

127. **Does thimerosal cause autism?**
In the totality of studies to date, there is no compelling evidence that thimerosal causes autism, attention-deficit/hyperactivity disorder, or other neurodevelopmental disorders.

Tozzi AE, Bisiacchi P, Tarantino V, et al: Neuropsychological performance 10 years after vaccination in infancy with thimerosal-containing vaccines, *Pediatrics* 123:475–482, 2009.

INFECTIONS WITH RASH

128. **What is the traditional numbering of the "original" six exanthemas of childhood, and when were they first described?**
   - **First disease:** Measles (rubeola), 1627
   - **Second disease:** Scarlet fever, 1627
   - **Third disease:** Rubella, 1881
   - **Fourth disease:** Filatov-Dukes disease (described in 1900 and though to be a distinct scarlatiniform type of rubella, attributed more recently to exotoxin-producing *S. aureus*; term is no longer used)
   - **Fifth disease:** Erythema infectiosum, 1905
   - **Sixth disease:** Roseola infantum (exanthem subitum), 1910

   Weisse ME: The fourth disease: 1900–2000, *Lancet* 357:299–301, 2001.

129. **What are the three Cs of measles?**
Cough, coryza, and conjunctivitis. After an incubation period of 4 to 12 days, these symptoms develop and are followed by an erythematous and maculopapular rash (typically on day 14 after exposure), which spreads from head to feet.

130. **What do Koplik spots look like?**
Koplik spots are thought to be pathognomonic for measles. They are punctate white-gray papules that occur on a red background, initially opposite the lower molars, but they may spread to involve other parts of the mucosa. However, they may be present for a day or less and should not be relied on for the diagnosis.

131. **What is "atypical" about atypical measles?**
   - Koplik spots are rarely present.
   - Conjunctivitis and coryza are not part of the prodrome.
   - Rash begins on the distal extremities and spreads toward the head (opposite what is seen in typical measles).
   - Hepatosplenomegaly is common.
   - Respiratory distress with clinical and radiographic signs of pneumonia and pleural effusions are increased in frequency.

   Atypical measles occurs primarily in patients who have received inactivated measles vaccine, which was used in the United States from 1963 to 1968. Therefore, atypical measles in more commonly seen in adults.

132. **Why is postmeasles blindness so common in underdeveloped countries?**
As many as 1% of all patients with measles in underdeveloped regions experience the progression of keratitis to blindness. By contrast, measles keratitis in developed countries is usually self-limited and benign. There are two principal reasons for the progression to blindness among patients with measles in underdeveloped countries:
- **Vitamin A deficiency:** Vitamin A is needed for corneal stromal repair, and a deficiency allows epithelial damage to persist or worsen. Many malnourished children have accompanying vitamin A deficiency, and vitamin A supplements may be of benefit during active illness.
- **Malnutrition:** Malnutrition may predispose a patient to corneal superinfection with HSV.

133. **What are the most feared neurologic complications of measles?**
- **Acute encephalitis:** Occurring in about 1 in every 1000 cases with permanent sequelae in a significant number of cases
- **Subacute sclerosing panencephalitis:** A rare progressive neurodegenerative CNS disease with seizures and intellectual deterioration that occurs on a delayed basis (average time of 11 years) following measles in unvaccinated children

Perry RT, Halsey NA: The clinical significance of measles: a review, *J Infect Dis* 189:S4–S16, 2004.

134. **How common is human herpesvirus type-6 (HHV-6) infection in children?**
Infection with HHV-6 is ubiquitous and occurs with high frequency in infants, 65% of whom have serologic evidence of primary infection by their first birthday. Nearly all children are seropositive by age 4 years. HHV-6 infection results in typical cases of roseola and is also associated with a number of other common pediatric problems, including "fever without localizing findings," nonspecific rash, and EBV-negative mononucleosis. In a study by Hall and colleagues, up to one third of all febrile seizures in children younger than 2 years were the result of HHV-6 infections. On rare occasions, the virus has been associated with fulminant hepatitis, encephalitis, and a syndrome of massive lymphadenopathy called *Rosai-Dorfman disease*.

Hall CB, Long CE, Schnabel KC, et al: Human herpesvirus-6 infection in children, *N Engl J Med* 331:432–438, 1994.

135. **What are the etiologic agents of exanthem subitum (roseola)?**
Multiple agents are likely. HHV-6 was discovered in 1986, and, in 1988, Japanese investigators isolated it from four children with exanthem subitum. In 1994, HHV-7 was also isolated from children with the clinical features of roseola. *Roseola-like* illnesses are also noted with various echoviruses (including Coxsackie viruses A and B), parainfluenza virus, and adenoviruses.

136. **What are the typical features of roseola?**
Roseola occurs most commonly between ages 6 and 24 months. Most children have an abrupt onset of high fever (>39°C) with no prodrome. Fever usually lasts 3 to 4 days but can range from 1 to 8 days. Within 24 hours of defervescence, a discrete erythematous macular or maculopapular rash appears on the face, neck, and/or trunk. Erythematous papules (Nakayama spots) may be noted on the soft palate and the uvula in two thirds of patients. Other common findings on examination include mild cervical lymph node enlargement, edematous eyelids, and a bulging anterior fontanelle in infants. A variety of symptoms can accompany the fever, including diarrhea, cough, coryza, and headache.

Caserta MT, Hall CB, Schnabel K, et al: Primary human herpesvirus 7 infection: a comparison of human herpesvirus 7 and human herpesvirus 6 infections in children, *J Pediatr* 133:386–389, 1998.

137. **What is the spectrum of disease caused by parvovirus B19?**
- Erythema infectiosum (most common; a childhood exanthem, also called *fifth disease* or "slapped-cheek disease" because of the classic appearance of the rash)

- Papular-purpuric gloves and socks syndrome (self-limited condition of edematous plaques with petechial purpura over the palms and soles)
- Arthritis and arthralgia (most common in immunocompetent adults)
- Intrauterine infection with hydrops fetalis
- Transient aplastic crisis in patients with underlying hemolytic disease
- Persistent infection with chronic anemia in patients with immunodeficiencies
- No symptoms

138. **Describe the characteristic rash of Rocky Mountain spotted fever (RMSF).**
    - Usually seen by day 3 of illness (5 to 11 days after tick bite), but may not appear until day 6
    - Begins as blanching red macules and maculopapules, which evolve into petechiae in 1 to 3 days
    - Begins on flexor surfaces of wrists and ankles and spreads to extremities face and trunk within hours
    - As rash progresses, may become pigmented with areas of desquamation
    - Involves palms and soles

    Dantas-Torres F: Rocky Mountain spotted fever, *Lancet Infect Dis* 7:724–732, 2007.

139. **How many patients with RMSF do not develop a rash?**
    10% to 20%. Because of the relatively common lack of classic features and the importance of early treatment, RMSF should be considered in the differential diagnosis of any patient in an endemic area who presents with fever, myalgia, severe headache, nausea, and vomiting *without* rash. Presumptive empirical therapy can be begun pending diagnostic studies (biopsy or serology). Risk for death increases when therapy is delayed for more than 5 days.

140. **Why is doxycycline recommended for *all* ages in patients with suspected RMSF?**
    Alternatives for older individuals could include tetracycline, chloramphenicol, or a fluoroquinolone, but doxycycline is advised even in younger patients for the following reasons:
    - Tetracycline at the recommended dose is associated with dental staining in children younger than 8 years.
    - Doxycycline at the recommended dose is unlikely to cause dental staining in younger children.
    - Doxycycline is effective against ehrlichiosis, which can mimic RMSF, and chloramphenicol may not be effective.
    - Fluoroquinolones may cause cartilage damage in juvenile animal models, and their use is not recommended for children.
    - Chloramphenicol may have serious adverse effects (e.g., aplastic anemia), no oral preparation is available in the United States, and it may be less effective for RMSF than doxycyclinie.

    American Academy of Pediatrics: Rocky Mountain spotted fever. In Pickering LK, editor: *2009 Red Book: Report of the Committee on Infectious Diseases*, ed 28, Elk Grove Park, IL, 2009, American Academy of Pediatrics, pp 575.

    Lochary ME, Lockhart PB, Willliams WT Jr: Doxycycline and staining of permanent teeth, *Pediatr Infect Dis J* 17:429–431, 1998.

141. **What conditions can mimic RMSF?**
    - Human monocytic ehrlichiosis
    - Drug hypersensitivity
    - Meningococcemia
    - Immune thrombocytopenic purpura
    - Enteroviral infection

- Henoch-Schönlein purpura
- Staphylococcal sepsis
- Infectious mononucleosis
- Toxic shock syndrome
- Kawasaki disease
- Adenovirus infection

Razzaq S, Schutze GE: Rocky mountain spotted fever, *Pediatr Rev* 26:125–129, 2005.

142. **How are the human ehrlichioses distinguished clinically from RMSF?**
The two most commonly described ehrlichioses—human monocytic ehrlichiosis (HME) and human granulocytic anaplasmosis (HGA)—present like RMSF as an acute, systemic, febrile illness but differ in a number of ways:
    - RMSF is a vasculitis, whereas HME and HGA target macrophages and neutrophils, respectively.
    - Elevated transaminases are more common in the ehrlichioses.
    - HGA and HME have leukopenia and thrombocytopenia; WBC count is often normal in RMSF.
    - Rash occurs more commonly in RMSF; it occurs in only 66% of children with HME and in less than 10% with HGA.

Rim JY, Eppes S: Tick-borne diseases, *Pediatr Ann* 36:390–403, 2007.

143. **How long after exposure to chickenpox (varicella) do symptoms develop?**
Ninety-nine percent of patients develop symptoms between 11 and 20 days after exposure.

144. **Should "well" children with varicella be treated with acyclovir?**
Studies have shown that oral acyclovir therapy (20 mg/kg, up to 800 mg) four times daily for 5 days, initiated within 24 hours after the onset of rash, decreases the maximal number of lesions by 15% to 30%, shortens the duration of the development of new lesions, and shortens the duration of fever by 1 day. The American Academy of Pediatrics Committee on Infectious Diseases opted not to recommend acyclovir for routine use in uncomplicated varicella for otherwise healthy children younger than 13 years because of "marginal therapeutic effect, the cost of the drug, feasibility of drug delivery in the first 24 hours of illness, and the currently unknown and unforeseen possible dangers of treating as many as 4 million children each year."

American Academy of Pediatrics: Varicella-zoster infections. In Pickering LK, editor: *2006 Red Book, Report of the Committee on Infectious Diseases*, ed 27, Elk Grove Village, IL, 2006, American Academy of Pediatrics, p 674.

145. **What is the risk for varicella-associated complications in normal children 1 to 14 years old?**
The most common complications of varicella-zoster virus infection include secondary bacterial skin infections (generally due to streptococci or staphylococci), neurologic syndromes (cerebellitis, encephalitis, transverse myelitis, and Guillain-Barré syndrome), and pneumonia. Thrombocytopenia, arthritis, hepatitis, and glomerulonephritis occur less commonly. Myocarditis, pericarditis, pancreatitis, and orchitis are described but are rare.
    The frequency of these complications in normal children is not precisely known, but it is estimated to be low on the basis of hospitalization and mortality data. Before the introduction of the varicella vaccine in 1995, about 4 million cases of chickenpox occurred in the United States each year, resulting in roughly 10,000 hospitalizations and 100 deaths. Since the introduction of routine immunization against varicella, rates of infection have decreased by more than 95%.

Watson B: Varicella: a vaccine preventable disease—a review, *J Infect* 44:220–225, 2002.

146. How common are second episodes of varicella after natural infection?
About 1 in 500 cases involve a second episode. These are more likely to occur in children who develop their first episode during infancy or whose first episode is subclinical or very mild.

Gershon A: Second episodes of varicella: degree and duration of immunity, *Pediatr Infect Dis J* 9:306, 1990.

147. What are shingles?
Reactivated varicella-zoster virus infection.
After the primary infection of chickenpox, the virus establishes a latent infection in the dorsal root ganglion. When reactivation occurs, the virus spreads to the skin through nerves, and a typical vesicular pattern along dermatomal lines occurs (Fig. 11-1). In its primary form, the infection is varicella; in its recurrent form, it is zoster.

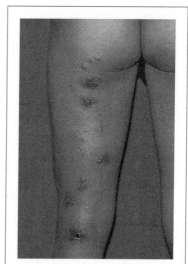

Figure 11-1. Herpes zoster with distribution along the S1 dermatome. (From Lissauer T, Clayton G: Illustrated Textbook of Pediatrics, 2nd ed. London, Mosby, 2001, p 193.)

148. In children with herpes zoster, what is the distribution of the rash?
Compared with adults, children have relatively more cervical and sacral involvement with resultant extremity and inguinal lesions:

- 50% thoracic
- 20% cervical
- 20% lumbosacral
- 10% cranial nerve

If there are lesions on the tip of the nose, herpes zoster keratitis is more likely because of possible involvement of the nasociliary nerve. When the geniculate ganglion is involved, there is risk for developing the Ramsay Hunt syndrome, which consists of ear pain with auricular and periauricular vesicles and facial nerve palsy.

Feder HM Jr, Hoss DM: Herpes zoster in otherwise healthy children, *Pediatr Infect Dis J* 23:451–457, 2004.

149. Should children with zoster be treated with antiviral agents?
Routine antiviral therapy is **not indicated.** In general, the prognosis for children with herpes zoster is very good, with extremely low probabilities of postherpetic neuralgia or of associations with undiagnosed malignancy.

150. Who gets herpes gladiatorum?
Herpes gladiatorum is a term used to describe ocular and cutaneous infection with HSV-1, which occurs in wrestlers and rugby players. The infection is transmitted primarily by direct skin-to-skin contact and is endemic among high school and college wrestlers.

151. What is the Tzanck prep?
It is a cytodiagnostic method that is used to examine blistering lesions for herpes simplex, herpes zoster, and varicella. A blister is unroofed, and scrapings of the base are placed and stained on a slide. The presence of multinucleated giant cells is diagnostic of one of those conditions (Fig. 11-2).

152. **What is hand-foot-and-mouth disease?**
Hand-foot-and-mouth disease is an illness that is caused most commonly by Coxsackie A viruses (especially A16) or enterovirus 71. It is associated with a petechial or vesicular exanthem involving the hands, the feet, and the oral mucosa.

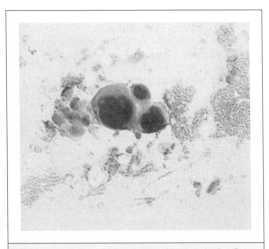

Figure 11-2. Tzanck preparation with multinucleated cells. (From Zitelli BJ, Davis HW: Atlas of Pediatric Physical Diagnosis, 4th ed. St. Louis, Mosby, 2002, p 277.)

INFLUENZA

153. **What are the types of influenza viruses?**
   - **Influenza A:** Infects many species, including humans, pigs, horses, and birds. It is subtyped on the basis of two surface glycoprotein antigens: *hemagglutinin* (three major subtypes: H1, H2, H3, but up to six subtypes isolated from humans) and *neuraminidase* (two major subtypes in humans: N1, N2). Overall, 16 different hemagglutinin and 9 different neuraminidase types have been identified; these can be independently reassorted to produce different subtypes. Influenza A can cause pandemics.
   - **Influenza B:** Infects only humans. The disease is generally less severe than influenza A, and the virus is not subtyped. It can cause seasonal outbreaks and epidemics, but no pandemics.
   - **Influenza C:** Causes very mild disease and has limited public health significance

154. **What are the functions of hemagglutinin and neuraminidase?**
Hemagglutinin is a glycoprotein necessary for the initiation of infection because it allows viral binding to sialic acid residues on the respiratory epithelial cells. Progeny virions result after viral replication and bind to the epithelial cells. *Neuraminidase* cleaves sialic acid residue, which permits release of progeny virions into the respiratory tree.

155. **What clinical features typically distinguish an infection with an influenza virus from the common cold?**
See Table 11-6.

156. **What is the difference between "antigenic shift" and "antigenic drift"?**
   - **Antigenic drift:** A subtle change in the surface glycoprotein (either hemagglutinin or neuraminidase) caused by a point mutation or deletion in the viral gene. This results in a new strain that requires yearly reformulation of the seasonal influenza vaccine.
   - **Antigenic shift:** Much less frequent than antigenic drift (occurring only in influenza A), it involves a profound change in the virus with a new hemagglutinin or neuraminidase type produced, possibly from another species; for example, simultaneous infection of a host with a human and avian influenza strain can result in genetic reassortment and a novel virus.

TABLE 11-6. INFLUENZA VERSUS COLD SYMPTOMS

Signs and Symptoms	Influenza	Cold
Onset	Sudden	Gradual
Fever	>38.3°C (101°F) lasting >3 days	Rare
Cough	Can become severe	Less common
Headache	Prominent	Rare
Myalgia	Severe	Slight
Fatigue	Fatigue lasting >1 wk	Mild
Extreme exhaustion	Early and prominent	Rare
Chest discomfort	Common	Mild
Stuffy nose	Sometimes	Common
Sneezing	Sometimes	Common
Sore throat	Sometimes	Common

From Meissner HC: Reducing the impact of viral respiratory infections in children. Pediatr Clin N Am 52:700, 2005.

157. **What two mechanisms are most likely to cause a pandemic?**
The influenza virus, an orthomyxovirus, contains eight segments of RNA and has a high intrinsic mutation rate.
■ **Adaptation:** Through genetic mutations, a virulent nonhuman virus can adapt to humans. Studies of the virus causing the 1918 influenza pandemic (the so-called Spanish influenza) have found that all eight viral gene segments were most closely related to avian influenza viruses. This suggested that the avian virus had adapted or "jumped" species. This then permitted person-to-person transmission. An estimated 40 to 50 million people died during that pandemic. In 1997, a highly pathogenic avian influenza A virus (H5N1, or "bird flu") was found to infect humans in Hong Kong. Fortunately, transmission rates have remained very limited. The mechanisms permitting adaptation remain unclear.
■ **Recombination:** A nonhuman influenza virus and a human influenza virus recombine to create a novel pathogenic virus. In the 1957 pandemic ("Asian flu") and the 1968 pandemic ("Hong Kong flu"), human and avian viruses reassorted. These pandemics resulted in estimated worldwide deaths of 2 million and 1 million, respectively.

158. **What makes the H1N1 of 2009 so novel?**
The pandemic H1N1, the cause of a worldwide problem that began in early 2009, is thought to be a quadruple reassortment of an influenza A virus involving two swine strains, one human strain, and one avian strain, which likely recombined through pigs as an intermediate mammalian host. About one half of the genetic component is from swine, one third is of avian origin, and slightly less than one fifth of human origin. Transmissibility rates are extremely high.
Pigs first became infected with the influenza virus in 1918, and the first swine virus was found in humans in 1974. Components of the 2009 pandemic virus are thought to have derived from the 1918 influenza pandemic.

Zimmer SM, Burke DS: Historical perspective—emergence of influenza A (H1N1) viruses, *N Engl J Med* 361:279–285, 2009.

Morens DM, Taubenberger JK, Fauci AS: The persistent legacy of the 1918 influenza virus, *N Engl J Med* 361:225–229, 2009.

159. **Which patients should not receive the live-attenuated influenza vaccine?**
Patients who:
- Are receiving **salicylates**
- Have known or suspected **immunodeficiency**
- Have a history of **Guillain-Barré syndrome**
- Have a history of **anaphylactic reaction to egg protein**
- Have **reactive airway disease**
- Have **other conditions** considered high risk for severe influenza (chronic pulmonary or cardiac disorders, pregnancy, chronic metabolic disease, renal dysfunction, hemoglobinopathies, or immunosuppressive therapy)

160. **What are the main antiviral medications used as treatment for influenza?**
- **Neuraminidase inhibitors:** Oseltamivir and zanamivir. These prevent release of virions from the host cell. Zanamivir is delivered by inhalation. These inhibitors are used against influenza B and A, including pandemic H1N1.
- **Adamantanes (M2 inhibitors):** Amantadine and rimantadine. These target the M2 protein of influenza A, which is involved in ion channels of the viral membrane essential for viral replication. Adamantanes are not effective against influenza B or pandemic H1N1.

Moscona A: Neuraminidase inhibitors for influenza, *N Engl J Med* 353:1363, 2005.

161. **What bacterial coinfection is most commonly identified in influenza-associated pediatric deaths?**
Methicillin-resistant *Staphylococcus aureus* (MRSA). In children in the United States, most deaths associated with influenza tend to result either from an exacerbation of an underlying medical condition or invasive coinfection from another pathogen. As the percentage of children colonized with MRSA has increased, this bacterium has assumed a greater role in coinfecting lungs after the influenza virus has damaged the tracheobronchial tree. In a child with a suspected secondary pneumonia during influenza season, coverage for a possible MRSA infection should be considered.

Finelli L, Fiore A, Dhara R, et al: Influenza-associated pediatric mortality in the United States: increase of *Staphylococcus aureus* coinfection, *Pediatrics* 122:805–811, 2008.

162. **What nonrespiratory complications can be associated with influenza infections?**
- Otitis media
- Myositis (particularly with influenza B)
- Febrile seizures
- Encephalitis, encephalopathy
- Reye syndrome
- Guillain-Barré syndrome
- Transverse myelitis
- Myocarditis, pericarditis

163. **Can the swine flu be contracted by eating pork?**
No. Epidemic H1N1 (swine flu) is contacted mainly through person-to-person transmission, particularly from coughing or sneezing. Properly cooked pork (to an internal temperature of 71°C [160°F]) kills bacteria and viruses, including H1N1.

LYMPHADENITIS AND LYMPHADENOPATHY

164. **What are the most common causes of acute unilateral lymphadenitis in normal, otherwise healthy children?**
S. aureus and *Streptococcus pyogenes* (group A streptococci) account for more than 80% of cases.

165. **What are the most common causes of chronic infectious lymphadenitis in children?**
Nontuberculous mycobacteria and *Bartonella henselae* (cat-scratch disease).

166. **An intensely erythematous but nontender submandibular or anterior-superior cervical node is most suggestive of what infectious process?**
Nontuberculous mycobacterial infection. A grouping of these nodes, which increase in size, coalesce, and eventually spontaneously rupture to form sinus tracts, previously was called *scrofula*.

167. **How is the diagnosis of nontuberculous mycobacterial disease made?**
Definitive diagnosis of nontuberculous mycobacterial infection depends on culture and isolation of the organism from infected tissue. Histopathologic examination of the tissue cannot adequately differentiate nontuberculous mycobacterial infection from tuberculosis. Skin test antigens specific for nontuberculous mycobacteria are of limited usefulness as a result of cross-reactivity with antigens of *Mycobacterium tuberculosis*. Suggestive clinical features include adenopathy with minimal warmth and tenderness together with induration in response to PPD skin testing and a negative chest radiograph.

168. **How is nontuberculous mycobacterial disease treated?**
Most experts recommend excision of the infected lymph node. Clarithromycin, rifampin, and ethambutol are effective against many strains of nontuberculous mycobacteria and are generally used when excision is incomplete because of nearby nervous tissue or vascular structures or when surgery is contraindicated.

169. **Swollen, tender pectoral nodes are most suggestive of what infection?**
Cat-scratch disease.

170. **What is the etiologic agent of cat-scratch disease?**
The cause of cat-scratch disease is *B. henselae*, which is detected in most cases by serologic tests and occasionally by polymerase chain reaction or culture. It is a fastidious, slow-growing, gram-negative bacillus found in the oral flora of cats and kittens. This organism was first isolated in 1991 and has also been associated with bacillary angiomatosis and peliosis hepatis, which occur primarily in adults with HIV infection.

171. **What is the typical course of the lymphadenitis in cat-scratch disease?**
An otherwise healthy child or adolescent presents with symptoms of regional lymphadenopathy that begin 1 to several weeks after a scratch (unrecalled by many patients). The lymph nodes are usually moderately tender and are associated with overlying erythema and fluctuance. About 10% to 30% eventually suppurate. The lymph nodes most commonly involved are axillary and cervical, but epitrochlear, submandibular, inguinal, and preauricular nodes may be enlarged. Enlarged pectoral nodes are highly suggestive of cat-scratch disease. Fever is usually absent or low grade, but temperatures as high as 40°C have been described in 30% to 50% of cases.

English R: Cat-scratch disease, *Pediatr Rev* 27:123–127, 2006.

172. **How commonly does cat-scratch disease manifest with presentations other than lymphadenopathy?**
In 20% to 25% of cases. Atypical forms include Parinaud oculoglandular syndrome (conjunctivitis, ipsilateral preauricular lymphadenopathy), prolonged fever of unknown origin, encephalitis, osteolytic bone lesions, neuroretinitis, visceral organ involvement (especially hepatosplenic), and erythema nodosum.

173. **What are the common presentations of EBV infection?**
EBV infection is frequently asymptomatic in young children. In adolescents and young adults, infection typically results in infectious mononucleosis, which is characterized as follows:
- **Clinical:** Fever, pharyngitis, lymphadenopathy (75% to 95%), splenomegaly (50%)
- **Hematologic:** More than 50% mononuclear cells, more than 10% atypical lymphocytes
- **Serologic:** Transient appearance of heterophil antibodies; emergence of persistent antibodies to EBV
A wide variety of symptoms (e.g., malaise, headache, anorexia, myalgias, chills, nausea) can occur. Neurologic presentations are rare but can include encephalitis, meningitis, myelitis, Guillain-Barré syndrome, and cranial or peripheral neuropathies.

174. **How was the monospot test developed?**
In 1932, Paul and Bunnell observed that patients with infectious mononucleosis make antibodies that agglutinate sheep RBCs. These antibodies are referred to as *heterophil antibodies* and serve as the basis for the monospot test, which is a rapid slide agglutination test. Today, horse or beef RBCs are usually used because they are more sensitive to agglutination than are sheep RBCs. Heterophil antibodies can also occur in serum sickness and as a normal variant. If there is clinical confusion, differential absorption can pinpoint the cause. Heterophil antibodies in infectious mononucleosis do not react with guinea pig kidney cells, whereas those of serum sickness do. Normal variant heterophil antibodies do not react with beef RBCs.

Durbin WA, Sullivan JL: Epstein-Barr virus infections, *Pediatr Rev* 15:63–68, 1994.

175. **How common are heterophil antibodies in infectious mononucleosis?**
In typical infectious mononucleosis with fever, tonsillopharyngitis, and lymphadenopathy, 75% of older children and adolescents have heterophil antibodies by the end of the first week of illness, and 85% to 90% have heterophil antibodies by the third week. These percentages are much lower in infants and children younger than 4 years, and false-negative screening with the monospot test is common in these groups and in patients without classic infectious mononucleosis.

176. **What is the natural course of serologic responses to EBV infection?**
A variety of distinct EBV antigens, including viral capsid antigen, early antigen, and nuclear antigen, can elicit antibody responses. Acute infection is best characterized by the presence of anti-viral capsid antigen immunoglobulin M.

Luzuriaga K, Sullivan JL: Infectious mononucleosis, *N Engl J Med* 362:1993–2000, 2010.

177. **When are steroids indicated for children with EBV infection?**
Among patients with acute EBV infection, steroids should be considered for the relief of respiratory obstruction as a result of enlarged tonsils. Some authorities have also advocated their use for severe autoimmune hemolytic anemia, aplastic anemia, neurologic disease, and severe life-threatening infection (e.g., liver failure).

178. **Which other organisms can cause an infectious mononucleosis-like picture?**
CMV, *Toxoplasma gondii*, HHV-6, adenovirus, HIV, and rubella.

179. **What are the clinical presentations of acquired CMV infection?**
In normal hosts who develop symptomatic acquired CMV infection, clinical manifestations include fever, malaise, and nonspecific aches and pains. The peripheral blood smear reveals an absolute lymphocytosis and many atypical lymphocytes. In contrast with EBV-infectious mononucleosis, exudative pharyngitis is not prominent. Liver involvement is very common, and liver function tests are usually abnormal. Like EBV disease, CMV mononucleosis can persist for several weeks.

180. **What is the most common form of tularemia?**
Ulceroglandular. Of six clinical forms of tularemia described, ulceroglandular tularemia constitutes about 75%. Three to 6 days after exposure, fever, myalgia, headaches, and regional lymphadenopathy develop. The original lesion is a papule, which ulcerates at the site of entry. Bacteremia may result in multiorgan involvement.

Eliasson H, Broman T, Forsman M, et al: Tularemia: current epidemiology and disease management, *Infect Dis Clin N Am* 20:289–311, 2006.

181. **What vectors are commonly associated with tularemia?**
Ticks, rabbits, deer, and muskrats have been associated with outbreaks of tularemia, although *Francisella tularensis* (the causative agent) has also been isolated from other mammals and invertebrates (e.g., horseflies, mosquitoes).

182. **When should an enlarged lymph node be considered suspicious for malignancy?**
■ Lymphadenopathy does not improve with antibiotic therapy and no regression by 4 to 6 weeks
■ Lack of associated infectious symptoms (e.g., fever, tenderness)
■ Risk of malignancy increases with nodes larger than 2 cm
■ Nodes that are hard, firm, rubbery, fixed (or matted) to each other
■ Supraclavicular nodes have a higher likelihood of malignancy
■ Generalized lymphadenopathy, especially with pallor, bruising, hepatosplenomegaly, 10% weight loss

Friedmann AM: Evaluation and management of lymphadenopathy in children, *Pediatr Rev* 29:53–59, 2008.

MENINGITIS

183. **What are the most common signs and symptoms of meningitis in infants younger than 2 months?**
In general, the findings among neonates and young infants with meningitis are minimal and often subtle. Temperature instability (fever or hypothermia) occurs in about 60% of infected infants; increasing irritability is present in about 60%, poor feeding or vomiting in roughly 50%, and seizures in about 40%. Lethargy, respiratory distress, and diarrhea are frequent nonspecific manifestations of meningitis in this patient group. On physical examination, about 25% of newborns and young infants have a bulging fontanelle, and only 13% have nuchal rigidity. The diagnosis of meningitis cannot be excluded on the basis of the absence of these physical findings in infants.

Pong A, Bradley JS: Bacterial meningitis and the newborn infant, *Infect Dis Clin North Am* 13:711–733, 1999.

184. **What percentage of neonates with bacterial sepsis and positive blood cultures have meningitis?**
Up to 25% of infants younger than 28 days with bacterial sepsis and positive blood cultures will have culture-confirmed meningitis.

185. **What is the most common cause of aseptic meningitis?**
Aseptic meningitis is defined as clinical and laboratory evidence of inflammation of the meninges (e.g., CSF pleocytosis and increased protein) without evidence of bacterial infection on Gram stain or culture. More than 80% of infectious cases are caused by enteroviruses (i.e., Coxsackie virus, enterovirus, echovirus, and, rarely, poliovirus). West Nile virus is an increasingly common cause of aseptic meningitis, especially in the late summer and early fall.

186. **What is the diagnostic test of choice for enteroviral meningitis?**
Polymerase chain reaction is highly sensitive and specific, and it is more rapid than viral cultures, which typically take 2 to 5 days to become positive.

187. **What is the major vector-borne virus in the United States?**
West Nile virus. First noted in the United States in the Queens borough of New York City in 1999, West Nile virus was originally discovered in Uganda in 1937 and is widely distributed throughout the world. Mosquitoes are the primary vector, with a variety of birds (e.g., crows, jays, sparrows) known to serve as hosts. Significant avian mortality is often the first sign of significant West Nile virus activity in a locale. No-vector-borne transmission (e.g., contaminated blood products, organ transplantation) has been described.

Truemper EJ, Romero JR: West Nile virus, *Pediatr Ann* 36:414–422, 2007.

188. **Is intracranial pressure elevated in patients with meningitis?**
In acute bacterial meningitis, pressure is elevated in up to 95% of cases. Elevation is also common among patients with tuberculous or fungal meningitis. The frequency of elevation in patients with viral meningitis is less well studied.

189. **Should computed tomography (CT) scans be performed before an LP during the evaluation of possible meningitis?**
CT scans are not routinely indicated before LP, unless one of the following is present:
- Signs of herniation (rapid alteration of consciousness, abnormalities of pupillary size and reaction, absence of oculocephalic response, fixed oculomotor deviation of eyes)
- Papilledema
- Abnormalities in posture or respiration
- Generalized seizures (especially tonic), which are often associated with impending cerebral herniation
- Overwhelming shock or sepsis
- Concern about a condition mimicking bacterial meningitis (e.g., intracranial mass, lead intoxication, tuberculous meningitis)

Haslam RH: Role of CT in the early management of bacterial meningitis, *J Pediatr* 119:157–159, 1991.

190. **What is the range of values found in CSF of infants and children who do not have meningitis?**
- **Term newborn infants:** WBC count, 0 to 19/mm^3; protein, 30 to 150 mg/dL; glucose, 30 to 120 mg/dL

■ **Infants and children:** WBC count, 0 to 9/mm^3; protein, 20 to 40 mg/dL; glucose, 40 to 80 mg/dL

Mann K, Jackson A: Meningitis, *Pediatr Rev* 29:425, 2008.

Kestenbaum LA, Ebberson J, Zorc JJ, et al: Defining cerebrospinal fluid white blood cell count reference values in neonates and young children, *Pediatrics* 125:257–264, 2010.

191. **If bloody CSF is collected during LP, how is CNS hemorrhage distinguished from a traumatic artifact?**
Most often, the blood is a result of the traumatic rupture of small venous plexuses that surround the subarachnoid space, but pathologic bloody fluid can be seen in multiple settings (e.g., subarachnoid hemorrhage, herpes simplex encephalitis). Distinguishing features that suggest pathologic bleeding include the following:
■ Bleeding that does not lessen during the collection of multiple tubes
■ Xanthochromia of the CNS supernatant
■ Crenated RBCs noted microscopically

192. **How is a traumatic LP interpreted?**
A "bloody tap" is a common result of an unsuccessful LP. Numerous formulas have been devised to craft a method to adjust leukocyte totals in blood-contaminated CSF to determine whether CSF pleocytosis (and thus possible meningitis) is present. Some rules have used the ratio of WBC to RBC counts in the peripheral blood to predict the expected WBC count in bloody CSF fluid and then compared this result to the observed WBC CSF count. Others have used ratios of 1:500 or 1:1000 RBCs to 1 WBC in the CSF to derive a "corrected" WBC count. However, no formulas in neonates or older children have been found sufficiently helpful to guide clinical decisions about bacterial meningitis.

Greenberg RG, Smith PB, Cotten CM, et al: Traumatic lumbar punctures in neonates, *Pediatr Infect Dis J* 27:1047–1051, 2008.

Bonsu BK, Harper MB: Corrections for leukocytes and percent of neutrophils do not match observations in blood-contaminated cerebrospinal fluid and have no value over uncorrected cells for diagnosis, *Pediatr Infect Dis J* 25:8–11, 2006.

193. **What two modifiable factors may reduce the risk for traumatic or unsuccessful LPs?**
■ **Use of a local anesthetic:** Decreased patient movement from the anesthetic appears to outweigh any possible obscuring of landmarks that might hinder a successful LP
■ **Early stylet removal:** The main purpose of the stylet in the spinal needle is to prevent the introduction of a small plug of skin into the subarachnoid space, which might result in formation of an epidermal tumor. Removing the stylet after introduction may allow better assessment of CSF flow and prevent advancement of the needle beyond the subarachnoid space.

Nigrovic LE, Kuppermann N, Neuman MI: Risk factors for traumatic or unsuccessful lumbar punctures in children, *Ann Emerg Med* 49:762–771, 2007.

Baxter AL, Fisher RG, Burke BL, et al: Local anesthetic and stylet styles: factors associated with resident lumbar puncture success, *Pediatrics* 117:876–881, 2006.

194. **How do the CSF findings vary in bacterial, viral, fungal, and tuberculous meningitis in children beyond the neonatal period?**
Although a large overlap is possible (e.g., bacterial meningitis can be associated with a low WBC count early in the illness, or viral meningitis can often be associated with a predominance of neutrophils early or even persistently in the illness). The usual findings are summarized in Table 11-7.

TABLE 11-7. TYPICAL FINDINGS IN BACTERIAL, VIRAL, FUNGAL, AND TUBERCULOUS MENINGITIS			
Cerebrospinal Fluid Findings	Bacterial	Viral	Fungal, Tuberculous
White blood cells per mm^3	>500	<500	<500
Polymorphonuclear neutrophils	>80%	<50%	<50%
Glucose (mg/dL)	<40	>40	<40
Cerebrospinal fluid–to-blood ratio	<30%	>50%	<30%
Protein (mg/dL)	>100	<100	>100

195. **What is the value of the CSF absolute neutrophil count (ANC) in the diagnosis of bacterial versus aseptic meningitis?**

In a study that derived prediction rules for children to determine which group with CSF pleocytosis were most likely to have bacterial rather than aseptic meningitis, five high-risk criteria were defined that, if all were absent, identified 100% of children who did not have bacterial meningitis (100% negative-predictive value).

- Positive CSF gram stain
- CSF ANC ≥1000 cells/μL
- CSF protein ≥80 mg/dL
- Peripheral blood ANC ≥10,000 cells/μL
- Presence of a seizure at or before presentation

Nigrovic LE, Malley R, Kuppermann N: Cerebrospinal fluid pleocytosis in children in the era of bacterial conjugate vaccines, *Pediatr Emerg Care* 25:112–120, 2009.

196. **When is the best time to obtain a serum glucose level in an infant with suspected meningitis?**

Because the stress of an LP can elevate serum glucose, the serum sample is ideally obtained just before the LP. When the blood glucose level is elevated acutely, it can take at least 30 minutes before there is equilibration with the CSF.

197. **How often does bacterial meningitis appear in younger patients with normal findings on the initial CSF examination?**

In up to 3% of cases in children between the ages of 3 weeks and 18 months with positive bacterial cultures of the CSF, the initial CSF evaluation (i.e., cell count, protein and glucose concentrations, and Gram stain) can be normal. Of note is that, in almost all of these cases, physical examination reveals evidence of meningitis or suggests serious illness and the need for empirical antibiotics.

Polk DB, Steele RW: Bacterial meningitis presenting with normal cerebrospinal fluid, *Pediatr Infect Dis J* 6:1040–1042, 1987.

198. **Does antibiotic therapy before LP affect CSF indices?**

Many children are begun on antibiotic therapy before an LP for presumptive meningitis or if a delay is anticipated in doing the LP. Prior administration of antibiotics does increase the number of falsely negative CSF cultures in patients with bacterial meningitis. Latex agglutination tests to detect bacterial capsular antigen have not been found to be helpful in pretreated individuals. In most cases, shortly after the initiation of antibiotics, the CSF Gram stain still demonstrates bacteria with typical staining properties. Prior antibiotic use decreases the CSF protein concentration and increases the CSF glucose concentration. However, it does not substantially affect the CSF WBC or CSF ANC counts. Care must be exercised in using prediction rules based on CSF profiles that are used to distinguish viral from bacterial infections.

Nigrovic LE, Malley R, Macias CG, et al: Effect of antibiotic pretreatment on cerebrospinal fluid profiles in children with bacterial meningitis, *Pediatrics* 122:726–730, 2008.

Nigrovic LE, Kuppermann N, McAdam AJ, Malley R: Cerebrospinal latex agglutination fails to contribute to the microbiologic diagnosis of pretreated children with meningitis, *Pediatr Infect Dis J* 23:786–788, 2004.

199. **What are the most common organisms responsible for bacterial meningitis in the United States?**
0 to 1 month old
- Group B streptococci (*Streptococcus agalactiae*)
- *E. coli*
- *Listeria monocytogenes*
- *S. pneumoniae*
- Miscellaneous Enterobacteriaceae
- Coagulase-negative staphylococci (in hospitalized preterm infants)

1 to 3 months old
- *S. pneumoniae*
- *Neisseria meningitidis*
- Group B streptococci
- *H. influenzae* (especially other than type b)
- *E. coli*

3 months to 2 years
- *S. pneumoniae*
- *N. meningitidis*
- *H. influenzae* (especially other than type b)

2 to 18 years old
- *S. pneumoniae*
- *N. meningitidis*

200. **Why are *H. influenzae* type B strains more virulent than nontypeable *Haemophilus* strains?**
H. influenzae type b expresses the type b polysaccharide capsule, which is a polymer of ribose and ribitol-5 phosphate. In the absence of type-specific antibody, the type b capsule promotes intravascular survival by preventing phagocytosis and complement-mediated bactericidal activity. It is likely that other factors also contribute to the unique virulence of *H. influenzae* type b.

201. **What are the drugs of choice for the empirical treatment of bacterial meningitis in children older than 1 month?**
In cases of suspected bacterial meningitis, both vancomycin and a third-generation cephalosporin (e.g., cefotaxime, ceftriaxone) are recommended for empirical therapy because resistance to penicillin and cephalosporins is present in 15% to greater than 50% of *S. pneumoniae* isolates. These agents also provide excellent coverage against *N. meningitidis* and *H. influenzae*. The exception is when the Gram stain suggests another etiology (e.g., gram-negative diplococci). Treatment failures have been reported when the dosage of vancomycin is less than 60 mg/kg per day. Vancomycin should not be used alone to treat *S. pneumoniae* meningitis because data from animal models indicate that bactericidal levels may be difficult to maintain. The combination of vancomycin plus cefotaxime or ceftriaxone has been shown to produce a synergistic effect *in vitro*, in animal models, and in the CSF of children with meningitis.

Alter SJ: Pneumococcal infections, *Pediatr Rev* 30:155–164, 2009.

Mann K, Jackson MA: Meningitis, *Pediatr Rev* 29:417–429, 2008.

202. **How quickly is the CSF sterilized in children with meningitis?**
In successful therapy, the CSF is usually sterile within 36 to 48 hours of the initiation of antibiotics. In patients with meningococcal meningitis, CSF is typically completely sterile no longer than 2 hours after starting treatment. With other organisms, the time until sterilization is generally at least 4 hours.

Kanegaye JT, Soliemanzadeh P, Bradley JS: Lumbar puncture in pediatric bacterial meningitis: defining the time interval for recovery of cerebrospinal fluid pathogens after parenteral antibiotic pretreatment, *Pediatrics* 108:1169–1174, 2001.

203. **How long after treatment has been initiated must individuals with meningitis remain in respiratory isolation?**
24 hours. Respiratory isolation is recommended for patients with suspected *H. influenzae* type b or meningococcal meningitis, but it can be discontinued after 24 hours of therapy.

204. **What is the accepted duration of treatment for bacterial meningitis?**
The duration of antibiotic treatment is based on the causative agent and clinical course. In general, a minimum of 7 days of therapy is required for meningococcal meningitis, 7 to 10 days for *H. influenzae* meningitis, and 10 days for pneumococcal meningitis. Disease as a result of group B streptococci or *L. monocytogenes* should be treated for 14 to 21 days, and meningitis caused by gram-negative enteric bacilli should be treated for a minimum of 21 days after the CSF has become sterile. Among patients with complications such as brain abscess, subdural empyema, delayed CSF sterilization, persistence of meningeal signs, or prolonged fever, the duration of therapy may need to be extended and should be individualized.

205. **What is the role of corticosteroids in the treatment of bacterial meningitis?**
The inflammatory response plays a critical role in producing the CNS pathology and resultant sequelae of bacterial meningitis. Several studies have demonstrated that treatment with dexamethasone reduces the incidence of hearing loss and other neurologic sequelae in infants and children with *H. influenzae* meningitis. For cases of meningitis caused by pathogens other than *H. influenzae*, the current recommendations by the American Academy of Pediatrics are to "consider" the use of dexamethasone with or shortly before the first dose of antimicrobial therapy. The role of steroids in meningitis caused by other bacterial pathogens (particularly *S. pneumoniae*) remains controversial. In adults, adjuvant corticosteroids decrease mortality in patients with pneumococcal meningitis, but this does not appear to be the case in children.

American Academy of Pediatrics: Pneumococcal infections. In Pickering LK, editor: *2009 Red Book, Report of the Committee on Infectious Diseases*, ed 28, Elk Grove Village, IL, 2009, American Academy of Pediatrics, p 528.

Mongelluzzo J, Mohamad Z, Ten Have TR, Shah S: Corticosteroids and mortality in children with bacterial meningitis, *JAMA* 299:2048–2055, 2008.

Greenwood BM: Corticosteroids for acute bacterial meningitis, *N Engl J Med* 357:2507–2509, 2007.

206. **Should children receiving therapy for bacterial meningitis undergo repeat LP?**
A repeat LP should be considered for patients with meningitis caused by penicillin-nonsusceptible *S. pneumoniae*, in children who show no clinical response to therapy within 24 to 36 hours, and in patients who have received dexamethasone because this might

interfere with the ability to interpret clinical changes (e.g., fever). In addition, repeat LP should be considered for patients with prolonged or recurrent fever, for patients with recurrent meningitis, and for immunocompromised hosts. Some experts also recommend repeat LP in neonates with meningitis because of the greater difficulty of tracking the infant's clinical course as a measure of CSF sterilization and because of the variable response of the immature neonatal immune system. An end-of-treatment LP is sometimes considered for neonates; the purpose of this is to provide a baseline if a subsequent febrile illness develops and reevaluation for sepsis and meningitis is performed.

207. **In a patient with meningitis, what are the indications for CT or magnetic resonance imaging?**
The following suggest the presence of an intracranial complication and should prompt a neuroimaging study:
- Prolonged obtundation
- Prolonged irritability
- Seizures developing after day 3 of therapy
- Focal seizures
- Focal neurologic deficits
- Increasing head circumference
- Persistent elevation of CSF protein or neutrophil count
- Recurrence of disease

   Wubbel L, McCracken GH: Management of bacterial meningitis, *Pediatr Rev* 19:78–84, 1998.

208. **What are the most common causes of prolonged fever in patients with meningitis?**
- Disease at other foci (e.g., arthritis)
- Nosocomial infection
- Thrombophlebitis (related to intravenous catheters and infusates)
- Sterile or infected abscesses from intramuscular injections
- Drug fever

   Subdural effusions have also been associated with prolonged fever, but these occur commonly among children with meningitis and are probably not a cause of fever.

209. **How commonly are subdural effusions noted in patients with bacterial meningitis?**
Subdural effusions are common in bacterial meningitis and should be considered part of the disease rather than a complication. Estimates of their incidence vary from 10% to 50%. The incidence is highest in young infants and in patients with *H. influenzae* and *S. pneumoniae* meningitis. About 1% of patients with meningitis have a subdural empyema; the typical presentation is fever, irritability, and meningeal signs. Subdural empyema can be diagnosed by CT and requires drainage and prolonged antibiotic therapy.

210. **If a child develops bacterial meningitis, what should the parents be told about long-term outcomes?**
Disease resulting from *S. pneumoniae* is associated with considerably more mortality and morbidity than is infection caused by *N. meningitidis* or *H. influenzae*. The mortality ranges from 8% to 15%. A 3-year multicenter surveillance study of invasive pneumococcal infections examined outcomes of meningitis caused by *S. pneumoniae* in 180 children. Twenty-five percent of children had evidence of neurologic sequelae at the time of hospital discharge, and 32% had unilateral or bilateral deafness. Predictors of mortality included coma on admission, requirement for mechanical ventilation, and shock. Hearing loss occurs in 5% to 10% of patients with *H. influenza* and *N. meningitidis* meningitis.

Koomen I, Grobbee DE, Roord JJ, et al: Hearing loss at school age in survivors of bacterial meningitis: assessment, incidence, and prediction, *Pediatrics* 112:1049–1053, 2003.

Arditi M, Mason EO Jr, Bradley JS, et al: Three-year multicenter surveillance of pneumococcal meningitis in children: clinical characteristics and outcome related to penicillin susceptibility and dexamethasone use, *Pediatrics* 102:1087–1097, 1998.

211. **How should contacts of children with *N. meningitidis* disease be managed?**
Antibiotic prophylaxis is indicated for household and day care or nursery school contacts in the previous 7 days of patients with invasive meningococcal disease. The attack rate of secondary cases among household contacts of an index patient is 500 to 800 times that of the general population. Only those medical personnel who have had intimate contact with the patient (e.g., through intubation or mouth-to-mouth resuscitation) require antibiotic prophylaxis. Another indication is for any passenger seated next to an index patient on a flight lasting more than 8 hours. For children, the drug of choice is rifampin given twice daily for two days. Other options for chemoprophylaxis include intramuscular ceftriaxone and oral ciprofloxacin (for those ≥18 years of age). Prophylaxis is not recommended for casual contacts at school, work, or hospital setting without exposure to the index patient's oral secretions.

American Academy of Pediatrics: Meningococcal infections. In Pickering LK, editor: *2009 Red Book: Report of the Committee on Infectious Diseases*, ed 28, Elk Grove Village, IL, 2009, American Academy of Pediatrics, pp 458–460.

212. **What is the most common parasitic infection of the CNS?**
Neurocysticercosis. This is a tapeworm disease that is most commonly initiated by the ingestion of undercooked pork containing *Taenia solium* larvae. After these larvae mature, eggs from adult tapeworms are then acquired by fecal-oral transmission among humans or autoinoculation. If hematogenous spread of these eggs to the brain occurs, cysts form that can result in seizures or other neurologic manifestations. Magnetic resonance imaging can demonstrate the ring-enhancing cysts characteristic of the disease.

OCULAR INFECTIONS

213. **Among neonates with conjunctivitis, what is the timing for the various etiologies?**
 - Chemical: Onset in less than 2 days
 - *Neisseria gonorrhoeae*: Onset in 2 to 7 days
 - *C. trachomatis*: Onset in 5 to 14 days
 - HSV: Onset in 6 to 14 days

214. **What is the best method of prophylaxis for ophthalmia neonatorum?**
Ophthalmia neonatorum is conjunctivitis in the first month of life with particular concerns regarding *C. trachomatis* and *N. gonorrhoeae* acquisition at birth. Other bacterial microbes and HSV can be pathogens. Chlamydia is now the more predominant etiology of neonatal conjunctivitis in the United States. As a consequence, erythromycin 0.5% ophthalmic ointment and tetracycline 1.0% ophthalmic ointment are now used routinely in nurseries in the United States to prevent conjunctivitis, although their efficacy for preventing chlamydial disease (primarily pneumonia) remains unclear. Worldwide, other methods are used, including 2.5% povidone-iodine ophthalmic solution and silver nitrate drops.

215. **Can newborns with chlamydial conjunctivitis be treated with topical therapy alone?**
No. Newborns diagnosed with chlamydial conjunctivitis should receive systemic therapy with oral erythromycin for 14 days. Topical therapy will not eradicate the organism from the upper

respiratory tract, and it fails to prevent the development of chlamydial pneumonia. Close follow-up evaluation is indicated to ensure the absence of relapse.

216. **In children with conjunctivitis and otitis media, what is the most likely etiologic agent?**
Nontypeable *H. influenzae* is the most common cause of the so-called conjunctivitis-otitis syndrome, which is characterized by concurrent conjunctivitis and otitis media.

217. **Can bacterial conjunctivitis be distinguished from viral conjunctivitis on clinical grounds alone?**
Classically, bacterial conjunctivitis is more common in infants and young children, with the discharge being purulent or mucopurulent. A history of sticky eyelids with eyelash closure on waking up is predictive of a bacterial etiology. The most common implicated organism is nontypeable *H. influenzae*. Viral conjunctivitis is accompanied by a serous exudate in children of all ages. Bacterial infections are more commonly associated with otitis media, and otoscopy should be performed on all patients. However, clinical findings can overlap. Both bacteria and viruses can cause unilateral or bilateral symptoms.

Aside from culture, another way to distinguish the culprit is by Giemsa stain of a conjunctival scraping. Neutrophils predominate in bacterial infections, lymphocytes in viral infections, and eosinophils in allergic conjunctivitis.

Patel PB, Diaz MC, Bennett JE, et al: Clinical features of bacterial conjunctivitis in children, *Acad Emerg Med* 14:1–5, 2007.

Richards A, Guzman-Cottrill JA: Conjunctivitis, Pediatr Rev 31:196-208, 2010.

218. **What is keratoconjunctivitis?**
Keratoconjunctivitis is an inflammatory process that involves both the conjunctiva and the cornea. Superficial inflammation of the cornea (keratitis) occurs commonly in association with viral and bacterial conjunctivitis, particularly in adults. Hence, many cases of conjunctivitis are more correctly called *keratoconjunctivitis*.

Epidemic keratoconjunctivitis is caused by adenovirus serotypes 8, 19, and 37. Some organisms, including *P. aeruginosa*, *N. gonorrhoeae*, and HSV, have a propensity to cause more severe infection of the cornea. Infection as a result of these pathogens must be recognized early to prevent corneal scarring with subsequent vision loss.

219. **When are topical antibiotics not sufficient for treating acute conjunctivitis?**
Topical therapy for neonatal chlamydial conjunctivitis should never be used as sole therapy because of the high likelihood of concomitant respiratory tract colonization (which can eventually progress to pneumonia). Infections resulting from *N. gonorrhoeae*, *P. aeruginosa*, *H. influenzae* type b, and *N. meningitidis* require systemic therapy to prevent the serious complications seen with these organisms. Of course, viral conjunctivitis does not respond to topical antibiotics.

220. **Are ophthalmic solutions better than ophthalmic ointments for eradicating conjunctivitis?**
Ophthalmic ointments are usually preferred for infants and young children because they can be instilled more reliably and remain in the eye for a longer time. In older children, ophthalmic solutions may be preferred to prevent the blurring of vision that occurs with ointments. In general, the efficacy of ophthalmic ointments is presumed to be superior to that of solutions. However, several antibiotics are available in high-concentration solutions. These "fortified" formulations have not been compared prospectively with other preparations, but they are widely used because of their presumed enhanced efficacy.

221. **What is the most common cause of Parinaud oculoglandular syndrome?**
Parinaud syndrome is characterized by granulomatous or ulcerating conjunctivitis and prominent preauricular or submandibular adenopathy. The most common cause is **cat-scratch disease**, but other causes include tularemia, sporotrichosis, tuberculosis, syphilis, and infectious mononucleosis.

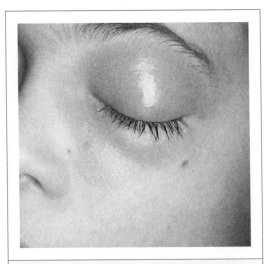

Figure 11-3. Periorbital cellulitis. (From Zitelli BJ, Davis HW: Atlas of Pediatric Physical Diagnosis, 4th ed. St. Louis, Mosby, 2002, p 848.)

222. **How is orbital cellulitis distinguished from periorbital (or preseptal) cellulitis?**
Periorbital cellulitis involves the tissues anterior to the eyelid septum (Fig. 11-3), whereas *orbital cellulitis* involves the orbit and is sometimes associated with abscess formation and cavernous sinus thrombosis. Distinction between these processes requires assessment of *ocular mobility*, *pupillary reflex*, *visual acuity*, and *globe position* (e.g., proptosis), which are normal in periorbital cellulitis but may be abnormal in orbital cellulitis. An abnormality in any of these four areas mandates radiologic evaluation (usually CT scan of the orbit) and possible surgical drainage.

223. **What are the causes that lead to periorbital and orbital cellulitis?**
- **Orbital:** Most cases originate in nearby paranasal sinuses (especially ethmoid) as a **complication of sinusitis.** The walls (lamina papyracea) of the ethmoid and sphenoid sinuses are paper thin with natural bony dehiscences that allow spread of infection. In addition, orbital and sinus veins anastomose and are valveless, which allows communicating blood flow and easier spread of infection.
- **Periorbital:** May result from **direct inoculation** of infection or inflammation in and around the eyelid, **trauma** (blunt or penetrating), and **spread of microorganisms** from the sinuses or nasopharynx into the preseptal space.

Sethuraman U, Kamat D: The red eye: evaluation and management, *Clin Pediatr* 48:588–600, 2009.

224. **What is the difference between a hordeolum, a stye, and a chalazion?**
- A **hordeolum** is a purulent infection of any one of the sebaceous or apocrine sweat glands of the eyelid, including the glands of Moll and Zeis, which drain near the eyelash follicle, and the meibomian glands, which drain nearer the conjunctiva. Clinically, a hordeolum is recognized as a red, tender swelling. It is usually caused by *S. aureus*.
- A **stye** is an external hordeolum, on the skin side of the eyelid.
- A **chalazion** is an internal hordeolum, on the conjunctival side of the eyelid.
  In all cases, these lesions are treated with warm compresses and topical antibiotic drops or ointment (although their value is debatable) and usually resolve within 7 days.

Intralesional triamcinolone injection can be beneficial for a chalazion. A chalazion is more likely to become chronic and require surgical excision.

225. **Why is the "ciliary flush" particularly worrisome when evaluating a patient with a pink or red eye?**
Ciliary flush refers to circumcorneal hyperemia in which conjunctival redness is concentrated in the area adjacent to the cornea (limbus). This can be a sign of significant ocular pathology (e.g., keratitis, anterior uveitis, acute angle-closure glaucoma) and requires hastened referral to an ophthalmologist.

OTITIS MEDIA

226. **How commonly does cerumen obscure the diagnosis of otitis media?**
As many as 30% of cases of otitis media are obscured by this waxy roadblock.

Schwartz RH, Rodriguez WJ, McAveney W, Grundfast KM: Cerumen removal: how necessary is it to diagnose acute otitis media? *Am J Dis Child* 137:1065–1068, 1983.

227. **Is ear pulling a reliable sign of infection?**
In the absence of other signs or symptoms (e.g., fever, upper respiratory infection symptoms), ear pulling alone is a very poor indicator of acute otitis media.

Baker RB: Is ear pulling associated with ear infection? [letter], *Pediatrics* 90:1006–1007, 1992.

228. **What are the landmarks of the tympanic membrane?**
See Fig. 11-4.

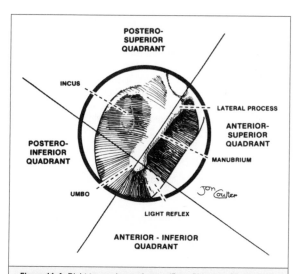

Figure 11-4. Right tympanic membrane. (From Bluestone CD, Klein JO: Otitis Media in Infants and Children. Philadelphia, WB Saunders, 1988, p 76.)

229. **What are the most reliable ways, on physical examination, to accurately diagnosis acute otitis media?**
Good visualization of the tympanic membrane (TM) and the use of a pneumatic otoscope are key.
- **Visualization of position:** Bulging of the TM implies fluid under pressure, whereas retraction is more commonly seen with effusion rather than suppuration.
- **Color and translucence:** Normal TM color is pearly gray and translucent; cloudiness implies suppuration; distinct redness defined as hemorrhagic, strongly or moderately red (especially if unilateral) can indicate infection but can be seen in other settings, particularly with high fever. Marked redness without TM bulging is unusual in acute otitis media.
- **Mobility:** Impaired mobility of the TM to positive pressure by pneumatic otoscopy implies a fluid-filled space.

   Rothman R, Owens T, Simel DL: Does this child have acute otitis media? *JAMA* 290:1633–1640, 2003.

230. **How often will acute otitis media resolve spontaneously without antibiotics?**
In 60% of cases or more. The likelihood of spontaneous resolution depends on the microbiologic etiology and is estimated at 20% with *S. pneumoniae*, 50% with *H. influenzae*, 80% with *M. catarrhalis*, and 100% with respiratory viruses.

231. **Should all children with acute otitis media be treated with antibiotics?**
Because of the high rate of spontaneous improvement, some suggest that children may not require antibiotic therapy for uncomplicated otitis media. However, placebo-controlled trials have demonstrated that treatment with an antimicrobial agent shortens the duration of symptoms and reduces the likelihood of persistent infection, especially in children younger than 2 years. The American Academy of Pediatrics and the American Academy of Family Practitioners recommend that decisions about antibiotic treatment should be based on diagnostic certainty, age, illness severity, and assurance of follow-up. In particular, antibiotic treatment should be seriously considered for all infants younger than 6 months, for children between 6 months and 2 years old with a certain diagnosis of otitis media or severe illness, and for children older than 2 years with a certain diagnosis of otitis media and severe illness. Severe illness is defined as moderate to severe otalgia or temperature of 39°C or higher in the previous 24 hours.

   Gloud JM, Matz PS: Otitis media, *Pediatr Rev* 31:102-115, 2010.

232. **What is the "wait and see" approach for otitis media?**
This is the observational option ("watchful waiting") for patients older than 2 years for whom the diagnosis of otitis media is certain but the illness is not severe. Anticipating a high percentage of spontaneous improvement, clinicians defer antibiotic therapy. If the patient does not improve with observation for 48 to 72 hours, antibiotics are initiated. The intent is to reduce potentially unnecessary antibiotics. When using this option, reliable follow-up should be ensured.

   Spiro DM, Tay KY, Arnold DH, et al: Wait-and-see prescription for the treatment of acute otitis media: a randomized controlled trial, *JAMA* 296:1235, 2006.

   American Academy of Pediatrics: Diagnosis and management of acute otitis media, *Pediatrics* 113:1451–1465, 2004.

233. **After an acute episode of otitis media, how long does the middle ear effusion persist?**
About 70% of patients will continue to have an effusion at 2 weeks, 40% at 1 month, 20% at 2 months, and 5% to 10% at 3 months.

   Teele DW, Klein JO, Rosner BA: Epidemiology of otitis media in children, *Ann Otol Rhinol Laryngol Suppl* 89:5, 1980.

KEY POINTS: DURATION OF MIDDLE EAR EFFUSION PERSISTENCE AFTER OTITIS MEDIA

1. Two weeks: 70%

2. One month: 40%

3. Two months: 20%

4. Three months: 5%-10%

234. **What are the most common viral and bacterial agents that cause otitis media?**
Tympanocentesis yields positive bacterial cultures in 65% to 90% of cases of acute otitis media. Virus or viral antigen is detected from middle ear fluid in 10% to 25% of cases (Table 11-8). The significance of virus in middle ear fluid is debated, although it seems clear that antecedent viral

TABLE 11-8. COMMON BACTERIA AND VIRUSES IDENTIFIED IN MIDDLE EAR FLUID			
Bacterial Isolates		**Viral Isolates***	
Streptococcus pneumoniae	43%	Respiratory syncytial virus	7%
Moraxella catarrhalis	21%	Rhinovirus	3%
Haemophilus influenzae	18%	Influenza virus	2%
Streptococcus pyogenes	4%	Adenovirus	2%
Other	4%	Parainfluenza virus	2%

*Viruses are given as the percentage of total aspirates.

infection is an important factor in the pathogenesis of otitis media and that concomitant viral infection may prolong the course of bacterial otitis media and lead to treatment failures.

Heikkinen T, Chonmaitree T: Increasing importance of viruses in acute otitis media, *Ann Med* 32:157–163, 2000.

235. **Among patients with otitis media, what are the indications for tympanocentesis?**
   - A toxic-appearing child
   - An unsatisfactory response to antibiotics
   - A suppurative complication
   - Underlying immunosuppression

   Some experts would also consider tympanocentesis in newborn infants with otitis media because the spectrum of potential pathogens may be broader than that seen in an older child.

236. **When should prophylactic antibiotics be considered for children with recurrent otitis media?**
Preventive antibiotic therapy (i.e., chemoprophylaxis) for otitis-prone children must be weighed against the potential for the development of nasopharyngeal colonization with

antibiotic-resistant organisms. Benefits with the use of amoxicillin or sulfisoxazole have been shown to be modest but greatest in children younger than 2 years and in those whose first episode occurred before 6 months of age. Chemoprophylaxis for recurrent otitis should be reserved for patients with three or more distinct and well-documented episodes in 6 months or four or more episodes in 12 months.

American Academy of Pediatrics: Antimicrobial prophylaxis. In Pickering LK, editor: *2009 Red Book: Report of the Committee on Infectious Diseases*, ed 28, Elk Grove Village, IL, 2009, American Academy of Pediatrics, p 819.

237. **What is the most common reason for general anesthesia in children?**
Placement of tympanostomy tubes. In one cohort study of more than 2200 children followed from birth, 6% had received tympanostomy tubes by their second birthday.

Paradise JL, Rockette HE, Colborn DK, et al: Otitis media in 2253 Pittsburgh-area infants: prevalence and risk factors during the first two years of life, *Pediatrics* 99:318–333, 1997.

238. **What are the indications for tympanostomy tubes?**
Tympanostomy tubes are most commonly inserted for the treatment of otitis media with effusion (OME) or for prophylaxis against recurrent otitis media.

Ongoing studies from the University of Pittsburgh have demonstrated that the presence of middle ear effusions for extended periods in otherwise well children with normal hearing do not negatively affect developmental outcomes. A child with OME that lasts 3 months or longer or that is associated with suspected hearing loss, language delay, or learning problems should undergo hearing evaluation. If significant hearing impairment is detected (>30 dB), placement of tympanostomy tubes should be considered after a child has had a speech-language evaluation. Tympanostomy tubes have been shown to improve hearing during the initial 6 months after the procedure. If hearing is normal or mildly abnormal (≤30 dB), the child should be monitored every 3 to 6 months. During this period of watchful waiting, periodic hearing testing should be done. Tympanostomy tubes could be considered for a child with 9 to 12 months of continuous bilateral middle ear effusion or 12 to 18 months of continuous unilateral middle ear effusion.

For patients with recurrent otitis media, the benefit of tube placement is modest and must be weighed against the risk for complications, which include sclerosis, retraction, and atrophy of the eardrum.

Feldman HM, Paradise JL: OME and child development, *Contemp Pediatr* 26:40–41, 2009.

Paradise JL, Feldman HM, Campbell TF, et al: Tympanostomy tubes and developmental outcomes at 9 to 11 years of age, *N Engl J Med* 356:248–261, 2007.

239. **What are the potential complications of tympanostomy tubes?**
- Residual **perforation** of the eardrum (2%)
- **Myringosclerosis** (white calcific plaques on the tympanic membrane; 30% to 50%)
- Segmental **atrophy** (localized areas of thinning of the tympanic membrane)
- **Retraction pockets** (25% to 50%)
- **Tube otorrhea** (75% after 12 months, 83% after 18 months)
- **Cholesteatoma** (0.7%)
- **Hearing loss** (near term: generally no reductions in hearing acuity; longer term: unclear)

Feldman HM, Paradise JL: OME and child development, *Contemp Pediatr* 26:40–41, 2009.

240. **Should a child with tympanostomy tubes be allowed to swim?**
Otolaryngologists differ widely in their guidance to parents about issues of swimming and bathing. Controlled studies have shown that the rate of otorrhea is similar between nonswimmers (15%) and surface swimmers without earplugs (20%). If diving or underwater

swimming is planned, fitted earplugs are recommended. Bath water with shampooing can cause inflammatory changes in the middle ear, and thus earplugs should be used if head dunking is anticipated during bathing. An *in vitro* study (using a head model) found water entry greatest with submersion in soapy water and with deeper swimming.

Hebert RL II, King GE, Bent JP III: Tympanostomy tubes and water exposure: a practical model, *Arch Otolaryngol Head Neck Surg* 124:1118–1121, 1998.

Isaacson G, Rosenfeld RM: Care of the child with tympanostomy tubes: a visual guide for the pediatrician, *Pediatrics* 93:924–929, 1994.

241. **A child with the acute onset of ear pain and double vision likely has what condition?**
     Gradenigo syndrome is an acquired paralysis of the abducens muscle with pain in the area that is served by the ipsilateral trigeminal nerve. It is caused by inflammation of the sixth cranial nerve in the petrous portion, with involvement of the gasserian ganglion. The inflammation is usually the result of infection from otitis media or mastoiditis. Symptoms may include weakness of lateral gaze on the affected side, double vision, pain, photophobia, tearing, and hyperesthesia.

242. **What are differences between acute and chronic mastoiditis?**
     - **Acute mastoiditis:** Presents as complication of acute otitis media with retroauricular inflammation (swelling and tenderness) and protrusion of the auricle; patients are younger; most likely causes are *S. pneumoniae* and *S. pyogenes*
     - **Chronic mastoiditis:** Typically with more extensive history of otitis media, including tympanostomy tubes; less than 50% with retroauricular swelling and tenderness; patients are older; most likely cause is *P. aeruginosa*

Lin HW, Shargorodsky J, Gopen Q: Clinical strategies for the mangegement of acute mastoiditis in the pediatric population, *Clin Pediatr* 49:110-115, 2010.

Stähelin-Massik J, Podvinec M, Jakscha J, et al: Mastoiditis in children: a prospective, observational study comparing clinical presentation, microbiology, computed tomography, surgical findings and histology, *Eur J Pediatr* 167:541–548, 2008.

243. **What are the potential complications of mastoiditis?**
     Epidural abscess, brain abscess, cervical abscess, sinus vein thrombosis, cervical vein thrombosis, and sensorineural hearing loss.

PHARYNGEAL AND LARYNGEAL INFECTIONS

244. **Can group A β-hemolytic streptococcal (GAS) pharyngitis reliably be distinguished from viral causes?**
     Streptococcal pharyngitis is a disease with variable clinical manifestations. Clues that suggest streptococcal disease include the abrupt onset of headache, fever, and sore throat with the subsequent development of tender cervical lymphadenopathy, tonsillar exudate, and palatal petechiae in the winter or early spring. The presence of concurrent conjunctivitis, rhinitis, cough, or diarrhea suggests a viral process. The physical findings are by no means diagnostic and, when present, are more commonly found in children older than 3 years. Even the most skilled clinician cannot exceed an accuracy rate of about 75%. A throat culture or a rapid antigen test is essential for confirming streptococcal infection.

245. **What is the typical rash of scarlet fever?**
     The rash, which is caused by a streptococcal pyrogenic exotoxin, usually begins on the neck, face, and upper trunk and generalizes to the remainder of the body over 1 to 2 days.

Palms and soles are usually spared. The rash has a sandpaper-like texture—pinpoint, erythematous, blanchable papules. The erythema (and some petechiae from fragile capillaries) may be prominent in skin folds (Pastia lines). Over 5 to 7 days, the rash fades and later is followed by desquamation, particularly on the hands, feet, axillae, and groin.

246. **Why is a throat culture for GAS advised if a rapid antigen detection test is negative?**
A variety of antigen detection tests are available. They have a high degree of specificity, but a lower sensitivity. Thus, a negative test does not exclude the possibility of GAS and a throat culture is recommended. Newer, more sensitive antigen detection tests may eliminate the need for culture in children when future studies are done. In adults, however, because of the low incidence of GAS infections and the extremely low risk for acute rheumatic fever, the American Heart Association advises that diagnosis can be made on the basis of antigen detection testing alone without confirmation of a negative antigen test by a negative throat culture.

Gerber MA, Baltimore RS, Eaton CB, et al: Prevention of rheumatic fever and diagnosis and treatment of acute streptococcal pharyngitis, *Circulation* 119:1154–1551, 2009.

247. **What is the rationale for the treatment of GAS pharyngitis?**
   - To prevent acute rheumatic fever (even though there is a low incidence of acute rheumatic fever in the United States, worldwide rheumatic heart disease is the leading cause of cardiovascular death during the first five decades of life)
   - To shorten the course of the illness, including headache, sore throat, and lymph node tenderness
   - To reduce the spread of infection and prevent suppurative complications
   - To prevent some cases of acute glomerulonephritis

248. **What is the recommended treatment for GAS pharyngitis?**
Except in a patient with a history of penicillin allergy, the recommended therapy is intramuscular benzathine G or oral penicillin V. Amoxicillin suspension is often prescribed rather than penicillin suspension because of better taste. Penicillin-allergic patients may take narrow-spectrum cephalosporins (cephalexin, cefadroxil), clindamycin, or macrolides (azithromycin, clarithromycin). Tetracyclines, trimethoprim-sulfamethoxazole, and older fluoroquinolones (e.g., ciprofloxacin) are not recommended.

Gerber MA, Baltimore RS, Eaton CB, et al: Prevention of rheumatic fever and diagnosis and treatment of acute streptococcal pharyngitis, *Circulation* 119:1154–1551, 2009.

249. **Why do some clinicians use treatments other than penicillins for GAS pharyngitis?**
Although 100% of GAS have demonstrated *in vitro* susceptibility to penicillins, treatment failures have been found to occur twice as frequently and bacterial failures three times more frequently after treatment for GAS pharyngitis with penicillin than with oral cephalosporins. Relapse rates occur more commonly as well (6% to 8% after 10 days of penicillin or amoxicillin) versus 2% for first-generation cephalosporins and 1% for second-generation and third-generation cephalosporins. One theory for these failures, despite the absence of penicillin resistance *in vitro*, is that normal flora (including *S. aureus* and *Moraxella catarrhalis*) may produce β-lactamases that can inactivate penicillin and amoxicillin in the local oral environment. Other factors, including tolerability, cost, and prior responses to treatment, are also involved in the choice of antibiotics.

Casey JR, Kahn R, Gmoser D, et al: Frequency of symptomatic relapses of group A β-hemolytic streptococcal tonsillopharyngitis in children from 4 pediatric practices following penicillin, amoxicillin and cephalosporin antibiotic treatment, *Clin Pediatr* 47:549–554, 2008.

Casey JR: Selecting the optimal antibiotic in the treatment of group A β-hemolytic streptococcal pharyngitis, *Clin Pediatr* 46:25S–35S, 2007.

250. **How does one differentiate a patient with a sore throat who is a streptococcal carrier with an intercurrent viral pharyngitis from one who is having repeated episodes of GAS pharyngitis?**

Streptococcal carrier
- Signs and symptoms of viral infection (rhinorrhea, cough, conjunctivitis, diarrhea)
- Little clinical response to antibiotics (sometimes difficult to assess because of the self-resolving nature of viral infections)
- Group A streptococcus present on cultures between episodes
- No serologic response to infection (i.e., anti-streptolysin O, anti-DNase B)
- Same serotype of group A streptococcus in sequential cultures

Recurrent group A streptococcal pharyngitis
- Signs and symptoms consistent with group A streptococcal infection
- Marked clinical response to antibiotics
- No group A streptococcus on cultures between episodes
- Positive serologic response to infection
- Different serotypes of group A streptococcus on sequential cultures

Gerber MA: Diagnosis and treatment of pharyngitis in children, *Pediatr Clin N Am* 52:729–747, 2005.

Hill HR: Group A streptococcal carrier versus acute infection: the continuing dilemma, *Clin Infect Dis* 50:491-492, 2010.

251. **When can children treated for positive streptococcal throat cultures return to school or day care?**
Although clinical improvement often occurs promptly, most patients remain culture positive 14 hours after the initiation of antibiotics. However, by 24 hours, nearly all patients are culture negative. To minimize contagion, children should receive a full 24 hours of antibiotic therapy before returning to school or child care.

Snellman LW, Stang HJ, Stang JM, et al: Duration of positive throat cultures for group A streptococci after initiation of antibiotic therapy, *Pediatrics* 91:1166–1170, 1993.

252. **How commonly do toddlers younger than 2 years develop GAS pharyngitis?**
Traditional teaching has been that toddlers rarely develop streptococcal pharyngitis. Studies indicate that the incidence of infection and the prevalence of carriage are greater than previously thought. In studies of patients younger than 2 years with fever and clinical pharyngitis, the range of group A β-hemolytic streptococcus positivity was 4% to 6%; among well children, the carrier rate is about 6%. The rate of rheumatic fever is exceedingly low in children younger than 3 years.

Berkovitch M, Vaida A, Zhovtis D, et al: Group A streptococcal pharyngotonsillitis in children less than 2 years of age—more common than is thought, *Clin Pediatr* 38:365–366, 1999.

Nussinovitch M, Finkelstein Y, Amir J, Varsano I: Group A beta-hemolytic streptococcal pharyngitis in preschool children aged 3 months to 5 years, *Clin Pediatr* 38:357–360, 1999.

253. **How long after the development of streptococcal pharyngitis can treatment be initiated and still effectively prevent rheumatic fever?**
Treatment should be started as soon as possible, but little is lost in waiting for throat culture results to establish the diagnosis. Antibiotic treatment prevents acute rheumatic fever even when therapy is initiated as long as **9 days** after the onset of the acute illness.

Catanzaro FJ, Stetson CA, Morris AJ, et al: The role of the streptococcus in the pathogenesis of rheumatic fever, *Am J Med* 17:749–756, 1954.

KEY POINTS: PHARYNGITIS

1. Clinical pictures of viral and streptococcal pharyngitis have significant clinical overlap.

2. Tetracyclines, trimethoprim-sulfamethoxazole, and older fluoroquinolones (e.g., ciprofloxacin) are not recommended for the treatment of group A β-hemolytic streptococcal pharyngitis.

3. About 6% of children are streptococcus carriers and will have positive cultures between episodes of pharyngitis.

4. Antibiotic treatment prevents acute rheumatic fever even when therapy is initiated as long as 9 days after the onset of acute illness.

5. Although the incidence of rheumatic fever is low in the United States, worldwide it is the leading cause of cardiovascular death during the first five decades of life.

254. **What diagnosis should be suspected in a teenager with pharyngitis followed by multifocal pneumonia and sepsis?**
Lemierre syndrome. This is a septic thrombophlebitis of the internal jugular vein that is typically caused by the anaerobic gram-negative rod *Fusobacterium necrophorum*. The illness begins as a pharyngitis or tonsillitis, thrombophlebitis develops, and there is seeding of multiple organs with septic emboli. Pneumonia may lead to respiratory failure in untreated cases. Anaerobic blood cultures, ultrasonography of the jugular vessels, and CT scan of the chest are helpful for establishing the diagnosis.

255. **What is the difference between herpangina and Ludwig angina?**
- **Herpangina** is a common viral infection during the summer and fall and is characterized by posterior pharyngeal, buccal, and palatal vesicles and ulcers. Coxsackie viruses A and B and echoviruses are the most common causative agents. In young children, it is often accompanied by a high temperature (39.4° to 40°C [103° to 104°F]). Herpangina is distinguished from HSV infections of the mouth, which are more anterior and involve the lips, tongue, and gingiva.
- **Ludwig angina** is an acute diffuse infection (usually bacterial due to mixed anaerobes) of the submandibular and sublingual spaces with brawny induration of the floor of the mouth and tongue. Airway obstruction can occur. The infections usually follow oral cavity injuries or dental complications (e.g., extractions, impactions).

Lin HW, O'Neill A, Cunningham MJ: Ludwig's angina in the pediatric population, *Clin Pediatr* 48: 583–587, 2009.

256. **What is quinsy?**
Peritonsillar abscess (from the lower Latin for "an inflammation of the throat").

257. **How is a peritonsillar abscess distinguished from peritonsillar cellulitis?**
A *peritonsillar abscess* is diagnosed when a discrete mass is palpated, usually in school-aged children and adolescents. The bulging abscess causes lateral displacement of the uvula. Trismus, due to spasm of masticator muscles, occurs more commonly in the setting of abscess than does simple cellulitis, which is characterized by signs of diffuse inflammation only. Many patients have a "hot potato" voice, which is a muffled voice caused by palatal edema and spasm of the internal pterygoid muscle that elevates the palate.

Galioto NJ: Peritonsillar abscess, *Am Fam Physician* 77:199–209, 2008.

258. **What radiographic features suggest the diagnosis of a retropharyngeal abscess?**

When a patient's neck is extended, a measurement of the prevertebral space that exceeds two times the diameter of the C2 vertebra suggests an abscess (Fig. 11-5). Pockets of air in the prevertebral space also suggest abscess. The retropharynx extends to T1 in the superior mediastinum, so empyema or mediastinitis is also possible whenever a retropharyngeal abscess is identified. CT scanning can delineate the extent of these deep neck infections.

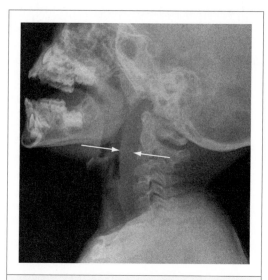

Figure 11-5. Thickening of the prevertebral soft tissues (*white arrows*) in a 3-year-old boy with neck stiffness due to a retropharyngeal abscess. (From Taussig LM, Landau LI [eds]: Pediatric Respiratory Medicine, 2nd ed. Philadelphia, Mosby, 2008, p 147.)

259. **Which age group is most susceptible to retropharyngeal abscess?**

This disease is most common in children between the ages of 1 and 6 years. There are several small lymph nodes in the retropharynx that usually disappear by the age of 4 or 5. These lymph nodes drain the posterior nasal passages and nasopharynx, and they may become involved if those sites are infected.

260. **What are the indications for removing adenoids?**
- Obstructive sleep apnea due to adenotonsillar hypertrophy
- Chronic adenoiditis
- Chronic sinusitis
- Repeat surgery for otitis media with effusion

   Gigante J: Tonsillectomy and adenoidectomy, *Pediatr Rev* 26:199–202, 2005.

261. **What are the indications for removing the tonsils?**
Absolute
- Obstructive sleep apnea syndrome due to adenotonsillar hypertrophy
- Suspected malignancy
- Recurrent hemorrhage

Relative
- Recurrent acute tonsillitis: the number of throat infections that might warrant a tonsillectomy to reduce subsequent episodes remains controversial. Guidelines from different organizations range from three to seven infections per year despite medical treatment. In general, the less severe the history of recurrent tonsillitis, the more marginally beneficial is the surgery.

■ Recurrent peritonsillar abscess

Gigante J: Tonsillectomy and adenoidectomy, *Pediatr Rev* 26:199–202, 2005.

262. **How should children with epiglottitis be managed?**
Acute epiglottitis is a medical emergency, and all children should be assumed to have a critical airway (i.e., or the potential for imminent occlusion exists). Because of the risk for airway obstruction upon agitation, the patient should be allowed to remain with parents, free from restraint. Examination should be performed as cautiously as possible. Continuous observation regardless of the setting (e.g., radiology suite), avoidance of supine positioning, and arrangements for admission to an intensive care unit are mandatory. Ideally, the epiglottis is visualized directly in an operating room, and the child is intubated immediately afterward.

Previously, more than 90% of cases were caused by *H. influenzae* type b. However, because of the routine use of *H. influenzae* type b vaccines in infants beginning in 1989 and 1990, the incidence of epiglottitis has decreased dramatically. Pneumococci, staphylococci, and streptococci (group A) now account for a relatively large percentage of cases.

263. **How is epiglottitis distinguished clinically from croup?**
See Table 11-9.

TABLE 11-9.	CLINICAL DISTINCTIONS BETWEEN CROUP AND EPIGLOTTITIS	
	Croup	**Epiglottitis**
Age	Younger (6 mo-3 yr)	Older (3-7 yr)
Onset of stridor	Gradual (24-72 hr)	Rapid (8-12 hr)
Symptoms	Prodromal upper respiratory infection	Minimal rhinitis
	Harsh, brassy cough	Little coughing
	Hoarseness	Muffled voice
	Slightly sore throat	Pain in throat
Signs	Mild fever	High body temperature ($>39°C$)
	Not toxic	Toxic appearance
	Variable distress	Severe distress; sits upright; may drool
	Harsh inspiratory stridor	Low-pitched inspiratory stridor
	Expiratory sounds uncommon	May have a low-pitched expiratory sound
Radiology	Subglottic narrowing	Edema of epiglottis and aryepiglottic folds (positive thumb sign)

264. **What are the criteria for the admission of a child with viral croup?**
■ *Clinical signs of impending respiratory failure:* Marked retractions, depressed level of consciousness, cyanosis, hypotonicity, and diminished or absent inspiratory breath sounds
■ *Laboratory signs of impending respiratory failure:* Pco_2 more than 45 mm Hg, Pao_2 less than 70 mm Hg in room air

- *Clinical signs of dehydration*
- *Social considerations:* Unreliable parents, excessive distance from hospital
- *Historic considerations:* High-risk infant with history of subglottic stenosis or prior intubations

Bjornson CL, Johnson DW: Croup, *Lancet* 371:329–339, 2008.

265. **Are steroids efficacious for the treatment of croup?**
The use of corticosteroids (including oral and intramuscular dexamethasone and nebulized budesonide) has been shown to be beneficial in treating croup. In particular, corticosteroid treatment reduces the incidence of intubation and results in more rapid respiratory improvement. In addition, among patients with mild or moderate croup, corticosteroids appear to reduce the use of nebulized racemic epinephrine, the need for return visits, and the need for hospitalization. Optimal doses are not clearly established. Dosing of dexamethasone is often based on the severity of croup ranging from mild croup with oral dosing (0.3 to 0.6 mg/kg up to 10 mg) to severe croup with intravenous or intramuscular dosing (0.6 mg/kg up to 15 mg).

Baumer JH: Glucocorticoid treatment in croup, *Arch Dis Child Educ Pract Ed* 91:ep58–ep60, 2006.

266. **If a child has received racemic epinephrine as a treatment for croup, is hospitalization required?**
In earlier days, children treated with racemic epinephrine were routinely hospitalized to observe for potential rebound mucosal edema and airway obstruction, regardless of how they appeared clinically. However, a number of recent studies have shown that children who are free of significant stridor or retractions at rest 2 hours after the administration of racemic epinephrine can be safely discharged, provided that adequate follow-up is ensured. In most of these studies, oral or intramuscular dexamethasone (0.6 mg/kg) was also administered.

Cherry JD: Croup, *N Engl J Med* 358:384–391, 2008.

267. **Is a cool-mist vaporizer truly of benefit for patients with croup?**
The usual advice for the home management of croup includes the use of a cool-mist vaporizer. The theory is that the coolness serves as a vasoconstrictor and that the humidified mist serves to thin respiratory secretions. Although this therapy remains time honored, it is largely unproven. The calming effects of being held by a parent during the mist treatment may have greater impact.

Cherry JD: Croup, *N Engl J Med* 358:384–391, 2008.

268. **What are membranous and pseudomembranous croup?**
Membranous croup is the historical term for diphtheria, and *pseudomembranous croup* is the historical term for bacterial tracheitis.
Bacterial tracheitis is usually caused by *S. aureus* and may occur after trauma to the neck or trachea or after a viral respiratory tract infection such as croup. The presentation of bacterial tracheitis is similar to that of severe croup or epiglottitis, and consequently a lateral neck radiograph is frequently obtained. In bacterial tracheitis, this study often reveals narrowing of the tracheal lumen as the result of a thick, purulent exudate that can extend into both mainstem bronchi.

269. **What is spasmodic croup?**
Spasmodic croup is a poorly understood cause of recurrent stridor in young children (usually 1 to 3 years old) and resembles acute infectious laryngotracheobronchitis in many respects. However, unlike infectious croup, a prodrome of upper respiratory symptoms is usually absent, and the patient is usually afebrile. The onset is sudden,

typically at night, with inspiratory stridor and a brassy cough that responds to therapies used for infectious croup (e.g., cool mist, racemic epinephrine, corticosteroids). Recurrence is common. The pathogenesis is unclear, but allergic and hypersensitivity components are suspected. In the rare patient who requires intubation, the typical finding is the pale and boggy mucosa of allergy and not the inflamed swelling of a primary infection.

SINUSITIS

270. **When do the sinuses develop during childhood?**
The maxillary and ethmoid sinuses are present at birth. Pneumatization of the sphenoid sinuses begins at about 2 to 3 years of age and is usually complete by about age 5. Frontal sinus pneumatization varies considerably, beginning at about 3 to 7 years of age and finishing by age 12 years.

KEY POINTS: PNEUMATIZATION OF THE PARANASAL SINUSES

1. Maxillary and ethmoid: Present at birth

2. Sphenoid: Begins at 2-3 years of age, complete by age 6 years

3. Frontal: Begins at 3-7 years of age, complete by age 12 years

4. Front sinus pneumatization is absent in 1% to 4% of the population

271. **What percentage of teenagers do not have frontal sinuses when radiographs are obtained?**
Frontal sinus pneumatization is absent in about 1% to 4% of the normal population due to agenesis. About 15% have unilateral frontal sinus hypoplasia.

272. **Does a thick, green nasal discharge on day 2 of a respiratory illness indicate a bacterial sinus infection?**
No. The character of nasal secretions (e.g., purulent, discolored, tenacious) does not distinguish viral from bacterial. Mucopurulent rhinitis commonly accompanies the common cold. Early treatment (<7 to 10 days) of purulent nasal discharge is a common cause of antibiotic overuse.

273. **What is the typical presentation of sinusitis in children?**
Unlike adults who may present with fever and localized pain, children have **persistent nasal symptoms** (anterior or posterior discharge, obstruction, or congestion) without improvement for 10 to 14 days or worsening after 5 to 7 days with or without daytime cough (which may worsen at night). The more acute presentation, less common, involves temperature of 39°C or higher and purulent nasal discharge occurring for at least 3 days in a patient who appears ill. Headache and facial pain are uncommon in younger patients with sinusitis but are seen more commonly in older children and teenagers who have had increased sinus pneumatization.

American Academy of Pediatrics: Appropriate use of antimicrobial agents. In Pickering LK, editor: *2009 Red Book: Report of the Committee on Infectious Diseases*, ed 28, Elk Grove Village, IL, 2009, American Academy of Pediatrics, p 741.

274. **Is transillumination helpful for diagnosing sinusitis in children?**
In general, transillumination of the sinuses is of very limited value in the diagnosis of acute sinusitis in young children.

275. **What is the role of plain radiographs in the diagnosis of sinusitis?**
Radiographs are not recommended for children 6 years of age and younger. Viral URIs often have features of rhinosinusitis, and false-positive rates are unacceptably high. Abnormal radiographs cannot distinguish bacterial or viral causes of sinusitis. In patients older than 6 years, it is controversial whether confirmatory radiographs before initiation of therapy are indicated. Most clinicians treat a patient with a suspected first-time acute sinusitis empirically without performing imaging studies.

276. **Which radiographic views are potentially useful for evaluating sinusitis?**
In children younger than 6 years, only the maxillary and ethmoid sinuses are clinically important, and 80% of children in this age group with acute sinusitis will have both sets of sinuses involved. Caldwell (anteroposterior) and Waters (occipitomental) views are necessary to assess these sinuses. To evaluate the frontal and sphenoid sinuses of older children, a lateral view is most informative.

277. **What constitutes an abnormal sinus radiograph?**
- Complete opacification of a sinus cavity
- Mucosal thickening of at least 4 mm
- Presence of an air-fluid level

Although these findings are not specific for sinusitis, they are helpful for confirming a diagnosis of acute sinusitis in patients with suggestive signs and symptoms (i.e., nasal discharge and cough persisting for more than 10 days without improvement or high fever and purulent nasal discharge for more than 3 days).

278. **When should CT scans be considered for the diagnosis of sinusitis?**
In most cases, a sinus CT scan is unnecessary. CT scans are more sensitive than sinus radiographs but also suffer from a lack of specificity. Scenarios that might warrant the use of CT scanning include the following:
- Complicated sinus disease with either orbital or CNS abnormalities
- Multiple recurrences
- Prolonged symptoms that are unresponsive to treatment and that suggest possible anatomic abnormalities, thereby raising sinus surgery as a consideration

Nash D, Wald ER: Sinusitis, *Pediatr Ann* 22:111–117, 2001.

279. **Which organisms are responsible for acute and chronic sinusitis in the pediatric age group?**
In **acute, uncomplicated sinusitis**, the etiologic organisms closely parallel those associated with acute otitis media: *S. pneumoniae, H. influenzae*, and *M. catarrhalis*. In patients with **chronic sinusitis**, the most common pathogens remain *S. pneumoniae, H. influenzae*, and *M. catarrhalis*, along with *S. aureus* and anaerobes. Fungal infection with zygomycosis (mucormycosis) is an important concern in immunosuppressed patients. *P. aeruginosa* must always be considered in patients with cystic fibrosis.

280. **What are indications for antibiotic therapy for children with sinusitis?**
This is an area of contention in an age of antibiotic overuse. Similar to otitis media, a large percentage (up to 60%) of children with clinically diagnosed sinusitis based on persistent symptoms will resolve without antibiotics. Most common colds are resolving without treatment within 7 to 10 days, but lingering (albeit improving) symptoms can commonly

persist beyond 10 days. The definitive study to evaluate the benefits of antibiotics—a randomized, placebo-controlled trial with pretreatment and posttreatment cultures from sinus aspirates—has not been done. Treatment is empirical and is recommended for severe symptoms in the early stages or clear persistence without improvement beyond 10 to 14 days to hasten recovery and prevent suppurative complications.

Pappas DE, Hendley JO, et al: Symptom profile of common colds in school-aged children, *Pediatr Infect Dis J* 27:8–11, 2008.

American Academy of Pediatrics Subcommittee on Management of Sinusitis: Clinical practice guideline: management of sinusitis, *Pediatrics* 108:798–808, 2001.

281. **For how long should sinus infections be treated?**
The duration of therapy for acute sinusitis in children has not been studied systematically. However, for patients whose symptoms improve dramatically within 3 to 4 days of initiating treatment, a 10-day course of therapy is usually effective. For patients who respond more slowly to antibiotics, treatment until symptoms resolve plus another 7 days is reasonable. Often, 3 weeks of treatment are required.

282. **List the predisposing factors for the development of chronic sinusitis.**
- Allergic rhinitis
- Anatomic abnormalities (e.g., polyps, enlarged adenoids)
- Impairment of mucociliary clearance (e.g., cystic fibrosis, primary ciliary dyskinesia)
- Foreign bodies (e.g., nasogastric tube)
- Abnormalities in immune defense

TUBERCULOSIS

283. **When are the various strengths of tuberculosis skin tests (TST) used?**
The standard-strength PPD (Mantoux test) contains 5 tuberculin units (TU) of purified protein derivative and is designated intermediate strength. This preparation is used for routine skin test screening. PPD is also available in 1-TU and 250-TU strengths, but these preparations are not generally recommended.

284. **How is the Mantoux test interpreted in children?**
The Mantoux test is interpreted in the context of clinical signs and symptoms and epidemiologic risk factors (e.g., known exposure). Positive tests are defined as follows:
Reaction of ≥5 mm
- Children in close contact with confirmed or suspected cases of tuberculosis
- Children with radiographic or clinical evidence of tubercular disease
- Children receiving immunosuppressive therapy
- Children with immunodeficiency disorders, including HIV infection
Reaction of ≥10 mm
- Children younger than 4 years
- Children with Hodgkin disease, lymphoma, diabetes mellitus, chronic renal failure, or malnutrition
- Children born in high-prevalence regions of the world, whose parents were born in such areas, or who have traveled to such areas
- Children frequently exposed to adults who are infected with HIV, homeless, incarcerated, illicit drug users, or migrant farm workers
Reaction of ≥15 mm
- Children 4 years or older with no risk factors

American Academy of Pediatrics: Tuberculosis. In Pickering LK, editor: *2009 Red Book Report of the Committee on Infectious Diseases*, ed 28, Elk Grove Village, 2009, IL, American Academy of Pediatrics, p 681.

285. **What are the reasons for a false-negative TST?**
About 10% to 20% of patients with culture-documented disease will have an initial TST that is negative. Reasons include:
■ Testing during the incubation period (2 to 10 weeks)
■ Young age
■ Problems with the administration technique
■ Severe systemic tuberculosis infection (miliary or meningitis)
■ Immunosuppression, malnutrition, or immunodeficiency
■ Concurrent infection: Measles, varicella, influenza, HIV, EBV, mycoplasma, mumps, rubella

286. **Should anergy panels be obtained for patients with negative tuberculosis testing?**
Anergy testing, the process of testing cutaneous reactions to a panel of unrelated antigens (such as tetanus, mumps, or candida), has in the past been used as an adjunct to assess immune function if TST is negative. However, anergy panels have not been shown to improve the reliability of negative TST. They are not recommended by most pediatric infectious disease experts.

287. **Why is a multiple puncture test (tine test) not considered an ideal test for tuberculosis?**
■ The exact dose of antigen (either PPD or old tuberculin) cannot be standardized, and thus interpretation is difficult. As a result, any positive test must be confirmed with a Mantoux test.
■ In a patient with a positive tine test, the need for a follow-up Mantoux test can lead to a booster phenomenon if the patient has had a previous bacille Calmette-Guérin (BCG) vaccine or infection with nontuberculous mycobacteria, again making interpretation difficult.
■ Significant variability exists among false-negative rates and especially among false-positive rates.
■ The use of tine tests has a tendency to result in parental reporting, which can be very unreliable.

288. **What is the role of interferon-release assays (IGRAs) in the diagnosis of tuberculosis in children?**
IGRA assays rely on interferon-γ produced by lymphocytes sensitized by antigens specific to *M. tuberculosis*. These antigens are not found in the BCG vaccine or in environmental mycobacteria. A whole-blood enzyme-linked immunoabsorbent assay (ELISA) can measure the interferon-γ concentration after incubation with antigen. The use of IGRA is an exciting development in the diagnostic methodology for tuberculosis but does require more study regarding its role as a solo test, adjunct to skin TST, and aspects of cost. QuantiFERON-TB Gold (QFT) is an IGRA assay approved by the FDA for use in adults, but data in children are limited.

Taylor REB, Cant AJ, Clark JE: Potential effect of NICE tuberculosis guidelines on paediatric tuberculosis screening, *Arch Dis Child* 93:200–203, 2008.

Shingadia D, Novelli V: The tuberculin skin test: a hundred, not out, *Arch Dis Child* 93:189–190, 2008.

289. **How should a patient with a positive TST be evaluated?**
History should search for clues that are suggestive of active infection, such as recurrent fevers, weight loss, adenopathy, or cough. A history of recurrent infections in the patient or

a family member may be suggestive of HIV infection, which is a risk factor for infection with *M. tuberculosis*. Information from previous tuberculin skin testing is invaluable. Epidemiologic information includes an evaluation of possible exposure to tuberculosis. A family history is obtained, including questions pertaining to chronic cough or weight loss in a family member or other contact. Travel history and current living arrangements should be elucidated. If the patient has immigrated to North America, a history of BCG vaccination should be ascertained.

Physical examination should focus on pulmonary, lymphatic, and abdominal systems. Examination should corroborate a history of BCG vaccination.

Laboratory evaluation, including a chest radiograph with a lateral film, is the next stage. Family members and close contacts should undergo skin testing. In certain circumstances, chest radiographs should be performed on the child's contacts.

If any of the preceding evaluation suggests active infection, sputum, gastric aspirates, and other appropriate specimens (e.g., lymph node tissue) should be obtained for mycobacterial culture and Ziehl-Neelsen or auramine-rhodamine staining.

290. **In a child with latent tuberculosis infection (LTBI), how effective is therapy in preventing the development of disease?**
A patient with a positive TST who has no clinical or radiographic abnormalities suggesting tuberculosis disease is thought to have LTBI. If a patient has never received antituberculous medication and has not had a known exposure to a person with isoniazid-resistant tuberculosis, that patient should be treated with isoniazid, once daily, for 9 months. Adherence to this regimen has been found to have an efficacy near 100% in preventing disease.

291. **In a younger child suspected of having tuberculosis disease, how should gastric aspirates be obtained?**
Because children younger than 10 years rarely produce sputum, gastric aspirates are a better source for the culture of mycobacteria in these patients, yielding the organism in up to 40% of cases. The aspirate should be obtained early in the morning as the child awakens to sample the overnight accumulation of respiratory secretions. The sample should be collected in a saline-free fluid, and the pH should be neutralized if any delay in processing is anticipated because *M. tuberculosis* does not tolerate acid environments.

292. **How do the manifestations of active pulmonary tuberculosis on chest radiograph differ between adults and children?**
Adults more commonly present with cavitary disease compared with children who have hilar adenopathy. Children older than 5 years tend to be asymptomatic, whereas infants with hilar adenopathy have air trapping and wheezing thought to result from the smaller bronchi being more easily compressed by enlarging lymph nodes.

Janner D: *A Guide to Pediatric Infectious Disease*, Philadelphia, 2005, Lippincott Williams & Wilkins, p 126.

293. **How are children with active pulmonary tuberculosis treated?**
Recommendations for the treatment of active tuberculosis in children have evolved over the past several years. Previously, therapy for at least 9 months was suggested for uncomplicated pulmonary disease. Studies in adults and children have demonstrated that 6 months of combined antituberculous therapy (short-course therapy) is as effective as 9 months of therapy. To date, the combined results of multiple studies in pediatric patients have demonstrated the efficacy of 6 months of therapy to be more than 95%.

The current standard regimen for active pulmonary tuberculosis in children consists of 2 months of daily isoniazid, rifampin, and pyrazinamide followed by 4 months of isoniazid and rifampin (daily or twice weekly). If drug resistance is a concern, either ethambutol or streptomycin is added to the initial three-drug regimen until drug susceptibilities are determined.

294. **What is the importance of DOT in the treatment of tuberculosis?**
Directly observed therapy (DOT), administration of medication by a third party (either a health care professional or a trained unrelated individual), has been found to be a valuable approach to the treatment of children and adolescents with tuberculosis disease. Failure to properly take chronic medications increases the likelihood of relapse and the development of resistance. DOT increases adherence and thus lowers rates of relapse, treatment failures, and drug resistance.

295. **Why are multiple antibiotics used for the treatment of tuberculosis disease?**
Compared with a patient with only a positive test but no disease, two features of *M. tuberculosis* make the organism difficult to eradicate after infection has been established. First, mycobacteria replicate slowly and may remain dormant for prolonged periods, but they are susceptible to drugs only during active replication. Second, drug-resistant organisms exist naturally within a large population, even before the initiation of therapy. These features render the organism—when it is present in significant numbers—extremely difficult to eradicate with a single agent.

296. **Why is pyridoxine supplementation given to patients who are receiving isoniazid?**
Isoniazid interferes with pyridoxine metabolism and may result in peripheral neuritis or convulsions. The administration of pyridoxine is generally not necessary for children who have a normal diet because they have adequate stores of this vitamin. Children and adolescents with diets deficient in milk or meat, exclusively breastfed infants, symptomatic HIV-infected children, and pregnant women should receive pyridoxine supplementation during isoniazid therapy.

297. **How effective is BCG vaccination?**
The BCG vaccines are among the most widely used in the world at present and are also perhaps the most controversial. The difficulties stem from the marked variation in reported efficacy of BCG against *M. tuberculosis* and *Mycobacterium leprae* infections. Depending on the population studied, efficacy against tuberculosis has ranged from 0% to 80%. Similarly, the efficacy against leprosy has ranged from 20% to 60% in prospective trials.
   The vaccines were derived from a strain of *Mycobacterium bovis* in 1906 and were subsequently dispersed to several laboratories around the world, where they were propagated under nonstandardized conditions. Hence, the vaccines in use today cannot be considered homogeneous. This may explain the observed variation in efficacy.

298. **How does BCG immunization influence tuberculosis skin testing?**
Generally, the interpretation of PPD tests is the same in BCG recipients as it is in nonvaccinated children. If positive, consideration should be given to several factors when deciding who should receive antituberculous therapy. These factors include time since BCG immunization, number of doses received, prevalence of tuberculosis in the country of origin, contacts in the United States, and radiographic findings.

299. **Why do children with tuberculosis rarely infect other children?**
Tuberculosis is transmitted by infected droplets of mucus that become airborne when an individual coughs or sneezes. As compared with adults, children with tuberculosis have several factors that minimize their contagiousness:
- Low density of organisms in sputum
- Lack of cavitations or extensive infiltrates on chest radiograph

- Lower frequency of cough
- Lower volume and higher viscosity of sputum
- Shorter duration of respiratory symptoms

Starke JR: Childhood tuberculosis during the 1990s, *Pediatr Rev* 13:343–353, 1992.

300. **In addition to tuberculosis, what other airborne microbes can cause respiratory disease?**
See Table 11-10.

TABLE 11-10. AIRBORNE MICROBIAL DISEASES	
Disease	Airborne Source
Aspergillosis	Conidia spores from decaying vegetation and soil
Brucellosis	Aerosolized from carcasses of domestic and wild animals
Chickenpox	Aerosolized from respiratory secretions
Coccidioidomycosis	Arthroconidia from soil and dust
Cryptococcosis	Aerosolized from bird droppings
Histoplasmosis	Conidia spores from bat or bird droppings
Legionnaires disease	Aerosolized contaminated water, especially from air-conditioning cooling towers
Measles	Aerosolized respiratory secretions
Mucormycosis	Spores from soil
Psittacosis	*Chlamydia psittaci* from birds
Q fever	*Coxiella burnetii* from a variety of farm and other animals
Tularemia	Aerosolized from multiple wild animals, especially rabbits

ACKNOWLEDGMENT

The editors gratefully acknowledge contributions by Drs. Alexis M. Elward, David A. Hunstad, and Joseph W. St. Geme III that were retained from previous editions of *Pediatric Secrets*.

CHAPTER 12

NEONATOLOGY

Philip Roth, MD, PhD

CLINICAL ISSUES

1. **Should an asymptomatic infant with a single umbilical artery have a screening ultrasound done for renal anomalies?**

   This point has been argued for years. A single umbilical artery is a rare phenomenon. In one study of nearly 35,000 infants, examination of the placenta showed that only 112 (0.32%) had a single umbilical artery. In a recent study, a single umbilical artery was detected in 2% of fetuses. Fetuses with a single umbilical artery had significantly more chromosomal (10.3%) and congenital anomalies (27%) than those with two umbilical arteries. However, isolated single umbilical artery in an otherwise normal infant is associated with a low incidence of renal and urinary tract anomalies, most of which are transient or mild. Screening is therefore best reserved for those who have other anomalies.

   Bourke WG, Clarke TA, Mathews TG, et al: Isolated single umbilical artery: the case for routine renal screening, *Arch Dis Child* 68:600–601, 1993.

   Doornebal N: Screening infants with an isolated single umbilical artery for renal anomalies: nonsense? *Early Hum Dev* 83:567–570, 2007.

   Rittler M et al: Single umbilical artery and associated malformations in over 5,500 autopsies. Relevance for perinatal management, *Pediatr Dev Pathol EPub* May 19, 2010.

2. **How does the handling of the umbilical cord at birth affect neonatal hemoglobin concentrations?**

   At the time of birth, the placental vessels may contain up to 33% of the fetal-placental blood volume. Constriction of the umbilical arteries limits blood flow from the infant, but the umbilical vein remains dilated. The extent of drainage from the placenta to the infant through the umbilical vein is very dependent on gravity. The recommendation is to keep the baby at least 20 to 40 cm below the placenta for about 30 to 60 seconds before clamping the cord. More elevated positioning or rapid clamping can minimize the placental transfusion and decrease red blood cell (RBC) volume. Delayed clamping (>1 minute) resulted in short-term increases in hemoglobin, jaundice requiring phototherapy, and higher ferritin levels at 6 months.

   Neilson JP: Cochrane update: effect of timing of umbilical cord clamping at birth of term infants on mother and baby outcomes, *Obstet Gynecol* 112:177–178, 2008.

   Brugnara C, Platt OS: The neonatal erythrocyte and its disorders. In Nathan DG, Orkin SH, Ginsburg D, Look AT, editors: *Nathan and Oski's Hematology of Infancy and Childhood*, ed 6, Philadelphia, 2003, WB Saunders, pp 30–31.

3. **What is the best method of umbilical cord care during the immediate neonatal period?**

   No single method of cord care has been determined to be superior for preventing colonization and infections. Antimicrobial agents, such as bacitracin or triple dye, are commonly used, but there are no efficacy data (other than reduced colonization). Alcohol accelerates the drying of the cord, but it has not been shown to reduce the rates of colonization or omphalitis. The use of topical antibiotics has been shown to delay cord separation. Therefore, simply cleaning with normal saline and allowing the cord to dry normally appears to be as safe and effective as using antibiotics.

Zupan J, Garner P, Omari AA: Topical umbical cord care at birth, *Cochrane Database Syst Rev* 3: CD001057, 2004.

Mullany LC, Darmstadt GL, Tielsch J: Role of antimicrobial applications to the umbilical cord in neonates to prevent bacterial colonization and infection: a review of the evidence, *Pediatr Infect Dis J* 11:996–1002, 2003.

4. **When should a parent begin to worry if an umbilical cord has not fallen off?**
   The umbilical cord generally dries up and sloughs by 2 weeks of life. Delayed separation can be normal up to 45 days. However, because neutrophilic and monocytic infiltration appear to play a major role in autodigestion, persistence of the cord beyond 30 days should prompt consideration of an underlying functional abnormality of neutrophils (leukocyte adhesion deficiency) or neutropenia.

Roos D, Laws SK: Hematologically important mutations: leukocyte adhesion deficiency, *Blood Cell Mol Dis* 6:1000–1004, 2001.

Kemp AS, Lubitz L: Delayed cord separation in alloimmune neutropenia, *Arch Dis Child* 68:52–53, 1993.

5. **How do you estimate the insertion distance necessary for umbilical catheters?**
   Measuring the distance from the umbilicus to the shoulder (lateral end of clavicle) allows for an estimation of desired length (Table 12-1). Alternatively, insertion distance in centimeters for the following situations is given below:
   - "High" umbilical artery catheter = [3 × weight (kg)] + 9
   - Umbilical venous catheter = [½ × UAC insertion distance] + 1

TABLE 12-1. INSERTION DISTANCE FOR UMBILICAL CATHETERS

Shoulder to Umbilicus (cm)	Aortic Catheter to Diaphragm (cm)	Aortic Catheter to Aortic Bifurcation (cm)	Venous Catheter to Right Atrium (cm)
9	11	5	6
10	12	5	6-7
11	13	6	7
12	14	7	8
13	15	8	8-9
14	16	9	9
15	17	10	10
16	18	10-11	11
17	20	11-12	11-12

Data from Dunn PM: Localization of umbilical catheters by post mortem measurement. Arch Dis Child 41:69-75, 1966.

6. **What is the appropriate position of a peripherally inserted central catheter (PICC)?**
   The tip of a PICC should be placed and positioned in as large a vein as possible, preferably the superior or inferior vena cava, but not in the right atrium, owing to the risk for perforation or pericardial effusions. Because of secondary migration, the catheter tip should be at least 1 cm from the cardiac silhouette in preterm infants and 2 cm in full-term infants. Catheters inserted through the basilic or cephalic veins will migrate toward the heart with flexion of the elbow, whereas adduction of the shoulder results in migration toward the heart if inserted in the former and away if inserted in the latter. After insertion, catheter placement should be determined radiographically.

Nadroo AM, Gless RB, Lin J, et al: Changes in upper extremity position causes migration of peripherally inserted central catheters in neonates, *Pediatrics* 110:131–136, 2002.

Darling JC, Newell SJ, Mohamdee O, et al: Central venous catheter tip in the right atrium: a risk factor for neonatal cardiac tamponade, *J Perinatol* 21:461–464, 2001.

7. **What are the increased risks of twin pregnancies?**
   - Premature delivery
   - Intrauterine growth restriction, including discordant growth (which may occur in up to one third of twin pregnancies)
   - Increased perinatal mortality, especially for premature, monozygotic, and discordant twins
   - Spontaneous abortion
   - Birth asphyxia
   - Fetal malposition
   - Placental abnormalities (abruptio placentae, placenta previa)
   - Polyhydramnios

8. **Why are monozygotic twins considered higher risk than dizygotic twins?**
   Monozygotic twins (identical twins) arise from the division of a single fertilized egg. Depending on the timing of the division of the single ovum into separate embryos, the amnionic and chorionic membranes can either be shared (if division occurs >8 days after fertilization), separate (if division occurs <72 hours after fertilization), or mixed (separate amnion, shared chorion if division occurs 4 to 8 days after fertilization). Sharing of the chorion and/or amnion is associated with potential problems of vascular anastomoses (and possible twin-twin transfusions), cord entanglements, and congenital anomalies. These problems increase the risk for intrauterine growth restriction and perinatal death. **Dizygotic twins**, however, result from two separately fertilized ova and, as such, usually have a separate amnion and chorion.

9. **How extensive is insensible water loss in preterm infants?**
   Insensible water loss is the loss of water through the lungs during respiration and from the skin by evaporation. A rough guide to the amount of insensible loss in milliliters per kilogram per day (mL/kg/day) for infants in humidified isolettes is given in Table 12-2.

TABLE 12-2. INSENSIBLE LOSS (ML/KG/DAY) FOR INFANTS IN HUMIDIFIED ISOLETTES

Age (days)	Body Weight (g)					
	500-750	751-1000	1001-1250	1251-1500	1501-1750	1751-2000
0-7	100	65	55	40	20	15
7-14	80	60	50	40	30	20

Data from Avery GB, Fletcher MA, MacDonald MG: Neonatology: Pathophysiology and Management of the Newborn. Lippincott Williams & Wilkins, Philadelphia, 1999, p 348.

10. **What factors affect insensible water loss?**
    - **Increase:** Prematurity, activity, fever, radiant warmer, phototherapy, and skin breakdown or defect
    - **Decrease:** Topical emollients, high humidity and mechanical ventilation (with humidified air)

11. **Do infants receiving phototherapy require additional fluids?**
    Unless there is evidence of dehydration, routine intravenous fluid or other supplementation of term and near-term infants is not necessary. Preterm infants weighing less than 1500 g should receive a 25% increment while receiving phototherapy.

    Subcommittee on Hyperbilirubinemia: Management of hyperbilirubinemia in the newborn infant 35 or more weeks of gestation, *Pediatrics* 114:297–316, 2004.

12. **Which infants require ophthalmologic evaluation for retinopathy of prematurity (ROP)?**
    The American Academy of Pediatrics recommends that an individual experienced in neonatal ophthalmology and indirect ophthalmoscopy examine the retinas of all neonates with a birthweight of less than 1500 g or a gestational age of less than 32 weeks, and of those selected infants weighing between 1500 and 2000 g who have had unstable clinical courses, including those requiring cardiorespiratory support, placing them at increased risk. The timing of the first examination should be based on gestational age at birth according to Table 12-3.

TABLE 12-3. TIMING OF FIRST EYE EXAMINATION BASED ON GESTATIONAL AGE AT BIRTH

Gestational Age at Birth (wk)	Age at Initial Examination (wk)	
	Postmenstrual	Chronologic
22	31	9
23	31	8
24	31	7
25	31	6
26	31	5
27	31	4
28	32	4
29	33	4
30	34	4
31	35	4
32	36	4

American Academy of Pediatrics: American Academy of Ophthalmology American Association for Pediatric Ophthalmology and Strabismus: Screening examination of premature infants for retinopathy of prematurity, Pediatrics 117:572–576, 2006.

13. **What are the stages of ROP?**
    - **Stage I:** Line of demarcation separates vascular and avascular retina
    - **Stage II:** Ridging of line of demarcation as a result of scar formation
    - **Stage III:** Extraretinal fibrovascular proliferation present (in addition, in stages II and III, the term plus disease refers to active inflammation as manifested by tortuosity of retinal vessels, which increases the risk for progression of ROP)
    - **Stage IV:** Subtotal retinal detachment
    - **Stage V:** Complete retinal detachment

14. **What are the indications for cryotherapy or laser therapy among patients with ROP?**
Based on the results of the Early Treatment for Retinopathy of Prematurity randomized trial, the threshold for treatment has changed and should be initiated for the following retinal findings:
- **Zone I ROP:** Any stage with plus disease
- **Zone I ROP:** Stage III with no plus disease
- **Zone II ROP:** Stage II or III with plus disease
The number of "clock-hours" of disease may no longer be the deciding factor in the decision to perform ablative treatment.

Section on Ophthalmology, American Academy of Pediatrics, American Academy of Ophthalmology, American Association for Pediatric Ophthalmology and Strabismus: Screening examination of premature infants for retinopathy of prematurity, *Pediatrics* 117:572–576, 2006.

Early Treatment for Retinopathy of Prematurity Cooperative Group: Revised indications for treatment of retinopathy of prematurity: results of the early treatment for retinopathy of prematurity randomized trial, *Arch Ophthalmol* 121:1684–1694, 2003.

15. **If maternal drug abuse is suspected, which specimen from the infant is most accurate for detecting exposure?**
Although urine has traditionally been tested when maternal drug abuse is a possibility, **meconium** has a greater sensitivity than urine and positive findings that persist longer. It may contain metabolites gathered over as much as 20 weeks, compared with urine, which represents more recent exposure. Recent studies show that umbilical cord tissue is as equally sensitive in the detection of fetal drug exposure as meconium, which in some cases may be passed in utero and in others not for several days. It is important to remember that maternal self-reporting is notoriously inaccurate as an indicator of drug use.

Montgomery D: Testing for fetal exposure to illicit drugs using umbilical cord tissue vs. meconium, *J Perinatol* 26:11–14, 2006.

16. **What are the manifestations of drug withdrawal in the neonate?**
The signs and symptoms of drug withdrawal in the neonate can be remembered by using the acronym **WITHDRAWAL**:
- **W**akefulness
- **I**rritability
- **T**remulousness, temperature variation, tachypnea
- **H**yperactivity, high-pitched persistent cry, hyperacusis, hyperreflexia, hypertonus
- **D**iarrhea, diaphoresis, disorganized suck
- **R**ub marks, respiratory distress, rhinorrhea
- **A**pneic attacks, autonomic dysfunction
- **W**eight loss or failure to gain weight
- **A**lkalosis (respiratory)
- **L**acrimation

Committee on Drugs: Neonatal drug withdrawal, *Pediatrics* 72:896, 1983.

17. **Does in utero exposure to selective serotonin reuptake inhibitors (SSRIs) result in neonatal withdrawal?**
SSRIs are being prescribed with increasing frequency to pregnant women with depression. Recent data suggest that within days of birth, infants experience withdrawal symptoms, including irritability, crying, hypertonia, and seizures. The drug that figures most prominently is paroxetine (Paxil), but similar symptoms have been reported with fluoxetine (Prozac), sertraline (Zoloft), and citalopram (Celexa).

Alwan S and Friedman JM: Safety of selective serotonin uptake inhibitors in pregnancy. *CNS Drugs* 23:493–509, 2009.

Nordeng H: Neonatal withdrawal symptoms after in utero exposure to selective serotonin reuptake inhibitors, *Acta Paediatr* 90:288–291, 2001.

Sanz EJ: Neonatal withdrawal symptoms after in utero exposure to selective serotonin reuptake inhibitors in pregnant women and neonatal withdrawal syndrome: a database analysis, *Lancet* 365:482–487, 2005.

18. **Does maternal smoking in pregnancy result in nicotine withdrawal in newborn infants?**
Infants exposed to nicotine before birth as demonstrated by elevated levels of cotinine in blood, urine, and saliva demonstrate increased irritability, tremors, and sleep disturbances during the first five days of life. Severity of symptoms correlates with levels of markers for exposure.

Godding V, Bonnier C, Fiasse L, et al: Does in utero drug exposure to heavy maternal smoking induce nicotine withdrawal symptoms in neonates? *Pediatric Res* 55:645–651, 2004.

19. **What bone is the most frequently fractured in the newborn?**
The clavicle. This injury, which stems from excessive traction during delivery, generally results in a greenstick fracture (Fig. 12-1).

20. **What are the two most common causes of fetal death?**
Chromosomal abnormalities (especially during early pregnancy) and **congenital malformations.**

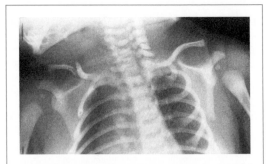

Figure 12-1. Radiograph of right clavicular fracture. (From Clark DA: Atlas of Neonatology. Philadelphia, WB Saunders, 2000, p 8.)

21. **With the recent increase in late preterm births (33 to 36 weeks), what are the most common causes for hospital readmission of these patients?**
Late preterm infants, who account in large part for the recent increase in prematurity in the United States, are more than twice as likely as their full-term counterparts to be readmitted to the hospital. The most common admission diagnoses are hyperbilirubinemia, feeding problems, respiratory difficulties, fever, and gastroesophageal reflux.

Braveman P, Kessel W, Egerter S, Richmond J: Early discharge and evidence-based practice: good science and good judgment, *JAMA* 278:334–336, 1997.

Maisels MJ, Kring E: Length of stay, jaundice, and hospital readmission, *Pediatrics* 101:995–998, 1998.

Tomashek KM et al: Early discharge among late preterm and term newborns and risk of neonatal morbidity, *Semin Perinatol* 30:61–68, 2006.

22. **With advances in reproductive technology, what have been the recent trends in the incidence of multiple births in the United States?**
In the past decade, for which there is complete data, the frequency of multiple births has increased by 30% to 33.8 per 1000 live births. If one looks at higher-order multiples (i.e., triplets and higher), the incidence increased by nearly 300% between 1985 and 1998 and has since stabilized at about 153 per 100,000 live births in 2006 (Fig. 12-2).

March of Dimes Peristats: http://www.marchofdimes.com/peristats, 2009.

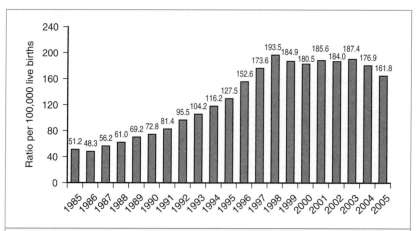

Figure 12-2. Incidence of higher-order multiple births in the United States. (Data from National Center for Health Statistics, final natality data. Retrieved from Peristats, March of Dimes, 2009.)

THE DELIVERY ROOM

23. **What is the clinical significance of fetal decelerations?**
The National Institute of Health recently convened a consensus conference to develop standardized definitions for fetal heart rate (FHR) patterns. Emphasis was placed on assessment of decelerations in the context of baseline FHR variability. Category III tracings with absence of baseline variability and either recurrent variable decelerations or bradycardia (baseline FHR <110 beats/minute) are predictive of abnormal fetal acid-base status at the time of observation. Consequently, prompt evaluation and interventions, including oxygen, change in position, treatment of hypotension, and discontinuation of drugs that stimulate uterine contractions, are indicated.

Macones GA, Hankins GD, Spong CV, et al: The 2008 National Institute of Child Health and Human Development workshop report on Electronic Fetal Monitoring: update on definitions, interpretation and research guidelines, *Obstet Gynecol* 112:661, 2008.

24. **How sensitive is FHR monitoring for detecting fetal asphyxia?**
The primary goals of FHR monitoring are to identify hypoxemic and acidotic fetuses in a timely manner that will prevent death or neurologic injury. Because most abnormal FHR tracings are not associated with fetal acidosis or hypoxia, and most episodes of acidosis and hypoxia do not result in neurologic disability, neither objective has been achieved. Nonetheless, FHR monitoring remains the standard in the United States.

Alfirevic Z, Devane D, Gyte G: Continuous cardiotocography as a form of electronic fetal monitoring for fetal assessment during labor, *Cochrane Database Syst Rev* 3:CD006066, 2006.

25. **What is an acceptable scalp pH for the fetus?**
Fetal scalp sampling to measure blood pH is used in conjunction with electronic FHR monitoring to assess fetal well-being during labor (Table 12-4). The range of acceptable values for fetal pH is broad. Clinically significant acidemia is defined as a scalp pH of less than 7.2. A scalp pH of more than 7.25 is considered normal. Values between 7.20 and 7.25 are considered borderline and warrant further sampling. A low pH does not predict subsequent cerebral palsy. Because of the cumbersome nature of this technique and discomfort to the patient, it is being performed with decreasing frequency.

TABLE 12-4. NORMAL FETAL SCALP BLOOD VALUES IN LABOR

	Early First Stage	Late First Stage	Second Stage
pH	7.33 ± 0.03	7.32 ± 0.02	7.29 ± 0.04
Pco_2 (mm Hg)	44 ± 4.05	42 ± 5.1	46.3 ± 4.2
Po_2 (mm Hg)	21.8 ± 2	21.3 ± 2.1	16.5 ± 1.4
Bicarbonate (mmol/L)	20.1 ± 1	19.1 ± 2.1	17 ± 2
Base excess (mmol/L)	3.9 ± 1.9	4.1 ± 2.5	6.4 ± 1.8

Data from Gilstrap LC: Fetal acid-base balance. In Creasy RK, Resnik R (eds): Maternal-Fetal Medicine, 4th ed. Philadelphia, WB Saunders, 2004, p 431.

26. **How long has meconium been present in the amniotic fluid if an infant has evidence of meconium staining?**
Gross staining of the infant is a surface phenomenon that is proportional to the length of exposure and meconium concentration. With heavy meconium, staining of the umbilical cord begins in as little as 15 minutes; with light meconium, it occurs after 1 hour. Yellow staining of the newborn's toenails requires 4 to 6 hours. Yellow staining of the vernix caseosa takes about 12 to 14 hours.

    Miller PW, Coen RW, Benirschke K: Dating the time interval from meconium passage to birth, *Obstet Gynecol* 66:459–462, 1985.

27. **Is meconium staining a good marker for neonatal asphyxia?**
No. Because 10% to 20% of all deliveries have in utero passage of meconium, meconium staining alone is not a good marker for neonatal asphyxia.

28. **If meconium is noted before or during the time of delivery, what is the recommended course of action?**
Although intrapartum nasopharyngeal and oropharyngeal suctioning by the obstetrician before the delivery of the thorax has been advocated for many years to reduce the incidence of meconium aspiration syndrome, recent data suggest that this may not be the case even in high-risk infants, that is, those with thick meconium, fetal heart rate decelerations, cesarean delivery, and/or need for delivery room resuscitation. However, once the baby is delivered, the next steps depend on whether the baby is vigorous as defined by good cry, respiratory effort, muscle tone, and heart rate of more than 100 beats/minute. If the baby is not vigorous, a laryngoscope should be inserted into the mouth, and a large bore catheter should be used to suction the mouth and posterior pharynx so that the glottis can be visualized. An endotracheal tube is then inserted into the trachea, connected to a suction source, and slowly withdrawn. The procedure is repeated until the trachea is clear of meconium or the baby develops bradycardia, requiring resuscitative measures to be initiated.

    Velaphi S, Vidyasagar D: Intrapartum and post delivery management of infants born to mothers with meconium stained amniotic fluid: Evidence based recommendations, *Clin Perinatal* 33:29–42, 2006.

29. **During asphyxia, how is primary apnea distinguished from secondary apnea?**
A regular sequence of events occurs when an infant is asphyxiated. Initially, gasping respiratory efforts increase in depth and frequency for up to 3 minutes, and this is followed by about 1 minute of primary apnea. If oxygen (along with stimulation) is provided during the apneic period, respiratory function spontaneously returns. If asphyxia continues, gasping then resumes for a variable period of time, terminating with the "last gasp" and followed by

secondary apnea. During secondary apnea, the only way to restore respiratory function is with positive-pressure ventilation (PPV) and high concentrations of oxygen. Thus, a linear relationship exists between the duration of asphyxia and the recovery of respiratory function after resuscitation. The longer the artificial ventilation is delayed after the last gasp, the longer it will take to resuscitate the infant. However, clinically, the two conditions are indistinguishable.

30. **How does one estimate the size of the endotracheal tube required for resuscitation?**
See Table 12-5.

TABLE 12-5. ENDOTRACHEAL TUBES NEEDED FOR RESUSCITATION		
Tube Size (Internal Diameter in mm)	Weight (g)	Gestational Age (wk)
2.5	<1000	<28
3.0	1001-2000	28-34
3.5	2001-3000	34-38
3.5-4.0	>3000	>38

Data from Hertz D: Principles of neonatal resuscitation. In Polin RA, Yoder MC, Burg FD (eds): Workbook in Practical Neonatology, 3rd ed. Philadelphia, WB Saunders, 2001, p 13.

31. **What is the "7-8-9" rule?**
The *7-8-9 rule* is an estimate of the length (in centimeters) that an oral endotracheal tube should be inserted into a 1-, 2-, or 3-kg infant, respectively. A variation of this rule is the tip-to-lip rule of adding 6 to the weight in kilograms of the infant to determine the insertion distance. With good visualization, the tube should be inserted 1 to 1.5 cm below the vocal cords. Tube placement should always be verified radiographically.

32. **When should epinephrine be given during a resuscitation in the delivery room?**
In a depressed infant with gasping or absent respirations, 100% oxygen should be given through PPV. Depending on the extent of asphyxia (and depression of heart rate to <60 beats/minute), cardiac compressions are usually initiated within 30 seconds. If there is no response (i.e., increased heart rate to >60 beats/minute) after at least 30 seconds of PPV with 100% oxygen and chest compressions, epinephrine is indicated. Epinephrine (1:10,000) can be given intravenously or through the umbilical vein at a dose of 0.1 to 0.3 mL/kg. If given endotracheally, usually a dose of 0.3 to 1.0 mL/kg should be considered.

33. **When is sodium bicarbonate administered in resuscitation?**
Recent review of the literature suggests that there are insufficient data to recommend the routine use of bicarbonate in neonatal resuscitation. The administration of bicarbonate may actually result in extracellular alkalosis and intracellular acidosis, which have adverse effects on both cardiac and cerebral function. In fact, it is even doubtful whether sodium bicarbonate should be used in treating neonatal metabolic acidosis other than in situations with ongoing losses from the kidneys or gastrointestinal tract. As a general principle, one should treat the underlying cause of acidosis and not the pH.

Aschner JL, Poland RL: Sodium bicarbonate: basically useless therapy, *Pediatrics* 122:831–835, 2008.

34. **Are there complications of sodium bicarbonate therapy in infants?**

    The relative risks of sodium bicarbonate therapy in infants are related to dosage (higher > lower), rapidity of administration (faster > slower), and osmolality (higher > lower). Physiologic complications include a transient increase in $Paco_2$ and fall in Pao_2. The sudden expansion of blood volume and an increase in cerebral blood flow may increase the risk for periventricular or intraventricular hemorrhage (IVH) in preterm infants (unproved). Furthermore, CO_2 produced from carbonic acid (derived from the reaction between protons and bicarbonate) rapidly diffuses into cells creating intracellular acidosis. This may impair cardiac function and output, which may already be compromised, thereby exacerbating venous hypercarbia. Remember, arterial pH values may not reflect the degree of intracellular acidosis and venous hypercarbia.

35. **When should a laryngeal mask airway (LMA) be used in neonatal resuscitation?**

    The LMA fits over the laryngeal inlet and may be used to effect ventilation when intubation is not feasible or is unsuccessful. The LMA should be considered when (1) anomalies of the lip, mouth, or palate make it impossible to achieve a good seal with the bag and mask; and (2) anomalies of the mouth, tongue, pharynx, mandible, or neck make visualization of the larynx with a laryngoscope impossible. Placement of the LMA does not require visualization and may be used to temporize while measures are taken to establish a more permanent airway (Fig. 12-3).

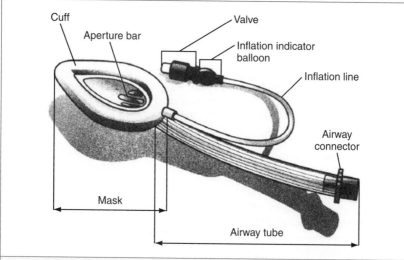

Figure 12-3. Laryngeal mask airway. (From Asensio JA, Trunkey DD [eds]: Current Therapy of Trauma and Surgical Critical Care. Philadelphia, Mosby, 2008.)

36. **Is there a role for CO_2 detectors in neonatal resuscitation?**

    After intubation, visualization of passage of the tube through the vocal cords, auscultation of breath sounds, and observation of chest movement are often used to ensure proper placement of the endotracheal tube in the trachea. However, these signs may be misleading and must be confirmed by rapid improvement in heart rate and/or detection of CO_2 following a few positive-pressure breaths. CO_2 detectors are available as either colorimetric devices or capnographs giving numeric CO_2 levels, with the former type the most commonly used. Beware, however, that patients with very low cardiac output such as those in cardiac arrest may have markedly diminished pulmonary blood flow resulting in failure to detect CO_2 despite tracheal placement of the endotracheal tube.

Leone TA et al: Disposable colorimetric carbon dioxide detector use as an indicator of a patent airway during non-invasive mask ventilation, *Pediatrics* 118:e202–e204, 2006.

37. **Should continuous positive airway pressure (CPAP) be administered in the delivery room to assist ventilation in the preterm infant?**
Because intermittent positive pressure breaths may be injurious to the immature preterm baby, administration of CPAP should be considered in infants with spontaneous respirations and a heart rate higher than 100 beats/minute who are showing signs of respiratory distress. Two recent trials comparing delivery room CPAP with intubation in infants born at 25 to 28 weeks' gestation showed no difference in the rate of death or bronchopulmonary dysplasia. Nonetheless, in the study by Morley et al, infants in the CPAP group required oxygen at 28 days of age less frequently and fewer days of intubation while experiencing a higher incidence of pneumothorax. In the study by Finer et al, infants who received CPAP treatment less frequently required intubation or postnatal steroids, required fewer days of mechanical ventilation and were more likely to be alive and free of mechanical ventilation at age 7 days.

Finer NN and SUPPORT study group early CPAP versus surfactant in extremely premature infants, *N Engl J Med* 362:2024–2026, 2010.

Morley CJ: Nasal CPAP or intubation at birth for very preterm infants, *N Engl J Med* 358:700–708, 2008.

38. **What techniques are available to keep preterm infants warm in the delivery room?**
Methods used in the delivery room to keep infants warm have included occlusive wrapping, heated mattresses, and kangaroo care (skin-to-skin contact). A number of studies have compared placement immediately after birth of preterm infants in a reclosable polyethylene bag without drying with standard drying after birth. A significantly higher neonatal intensive care unit (NICU) admission rectal temperature was observed in infants managed in this way, especially in those younger than 30 weeks' gestational age. A large multicenter trial is under way to confirm these results.

Watkinson M: Temperature control of preterm infants in the delivery room, *Chin Perinatol* 33:43–53, 2006.

Finer NN and the SUPPORT Study group Early CPAP versus surfactant in extremely premature infants, *N Engl J Med* 362:2024–2026, 2010.

39. **Should 100% O_2 or room air be used in neonatal resuscitation?**
The guidelines of the Neonatal Resuscitation Program (NRP) recommend use of 100% O_2 when PPV is required in the resuscitation of full-term infants. However, there is a growing body of data showing that 21% O_2 (room air) is just as effective as 100% O_2 and less likely to cause reperfusion injuries following asphyxia. Therefore, one may choose to start with 21% O_2 but be prepared to increase to 100% if the infant has not shown clinical improvement in 90 seconds. In the case of preterm infants, especially those born before 32 weeks' gestational age, who are especially vulnerable to hyperoxic injury, initial oxygen concentration for resuscitation should begin between 21% and 100% O_2—perhaps 30%—and be titrated based on achieving saturations higher than 85%, a rise toward 90% saturation over several minutes, and saturations that do not exceed 95%. Failure to achieve these goals and/or a rapid increase in heart rate to greater than 100 beats/minute should prompt the resuscitator to increase to 100% O_2 until adequate oxygenation is achieved.

Richmond S, Goldsmith JP: Air or 100% oxygen in neonatal resuscitation, *Clin Perinatol* 33:11–27, 2006.

Ten VS et al and Matsiukvich D: Room air or 100% oxygen for resuscitation of infants with perinatal depression, *Curr Opin Pediatr* 21:188–193, 2009.

40. **After a "traumatic" delivery, what are the commonly injured systems?**
- **Cranial injuries:** Caput succedaneum, subconjunctival hemorrhage, cephalohematoma, subgaleal hematoma, skull fractures, intracranial hemorrhage, cerebral edema
- **Spinal injuries:** Spinal cord transection
- **Peripheral nerve injuries:** Brachial palsy (Erb-Duchenne paralysis, Klumpke paralysis), phrenic nerve and facial nerve paralysis

- **Visceral injuries:** Liver rupture or hematoma, splenic rupture, adrenal hemorrhage
- **Skeletal injuries:** Fractures of the clavicle, femur, and humerus

41. **Who was Virginia Apgar, and how does one remember her score?**
    Virginia Apgar, an anesthesiologist at Columbia Presbyterian Medical Center in New York City, introduced the Apgar scoring system in 1953 to assess the newborn infant's response to the stress of labor and delivery. A pneumonic to help remember the components of the score is as follows:
    - **A**ppearance (pink, mottled, or blue)
    - **P**ulse (>100, <100, or 0 beats/minute)
    - **G**rimace (response to suctioning of the nose and mouth)
    - **A**ctivity (flexed arms and legs, extended limbs, or limp)
    - **R**espiratory effort (crying, gasping, or no respiratory activity)
      Each category is assigned a rating of 0, 1, or 2 points, with a total score of 10 indicating the best possible condition.

42. **Is a low Apgar score alone sufficient to diagnose a neonate as asphyxiated?**
    No. It is not acceptable to label an infant as asphyxiated simply because of a low Apgar score. Typically, a sentinel hypoxic event before or during labor is followed by fetal bradycardia or absent variability in the presence of variable and/or late decelerations. If asphyxiated, neonates typically have a profound metabolic acidosis and demonstrate abnormalities within 72 hours of birth in multiple organ systems. Signs referable to the central nervous system (CNS) are often most prominent. The cardinal features of hypoxic-ischemic encephalopathy include seizures, alterations of consciousness, and abnormalities of tone. Disorders of reflexes, respiratory pattern, oculovestibular responses, and autonomic function are less significant components of this entity. Early imaging studies may also show evidence of acute nonfocal cerebral abnormality.

    American Academy of Pediatrics Committee on Fetus and Newborn, American Academy of Obstetricians and Gynecologists and Committee on Obstetric Practice: The Apgar score, *Pediatrics* 117:1444–1447, 2006.

    Leuthner SR, Das U: Low Apgar scores and the definition of birth asphyxia, *Pediatr Clin North Am* 51:737–745, 2004.

    Hankins GDV, Speer M: Neonatal encephalopathy and cerebral palsy: defining the pathogenesis and pathophysiology, *Obstet Gynecol* 102:628–636, 2003.

43. **When should neonatal resuscitation be stopped?**
    Although each case should be considered individually, the discontinuation of efforts is generally appropriate after 10 minutes of absent heart rate despite adequate resuscitative measures. Current data suggest that asystole for longer than 10 minutes is highly unlikely to result in survival or survival without severe disability. Furthermore, more than 10 minutes may have elapsed if one considers time for assessment and optimization of resuscitative measures.

    American Heart Association: *Neonatal Resuscitation Textbook*, Dallas, 2006, American Heart Association, p 9–10.

KEY POINTS: DELIVERY ROOM AND RESUSCITATION

1. Infants born of multiple gestations contribute a disproportionate share of neonatal complications and neonatal intensive care unit admissions.
2. Apgar scores at 1 and 5 minutes do not predict long-term outcome.
3. Sodium bicarbonate should never be administered without first ensuring adequate ventilation, whether spontaneous or artificial.
4. Late preterm births (33-36 weeks) account for most of the recent increase in prematurity.

DEVELOPMENT AND GROWTH

44. **What is the best way to assess gestational age in the fetus?**
Nägele's rule, which dates pregnancy from the first day of the last menstrual period, has historically been the mainstay for assessment of gestational age. However, ultrasound measurements done between 5 and 20 weeks of gestation can predict gestational age quite accurately. Before 12 weeks of gestation, crown-rump length is the measurement of choice; beyond 12 weeks, biparietal diameter is the preferred study. During later gestation, the accuracy of fetal age determination is improved by the assessment of multiple variables (e.g., femur length, abdominal circumference, biparietal diameter) and by serial determinations. Maternal dates should always be used as the basis for gestational age determination unless ultrasound studies are highly discrepant. Estimates of uterine size, which approximate gestational age from 16 to 38 weeks, may also be clinically useful.

45. **What features constitute the biophysical profile?**
The biophysical profile is a scoring system that assesses fetal well-being before birth. Five variables are assessed:
1. Fetal breathing movements
2. Gross body movements
3. Fetal tone
4. Reactive fetal heart rate
5. Qualitative amniotic fluid volume
Normal results equate to 2 points per variable, for a possible total of 10 points.

46. **What factors influence biophysical profile performance?**
- Drugs (sedatives, theophylline, cocaine, and indomethacin)
- Cigarette smoking, hyperglycemia, and hypoglycemia
- Spontaneous premature rupture of membranes
- Fetal arrhythmia
- Periodic decelerations
- Acute disasters (e.g., abruptio placentae)

47. **What is the first bone in the human fetus to ossify?**
The clavicle. In the long bones, the process of ossification occurs in the primary centers of ossification in the diaphysis during the embryonic period of fetal development. Although the femora are the first long bones to show traces of ossification, the clavicles, which develop initially by intramembranous ossification, begin to ossify before any other bones in the body.

48. **What external characteristics are useful for estimating gestational age?**
See Table 12-6.

49. **At what gestational age does pupillary reaction to light develop?**
Pupillary reaction to light may appear as early as 29 weeks into gestation but is not consistently present until about 32 weeks.

50. **At what gestational age does a sense of smell develop?**
Although earlier responses are inconsistent, normal premature infants respond to concentrated odor after 32 weeks of gestation.

TABLE 12-6. EXTERNAL GESTATIONAL AGE CHARACTERISTICS

External Characteristics	Gestational Age			
	28 Weeks	32 Weeks	36 Weeks	40 Weeks
Ear cartilage	Pinna soft, remains folded	Pinna slightly harder but remains folded	Pinna harder, springs back	Pinna firm, stands erect from head
Breast tissue	None	None	1-2 mm nodule	6-7 mm nodule
Male genitalia	Testes undescended, smooth scrotum	Testes in inguinal canal, few scrotal rugae	Testes high in scrotum, more scrotal rugae	Testes descended, pendulous scrotum covered with rugae
Female genitalia	Prominent clitoris, small widely separated labia	Prominent clitoris, larger separated labia	Clitoris less prominent, labia majora covers labia minora	Clitoris covered by labia majora
Plantar surface	Smooth	1-2 anterior creases	2-3 anterior creases	Creases cover sole

From Volpe JJ Neurology of the Newborn, 5th ed. Philadelphia, WB Saunders, 2008, p 122.

51. **When does the fetal heart begin to contract in utero?**
    Contractions begin by the 22nd day of gestation. These contractions resemble peristaltic waves and begin in the sinus venosus. By the end of the fourth week, they result in the unidirectional flow of blood.

52. **How does fetal circulation differ from neonatal circulation?**
    - Intracardiac and extracardiac shunts are present (i.e., placenta, ductus venosus, foramen ovale, and ductus arteriosus).
    - The two ventricles work in parallel rather than in series.
    - The right ventricle pumps against a higher resistance than the left ventricle.
    - Blood flow to the lung is only a fraction of the right ventricular output.
    - The lung extracts oxygen from the blood instead of providing oxygen for it.
    - The lung continually secretes a fluid into the respiratory passages.
    - The liver is the first organ to receive maternal substances (e.g., oxygen, glucose, amino acids).
    - The placenta is the major route of gas exchange, excretion, and acquisition of essential fetal chemicals.
    - The placenta provides a low resistance circuit.

    Allen HD, Gutgesell HP, Clark EB, Driscoll DJ, editors: *Moss and Adams' Heart Disease in Infants, Children, and Adolescents*, ed 6, Baltimore, 2001, Williams & Wilkins, pp 41–63.

53. **How does postmaturity differ from dysmaturity?**
    - **Postmature:** An infant born of a postterm pregnancy (>42 weeks of gestation)
    - **Dysmature:** Features of placental insufficiency are present (e.g., loss of subcutaneous fat and muscle mass; meconium staining of the amniotic fluid, skin, and nails)

54. **What is the normal rate of head growth in the preterm infant?**
    The rate is about 0.5 to 1 cm/week during the first 2 to 4 months of life. An increase in the circumference of the head of about 2 cm in 1 week should raise a suspicion of CNS pathology, such as hydrocephalus. However, some premature infants may experience rapid "catch-up" head growth after significant early stress or illness. The ratio of body length to head circumference may be used to distinguish normal from abnormal head growth. A ratio of 1.42 to 1.48 is reportedly normal, whereas a low ratio of 1.12 to 1.32 indicates relative or absolute macrocephaly.

55. **How is the ponderal index used to classify growth-retarded infants?**

$$Ponderal\ index = \frac{weight(g)}{(length[cm])^3} \times 100$$

This index has been used to estimate the adequacy of intrauterine fetal nutrition. Values of less than 2.0 between 29 and 37 weeks of gestation and of 2.2 beyond 37 weeks of gestation have been associated with fetal malnutrition. Growth-restricted infants with low ponderal indices also appear to be at increased risk for the development of neonatal hypoglycemia. Maternal conditions associated with a low ponderal index (fetal malnutrition) include poor maternal weight gain, lack of prenatal care, preeclampsia, and chronic maternal illness.

56. **What morbidities (short- and long-term) are known to occur more frequently in growth-restricted babies?**
    - **Short-term morbidities:** Perinatal asphyxia, meconium aspiration, fasting hypoglycemia, alimented hyperglycemia, polycythemia-hyperviscosity, and immunodeficiency
    - **Long-term morbidities:** Poor developmental outcome and altered postnatal growth
      Most studies demonstrate normal intelligence and developmental quotients in infants who are small for gestational age (SGA), although there appears to be a higher incidence of behavioral and learning problems. The presence or absence of severe perinatal asphyxia is extremely important for predicting later intellectual and neurologic function. Recent population studies suggest that a complex interplay of genetics and the environment leads to an increased likelihood of hypertension, hypercholesterolemia, and diabetes mellitus in adulthood.

    Simmons R: Developmental origins of adult metabolic disease, *Endocrinol Metab Clin N Am* 35: 193–204, 2006.

    Tamashiro KL & Moran TH: Perinatal environment and its influences on metabolic programming of offspring, *Physiol Behav Epub* April 13, 2010.

57. **When do premature infants "catch up" on growth charts?**
    Most catch-up growth takes place during the first 2 years of life, with maximal growth rates occurring between 36 and 40 weeks after conception. Little catch-up growth occurs after the chronologic age of 3 years. About 15% of infants born prematurely remain below normal weight at 3 years of age.

58. **What is the outcome for extremely premature babies?**
    Although outcomes differ by centers, impairment-free survival in infants with extremely low birthweight has improved. With impairment defined as cerebral palsy, vision impairment, sensorineural hearing loss, seizures, and mental retardation, intact survival is seen in 67%, 61%, 73%, and 91% of infants born in the four gestational weeks from 24 to 27 weeks, respectively. Similar results have been extremely elusive at either 22 or 23 weeks. Despite the

apparent improvement in outcomes, neonates born before 29 weeks' gestation represent 30% of all cases of cerebral palsy despite representing less than 1% of all births.

BLISS: http://www.bliss.org.uk.

March of Dimes Birth Defects Foundation: http://www.modimes.org.

Parents of Premature Babies: http://www.preemie-l.org.

Robertson SMT, Watt M-J, Dinu IA: Outcomes for the extremely premature infant: what is new? And where are we going, *Pediatr Neurol* 40:189–196, 2009.

The Vermont Oxford: http://www.vtoxford.org.

GASTROINTESTINAL ISSUES

59. **When does the newborn infant's stomach begin to secrete acid?**
The pH of gastric fluid in newborns is usually neutral or slightly acidic and decreases shortly after birth. pH values are less than 3 by 6 to 8 hours of age and then increase again during the second week of life. Preterm infants frequently demonstrate gastric pH values greater than 7 for many days depending on the degree of prematurity.

60. **When is meconium usually passed after birth?**
Most infants pass some meconium during the first 12 hours of life. Overall, 99% of term infants and 95% of premature infants pass meconium by 48 hours of life. However, the smallest of premature infants may have a delayed passage of meconium as a result of the relative immaturity of rectal sphincteric reflexes.

61. **What differentiates meconium ileus from meconium plug syndrome?**
- **Meconium ileus:** Obstruction of the distal ileum occurs as a result of thick, tenacious concretions of inspissated meconium. A barium enema may reveal a microcolon, and 25% of cases have associated intestinal atresia as a result of intrauterine obstruction. Meconium ileus is a common presentation (10% to 20%) of cystic fibrosis during the newborn period. Obstruction can progress to volvulus, necrosis, and perforation.
- **Meconium plug syndrome:** This condition presents symptoms of either the delayed passage of meconium or intestinal obstruction. Barium enema usually demonstrates a normal-caliber colon with multiple filling defects proximal to the obstruction. Small preterm infants, infants of diabetic mothers, and infants born to mothers who received magnesium sulfate are especially likely to develop meconium plug syndrome, implicating hypoglycemia and hypermagnesemia in its pathogenesis. Among infants with meconium plug syndrome, there is also an increased frequency of cystic fibrosis (although much less than that seen among infants with meconium ileus) and Hirschsprung disease.

62. **After an asphyxial event, how long should feeding be delayed?**
During an asphyxial event, vasoconstriction of the mesenteric vessels can result in intestinal ischemia. Because of the relationship between ischemia and the incidence of necrotizing enterocolitis, feedings should be delayed for 2 to 3 days to allow for repair of the intestinal mucosa.

63. **How is gastroschisis differentiated from omphalocele in the newborn infant?**
Both are ventral wall defects, yet their pathogenesis and prognosis differ markedly (Table 12-7).

Chabra S, Gleason CA: Gastroschisis: embryology, pathogenesis, epidemiology, *NeoReviews* 6:e493–e499, 2005.

TABLE 12-7. DIFFERENCES BETWEEN GASTROSCHISIS AND OMPHALOCELE		
	Gastroschisis	Omphalocele
Incidence	1 in 10,000 (now increasing)	1 in 5000
Defect location	Right paraumbilical	Central
Covering sac	Absent	Present (unless sac ruptured)
Description	Free intestinal loops	Firm mass including bowel, liver, etc.
Associated with prematurity	50%-60%	10%-20%
Necrotizing enterocolitis	Common (18%)	Uncommon
Common associated anomalies	Gastrointestinal (10%-25%)	Trisomy syndromes (30%)
	Intestinal atresia	Cardiac defects (20%)
	Malrotation	Beckwith-Wiedemann syndrome
	Cryptorchidism (31%)	Bladder exstrophy
Prognosis	Excellent for small defect	Varies with associated anomalies
Mortality	5%-10%	Varies with associated anomalies (80% with cardiac defect)

From Chabra S, Gleason CA. Gastroschisis: Embryology, pathogenesis, epidemiology. NeoReviews 6: e493-e499, 2005.

64. **Which conditions are associated with intra-abdominal calcifications?**
Meconium peritonitis and intra-abdominal tumors are the most common disorders associated with intra-abdominal calcifications in the neonate. The calcifications of meconium peritonitis are streaky or plaquelike and occur over the abdominal surface of the diaphragm or along the flanks. Intraintestinal calcifications appear as small round densities that follow the course of the intestine and occur in association with intestinal stenoses, atresias, and aganglionosis. Intra-abdominal calcifications have also been observed in infants with adrenal hemorrhages and congenital infections.

65. **What is necrotizing enterocolitis (NEC)?**
NEC is a necrotizing inflammatory intestinal disorder that is the most common acquired gastrointestinal emergency in newborns. Signs and symptoms include abdominal distention, increasing gastric residuals, stool with blood, erythema of the abdominal wall, and lethargy. Positive blood culture is found in about 25% of cases at the time of diagnosis.

66. **What are the most important risk factors for NEC in preterm infants?**
In an analysis of 15,072 neonates born at 98 centers over a 2-year period, the most important variables associated with NEC were gestational age and birthweight. Apgar score was not related. Other variables associated with an increased risk for NEC included the use of a ventilator on the first day of life, exposure to both glucocorticoids and indomethacin during the first week of life, and symptomatic patent ductus arteriosus requiring surgery. Cesarean delivery and the use of breast milk were associated with a lower risk for surgical NEC. The impact of antenatal steroids has varied between studies.

Srinivasan PS, Brandler MD, D'souza A: Necrotizing enterocolitis, *Clin Perinatol* 35:251–272, 2008.

Guthrie SO, Gordon PV, Thomas V, et al: Necrotizing enterocolitis among neonates in the United States, *J Perinatol* 23:278–285, 2003.

67. **Is pneumatosis intestinalis pathognomonic for NEC?**
    No. Pneumatosis intestinalis can be seen in various other conditions, including Hirschsprung disease, **pseudomembranous** enterocolitis, neonatal ulcerative colitis, and ischemic bowel disease. However, it is a characteristic finding in 85% of patients with NEC. Dark, concentric rings within the bowel wall represent hydrogen as a byproduct of bacterial metabolism (Fig. 12-4).

68. **Is it safe to feed infants with umbilical, arterial, or venous catheters?**
    The association of umbilical arterial catheters with NEC is weak. In a recent survey of 549 NICUs, 92% of medical directors believed that it was safe to provide trophic feedings with an umbilical venous catheter in place, and 88% practiced this most of the time. Seventy-nine percent of medical directors used trophic feedings with an umbilical arterial catheter in place most or some of the time.

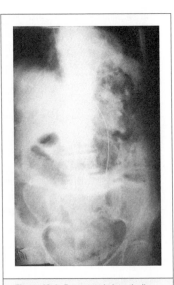

Figure 12-4. Pneumatosis intestinalis. Radiograph of the abdomen shows extensive changes of linear and bubbly forms. (From Katz DS, Math KR, Groskin SA: Radiology Secrets. Philadelphia, Hanley and Belfus, 1998, p 114.)

Tiffany KF, Burke BL, Collins-Odoms C, Oelberg DG: Current practice regarding the enteral feeding of high-risk newborns with umbilical catheters in situ, *Pediatrics* 112:20–23, 2003.

69. **How long should infants with NEC receive nothing by mouth?**
    Infants with true NEC (radiographic or surgical evidence) should continue to receive nothing by mouth for a minimum of 2 to 3 weeks. Infants in whom the diagnosis is suspected but not proved should be treated conservatively; many of these infants may be fed after 3 to 7 days.

70. **Does the feeding of immunoglobulin to infants as prophylaxis prevent NEC?**
    The evidence does not support the administration of oral immunoglobulin for the prevention of NEC. There are no randomized controlled trials of oral immunoglobulin A alone for the prevention of NEC.

Foster J, Cole M: Oral immunoglobulin for preventing necrotizing enterocolitis in preterm and low birth-weight neonates, *Cochrane Database Syst Rev* 1:CD001816, 2004.

71. **Does the prophylactic administration of antibiotics prevent NEC?**
    In a meta-analysis of five relevant trials, the administration of enteral antibiotics resulted in a statistically significant reduction in the incidences of NEC and NEC deaths. One study found an increased incidence of colonization with resistant bacteria. Because of the concerns about the development of resistant flora, enteral antibiotics should not be used at this time.

Bury RG, Tudehope D: Enteral antibiotics for preventing necrotizing enterocolitis in low birthweight or preterm infants, *Cochrane Database Syst Rev* 1:CD000405, 2001.

72. **Is there a role for probiotics in the prevention of NEC?**
    Probiotics are nonpathogenic bacteria that promote health when allowed to multiply within the gastrointestinal tract. They consist primarily of *Lactobacillus* and *Bifidobacterium* species.

A systematic review of multiple studies ($n = 1393$) revealed a reduction in the risk for NEC in infants less than 33 weeks' gestational age. Elucidation of short-term and long-term effects such as systemic infection following exposure and alterations in immune and gastrointestinal function await further studies.

Deshpande G et al: Updated meta-analysis of probiotics for preventing necrotizing enterocolitis, *Pediatrics* 125:921–930, 2010.

73. **Are trophic feedings beneficial to preterm infants?**
To prevent NEC, unstable and immature neonates are often not fed and are exclusively nourished with parenteral nutrition. In an effort to increase feeding tolerance and shorten hospital stay, trophic feeds consisting of less than 25 kcal/kg day given at the same rate for at least 5 days have been provided. A systematic review of studies that compared infants receiving no feedings to those given trophic feeds revealed that the latter required fewer days to reach full feeds and had a shorter hospital stay. However, there was a small but nonsignificant increase in the incidence of NEC. A much larger, multicenter trial would be required to accurately assess the true impact of trophic feeds on NEC and help guide the decision to feed infants in this manner.

Tyson JE: Trophic feedings for parenterally fed infants, *Cochrane Database Syst Rev* 3:CD000504, 2005.

74. **How is NEC classified?**
See Table 12-8.

TABLE 12-8. CLASSIFICATION OF NECROTIZING ENTEROCOLITIS (NEC)

Stage	Classification	Clinical Signs	Radiologic Signs
I	Suspected NEC	Abdominal distention Bloody stools Emesis, gastric residuals Apnea, lethargy	Ileus, dilation
II	Proven NEC	As in stage I, plus: Abdominal tenderness $\pm$ metabolic acidosis, thrombocytopenia	Pneumatosis intestinalis and/or portal venous gas
III	Advanced NEC	As in stage II, plus: Hypotension Significant acidosis Thrombocytopenia, disseminated intravascular coagulation Neutropenia	As in stage II, with pneumoperitoneum

Modified from Walsh MC, Kliegman RM: Necrotizing enterocolitis: treatment based on staging criteria. Pediatr Clin North Am 33:179, 1986.

Caplan M: Neonatal necrotizing enterocolitis. In Martin RJ, Fanaroff AA, Walsh MC, editors: *Fanaroff and Martin's Neonatal-Perinatal Medicine*, ed 8, Philadelphia, 2006, Mosby.

Walsh MC, Kliegman RM: Necrotizing enterocolitis: treatment based on staging criteria, *Pediatric Clin North Am* 33:179, 1986.

75. **Does the rapid advancement of feedings cause NEC?**
Retrospective studies suggest an association in contrast to a prospective trial by Rayyis and colleagues comparing 15 cc/kg per day with 35 cc/kg per day, which did not demonstrate increased risk. Berseth and colleagues compared infants maintained on trophic feeds (20 mL/kg for 10 days) with those advanced on feeds (20 mL/kg/day) and demonstrated a higher risk for NEC in the latter group. A recent case-control study revealed that infants with NEC reached full feeds faster than controls (9.9 versus 14.3 days).

Henderson G: Enteral feeding regimens and necrotizing enterocolitis in preterm infants: a multicentre case-controlled study, *Arch Dis Child Fetal Neonatal Ed* 94:120–123, 2009.

Berseth CL, Bisquera JA, Paje VU: Prolonging small feeding volumes early in life decreases the incidence of necrotizing enterocolitis in very low birth weight infants, *Pediatrics* 111:529–534, 2003.

Rayyis SF, Ambalavanan N, Wright L, Carlo WA: Randomized trial of "slow" versus "fast" feed advancements on the incidence of necrotizing enterocolitis in very low birth weight infants, *J Pediatr* 134:293–297, 1999.

76. **How is the volume of gastric aspirate helpful for the diagnosis of intestinal obstruction in a newborn?**
A large aspirate during the first 15 minutes after birth suggests obstruction. In normal-term newborns, the mean gastric aspirate is about 5 mL. In newborns with obstruction (e.g., duodenal atresia, jejunal atresia, annular pancreas), the mean aspirate is about 60 mL. Any gastric aspirate of more than 20 mL should be viewed as suspicious.

Britton JR, Britton HL: Gastric aspirate volume at birth as an indication of congenital intestinal obstruction, *Acta Pediatr* 84:945–946, 1995.

HEMATOLOGIC ISSUES

77. **When does the switch from fetal to adult hemoglobin synthesis occur in the neonate?**
The switch from the production of hemoglobin F to hemoglobin A begins in a very programmed fashion in the fetus and neonate at about 32 weeks of gestation. At birth, about 50% to 65% of hemoglobin is type F.

78. **Does the definition of anemia vary by gestational age?**
For the term infant, most authorities consider a venous blood hemoglobin of less than 13 g/dL or a capillary hemoglobin of less than 14.5 g/dL as consistent with anemia. In preterm infants beyond 32 weeks of gestation, hematologic values differ only minimally from those of full-term infants, and therefore the same values may be used.

79. **Describe the changes in hemoglobin concentration seen during the first few days of life.**
In all newborn infants, hemoglobin levels rise slightly during the first few hours of life (because of hemoconcentration) and then fall somewhat during the remainder of the first day. In healthy full-term infants, the hemoglobin concentration then stays relatively constant for the rest of the first week of life. However, appropriate-for-gestational-age infants of less than 1500-g birthweight may show a decline of 1 to 1.5 g/day during this same period.

80. **What are the indications for RBC transfusions in premature infants?**
In recent years, the pendulum has swung toward more restrictive transfusion guidelines. Adoption of these guidelines has not shown adverse effects on outcomes like death, chronic lung disease, and developmental disability, while simultaneously reducing donor exposures (Table 12-9).

TABLE 12-9. TRANSFUSION CRITERIA THEN AND NOW

Typical RBC Transfusion Criteria for Infants with Very Low Birthweight before 1990
Indications for transfusion:

- When 5%-10% of the infant's blood volume has been removed in a period of <48 hr, it should be replaced with packed RBCs.
- In infants weighing <1500 g, hemoglobin values should be maintained in excess of 13 g/dL during the first week of life.
- In convalescent infants (3-8 wk of age), clinical symptoms and signs (persistent tachycardia or tachypnea, lethargy, easy fatigue with feedings, poor weight gain, central venous oxygen tension lower than 25 mm Hg) are indications for transfusion.

Current Conservative RBC Transfusion Criteria for Infants with Very Low Birthweight

1. For infants requiring moderate or significant ventilation (defined as mean airway pressure >8 cm H_2O and fraction of inspired oxygen [Fio_2] >0.40): Transfuse if hematocrit ≤35% (hemoglobin ≤11 g/dL).
2. For infants requiring minimal mechanical ventilation (defined as all other infants requiring a) positive-pressure ventilation or b) continuous positive airway pressure [endotracheal or nasal continuous positive airway pressure] of ≥6 cm H_2O and Fio_2 >0.40): Transfuse if hematocrit is ≤30% (hemoglobin ≤10 g/dL).
3. For infants receiving supplemental oxygen who do not require mechanical ventilation: Transfuse if hematocrit is ≤25% (hemoglobin ≤8 g/dL) and one or more of the following is present:
   - Tachycardia (heart rate >180 beats/min) or tachypnea (respiratory rate >80 breaths/min) lasting more than 24 hr
   - An increased oxygen requirement from the previous 48 hr, defined as:
     - A fourfold or greater increase in nasal cannula flow (i.e., from 0.25 L/min to 1 L/min), *or*
     - An increase in nasal continuous positive airway pressure of 20% or more from previous 48 hr (i.e., from 5 to 6 cm H_2O), *or*
     - An absolute and sustained increase in Fio_2 of 0.10 or higher (via Oxy-Hood, nasal continuous positive airway pressure, or cannula)
   - Weight gain of <10 g/kg/day over the previous 4 days while receiving ≥100 kcal/kg/day
   - Multiple episodes of apnea and bradycardia (≥10 episodes in a 24-hr period or two or more episodes in a 24-hr period requiring bag-mask ventilation) while receiving therapeutic doses of methylxanthines
   - Undergoing surgery
4. For infants without any symptoms: Transfuse if hematocrit ≤20% (hemoglobin <7 g/dL) and the absolute reticulocyte count is <100,000 cells/μL (<2%).

RBC = red blood cell.
Adapted from von Kohorn I, Bhrenkranz R: Anemia in the preterm infant: erythropoietin versus erythrocyte transfusion—it's not that simple. Clin Perinatol 36:111–123, 2009.

Von Kohorn I, Ehrenkranz RA: Anemia in the preterm infant: erythropoietin vs. erythrocyte transfusion—it's not that simple, *Clin Perinatol* 36:111–123, 2009.

81. **When and at what dose should iron supplementation be initiated and for how long should it be maintained?**
The timing for initiation of iron supplementation in preterm infants has been a subject of controversy for decades. Recommendations of the AAP, Canadian Pediatric Society, and European Society of Pediatric Gastroenterology and Nutrition suggest that doses of 2 to 4 mg/kg per day of iron be initiated at 4 to 8 weeks of age and maintained for 12 to 15 months.

Rao R, Georgieff MK: Iron therapy for preterm infants, *Clin Perinatol* 36:27–42, 2009.

82. **Should erythropoietin be used in preterm infants?**
Despite many earlier studies demonstrating reticulocytosis and increased hematocrit following treatment with erythropoietin, the modest effect of treatment on the number of transfusions and volume transfused in milliliters has raised questions regarding its efficacy. Because the smallest, most immature infants are frequently transfused before the onset of the effects of erythropoietin, the patients may not experience any decrease in the number of donors to which they are exposed. Furthermore, recent data have raised the question of whether the promotion of neovascularization by erythropoietin could result in an increased incidence of retinopathy of prematurity. Therefore, at the present time, there is wide variation in the use of this hormone. Erythropoietin is currently being investigated as an adjunct therapy to prevent brain injury.

McPherson RJ and Juul SE. Erythropoietin for infants with hypoxic ischemic encephalopathy, *Curr Opin Pediatr* 22:139–145, 2010.

Von Kohorn I, Ehrankranz RA: Anemia in the preterm infant: erythropoietin vs erythrocyte transfusion—it's not that simple, *Clin Perinatol* 36:111–123, 2009.

83. **How can Rh disease be prevented?**
Unsensitized pregnant women who are Rh negative should have a repeat antibody screen at about 28 weeks of gestation and receive 300 mg of Rh immunoglobulin (RhoGAM) prophylactically. After delivery, if the infant is Rh positive, the mother should receive within 72 hours of delivery an additional dose of RhoGAM. At the time of delivery, the dose of RhoGAM may be increased if the fetomaternal hemorrhage is excessively large.

84. **Why is the direct Coombs test frequently negative or weakly positive in infants with ABO incompatibility?**
There are fewer A or B antigenic sites on the newborn RBC, and there is also a greater distance between antigenic sites compared with adult RBCs. Absorption of serum antibody by ABO antigens located on tissues throughout the body.

85. **If fetomaternal hemorrhage is suspected as a cause of neonatal anemia, how is this diagnosed?**
The Kleihauer-Betke test detects the presence of fetal cells in the maternal circulation. Because fetal hemoglobin is resistant to elution with acid, the treatment of a maternal blood smear with acid will result in darkly stained fetal cells among the maternal "ghost" cells. From the percentage of fetal RBCs and the estimated maternal blood volume, the size of the hemorrhage can be determined. One percent fetal cells in the maternal circulation indicates a bleed of about 50 mL.

86. **If a gastric aspirate contains blood shortly after birth, what test can determine whether the blood is swallowed maternal blood or fetal hemorrhage?**
The Apt test. This test relies on the increased sensitivity of adult hemoglobin to alkali as compared with fetal hemoglobin.

- **Method:** Mix the specimen with an equal quantity of tap water. Centrifuge or filter. Supernatant must have pink color to proceed. To five parts of supernatant, add one part of 0.25 N (1%) NaOH.
- **Interpretation:** A pink color persisting for more than 2 minutes indicates fetal hemoglobin. Adult hemoglobin gives a pink color that becomes yellow in 2 minutes or less, thereby indicating the denaturation of hemoglobin.

87. **How is polycythemia defined?**

Polycythemia is defined by a venous hematocrit of 65% because this exceeds the mean hematocrit found in normal newborns by two standard deviations. As the central venous hematocrit rises above 65%, there is an increase in viscosity. In neonates, some of the increase in viscosity with polycythemia is ameliorated by the lower viscosity of plasma. Because direct measurements of blood viscosity are not readily available in most laboratories, a high hematocrit level is thought to be the best indirect indicator of hyperviscosity.

88. **What are the clinical manifestations of polycythemia?**

In symptomatic infants, the most common presentations relate to CNS abnormalities, including lethargy, hypotonia, tremulousness, and irritability. With severe CNS involvement, seizures can result. Hypoglycemia is common. Other organ systems can be involved, including the gastrointestinal tract (vomiting, distension, NEC), the kidneys (renal vein thrombosis, acute renal failure), and the cardiopulmonary system (respiratory distress, congestive heart failure). However, infants with polycythemia are often asymptomatic.

89. **Which infants with polycythemia should be treated?**

Because polycythemia results from a diverse array of etiologies, it is difficult to determine whether outcome depends more on etiology or the chronic elevation of viscosity. There is controversy regarding guidelines for treatment. Many authorities recommend a partial exchange transfusion, regardless of symptoms, in infants with a central venous hematocrit level of at least 70% (because of the correlation with laboratory-measured hyperviscosity) or in those with a central hematocrit level of 65% or higher if there are signs and symptoms attributable to polycythemia.

90. **Describe the preferred method for partial exchange transfusions in polycythemic neonates.**

Partial exchange transfusions can be performed through an umbilical venous catheter, an umbilical arterial catheter, or a peripheral venous catheter. Aliquots equal to 5% of the estimated blood volume are withdrawn and historically have been replaced either with fresh-frozen plasma, Plasmanate, 5% albumin, or normal saline. Adult plasma poses the risk for transfusion-acquired infections and may actually raise neonatal blood viscosity, whereas albumin offers no proven benefit. Therefore, the amount of blood volume to be exchanged with readily available crystalloid may be calculated using the following formula:

$$\text{Blood volume to be exchanged} = \frac{\text{Observed hematocrit} - \text{desired hematocrit}}{\text{Observed hematocrit}} \times \text{blood volume} \times \text{weight (kg)}$$

91. **What is the definition of thrombocytopenia in the neonate?**

Based on numerous studies, a normal platelet count in neonates of any viable gestational age is defined as more than 150,000/mm^3. However, counts in the 100,000 to 150,000/mm^3 range are frequently seen in healthy newborns. Consequently, patients with counts in this latter category should have repeat counts as well as further studies if illness is suspected.

Roberts I, Stanworth S, Murray NA: Thrombocytopenia in the neonate, *Blood Rev* 22:173–186, 2008.

92. **At what platelet count should platelet transfusion be considered?**
Surveys of neonatologists reveal tremendous variability in the thresholds used for transfusion of platelets especially because most are given prophylactically and are given not to treat active bleeding. Because the risk for bleeding is greatest in the first week of life, consensus opinion offers the guidelines shown in Table 12-10.

TABLE 12-10. GUIDELINES FOR PLATELET TRANSFUSION			
Platelet Count × 10^9/L	Nonbleeding Neonate (1st Week of Life)	Nonbleeding Neonate (2nd Week and Onward)	Neonate with Major Bleeding
<30	Transfuse	Transfuse	Transfuse
30-49	Transfuse if <1000 g, clinically unstable, evidence of previous bleed, coagulopathy, and/or undergoing surgery	Do not transfuse	Transfuse
50-99	Do not transfuse	Do not transfuse	Transfuse

Adapted from Roberts I, Stanworth S, Murray NA: Thrombocytopenia in the neonate. Blood Rev 22:173-186, 2008.

93. **What features on physical examination suggest a specific cause of thrombocytopenia?**
   - "Blueberry-muffin rash" (**to**xoplasmosis **r**ubella **c**ytomegalovirus **h**erpes [TORCH] or viral infection)
   - Absence of radii (**t**hrombocytopenia **a**bsent **r**adii [TAR] syndrome)
   - Palpable flank mass and hematuria (renal vein thrombosis)
   - Hemangioma, large, often with bruit (Kasabach-Merritt syndrome)
   - Abnormal thumbs (Fanconi syndrome, albeit thrombocytopenia is less likely in newborns)
   - Markedly dysmorphic features (chromosomal abnormalities, particularly trisomy 13 or 18)

94. **What are the two main types of neonatal thrombocytopenia caused by maternal antibody?**
Transplacental passage of antibody from the mother to infant can be due to maternal idiopathic thrombocytopenic purpura (ITP), with the newborn a secondary target, and isoimmune thrombocytopenia, with the newborn a primary target. The diseases can have a similar clinical appearance. Babies generally appear well, do not have hepatosplenomegaly, and have thrombocytopenia that persists for 3 to 12 weeks postnatally.

95. **In the mother with new-onset thrombocytopenia during pregnancy, how can one determine the risk to the fetus?**
Because only a small percentage of infants born to mothers with ITP have severe thrombocytopenia, prediction of this outcome is highly challenging. There are conflicting

results regarding the predictive ability of platelet counts, platelet-associated immunoglobulin G (IgG), and circulating platelet autoantibodies. However, a previous history of an affected infant has been shown to be predictive in several studies. Although cordocentesis could provide direct data on the fetal platelet count, the risks of the procedure outweigh the risks of associated neonatal disease and thus cannot be justified.

Gill KK, Kelton JG: Management of idiopathic thrombocytopenia purpura in pregnancy, *Semin Hematol* 37:275–289, 2000.

Stavrou E, McCrae KR: Immune thrombocytopenia in pregnancy, *Hematol Oncil Clin North Amer* 23:1299–1316, 2009.

96. **When do the prothrombin time and partial thromboplastin time "normalize" to adult values?**
The prothrombin time reaches adult values at about 1 week of age, whereas the partial thromboplastin time does not attain adult values until 2 to 9 months of age.

97. **How is disseminated intravascular coagulation (DIC) diagnosed in the neonate?**
The laboratory findings of DIC include evidence of RBC fragmentation on peripheral smear; elevation of prothrombin time, partial thromboplastin time, and thrombin time; thrombocytopenia; decreased levels of factors V, VIII, and fibrinogen; and in some cases, the presence of fibrin split products.

98. **How should newborn infants with DIC be managed?**
Treatment should be directed primarily at the underlying disease rather than just at the coagulation defects. In many cases, treatment of the former makes specific treatment of the latter unnecessary. However, in cases in which the stabilization of coagulopathy is not imminent, treatment with fresh-frozen plasma and platelets is recommended. In cases in which fluid overload is a major concern, exchange transfusion with fresh whole blood may be used. However, this second approach is not superior to the first with respect to the resolution of DIC. The use of heparin in patients with DIC is currently reserved for cases of thrombosis of major vessels or purpura fulminans.

99. **What causes hemorrhagic disease of the newborn?**
For evolutionary reasons that are unclear, a newborn has only about 50% of the normal vitamin K–dependent cofactors. Unless vitamin K is given, these levels steadily decline during the first 3 days of life. In addition, breast milk is low in vitamin K. Early hemorrhagic disease can be observed during the first few days of life in infants who are exclusively breastfed and who do not receive vitamin K prophylaxis at birth; they may bleed from various sites (e.g., umbilical cord, circumcision). Infants born to mothers who have received medications that affect the metabolism of vitamin K (e.g., warfarin, antiepileptic medications, antituberculous drugs) are at risk for developing severe life-threatening intracranial hemorrhages at or shortly after delivery.

HYPERBILIRUBINEMIA

100. **What are the normal changes in bilirubin levels in full-term healthy newborns?**
All newborn infants exhibit a progressive rise in serum bilirubin concentrations following birth. Beginning with an average bilirubin in cord blood of 2 mg/dL, serum levels rise and peak at 5 to 6 mg/dL between 60 and 72 hours of life. The 97th percentile for bilirubin in healthy full-term infants is 12.4 mg/dL for bottle-fed infants and 14.8 mg/dL for breastfed infants. If untreated, at least 1% to 2% of newborns will develop bilirubin levels of 20 mg/dL.

101. **How should infants be assessed for jaundice before discharge?**
The American Academy of Pediatrics recommends two clinical options individually or in combination: a predischarge total serum bilirubin (or transcutaneous bilirubin) and/or assessment of clinical risk factors. Predischarge bilirubins should be plotted on the chart in Figure 12-5 to assess risk.

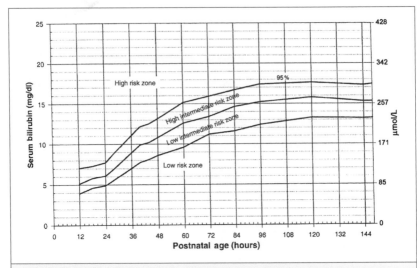

Figure 12-5. Assessment of jaundice. (From Subcommittee on Hyperbilirubinemia: Management of hyperbilirubinemia in the newborn infant 35 or more weeks of gestation. Pediatrics 114:297-316, 2004.)

102. **How soon should infants be evaluated for jaundice after discharge?**
All infants discharged before the age of 24 hours should be seen by 72 hours of age by a qualified health care professional. Infants discharged between 24 and 47.9 hours should be evaluated by 96 hours of age, and those discharged after 48 hours should be seen by 120 hours of age.

Subcommittee on Hyperbilirubinemia: Management of hyperbilirubinemia in the newborn infant 35 or more weeks of gestation, *Pediatrics* 114:297–316, 2004.

103. **What is believed to be the fraction of bilirubin that is toxic to the CNS?**
Routine clinical laboratory tests measure the total bilirubin and the conjugated bilirubin. Of the total unconjugated bilirubin, most is bound to albumin and thus cannot cross the blood-brain barrier. Although the free bilirubin is believed to cause neurotoxicity, routine measurement in clinical practice is not available. Measurement of the bilirubin (mg/dL)-to-albumin (g/dL) (B/A) ratio may be helpful in managing jaundiced infants by acting as a surrogate for free bilirubin. Patients are thought to be at increased risk for bilirubin toxicity if the ratio is 8.0 or higher in infants born at 38 weeks' gestation or later, at least 7.2 in infants 35 to 36$^6/_7$ weeks' gestation and well or at least 38 weeks' gestation and classified as high risk (e.g., sepsis, acidosis, hemolysis, glucose-6-phosphate dehydrogenase deficiency), or at least 6.8 in infants 35 to 36$^6/_7$ weeks' gestation and classified as high risk.

Ahlfors CE: Predicting bilirubin neurotoxicity in jaundiced infants, *Curr Opin Pediatr* 22:129–133, 2010.

American Academy of Pediatrics: Clinical practice guideline: management of hyperbilirubinemia in the newborn infant 35 or more weeks of gestation, *Pediatrics* 114:297–316, 2004.

104. **What are the risks and benefits of restrictive versus liberal transfusion criteria in preterm infants?**
Two recent studies that assigned preterm infants to liberal (10.0 to 15.3 Iowa trial; 8.5 to 13.5 PINT trial) compared with restrictive (7.3 to 11.3 Iowa trial; 7.5 to 11.5 PINT trial) hemoglobin thresholds depending on postnatal age and respiratory support, demonstrated a reduction in the number of transfusions (Iowa trial) and donor exposures (PINT trial) in the restrictive group. However, the Iowa trial, which aimed for higher hemoglobin levels in the liberal group, demonstrated a reduction in brain injury and the combined outcome of brain injury or death. Perhaps, until more data are available, attempts to further restrict transfusions should be undertaken cautiously, especially in infants born weighting less than 1000 g.

Crowley M and Kirpilani H: A rational approach to red blood cell transfusion in the newborn ICU, *Curr Opin Pediatr* 22:151–157, 2010.

Kirpilani H, Whyte RK, Andersen C, et al: A randomized controlled trial of a restrictive vs. liberal transfusion threshold for extremely low birth weight infants: the PINT study, *J Pediatr* 149: 301–307, 2006.

Bell EF, Strauss RG, Widness JA, et al: Randomized trial of liberal vs. restrictive guidelines for red blood cell transfusions in preterm infants, *Pediatrics* 115:1685–1691, 2005.

105. **What conditions are associated with increased erythrocyte destruction?**
In infants with onset of jaundice before age 24 hours, bilirubin rise greater than 0.5mg/dL per hour, decreasing hemoglobin, elevated reticulocyte count, pallor, and/or hepatosplenomegaly, consideration must be given to disease states associated with RBC destruction as noted below:
Isoimmunization
- Rh incompatibility
- ABO incompatibility
- Other blood group incompatibilities

Erythrocyte biochemical defects
- Glucose-6-phosphate dehydrogenase deficiency
- Pyruvate kinase deficiency
- Hexokinase deficiency
- Congenital erythropoietic porphyria
- Other biochemical defects

Structural abnormalities of erythrocytes
- Hereditary spherocytosis
- Hereditary elliptocytosis
- Infantile pyknocytosis
- Other

Infection
- Bacterial
- Viral
- Protozoal

Sequestered blood
- Subdural hematoma and cephalohematoma
- Ecchymoses
- Hemangiomas

From Martin RJ, Fanaroff AA, Walsh MC, editors: *Fanaroff and Martin's Neonatal-Perinatal Medicine*, ed 8, Philadelphia, 2006, Mosby, p 1428.

106. **Which infants are "set-ups" for ABO incompatibility?**
Infants who are type A or B and whose mothers are type O. In individuals with type A or B blood, naturally occurring anti-A and anti-B isoantibodies are primarily IgM and do not

cross the placenta. However, in type O individuals, isoantibodies are frequently IgG. These antibodies can cross the placenta and cause hemolysis. Although about 12% of maternal-infant pairs qualify as set-ups for ABO incompatibility, less than 1% of infants have significant hemolysis.

107. **What screening tests should pregnant women have to identify infants at risk for hyperbilirubinemia?**
All pregnant women should be tested for ABO and Rh(D) blood types and have a serum screen for unusual isoimmune antibodies.

> Subcommittee on Hyperbilirubinemia: Management of hyperbilirubinemia in the newborn infant 35 or more weeks of gestation, *Pediatrics* 114:297–316, 2004.

108. **What are the clinical features of bilirubin toxicity?**
The early clinical manifestations of bilirubin toxicity can be subtle. In addition, they can progress rapidly to severe and life-threatening manifestations. Acutely, toxicity is called *bilirubin-induced neurologic dysfunction* (BIND). For chronic cases, the term *kernicterus* is generally used. Using the BIND score, infants with subtle signs of bilirubin toxicity can be identified (Table 12-11).

TABLE 12-11. CLINICAL FEATURES OF BILIRUBIN-INDUCED NEUROLOGIC DYSFUNCTION (BIND)			
Signs	Mild	Moderate	Severe
Behavior	Too sleepy Decreased feeding Decreased vigor	Lethargy and/or irritability (depending on arousal state) Very poor feeding	Semicoma Apnea Extreme irritability Seizures Fever
Muscle tone	Slight but persistent decrease in tone	Mild to moderate hypertonicity Mild nuchal or truncal arching	Severe hypotonia or hypertonia Atonic Opisthotonus Posturing, bicycling
Cry pattern	High-pitched	Shrill and piercing (especially when stimulated)	Inconsolable, very weak, and cries only with stimulation

109. **When should phototherapy be instituted in infants who are at least 35 weeks of gestational age?**
The American Academy of Pediatrics guidelines for instituting phototherapy in term and near-term infants are shown in Figure 12-6.

110. **What distinguishes breastfeeding jaundice from breast-milk jaundice?**
Hyperbilirubinemia in breastfed infants during the first week of life is called **breastfeeding jaundice** and is thought to be the result of poor caloric intake and/or dehydration. Hyperbilirubinemia in breastfed infants after the first week of life is known as **breast-milk**

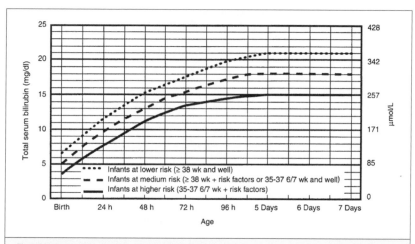

Figure 12-6. American Academy of Pediatrics guidelines for instituting phototherapy. (From Subcommittee on Hyperbilirubinemia: Management of hyperbilirubinemia in the newborn infant 35 or more weeks of gestation. Pediatrics 114:297–316, 2004.)

jaundice. The cause of breast-milk jaundice is uncertain; however, possible etiologies include an increased enterohepatic circulation of bilirubin as a result of the presence of β-glucuronidase in human milk and/or the inhibition of the hepatic glucuronosyl transferase by a factor such as free fatty acids in some human milk samples. The incidence and duration compared with physiologic jaundice are noted in Table 12-12.

TABLE 12-12. COMPARISON OF PHYSIOLOGIC, BREASTFEEDING, AND BREAST-MILK JAUNDICE

	Physiologic Jaundice	Breastfeeding Jaundice	Breast-Milk Jaundice
Time of onset (TSB >7 mg/dL)	After 36 hr	2-4 days	4-7 days
Usual time of peak bilirubin	3-4 days	3-6 days	5-15 days
Peak TSB	5-12 mg/dL	>12 mg/dL	>10 mg/dL
Age when total bilirubin <3 mg/dL	1-2 wk	>3 wk	9 wk
Incidence in full-term neonates	56%	12%-13%	2%-4%

TSB = total serum bilirubin.
From Gourley G: Pathophysiology of breast milk jaundice. In Polin RA, Fox W (eds): Fetal and Neonatal Physiology. Philadelphia, WB Saunders, 1992, p 1174.

111. **Why should infants at risk for breastfeeding jaundice be fed more frequently?**
Breastfed infants exhibit their maximal weight loss by day 3 of life and lose on average 6.1% ± 2.5% of their birthweight. Infants breastfed an average of more than 8 times per day during the first 3 days of life have significantly lower serum bilirubin concentrations than

those who are less frequently breastfed. This practice accelerates and enhances the acquisition of milk supply. With increased milk available, dehydration is less likely to occur, and the excretion of bilirubin by the gastrointestinal tract is more rapid. Infants with adequate intake should have four to six wet diapers per day.

112. **Should breastfeeding be discontinued in an infant with hyperbilirubinemia?**
   Only in rare metabolic disorders (e.g., galactosemia) should breastfeeding be permanently discontinued. In breastfed infants who require phototherapy, the American Academy of Pediatrics recommends that breastfeeding should be continued. However, an alternative option, which has been shown to decrease bilirubin and increase the efficacy of phototherapy, is to temporarily stop breastfeeding and feed formula in its place. In any case, about one third of healthy, breastfed infants will have persistent jaundice for 14 days. In contrast, this prolonged jaundice occurs in less than 1% of formula-fed infants.

113. **Where does bilirubin go when you turn on the lights?**
   It becomes lumirubin (through a "cyclization" reaction) and is rapidly excreted in bile, with a half-life of about 2 hours. In addition to the aforementioned principal pathway of bilirubin elimination, photoisomers are also formed, and because of their water solubility, they can be excreted in the urine.

114. **What are the factors that affect the efficacy of phototherapy?**
   - Spectrum of light emitted (blue-green is most effective)
   - Spectral irradiance (intensive phototherapy $= 30$ W/cm^2 per nm)
   - Spectral power (expose maximal surface area)
   - Cause of jaundice (phototherapy is less effective with hemolysis and cholestasis)
   - Total bilirubin at start (the higher the bilirubin, the greater the decline)

   Subcommittee on Hyperbilirubinemia: Management of hyperbilirubinemia in the newborn infant 35 or more weeks of gestation, *Pediatrics* 114:297–316, 2004.

115. **What are the contraindications to phototherapy?**
   Infants with a family history of light-sensitive porphyria should not receive phototherapy. The presence of direct hyperbilirubinemia is not considered a contraindication, but it will decrease the effectiveness of phototherapy may result in bronze baby syndrome.

116. **What are the common adverse effects of phototherapy?**
   Loose stools increased insensible water loss, skin rashes, overheating, and the potential for burns if the lights are placed too close to the infant's skin. If direct hyperbilirubinemia is present, the bronze baby syndrome can result.

   Maisels MJ, McDonagh AF: Phototherapy for neonatal jaundice, *N Engl J Med* 358:920–928, 2008.

117. **A newborn develops dark skin discoloration and dark urine after beginning phototherapy. What is the diagnosis?**
   Bronze baby syndrome. Infants who develop the syndrome typically have an elevated direct serum bilirubin concentration. The bronze baby syndrome results from the retention of photoproducts (e.g., lumirubin) that cannot be excreted in the bile. Most infants appear to recover without complications. Direct hyperbilirubinemia is not a contraindication to phototherapy.

KEY POINTS: HEMATOLOGY AND HYPERBILIRUBINEMIA

1. The switch from fetal to adult hemoglobin occurs in a preprogrammed manner.

2. Late preterm infants are at higher risk than term infants for bilirubin encephalopathy.

3. Although ABO incompatibility is common, sensitization and hemolysis are not.

4. Exchange transfusion for hyperbilirubinemia in healthy full-term infants without evidence of hemolysis is almost never required.

5. Every newborn infant should have a predischarge assessment of risk for the development of severe hyperbilirubinemia.

118. **What are the complications of exchange transfusions in the newborn?**
Acute
Hypocalcemia (as a result of the binding of calcium by citrate)
- Thrombocytopenia (as a result of the removal of platelets and the use of stored blood that may be low in platelets)
- Hyperkalemia (as a result of the higher potassium levels of stored blood)
- Hypovolemia (if blood replacement is inadequate)
- Diminished oxygen delivery (if blood stored for >5 to 7 days is used, the resultant loss of 2,3-diphophoglycerate may have deleterious effects on oxygen delivery)
Late
- Anemia (for unknown reasons)
- Graft-versus-host disease (as a result of the introduction of donor lymphocytes into a relatively immunocompromised neonatal host)

119. **What is the relationship between delayed neonatal jaundice and urinary tract infection (UTI)?**
Unexplained jaundice developing between 10 and 60 days of age can be associated with a UTI in infants. The typical patient is usually afebrile (in two thirds of cases) with hepatomegaly and minimal systemic symptoms. Hyperbilirubinemia is usually conjugated, and liver transaminases may be normal or mildly elevated. Treatment of the UTI (usually caused by *Escherichia coli*) results in reversal of the liver dysfunction, which is believed to be the result of endotoxins.

120. **Can transcutaneous bilirubin measurements be used in place of serum levels?**
Numerous devices have been developed that accurately measure bilirubin levels that are highly correlated with serum bilirubins. However, most studies show that the deviation of transcutaneous measurements is greatest (about 3 mg/dL) at the highest levels (>13 to 15 mg/dL). Therefore, many authorities recommend serum confirmation if the transcutaneous bilirubin is greater than the 75th percentile, more than 13 mg/dL, or if a level that is 3 mg/dL higher would be clinically meaningful. In any case, this methodology should lead to a sharp reduction in the need for blood measurements.

Grohmann K, Roser M, Rolinski B, et al: Bilirubin measurement for neonates: comparison of 9 frequently used methods, *Pediatrics* 117:1174–1183, 2006.

121. **What is the role of metalloporphyrins in the treatment of hyperbilirubinemia?**
Metalloporphyrins are inhibitors of the rate-limiting enzyme, heme oxygenase, in the pathway of heme degradation leading to bilirubin production. Tin mesoporphyrin (SnMP) has been most extensively studied in human infants and has been shown to reduce the need for phototherapy. However, this compound is phototoxic, contains a foreign metal that may be released, induces heme oxygenase, and can inhibit other enzymes such as nitric oxide synthase and soluble guanylate cyclase, whose products are required for important biologic functions. Thus, these compounds have not found widespread use in the treatment of hyperbilirubinemia. Advocates of "bloodless medicine" have promoted its use as a means of avoiding exchange transfusions.

Yaffe SJ, Aranda JV, editors: *Neonatal and Pediatric Pharmacology: Therapeutic Principles in Practice*, ed 3, Philadelphia, 2005, WB Saunders, pp 198–200.

122. **Who was Sister Ward?**
In the early 1950s, Sister Ward was the nurse in charge of the unit for premature infants at Rochford General Hospital in Essex, England. On warm summer days, Sister Ward would take her infants to the courtyard to give them a little fresh air and sunshine. It was after such an afternoon of sunshine that Sister Ward observed that sunlight was able to "bleach" the skin of jaundiced neonates. The account of her discovery, as recorded by R.H. Dobbs, follows:

One particularly fine summer's day in 1956, during a ward routine, Sister Ward diffidently showed us a premature baby, carefully undressed and with fully exposed abdomen. The infant was pale yellow except for a strongly demarcated triangle of skin very much yellower than the rest of the body. I asked her, "Sister, what did you paint it with—iodine or flavine—and why?" But she replied that she thought it must have been the sun. "What do you mean Sister? Suntan takes days to develop after the erythema has faded." Sister Ward looked increasingly uncomfortable, and explained that she thought it was a jaundiced baby, much darker where a corner of the sheet had covered the area. "It's the rest of the body that seems to have faded." We left it at that, and as the infant did well and went home, fresh air treatment of prematurity continued.

METABOLIC ISSUES

123. **How frequently are the various metabolic disorders detected by newborn screening?**
Although there is some variability in different populations, some of the commonly held frequencies are as follows:
- Biotinidase deficiency: 1 in 60,000
- Congenital adrenal hyperplasia: 1 in 16,000 (North America)
- Cystic fibrosis: 1 in 3,500 (whites), 1 in 15,000 (African Americans), 1 in 7000 (Hispanics)
- Galactosemia: 1 in 47,000
- Homocystinuria: 1 in 300,000
- Hypothyroidism: 1 in 3000 to 4000
- Maple syrup urine disease: 1 in 185,000
- Medium-chain acyl CoA dehydrogenase deficiency: 1 in 6400 to 46,000
- Phenylketonuria: 1 in 13,500 to 19,000
- Sickle cell disease: 1 in 2000 to 2500
- Tay-Sachs disease: 1 in 3000 (U.S. Jews)
- Tyrosinemia: 1 in 12,000 to 100,000

Kay CI: Committee on Genetics: Newborn screening fact sheets, *Pediatrics* 118:e934–e963, 2006.

124. **In what settings should inborn errors of metabolism be suspected?**
- Onset of symptoms that correlates with dietary changes
- Loss or leveling of developmental milestones
- Patient with strong food preferences or aversions
- Parental consanguinity
- Unexplained sibling death, mental retardation, or seizures
- Unexplained failure to thrive
- Unusual odor
- Hair abnormalities, especially alopecia
- Microcephaly or macrocephaly
- Abnormalities of muscle tone
- Organomegaly
- Coarsened facial features, thick skin, limited joint mobility, and hirsutism

   Levy PA: Inborn errors of metabolism, *Pediatr Rev* 30:131–138, 2009.

125. **What key urine odors are associated with inborn errors of metabolism?**
- Cabbage: Tyrosinemia, type I
- Cat urine: 3-methylcrotonyl-CoA carboxylase deficiency
- Fish: Trimethylaminuria
- Hops: Oasthouse urine disease
- Maple syrup: Maple syrup urine disease
- "Mousy" or musty: Phenylketonuria
- Sweaty feet or cheesy: Isovaleric acidemia; glutaric aciduria, type II

126. **What is the definition of neonatal hypoglycemia?**
Based on statistical definition, most authorities accept 40 mg/dL as the lower limit of normal during the first 24 hours of life. However, a normal glucose is that level which is needed to meet the requirements of cerebral energy metabolism, which cannot be readily measured.

127. **When is hypoglycemia most likely to occur in a neonate?**
During gestation, glucose is freely transferred across the placenta by the process of facilitated diffusion. However, after birth, the infant must adjust to the sudden withdrawal of this transplacental supply. In all infants, there is a nadir in blood sugar between 1 and 3 hours of life. During the first 12 to 24 hours of life, newborns are at increased risk for hypoglycemia because gluconeogenesis and especially ketogenesis are incompletely developed. These factors are accentuated in preterm infants, infants of diabetic mothers, infants with erythroblastosis fetalis, asphyxiated infants, and infants who are small or large for gestational age.

   Sperling MA, Menon RK: Differential diagnosis and management of neonatal hypoglycemia, *Pediatr Clin North Am* 51:703–723, 2004.

128. **How should hypoglycemia be treated?**
Both symptomatic and asymptomatic hypoglycemia should be treated. If an asymptomatic infant can take oral feedings, these may suffice initially. Otherwise, the infant should receive therapy based on his or her response:
- If an intravenous line is in place and the infant is asymptomatic, the glucose concentration infusion rate should be increased to 6 to 8 mg/kg per minute. Glucose should be rechecked within 15 minutes.

- If an infant is symptomatic (or asymptomatic and unresponsive to a glucose infusion rate of 6 to 8 mg/kg per minute), a bolus of intravenous glucose (200 mg/kg or 2 mL/kg of 10% dextrose water [$D_{10}W$]) should be given and followed by a glucose infusion of 6 to 8 mg/kg per minute (3.6 to 4.8 mL/kg/h of $D_{10}W$), with rechecking of glucose values within 15 minutes, frequent glucose-monitoring, and increases in infusion rates and concentrations as needed.
- Glucagon (0.02 to 0.03 mg/kg up to 1 mg intramuscularly) can be given as an anti-insulin measure until an intravenous line is established, but glucagon is not as helpful in the low-birthweight infant.
- If 15 to 20 mg/kg per minute of glucose is required, glucocorticoids (hydrocortisone, 5 mg/kg per day, or prednisone, 2 mg/kg per day) can enhance gluconeogenesis. Diazoxide (10 to 15 mg/kg per day) can suppress insulin secretion. For these therapies and others (e.g., somatostatin), an endocrinologist should be consulted.

129. **What features on physical examination suggest the etiology of hypoglycemia?**
    - **Macrosomia:** This occurs in infants of diabetic mothers, infants with severe congenital hyperinsulinism, and infants with Beckwith-Wiedemann syndrome; recall that insulin is a growth factor and that hyperinsulinism leads to macrosomia.
    - **Midline defects:** Congenital pituitary deficiency can be associated with midline defects such as cleft lip, cleft palate, single central incisor, and micro-ophthalmia.
    - **Micropenis:** Congenital gonadotropin deficiency and possible pituitary abnormalities cause this condition.
    - **Hepatomegaly:** This is associated with glycogen storage diseases and fatty acid oxidation disorders.

130. **Should insulin be used to treat preterm infants?**
    Review of studies comparing insulin treatment of hyperglycemia and reduction of glucose infusion rate shows no difference in mortality or morbidity, suggesting that the cause of hyperglycemia and not the blood sugar itself may determine the outcome. Furthermore, early institution of insulin therapy in infants with very low birthweight offers little benefit despite reducing episodes of hyperglycemia and facilitating the infusion of greater quantities of carbohydrate.

    Bottino M: *Cochrane Database Syst Rev* 1:CD007453, 2009.

131. **What are the manifestations of hypocalcemia in the neonate?**
    The major manifestations are jitteriness and seizures. Additional signs such as high-pitched cry, laryngospasm, Chvostek sign (facial muscle twitching on tapping), and Trousseau sign (carpopedal spasm) may be present, but more commonly these are absent during the neonatal period.

132. **What is the differential diagnosis of hypocalcemia in the neonate?**
    Early neonatal hypocalcemia (first 3 days of life)
    - Premature infants
    - Infants with birth asphyxia
    - Infants of diabetic mothers

    Late neonatal hypocalcemia (after the end of the first week of life)
    - High-phosphate cow milk formula
    - Intestinal malabsorption
    - Postdiarrheal acidosis
    - Hypomagnesemia

- Neonatal hypoparathyroidism
- Rickets
- Decreased ionized fraction of calcium (with either normal or decreased total calcium)
- Citrate (exchange transfusion)
- Increased free fatty acid (Intralipid)
- Alkalosis

133. **When should hypocalcemia be treated in the neonate?**
Hypocalcemia should be treated when it is associated with signs or symptoms or when the serum calcium level is less than 7.0 mg/dL or the ionized calcium level is less than 4 mg/dL. The first line of therapy generally consists of increasing the amount of calcium in the intravenous infusion to achieve 20 to 75 mg/kg per day of elemental calcium and evaluating serum levels every 6 to 8 hours. After normal calcium levels are achieved, the intravenous dose can be weaned over 2 to 3 days. The infusion of a bolus of intravenous calcium (10% calcium gluconate, 2 mL/kg) over 10 minutes should be reserved for the infant with seizures. In the asymptomatic infant, hypocalcemia most frequently resolves spontaneously without the need for further therapy.

134. **In which neonates should the serum magnesium concentration be measured?**
- Any hypocalcemic infant who is not responding to calcium therapy
- Hypotonic infants born to mothers who received magnesium sulfate therapy before delivery
- Infants with seizures of unknown etiology

135. **How is hypomagnesemia treated?**
Hypomagnesemic infants should be treated with 50% magnesium sulfate: 2-5 mg/kg of elemental magnesium, or 0.1-0.2 mmol/kg given IM or by slow intravenous infusion over 20 minutes. Magnesium levels are followed and the dosage repeated, if necessary.

NEONATAL SEPSIS

136. **Can sepsis be distinguished from other causes of respiratory distress in the neonate?**
Not reliably. Diagnosis is confirmed only by a positive blood, urine, or CSF culture.

137. **What laboratory tests can rule out sepsis on admission?**
None. Total white blood cell (WBC) counts, immature-to-total (I:T) ratios of neutrophils, and C-reactive protein are of limited value as single tests for the diagnosis of bacterial sepsis in the newborn. In one third of infants with proven bacterial disease, total WBC counts are normal, particularly early during the course of infection. The most sensitive neutrophil index for identifying septic infants is the I:T neutrophil ratio. An I:T ratio of more than 0.2 has been considered abnormal, although some studies have suggested that a ratio as high as 0.27 may be seen in healthy term newborns. Neutropenia (total WBC $<5000/mm^3$ or absolute neutrophil count $<1750/mm^3$) is the most specific indicator. The least sensitive neutrophil index is the absolute band count (normal, $<2000/mm^3$). Generally, abnormal neutrophil indices have low PPVs and therefore are not helpful as sole tests for clearly identifying which infants are infected. However, they have a much higher negative-predictive value, particularly if repeated 12 hours after birth, and thus they can be very helpful for determining which infants do not have infection.

138. **How should asymptomatic infants born to mothers with risk factors for infection be evaluated?**

The major risk factors for infection are prolonged rupture of membranes, signs or symptoms of chorioamnionitis, and colonization with group B streptococci. Figure 12-7 uses a "sepsis screen" to help identify patients, both preterm and term, who need treatment and for how long.

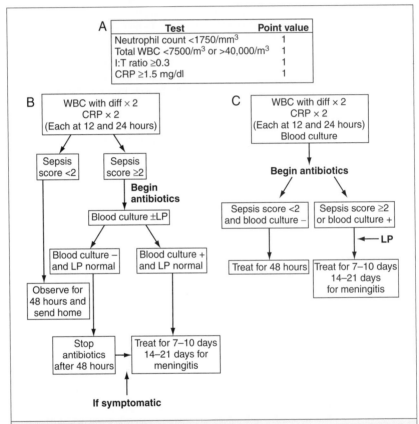

Figure 12-7. Evaluation of asymptomatic infants with one or more risk factors for neonatal sepsis. Sepsis screen **(A)** with algorithm to evaluate **(B)** term (≥ 35 weeks) and **(C)** preterm infants. CRP = C-reactive protein; LP = lumbar puncture; WBC = white blood count. (From Garber SJ, Harris MC: Neonatal sepsis. In Burg FD, Ingelfinger JR, Polin RA, Gershon AA [eds]: Current Pediatric Therapy, 18th ed. Philadelphia, WB Saunders, 2006, pp 296-300.)

From Garber SJ, Harris MC: Neonatal sepsis. In Burg FD, Ingelfinger JR, Polin RA, Gershon AA, editors: *Current Pediatric Therapy*, ed 18, Philadelphia, 2006, WB Saunders, pp 296–300.

139. **How should symptomatic infants be evaluated?**

Figure 12-8 uses a "sepsis screen" to identify symptomatic infants who do not require antibiotics or in whom antibiotics can be used.

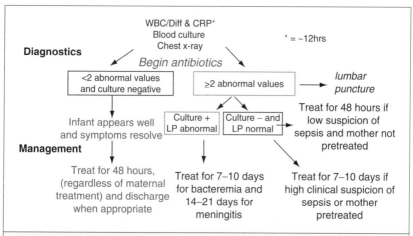

Figure 12-8. Evaluation of symptomatic infants for neonatal sepsis. (From Gerdes JS, Polin RA: Neonatal septicemia. In Burg FD, Ingelfinger JR, Polin RA, Gerschon AA [eds]: Current Pediatric Therapy, 17th ed. Philadelphia, WB Saunders, 2002, pp 347-351.)

140. **What are some newer markers that are useful in the diagnosis of neonatal sepsis?**
The ideal marker for sepsis provides high sensitivity and negative-predictive value (i.e., close to 100%) and good specificity and PPV (i.e., >80% or better). In addition, the marker should remain abnormal for a significant time (>24 hours) to allow detection in most clinical circumstances. In addition to WBC parameters and acute phase reactants, markers that show promise are the following:
  ■ CD11b, a neutrophil cell surface–associated molecule, which is rapidly upregulated following microbial exposure
  ■ CD64, a leukocyte surface antigen, which rapidly increases on neutrophils and persists for 0 to 24 hours
  ■ Interlukin-6, which increases rapidly and stimulates C-reactive protein production but has a relatively short half-life
  ■ Interleukin-8, a chemoattractant for neutrophils, which rises rapidly and is sustained for at least 24 hours
  These may be used individually or in combination, but as of now are not routinely available.

Ng PC, Lam HS: Diagnostic markers for neonatal sepsis, *Curr Opin Pediatr* 18:125–131, 2006.

141. **Should an LP be performed on all newborns as part of the sepsis evaluation?**
The need for LP as part of the sepsis evaluation of a newborn is controversial, with some authors suggesting its omission in asymptomatic infants. However, in symptomatic infants, an LP should be strongly considered because of the following: (1) bacterial meningitis can be present in newborns without CNS symptoms; (2) a significant number of infants (15% to 30%) can have meningitis without bacteremia, especially after the first week of life, and (3) meningitis can coexist in premature infants with suspected respiratory distress syndrome. The procedure should be postponed in an infant with cardiorespiratory instability or significant thrombocytopenia.

Stoll BJ, Hansen N, Fanaroff AA, et al: To tap or not to tap: high likelihood of meningitis without sepsis among VLBW infants, *Pediatrics* 113:1181–1186, 2004.

Wiswell TE, Baumgart S, Gannon CM, Spitzer AR: No lumbar puncture in the evaluation for early neonatal sepsis: will meningitis be missed? *Pediatrics* 95:803–806, 1995.

142. **List the contraindications to the performance of an LP.**
   - Uncorrected thrombocytopenia or bleeding diathesis
   - Infections in the skin or underlying structures adjacent to the puncture site
   - Lumbosacral anomalies
   - Cardiorespiratory instability
   - Increased intracranial pressure: Although the presence of open sutures reduces the likelihood of herniation, this remains a possibility. In the presence of a rapidly deteriorating level of consciousness, cranial nerve palsies, abnormal posturing, abnormalities of vital signs without other cause and/or a tense fontanelle, brain imaging (computed tomography or magnetic resonance imaging) should be obtained before performing an LP.

   MacDonald MG, Ramasethu J: *Atlas of Procedures in Neonatology*, ed 4, Philadelphia, 2007, Lippincott Williams & Wilkins.

143. **Are skin surface cultures helpful for the evaluation of suspected neonatal sepsis?**
   The theoretic value of these cultures is that they might help to identify the possible etiologic agents and thus guide therapy. However, an analysis of nearly 25,000 cultures in more than 3300 patients revealed that surface cultures correlated with urine, blood, or cerebrospinal fluid (CSF) cultures in only about 50% of cases. Based on these and more recent studies demonstrating poor PPV, most agree that surface cultures in this setting have little clinical value.

   Evans ME, Schaffner W, Federspiel CF, et al: Sensitivity, specificity, and predictive value of body surface cultures in a neonatal intensive care unit, *JAMA* 259:248–252, 1988.

   Fulginiti VA, Ray CG: Body surface cultures in the newborn infant: an exercise in futility, wastefulness, and inappropriate practice, *Am J Dis Child* 142:19–20, 1988.

144. **What is the preferred strategy for identifying women for intrapartum group B streptococcus (GBS) prophylaxis?**
   The initial guidelines from the Centers for Disease Control and Prevention recommended either late antenatal culture for GBS or a risk-based approach monitoring women with obstetric factors (e.g., maternal fever, rupture of membranes >18 hours). Despite a dramatic initial decline in the incidence of early-onset GBS disease, analysis revealed that the risk factor–based strategy identified <50% of affected infants' mothers compared with 85% to 90% with culture-based screening. On that basis, the latter became the recommended approach, resulting in an overall decline of 81% in early-onset GBS between 1993 and 2003.

   Schrag S, Schuchat A: Prevention of neonatal sepsis, *Clin Perinatol* 32:601–615, 2005.

145. **Do intrapartum antibiotics change the clinical presentation of early-onset GBS sepsis?**
   No. In a study of 319 infants with early-onset GBS disease, the administration of intrapartum antibiotics to the mother did not affect the constellation and timing of clinical signs of disease. All infants born to pretreated mothers became ill during the first 24 hours of life (80% within the first 6 hours of life).

   Bromberger P, Lawrence JM, Braun D, et al: The influence of intrapartum antibiotics on the clinical spectrum of early-onset group B streptococcal infection in term infants, *Pediatrics* 106:244–250, 2000.

KEY POINTS: SEPSIS

1. Because there are no reliable screening tests for sepsis, clinical judgment is paramount.

2. Screening cultures for group B streptococcus should be performed for all pregnant women at 35 to 37 weeks of gestation.

3. Coagulase-negative staphylococci are the most common bacterial pathogens responsible for nosocomial infections.

4. Neonatal meningitis can occur in the absence of a positive blood culture.

5. Fungal infection must be considered in sick preterm infants who are evaluated for sepsis.

146. **In cultures that are positive for coagulase-negative staphylococci, what distinguishes contamination from "true" infection?**
To help with the differentiation of a true coagulase-negative staphylococcal infection from blood-culture contamination (especially in infants with central catheters), blood cultures should be obtained from two different sites. In infants with infections, both cultures should grow coagulase-negative staphylococci with identical sensitivity patterns. If only a single blood culture is obtained, some authors have suggested that a colony count higher than 50 CFU/mL is suggestive evidence of true bacteremia. In clinical practice, however, that number of colony-forming units has a relatively poor predictive accuracy. See Figure 12.9.

147. **What are the most common pathogens that are responsible for late-onset sepsis in the newborn infant?**
   - Coagulase-negative staphylococci (48%)
   - *Staphylococcus aureus* (8%)
   - *Enterococcus* species (3%)
   - Gram-negative enterics (18%)
   - *Candida* species (10%)

   Stoll BJ, Hansen N, Fanaroff AA, et al: Late-onset sepsis in very low birth weight neonates: the experience of the NICHD Neonatal Research Network, *Pediatrics* 110:285–291, 2002.

148. **What are the major risk factors for nosocomial sepsis?**
   - Prematurity
   - Use of parenteral alimentation and central lines
   - Intravenous fat emulsions
   - H_2 blockers
   - Steroids for bronchopulmonary dysplasia (BPD)
   - Prolonged duration of mechanical ventilation
   - Overcrowding
   - Heavy staff workloads

149. **Is methicillin-resistant *S. aureus* (MRSA) a significant pathogen in the NICU?**
Although *S. aureus* accounts for 8% of late-onset sepsis in the NICU, the percentage of MRSA is not well established. Recent data suggest that a higher proportion of hospitalized patients with MRSA disease have community-acquired rather than hospital-acquired strains. In fact, about 3% of pregnant women had vaginal colonization with MRSA, which could be transmitted to their infants at the time of birth. Other reports have shown transmission of MRSA through breast milk. In NICUs with evidence of high rates of MRSA nasal colonization, treatment with nasal mupirocin is recommended by many authorities but unproven.

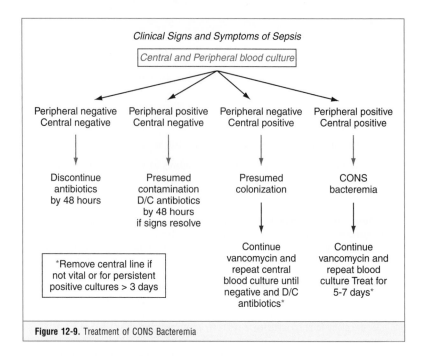

Figure 12-9. Treatment of CONS Bacteremia

150. **How is systemic candidiasis diagnosed in the neonate?**

By cultures of blood, urine, and CSF or other body fluids that are generally sterile. Because cultures are only intermittently positive, multiple systemic cultures should be obtained. A urinalysis demonstrating budding yeasts or hyphae should raise suspicion of systemic infection. Gram stains of buffy coat smears may also demonstrate organisms. An ophthalmologic examination may indicate the presence of candidal endophthalmitis. Renal and brain ultrasounds should be performed to look for characteristic lesions. In addition, echocardiography should be performed in infants with central catheters to rule out cardiac vegetations.

151. **Should preterm infants receive prophylaxis for the prevention of *Candida* infections?**

A number of studies have examined the role of fluconazole prophylaxis in reducing mortality, infections, and colonization among infants with very low birthweight. Although reduced mortality was not a consistent finding, decreased colonization and invasive infections were consistently seen. Although not seen as of yet, concerns remain that use of this high-cost treatment will increase fluconazole resistance and the emergence of *Candida glabrata* and *Candida krusei*, which are inherently less sensitive to the drug.

Carey AJ, Saiman L, Polin RA: Hospital-acquired infections in the NICU: epidemiology for the new millennium, *Clin Perinatol* 35:223–249, 2008.

NEUROLOGIC ISSUES

152. **What are normal CSF values for healthy neonates?**

Because of the frequent administration of intrapartum and in some cases postnatal antibiotics, current cutoffs for meningitis may differ from those frequently cited in the past. Using a CSF WBC count of 21/mm³ results in a sensitivity and specificity of 79% and 81%, respectively, for the diagnosis of meningitis. Although protein levels in term infants are generally below 100 mg/dL, levels in preterm infants are higher and vary inversely with gestational age. Normal values for glucose remain at 81% and 74%, respectively, of blood concentrations in term and preterm infants.

Garges HP, Moody MA, Cotton CM, et al: Neonatal meningitis: what is the correlation among CSF cultures, blood cultures and CSF parameters? *Pediatrics* 117:1094–1100, 2006.

153. **What is the risk for prenatal viral transmission in infants born to mothers with hepatitis B?**
If a mother is HBsAg and HBeAg positive, the risk for transmission is 70% to 90%. The risk is substantially lowered to 5% to 20% if the mother is HBsAg positive but HBeAg negative. Infants infected in the perinatal period have a greater than 90% chance of developing chronic hepatitis B infection, and of these, 25% go on to develop hepatocellular carcinoma.

154. **Should preterm infants receive hepatitis B vaccine during their newborn stay in the hospital?**
Because of the possibility of decreased immunologic response to vaccine at birth in preterm infants with birthweight of less than 2000 g, hepatitis B vaccine should be deferred until 1 month chronologic age. If medically stable, gaining weight consistently, and ready for discharge before 1 month of age, preterm infants may receive the first dose before discharge. Of course, if the infant's mother is HbsAg positive or status unknown, vaccine must be administered despite birthweight of less than 2000 g within 12 hours of birth along with HBIG.

155. **What regimen is recommended to prevent mother-to-infant transmission of HIV infection?**
Zidovudine therapy is administered in three phases beginning prenatally with oral treatment commencing between 14 and 34 weeks and continuing until birth, intravenous treatment during labor and delivery, and oral treatment to newborn infants for the first 6 weeks of life. Treatment during pregnancy is generally part of a combination treatment regimen. Even if the mother has received no treatment, initiation of zidovudine in her newborn before 48 hours of age will still result in reduction of transmission. Additional protection, especially in women with high viral loads, may be afforded by cesarean delivery before rupture of membranes and the onset of labor.

156. **After a difficult delivery, what three major forms of extracranial hemorrhage can occur?**
■ Caput succedaneum
■ Cephalhematoma
■ Subgaleal hemorrhage
Figure 12-10 and Table 12-13 characterize the major forms of extracranial hemorrhages.

From Volpe JJ, editor: *Neurology of the Newborn*, ed 5, Philadelphia, 2008, WB Saunders, p 960.

157. **If a cephalhematoma is suspected, should a skull radiograph be performed to evaluate for fracture?**
Cephalhematomas occur in up to 2.5% of live births. In studies, the incidence of associated fractures ranges from 5% to 25%. These fractures are almost always linear and nondepressed and do not require treatment. Thus, in an asymptomatic infant with a cephalhematoma over the convexity of the skull and without suspicion of a depressed fracture, radiographic imaging is not necessary. If the examination suggests cranial depression or neurologic signs are present, radiographic imaging is warranted.

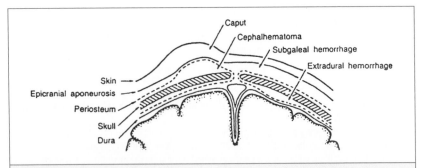

Figure 12-10. Major forms of extracranial hemorrhage. (From Volpe JJ [ed]: Neurology of the Newborn, 5th ed. Philadelphia, WB Saunders, 2008, p 960.)

TABLE 12-13. MAJOR VARIETIES OF TRAUMATIC EXTRACRANIAL HEMORRHAGE

Lesion	Features of External Swelling	Increases after Birth	Crosses Suture Lines	Marked Acute Blood Loss
Caput succedaneum	Soft pitting	No	Yes	No
Subgaleal hemorrhage	Firm, fluctuant	Yes	Yes	Yes
Cephalhematoma	Firm, tense	Yes	No	No

From Volpe JJ (ed): Neurology of the Newborn, 3rd ed. Philadelphia, WB Saunders, 1995, p 770.

158. **Should all preterm infants be examined by cranial ultrasound?**
Because of the relative noninvasiveness of ultrasound, most neonatologists recommend that a single cranial ultrasonogram be obtained during the first week of life in infants born before 35 weeks' gestational age.

159. **When screening for IVH, when is the best time to perform an ultrasound?**
In a series of infants studied by ultrasonography, about 50% had the onset of hemorrhage on the first day of life, 25% on the second day, and 15% on the third day. Thus, a single scan on the fourth day of life would be expected to detect more than 90% of IVHs. However, about 20% to 40% of hemorrhages show evidence of extension within 3 to 5 days after initial diagnosis, and thus a second scan is indicated to take place about 5 days after the first to determine the maximal extent of hemorrhage.

160. **How are IVHs classified?**
Most traditional systems of classification include a grading system that is in accordance with increasing severity:
- **Grade I:** Germinal matrix hemorrhage only
- **Grade II:** IVH without ventricular dilation
- **Grade III:** IVH with ventricular dilation
- **Grade IV:** Grade III hemorrhage plus intraparenchymal involvement

Some authorities have abandoned the grade IV classification in favor of "periventricular hemorrhagic infarction" to emphasize that these lesions have a different pathophysiology and are not simply extensions of germinal matrix or IVH into parenchymal tissue. As such, the extent of parenchymal involvement rather than the grade of hemorrhage is more important for determining prognosis.

161. **What is the cause of hydrocephalus after an intracranial hemorrhage?**
The acute hydrocephalus is believed to be a result of impairment of CSF absorption by the arachnoid membrane caused by the particulate blood clot. In subacute or chronic hydrocephalus, ventricular enlargement is the result of an obliterative arachnoiditis (likely a chemical inflammatory response from the continued presence of blood), which usually causes a communicating hydrocephalus. Less commonly, obstruction of the aqueduct of Sylvius can lead to a noncommunicating hydrocephalus.

162. **How common is progressive posthemorrhagic ventricular enlargement?**
The likelihood of this phenomenon depends on the extent of the initial hemorrhage, ranging from only about a 5% likelihood in patients with grade I IVH to 80% in those with grade IV IVH.

163. **Can serial LPs prevent posthemorrhagic hydrocephalus?**
No. Although LPs are useful for lowering increased intracranial pressure and for treating hydrocephalus after it has developed, they are of no benefit for preventing the onset. Infants with slowly progressive ventricular dilation and increasing head circumference, who do not show signs of spontaneous arrest and improvement within 4 weeks, should undergo a trial of serial LPs. Their effectiveness should be assessed with ultrasound. If there is no benefit, the placement of a ventriculoperitoneal shunt is necessary.

164. **How much fluid should be removed by LP in an infant with ventriculomegaly?**
Because the volume of CSF in the dilated ventricles of infants with posthemorrhagic hydrocephalus is large, the removal of a significant amount of fluid (10 to 15 mL/kg) is usually required.

165. **What factors predispose premature infants to the development of periventricular leukomalacia?**
Periventricular leukomalacia occurs primarily in the distribution of the end zones of deep penetrating arteries resulting in both focal (e.g., cysts) and more diffuse injury to white matter near the trigone of the lateral ventricles and around the foramen of Munro. Predisposing factors include the following:
- Cerebral ischemia due to phenomena like hypotension and hypocarbia occurring in infants with impaired cerebrovascular autoregulation and pressure-passive cerebral circulation
- Infection and inflammation due to intrauterine infection and fetal inflammatory responses resulting in the production of cytokines, excitotoxic molecules, and reactive oxygen and nitrogen species
- Vulnerability of pre-oligodendroglia to free radicals and excitotoxic molecules (e.g., glutamate)

166. **What modalities can be used to detect periventricular leukomalacia?**
The most common imaging technique used in the NICU is ultrasound, which is capable of detecting cystic periventricular leukomalacia. However, because overt cysts, which represent focal necrosis, are seen in only 3% or less of preterm infants, magnetic resonance imaging must be used to detect abnormal white matter signal, which may be seen in as many as 79% of preterm infants at term equivalent. What remains unclear is whether this observation represents noncystic periventricular leukomalacia or diffuse white matter gliosis. These entities may represent a spectrum of severity ranging from necrosis with cysts, to glial scars, to neither.

167. **What is the most common brachial plexus palsy?**
Erb palsy (Fig. 12-11). Neonatal brachial plexus injuries occur in less than 0.5% of deliveries and are often associated with shoulder dystocia and breech or forceps delivery.
- Involves upper plexus (C5, C6)
- In 50% of cases, C7 is affected
- Arm held limply adducted, internally rotated, and pronated with wrist flexed and fingers flexed ("waiter's tip" position)
- Biceps reflex absent, Moro reflex with hand movement but no shoulder abduction, palmar grasp present
- Ipsilateral diaphragmatic involvement in 5%

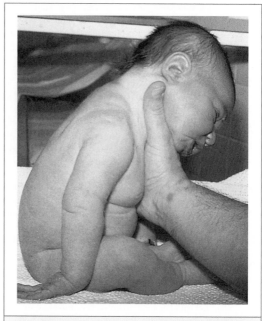

Figure 12-11. Erb palsy. Newborn demonstrating characteristic posture with the right arm limply adducted and internally rotated. (From Zitelli BJ, Davis HW: Atlas of Pediatric Physical Diagnosis, 5th ed. Philadelphia, Mosby, 2007, p 45.)

168. **What is Klumpke paralysis?**
A brachial plexus palsy involving injury to the lower plexus (C8, T1). It is associated with weakness of the flexor muscles of the wrist and the small muscles of the hand ("claw hand"). Up to one third of these patients have an associated Horner syndrome.

169. **How is brachial plexus injury treated?**
Therapy must be aimed at preventing contractures. For the first 7 to 10 days, the arm is gently immobilized against the abdomen to minimize further hemorrhage and/or swelling. After this initial period, passive range of motion exercises at the shoulder, elbow, wrist, and hand are performed. In addition, wrist splints to stabilize the fingers and avoid contractures should be used. Improvements in microsurgical techniques have increased interest in this modality if recovery is limited at 4 to 6 months, particularly in cases of nerve root avulsion. Surgical options include removal of fibrous tissue or neuroma, sural nerve graft, or local root grafts. Other therapies include the use of botulinum toxin with physical therapy if severe contractures have evolved.

Noetzel MJ, Park TS, Robinson S, Kaufman B: Prospective study of recovery following neonatal brachial plexus injury, *J Child Neurol* 16:488–492, 2001.

170. **What is the outcome of neonatal brachial plexus palsy?**
About 90% of patients have normal examinations by 12 months of age. Onset of recovery within 2 weeks and involvement of only the proximal upper extremity are both favorable prognostic signs. Infants who recovered completely regained antigravity movements of the biceps, triceps, and deltoids by 4.5 months, whereas those with mild weakness did so by 6 months. Infants who did not recover antigravity movement in the deltoid ($\pm$ the biceps and/or triceps) at 6 months are likely left with moderate weakness, whereas those with severe weakness showed minimal to no recovery in wrist extensors at the same age.

Hale HB, Bae DS, Walters PM: Current concepts in the management of brachial plexus palsy, *J Hand Surg Am* 35:322–331, 2010.

Noetzel MJ, Park TS, Robinson S, Kaufman B: Prospective study of recovery following neonatal brachial plexus injury, *J. Child Neurol* 16:488–492, 2001.

Strombeck C, Krumlinde-Sundholm L, Forssberg H: Functional outcome at 5 years in children with obstetrical brachial plexus palsy with and without microsurgical reconstruction, *Dev Med Child Neurol* 42:148–157, 2000.

KEY POINTS: NEUROLOGY

1. The major forms of neonatal extracranial hemorrhages can be distinguished clinically.

2. In more than 90% of cases, intraventricular hemorrhages in preterm infants occur during the first 3 days of life.

3. Posthemorrhagic hydrocephalus is most likely to occur after the most severe intraventricular hemorrhages.

4. Recovery occurs in about 90% of patients with brachial plexus injuries.

5. Periventricular leukomalacia and other forms of white matter injury play a major part in long-term disabilities in preterm newborns.

171. **In newborns with facial paralysis, how is peripheral nerve involvement distinguished from central nerve involvement?**
    - **Peripheral:** This usually results from compression of the peripheral portion of the nerve by prolonged pressure from the maternal sacral promontory. The use of forceps alone is not thought to be an important causative factor. Peripheral paralysis is unilateral. The forehead is smooth on the affected side, and the eye is persistently open.
    - **Central:** This type often results from contralateral CNS injury (temporal bone fracture and/or posterior fossa hemorrhage or tissue destruction). It involves only the lower half or two thirds of the face; the forehead and eyelids are not affected.
    In both forms of paralysis, the mouth is drawn to the normal side when crying, and the nasolabial fold is obliterated on the affected side.

172. **Is ankle clonus normal in the newborn infant?**
    Bilateral ankle clonus of 5 to 10 beats may be a normal finding, especially in infants who are crying, hungry, or jittery. This is particularly true if the clonus is neither accompanied by other signs of upper motor neuron dysfunction nor asymmetrical. Clonus should disappear at about 3 months of age.

173. **Do newborns prefer to turn their heads to the right or to the left?**
    Healthy neonates prefer to turn their heads to the right, which may reflect the normal asymmetry of cerebral function at this age. This preference has been observed as early as 28 weeks of gestation. By 39 weeks of gestation, 90% of newborn infants spend 80% of the time with their heads turned to the right side.

174. **Does hypothermia improve the outcomes of term infants following perinatal asphyxia?**
    Timely use of mild therapeutic hypothermia following intrapartum asphyxia results in reduction in the combined incidence of mortality and major neurodevelopmental disability at 18 months of age as well as in the incidence of these outcomes individually. Short-term adverse effects

were few (e.g., small increase in need for inotropic support, thrombocytopenia, and insignificant sinus bradycardia) and were outweighed by the benefits. The reduction in both of these outcomes is extremely reassuring in demonstrating that the increased survival does not result in more impaired infants.

Agostoni C: Role of long chain polyunsaturated fatty acids in the first year of life. *J Pediatr Gastroenterol Nutr* 47:S41–S44, 2008.

Barks JD: Current concepts in hypothermic neuroprotection, *Semin Fetal Neonatal Med* 13:30–34, 2008.

Jacobs S: Cooling for newborns with hypoxic-ischemic encephalopathy, *Cochrane Database Syst Rev* 4:CD003311, 2007.

175. **What methods are available for providing therapeutic hypothermia and which is preferable?**
The goal of hypothermia is to lower systemic temperature by 2° to 3°C. This can be accomplished by either whole-body cooling or selective head cooling. Both methods have been shown in randomized trials to lower mortality and reduce neurodevelopmental disabilities, including severe neuromotor abnormalities, mental retardation (MDI <70) and visual impairment. Additional trials are still needed to determine whether one method is preferable over the other.

NUTRITION

176. **How many calories are required daily for growth in a healthy, growing preterm infant?**
Preterm infants need about 120 cal/kg/day. About 45% of the caloric intake should be carbohydrate, 45% should be fat, and 10% should be protein. Infants who expend increased calories (e.g., those with chronic lung disease, fever, or cold stress) may need up to 150 cal/kg per day.

177. **How should enteral feedings be started in the preterm infant?**
Initiation of feedings in preterm infants frequently depends on their cardiorespiratory stability. There is great variability from study to study on the definition of "early" feedings ranging from 1 to 8 days. Minimal enteral feeds (trophic feedings) generally consist of breast milk or preterm infant formula at a volume of 12 to 24 mL/kg per day. The volume is held constant for anywhere from 5 to 10 days. Subsequently, feeds are advanced by about 20 mL/kg per day until a volume of 140 to 160 mL/kg per day is achieved. Although many reports suggest that infants receiving trophic feeds may reach full feeds sooner, have a shorter length of stay, and have a reduced incidence of NEC, they are limited by small cohorts of patient subjects, nonblinding of groups, and variability in feeding regimen parameters.

Tyson JE, Kennedy KA, Lucke JF, Pedroza C: Dilemmas initiating enteral feedings in high risk infants: how can they be resolved? *Semin Perinatol* 31:61–73, 2007.

178. **What are the documented medical benefits of breastfeeding?**
Proven benefits
   ■ Fewer episodes of otitis media and respiratory and gastrointestinal illness occur in breastfed infants.
   ■ Human milk facilitates the growth of beneficial, nonpathogenic flora compared with the pathogenic anaerobes and coliforms that predominate in infants who are fed formula.
   ■ Formula-fed infants have reduced quantities of host-defense proteins in the gastrointestinal tract (e.g., lactoferrin, secretory IgA).
Suggested but unproven benefits
   ■ Decreased incidence of neonatal sepsis and necrotizing enterocolitis in preterm infants
   ■ Enhancement of subsequent intelligence

- Reduction in incidence of atherosclerosis
- Reduction in incidence of diabetes mellitus

Hoddinott P, Tappin D, Wright C: Breast feeding. *BMJ* 336:881–887, 2008.

Laleche League, http://www.lalecheleague.org.

179. **How does maternal breast milk differ for a full-term versus a premature baby?**
The composition of human milk for preterm infants differs from that for term infants in a number of ways. For every 100 mL, it is higher in calories (67 to 72 kcal versus 62 to 68 kcal), higher in protein (1.7 to 2.1 g versus 1.2 to 1.7 g), higher in lipids (3.4 to 4.4 g versus 3.0 to 4.0 g), lower in carbohydrates, higher in multiple minerals and trace elements (especially sodium [Na], chloride [Cl], iron [Fe], Zinc [Zn], and copper [Cu]), and higher in vitamins (especially vitamins A and E). However, as breast milk becomes mature, many of these nutritional advantages are lost.

180. **How does colostrum differ from mature human breast milk?**
Colostrum is the thick, yellowish mammary secretion that is characteristic of the first postpartum week. It is higher in phospholipids, cholesterol, and protein concentration and lower in lactose and total fat composition than mature breast milk. Colostrum is particularly rich in immunoglobulins, especially secretory IgA.

181. **With regard to breastfeeding, how do fore milk and hind milk differ?**
The caloric density of human milk increases in a nonlinear fashion while the infant is breast feeding. Hind milk (produced at the end of the feeding) can have a fat content that is 50% higher than fore milk. In preterm infants with poor weight gain, hind milk may offer a nutritional advantage.

182. **What are contraindications to breastfeeding?**
- **Inborn errors of metabolism:** Galactosemia, phenylketonuria, and urea cycle defects
- **Infections**: Human immunodeficiency virus, tuberculosis (before treatment), human T-cell lymphotropic virus (HTLV) types I and II, cytomegalovirus (in preterm infants), and herpes simplex (when lesions are present on the breast)
- **Substance abuse or use:** Cocaine, narcotics, stimulants, and marijuana
- **Medications:** Sulfonamides (for ill, stressed, or preterm infants or infants with hyperbilirubinemia and glucose-6-phosphate dehydrogenase deficiency), radioactive medicines, chemotherapeutic agents (alkylating agents), bromocriptine (suppresses lactation), and lithium (in general, psychotropic drugs should be used with caution). Otherwise, most other medications are compatible with breastfeeding, or suitable substitutes exist.

American Academy of Pediatrics: *Pediatric Nutrition Handbook*, ed 6, Elk Grove Village, 2009, pp 39–40.

183. **What advice should be given to a mother who plans to express and save breast milk for later feedings?**
Ideally, she should collect the milk as cleanly as possible and then store it rapidly at 3° to 4°C or colder; the milk should then be used within 5 days. Alternatively, breast milk can be stored in the freezer compartment of a refrigerator for about 6 months. If more prolonged storage is necessary (12 months), the milk should be kept frozen at a temperature of −20°C or lower (usually in a separate freezer). After the milk has thawed, it should not be refrozen.

184. **Should mothers maintained on methadone breastfeed their babies?**
Numerous studies show that the amount of methadone transferred through milk is low across the range of doses typically used and not likely to result in toxicity to the infant. In fact,

some recent data suggest that breastfeeding in this instance may actually lessen the symptoms of neonatal abstinence.

Hale TW: *Medications and Mothers' Milk*, ed 13, Amarillo, TX, 2008, Hale Publishing.

185. **What are the advantages of a 60/40 whey-to-casein ratio in infant formulas?**
The term 60/40 refers to the percentage of whey (lactalbumin) and casein in human milk or cow milk formulas. This ratio makes for small curds and therefore easy digestibility by the infant. The 60/40 ratio is of particular advantage to the preterm infant because it is associated with lower levels of serum ammonia and a decreased incidence of metabolic acidosis. Only human milk or formulas that supply protein in this ratio provide adequate amounts of the amino acids cystine and taurine, which may be essential for the preterm infant.

186. **How much formula should an average infant drink per day?**
A healthy term newborn in the first 1 to 2 days of life may drink only 0.5 to 1 ounces every 3 to 4 hours. After feedings are well established, infants may ingest 200 mL/kg/day or more.

187. **"Low-iron" or "regular iron-fortified" formulas: which are preferred for infants?**
Generally, low-iron formula has 4 to 6 mg/L of elemental iron, whereas regular iron-fortified formula has 12 mg/L. Infants who are not breastfed should be placed on regular iron-fortified formula. Although a greater percentage of iron is absorbed from the ingested low-iron formula, the quantity may not be sufficient to protect against the development of iron-deficiency anemia. In addition, despite anecdotal experiences, the incidence of colic, constipation, vomiting, and fussiness does not vary among infants fed the two formulas. The American Academy of Pediatrics recommends that all formula fed to infants be iron fortified.

188. **Is vitamin supplementation necessary for exclusively breastfed term infants?**
As a result of the growing concerns about the relationship of sunlight exposure and skin cancer, the low concentration of vitamin D in breast milk, and the inability to predict adequate exposure as a result of diverse lifestyle and cultural practices, cases of rickets in breastfed infants have been reported. The following recommendations have therefore been made:
- Beginning in the first 2 months of life, all breastfed infants should be supplemented with 400 IU/day of vitamin D to prevent the occurrence of rickets.
- Malnourished mothers may need to supplement their breastfed babies with multivitamins.
- Mothers who are strict vegetarians may have low concentrations of B vitamins in their breast milk, and infants may need supplementation with vitamin B_{12}.

American Academy of Pediatrics: *Pediatric Nutrition Handbook*, ed 6, Elk Grove Village IL, 2009.

189. **If alimentation is being administered through a peripheral vein, is heparinization necessary?**
The administration of heparin to premature infants in a concentration of 0.5 to 1.0 U/mL has been shown to improve the clearance of lipids through the enhanced release of lipoprotein lipase. Therefore, heparin should be used whenever fats are being administered intravenously.

190. **What is nonnutritive sucking?**
Nonnutritive sucking is a mode of sucking that is unique to humans and that is characterized by a highly regular, burst-pause pattern. Nonnutritive sucking occurs in all sleep and awake states, although it is seen less often during quiet sleep and crying. It assumes a recognizable rhythmic pattern after 33 weeks of gestation.

191. **How do protein requirements vary with the mode of nutrient delivery (intravenous versus enteral)?**
Whether delivered intravenously or enterally, the protein requirements needed to achieve in utero accretion rates are similar. Preterm infants have slightly higher protein requirements (3.0 to 3.5 g/kg per day) than term infants (2.0 to 2.5 g/kg per day).

192. **Which fatty acids are essential for the neonate?**
Humans cannot synthesize fatty acids with double bonds in the ω-6 and ω-3 positions. Therefore, linoleic acid (ω-6) and linolenic acid (ω-3) must be provided in the diet to serve as precursors for fatty acids with these bonds. In infants weighing less than 1750 g who experience delay in or difficulty with maintaining full enteral feedings, arachidonic and docosahexaenoic acids, which are normally derived in utero from maternal plasma, may also be essential. These fatty acids are vital for normal brain development, myelination, cell proliferation, and retinal function. Fatty acids in human milk are composed of 12% to 15% linoleic acid.

193. **What are the proven advantages of supplementing formulas with long-chain polyunsaturated fatty acids?**
- Docosahexaenoic acid–supplemented infants transiently demonstrate higher behaviorally and electrophysiologically based measurements of visual acuity.
- The beneficial effects on visual function are inconsistent in meta-analysis.
- The effects on cognitive development are controversial but appear more compelling in preterm infants.

    Simmer K, Patole S: Long chain polyunsaturated fatty acid supplementation in preterm infants, *Cochrane Database Syst Rev* 1:CD000375, 2004.

    SanGiovanni JP, Parra-Cabrera S, Colditz GA, et al: Meta-analysis of dietary essential fatty acids and long-chain polyunsaturated fatty acids as they relate to visual resolution acuity in healthy preterm infants, *Pediatrics* 105:1292–1298, 2000.

194. **What are the manifestations of essential fatty acid deficiency?**
Scaly dermatitis, alopecia, thrombocytopenia (and platelet dysfunction), failure to thrive, and increased susceptibility to recurrent infection. To prevent and treat fatty acid deficiency, 4% to 5% of caloric intake should be provided as linoleic acid and 1% as linolenic acid. This requirement can be met by 0.5 to 1.0 g/kg per day of intravenous lipids.

195. **Why are nucleotides being added to a number of infant formulas?**
Dietary nucleotides may play a role during early neonatal life in the desaturation and elongation of essential fatty acids, which are necessary for brain and retinal development. The addition of nucleotides to formula (simulating the composition of breast milk) may be especially important during early development. Nucleotides are present in relatively large amounts in human milk, and several studies have suggested an important role for nucleotides in immune function, gastrointestinal function, and lipoprotein metabolism.

196. **What are the manifestations of vitamin E deficiency in the neonate?**
Hemolytic anemia (with reticulocytosis), **peripheral edema**, and **thrombocytosis**.
Vitamin E is important for stabilizing the RBC membrane, and a deficiency can result in a mild hemolytic anemia. The American Academy of Pediatrics recommends that 0.7 IU (international unit) of vitamin E per 100 kcal be present in feedings for preterm infants. There is current consensus that infants weighing less than 1000 g require 6 to 12 IU of vitamin E per kilogram per day and that this can generally be met by preterm formulas that provide 4 to 6 IU per 100 kcal.

KEY POINTS: GROWTH AND NUTRITION

1. Infants with late-onset in utero growth restriction have a low ponderal index.

2. Breast milk is protective against infection and may reduce the incidence of adult chronic diseases.

3. The presence of an umbilical artery catheter is not a contraindication to breastfeeding.

4. In infants who are not breast fed, intravenous amino acids should be started as soon as possible.

5. Long-chain polyunsaturated fatty acid supplementation in formula appears to enhance visual and cognitive function.

RESPIRATORY ISSUES

197. **What causes infants to grunt?**
Infants with respiratory disease tend to expire through closed or partially closed vocal cords to elevate transpulmonary pressure and to therefore increase lung volume. The latter effect results in an improved ventilation-to-perfusion ratio with better gas exchange. It is during the last part of expiration, when gas is expelled through the partially closed vocal cords, that the audible grunt is produced.

198. **What do hyperpnea and tachypnea signify in the neonate?**
- **Hyperpnea** refers to deep, relatively unlabored respirations at mildly increased rates. It is typical of situations in which there is reduced pulmonary blood flow (e.g., pulmonary atresia), and it results from the ventilation of underperfused alveoli.
- **Tachypnea** refers to shallow, rapid, and somewhat labored respirations, and it is seen in the setting of low lung compliance (e.g., primary lung disease, pulmonary edema).

199. **Until what age are infants obligate nose breathers?**
Although 30% of newborn infants breathe through their mouth or nose and mouth, the remaining 70% are obligate nose breathers until the third to sixth week of life.

200. **What are the effects of severe hypercarbia ($Pco_2 = 100$ mm Hg) if there is no associated hypoxia?**
There are few data about human newborns regarding the effects of isolated severe hypercarbia in the absence of hypoxia. However, results from animal studies and limited clinical observations in humans suggest that this condition can lead to a pressure-passive cerebral circulation and a possible increased risk for IVH. In addition, the high $Paco_2$ may disrupt the blood-brain barrier and enhance the deposition of molecules such as bilirubin in the CNS, thereby leading to kernicterus. Finally, on a more cellular level, data in animal model systems demonstrate alterations in brain cell membrane lipid peroxidation as well as Na^+,K^+-ATPase activity. The significance of these latter findings remains undetermined. Moderate degrees of hypercarbia may be neuroprotective, and it may decrease lung injury in ventilated neonates.

201. **In an infant who is receiving mechanical ventilation, what is an acceptable range for pH, Pco_2, and Po_2?**
- **Pao_2:** 50 to 70 mm Hg
- **$Paco_2$:** 50 to 70 mmHg (in term infants with PPHN: 35 to 45)
- **pH:** ≥ 7.2 (in term infants with PPHN: 7.3 to 7.4)

202. **What mechanical ventilator settings are likely to affect Po_2 and Pco_2?**
- **Pao_2 is *increased*** by raising the positive end-expiratory pressure (PEEP), the peak inspiratory pressure, the inspiratory-to-expiratory ratio, or the inspired oxygen concentration.
- **Pco_2 is *decreased*** by increasing the rate or peak inspiratory pressure. An increase in PEEP may increase the $Paco_2$ by decreasing the tidal volume.

203. **What are the physiologic effects of PEEP?**
PEEP can prevent alveolar collapse, maintain lung volume at end expiration, and improve ventilation-perfusion mismatch. However, an increase in PEEP may decrease tidal volume and impede CO_2 elimination. Elevations in PEEP to nonphysiologic values may decrease lung compliance, impair venous return, decrease cardiac output, and reduce tissue oxygen delivery.

204. **Is there a role for nasal ventilation?**
Although providing positive-pressure breaths in a noninvasive manner would potentially avoid the complications of intubation, there are no data to support the use of nasal ventilation as a primary treatment for pulmonary disorders. However, this type of ventilation has been successfully employed to prevent extubation failures, and shows a trend toward reduced apnea. The importance of synchronization with this modality is not established.

Barrington KJ, Bull D, Finer NN: Randomized trial of nasal synchronized intermittent mandatory ventilation compared with continuous positive airway pressure after extubation of very low birth weight infants, *Pediatrics* 107:638–641, 2001.

Davis PG, Lemyre B, de Paoli AG: Nasal intermittent positive pressure ventilation vs. nasal continuous positive airway pressure for preterm neonates after extubation, *Cochrane Database Syst Rev* 3:CD003212, 2001.

205. **How do high-frequency oscillatory ventilation and high-frequency jet ventilation differ?**
In general, high-frequency jet ventilation has been used more commonly to treat infants with severe air leak syndromes, whereas high-frequency oscillatory ventilation has been of greater value for infants with difficulties achieving adequate oxygenation and requiring "high" settings. Neither ventilator has been proved superior to conventional ventilation for the management of infants with uncomplicated respiratory distress syndrome (RDS) or as rescue therapy in preventing chronic lung disease (Table 12-14).

TABLE 12-14.	HIGH-FREQUENCY OSCILLATORY VENTILATION VERSUS HIGH-FREQUENCY JET VENTILATION	
	High-Frequency Oscillatory Ventilation	High-Frequency Jet Ventilation
Frequency	10-30 Hz	10-40 Hz
Total volume	Determined by oscillator	Increased by gas entrainment
I:E ratio	Constant	Variable
Expiratory phase	Active, less risk of gas trapping	Passive, more risk for gas trapping
Airway damage	Similar to IPPV	Necrotizing tracheobronchitis
May be used in combination with IPPV	Yes	Yes

I:E = inspiratory to expiratory; IPPV = intermittent positive-pressure ventilation.

Lampland AL, Mammel MC: The role of high frequency ventilation in neonates: evidence-based recommendations, *Clin Perinatol* 34:129–144, 2007.

Stark AR: High-frequency oscillatory ventilation to prevent bronchopulmonary dysplasia—are we there yet? *N Engl J Med* 347:682–683, 2002.

206. **Has nasal prong continuous positive airway pressure (CPAP) been proved to decrease the risk for BPD?**
In the largest trial to date, early administration of CPAP compared with intubation in infants born at 25 to 28 weeks' gestation does not reduce the incidence of death or chronic lung disease. The question still remains about whether significant reduction will be achieved by combining this treatment with early administration of surfactant.

Morley CJ, Davis PG, Doyle LW, et al: COIN trial investigators: nasal CPAP or intubation at birth for very preterm infants, *N Engl J Med* 358:700–708, 2008.

207. **Have antenatal steroids or surfactant been proved to decrease the risk for chronic lung disease?**
No. Because both treatments offer benefits with regard to preventing and treating RDS and increasing survival of extremely immature infants, it may not be surprising that neither one has been shown to lower the incidence of BPD.

Bhandari A, Bhandari V: Pitfalls, problems, and progress in bronchopulmonary dysplasia, *Pediatrics* 123:1562–1573, 2009.

Van Marter LJ, Allred EN, Leviton A, et al: Neonatology Committee for the Developmental Epidemiology Network: Antenatal glucocorticoid treatment does not reduce chronic lung disease among surviving preterm infants, *J Pediatr* 138:198–204, 2001.

208. **What is the function of surfactant?**
Surfactant is a surface-active material that is made up of a mixture that is rich in phosphatidylcholine (64%), phosphatidylglycerol (8%), and lesser amounts of proteins and other lipids. Surfactant acts as an antiatelectasis factor in the alveolar lining by lowering surface tension at diminished lung volumes and increasing it at high volumes. This allows for the maintenance of functional residual capacity, which acts as a reservoir to prevent wide fluctuation in arterial Po_2 and Pco_2 during respiration. In patients with RDS, surfactants have been shown to decrease the need for supplemental oxygen therapy, to lower mortality rates, and to decrease the incidence of air-leak syndromes. The incidence of BPD has not been substantially reduced owing to increased survival of extremely preterm infants, who are most likely to develop this disorder.

209. **Do the kinds of surfactants used to treat infants with RDS differ in effectiveness?**
Two general classes of surfactants are available for replacement therapy: natural surfactants prepared from mammalian lungs (e.g., Survanta, Infasurf, Curosurf) and synthetic surfactants (e.g., Exosurf, Surfaxin). Although natural surfactant extracts appear to have a better immediate effect (i.e., less supplemental oxygen required, fewer pneumothoraces), long-term clinical outcomes (e.g., chronic lung disease, death) with synthetic surfactants were not significantly different. Studies with Surfaxin, which contains a peptide with SP-B like functions, may be clinically comparable to natural surfactants.

Moya F, Maturana A: Animal-derived surfactants vs. past and current synthetic surfactants: current status, *Clin Perinatol* 34:145–177, 2007.

Soll RF, Blanco F: Natural surfactant extract versus synthetic surfactant for neonatal respiratory distress syndrome, *Cochrane Database Syst Rev* 2:CD000144, 2001.

210. **In surfactant therapy, is "prophylaxis" or "rescue" treatment better?**
Although some institutions administer surfactant as soon as possible after birth (preventilatory or within minutes of ventilation) as prophylaxis and others wait for the development of RDS to administer rescue therapy, earlier administration is advantageous, even with the latter approach. Early compared with late rescue treatment reduces the occurrence of pneumothorax, pulmonary intentional emphysema, mortality, and the combined outcome of death or chronic lung disease at 36 weeks' postmenstrual age. Recent data suggest that, for the most immature babies (<28 weeks or possibly <26 weeks), prophylaxis improves survival and lessens the severity of RDS, but it appears to not reduce the incidence of chronic lung disease.

Engle WA: Surfactant-replacement therapy for respiratory distress in the preterm and term neonate, *Pediatrics* 121:419–432, 2008.

Soll RF, Morley CJ: Prophylactic versus selective use of surfactant in preventing morbidity and mortality in preterm infants, *Cochrane Database Syst Rev* 2:CD000510, 2001.

211. **What are the adverse effects of prophylactically administering surfactant in the delivery room?**
■ About 20% to 60% of healthy infants whose gestational age is 30 weeks or more will be treated unnecessarily.
■ It imposes extra risks and unwarranted expenses.
■ The use of surfactant may lead to a transient decrease in oxygen saturation.
■ It delays resuscitation efforts and stabilization if administered before ventilation.

212. **What is the mechanism of action of inhaled nitric oxide (iNO) in the management of PPHN?**
Nitric oxide, produced endogenously in endothelial cells at the time of transition from fetal to neonatal life, diffuses to the vascular smooth muscle cell, where it increases the activity of soluble guanylate cyclase. This leads to the intraconversion of guanosine triphosphate to cyclic guanosine monophosphate (cGMP), which causes smooth muscle relaxation leading to pulmonary vasodilation. Similarly, exogenous iNO diffuses from the alveolus to the smooth muscle cells with similar effects. iNO is then rapidly bound and inactivated by reduced hemoglobin in the vascular space, thus avoiding concomitant reductions in systemic blood pressure.

213. **Should iNO be used in preterm infants?**
Trials of iNO in preterm infants were originally undertaken to improve cardiopulmonary outcome. However, recent data suggest that treatment of infants with severe RDS results in improved neurodevelopmental outcome. Although these effects may be mediated in part by a reduction in the incidence of chronic lung disease, severe IVH, and periventricular leukomalacia, iNO may exert a direct effect on the CNS.

Marks JD, Schreiber MD: Inhaled nitric oxide and neuroprotection in preterm infants, *Clin Perinatol* 35:793–807, 2008.

214. **Is there a role for sildenafil (Viagra) in the treatment of PPHN?**
Under normal conditions, vascular smooth muscle cGMP is degraded by phosphodiesterase-5 (PDE-5). As an inhibitor of PDE-5, sildenafil prolongs the half-life of cGMP and by so doing could prolong the vasodilating effects of nitric oxide (endogenous or exogenous). Trials to date assessing the effects of this drug, especially in settings in which iNO and high-frequency ventilation are unavailable because of their high costs, have demonstrated improved oxygenation and a possible reduction in mortality. Definitive data await trials with increased numbers of subjects and comparing sildenafil to other pulmonary vasodilators.

Steinhorn RH, Kinsella JP, Pierce C, et al: Intravenous sildenafil in the treatment of neonates with persistent pulmonary hypertension, *J Pediatr* 155:841–847, 2009.

215. **Which infants benefit most from extracorporeal membrane oxygenation (ECMO)?**
ECMO is prolonged cardiopulmonary bypass that is used to treat newborn infants (<1 week old) with reversible pulmonary disease that has been complicated by PPHN. Although overall survival is about 70% to 80%, it varies by diagnosis, with rates of more than 90% for meconium aspiration syndrome, 75% for sepsis, and about 50% for congenital diaphragmatic hernia. Use of iNO has reduced the need for ECMO.

216. **What are the risks for and contraindications to ECMO?**
The risk for thrombosis is an ever-present threat during ECMO therapy. Therefore, all infants receiving ECMO are heparinized. However, heparinization creates an increased risk for systemic bleeding and intracranial hemorrhage. Long-term morbidities are generally referable to the CNS. Contraindications to ECMO include uncontrolled bleeding, grade II or greater IVH, pulmonary hemorrhage, irreversible pulmonary disease, history of severe asphyxia, prolonged mechanical ventilation (>7 to 14 days), lethal genetic condition, and significant prematurity (birthweight <2000 g; gestational age <35 weeks).

217. **What is the most common type of congenital diaphragmatic hernia (CDH)?**
Bochdalek hernia, which accounts for 90% of all CDHs. This is a posterolateral hernia that most commonly (70% to 90%) occurs on the left side. The usual presentation is at birth with severe cardiorespiratory distress. Examination is characterized by a scaphoid abdomen and decreased breath sounds on the affected side. Radiographs reveal loops of bowel in the thoracic cavity (Fig. 12-12). Bag-mask ventilation should be minimized to avoid abdominal distention.

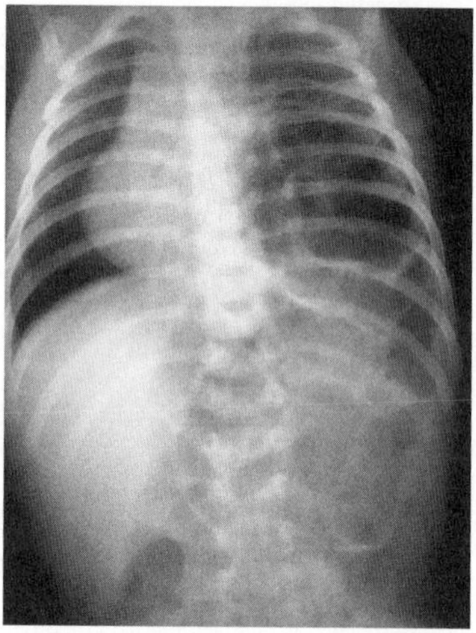

Figure 12-12. Chest radiograph of a newborn with Bochdalek hernia. Note the absence of the left diaphragmatic shadow, gas-filled loops of bowel in the left chest, and heart and mediastinum shifted to the right. (From Taussig LM, Landau LI [eds]: Pediatric Respiratory Medicine, 2nd ed. Philadelphia, Mosby, 2008, p 937.)

218. **What characterizes the diagnosis of BPD?**
In the postsurfactant era, pathologic changes in infants dying with BPD are characterized less by airway injury and fibrosis and instead are most notable for alveolar simplification and reduced septation. Clinical definitions have also varied and have been confounded by different target oxygen saturations in different NICUs. A recent consensus at the National Institutes of Health conference has attempted to create a consistent physiologic definition, as demonstrated in the figure for infants born before 32 weeks' gestation. For those born at 32 weeks' gestation or later, the same approach is used, but assessment is performed at 56 days rather than 36 weeks' postmenstrual age (Fig.12-13).

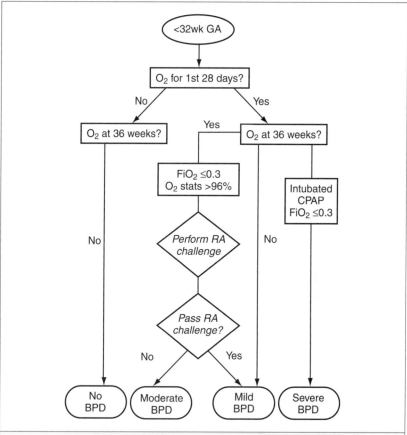

Figure 12-13. Physiologic definition of BPD. GA = gestational age; RA = room air. (From Aschner JL, Walsh MC. Long term outcomes: what should the focus be? Clin Perinatol 34:205-217, 2002.)

Aschner JL, Walsh MC: Long term outcomes: what should the focus be? *Clin Perinatol* 34:205–217, 2007.

Walsh MC, Szefler S, Davis J, et al: Summary proceedings from the bronchopulmonary dysplasia group, *Pediatrics* 117:S52–S56, 2006.

219. **What are the advantages and disadvantages of long-term diuretic therapy for BPD?**
Long-term diuretic therapy in infants with BPD improves pulmonary function, decreases airway resistance, increases pulmonary compliance, and allows for the weaning of supplemental oxygen. However, the duration of supplemental oxygen may not be shortened. Furthermore, the long-term effect on infant mortality is not entirely clear. Diuretic therapy is not without side effects, including electrolyte imbalance, nephrocalcinosis, bone demineralization, and ototoxicity.

Brion LP, Primhak RA: Intravenous or enteral loop diuretics for preterm infants with (or developing) chronic lung disease, *Cochrane Database Syst Rev* 1:CD001453, 2002.

KEY POINTS: RESPIRATORY SYSTEM

1. Hypercarbia is tolerated to avoid barotrauma and to minimize the occurrence of chronic lung disease.

2. Whether surfactant is administered as "prophylaxis" or "rescue," the earlier the time of administration, the more potent the effects.

3. Outside of clinical trials and clinical respiratory disease unresponsive to maximal support, postnatal steroids should not be administered to prevent chronic lung disease or to facilitate extubation.

4. In addition to treating apnea, caffeine reduces the incidence of chronic lung disease, death, and long-term disability.

5. Continuous positive airway pressure is used to prevent extubation failure and apnea but has not been shown to reduce the incidence of chronic lung disease or death.

220. **What is the role of vitamin A supplementation for preventing or reducing the severity of BPD?**
Because vitamin A is involved in the proliferation and differentiation of epithelial cells, it is thought to play an important role in the repair process in the lung after barotrauma and oxygen exposure. Although vitamin A deficiency has been associated with the development of BPD, studies examining the effects of vitamin A supplementation on the incidence of BPD have shown conflicting results. However, the most recent large multicenter trial has demonstrated a modest reduction in the incidence of chronic lung disease in infants with extremely low birthweight while reducing the biochemical evidence of vitamin A deficiency.

Tyson JE, Wright LL, Oh W, et al: Vitamin A supplementation for extremely-low-birth-weight infants. National Institute of Child Health and Human Development Neonatal Research Network, *N Engl J Med* 340:1962–1968, 1999.

221. **When should steroids be initiated in neonates with BPD?**
Studies of long-term follow-up have demonstrated an increased incidence of cerebral palsy and adverse neurodevelopmental sequelae in premature infants who have been treated with postnatal steroids. Consequently, this treatment should be limited to patients who are participating in controlled clinical trials or to those receiving maximal ventilatory and oxygen support who are showing no signs of progress and at significant risk for death.

American Academy of Pediatrics and Canadian Pediatric Society: Postnatal corticosteroids to treat or prevent chronic lung disease in preterm infants, *Pediatrics* 109:330–338, 2002.

222. **Why are infants with BPD at increased risk for poor neurodevelopmental outcome?**
- Recurrent episodes of hypoxia occurs as a result of chronic lung disease and BPD spells.
- BPD is associated with IVH and periventricular leukomalacia.
- Poor nutrition is an issue during periods of critical brain growth.
- Prolonged illness and hospitalization preclude normal stimulation and parent-infant interaction.
Using the physiologic definition of BPD, increased severity of disease was correlated with increased adverse neurodevelopmental outcomes.

Gerdes JS: Bronchopulmonary dysplasia. In Polin RA, Yoder MC, editors: *Workbook in Practical Neonatology*, ed 4, Philadelphia, 2007, Saunders, p 181.

Ehrenkrantz R, Walsh MC, Kohr B, et al: Validation of the NIH consensus definition of bronchopulmonary dysplasia, *Pediatrics* 116:1353–1360, 2005.

223. **What is the difference between apnea and periodic breathing?**
Apnea is the cessation of respiration for more than 20 seconds or for a shorter duration if it is associated with cyanosis and/or bradycardia. Periodic breathing is commonly seen in preterm infants, and it is defined as a pattern of three or more respiratory pauses of more than 3 seconds' duration with less than 20 seconds of respirations between pauses. Periodic breathing is not associated with bradycardia. Both apnea and periodic breathing reflect a lack of maturation of respiratory control centers in the preterm infant.

American Sleep Apnea Association: http://www.sleepapnea.org.

224. **When should apnea be treated?**
In all cases of apnea, an underlying cause should be sought and treated if found. In idiopathic apnea, therapy should be initiated when episodes do not resolve with gentle tactile stimulation and require vigorous stimulation or when patients have a frequency of more than four episodes in 8 hours.

225. **What methods are effective for treating apnea of prematurity?**
- Use of oscillating waterbeds
- Administration of CPAP (this is especially helpful in apnea with an obstructive component)
- Provision of supplemental oxygen (with or without CPAP). If supplemental oxygen is used, the Pao_2 must be carefully monitored either directly by arterial blood gases or indirectly by noninvasive oxygen monitoring devices (e.g., pulse oximetry).
- Administration of respiratory stimulants (primarily methylxanthines), of which caffeine is most commonly used

226. **Does caffeine therapy affect the incidence of chronic lung disease and other long-term outcomes?**
A large recent multicenter trial showed that treatment of infants who weigh less than 1250 g with caffeine reduced the incidence of chronic lung disease and led to weaning off positive pressure therapy 1 week sooner compared with placebo controls. In addition, the incidence of death or disability at 18 months was reduced in the caffeine compared with the placebo group.

Schmidt B, Roberts RS, Davis P, et al: Caffeine therapy of apnea of prematurity, *N Engl J Med* 354:2112–2121, 2006.

227. **What are the criteria for discontinuing the use of an apnea monitor or methylxanthines?**
Methylxanthines are usually discontinued after an apnea-free period of 4 to 8 weeks. Alternatively, 44 weeks' postconceptional age can be used as a milestone for the maturation of respiratory control in virtually all babies. The apnea monitor is then discontinued 4 to 8 weeks later if there is no recurrence of symptomatic apnea. A home pneumogram or downloading of the data stored in the home "smart monitor" should be recorded before monitor discontinuance.

228. **Do home apnea monitors help prevent sudden infant death syndrome (SIDS)?**
Epidemiologic studies have not been able to demonstrate an impact of home monitoring on the incidence of SIDS. On that basis, the American Academy of Pediatrics recommends that home monitors not be prescribed to prevent SIDS. Indications for monitoring include the following:
- Premature infants with persistent apnea and bradycardia
- Technology-dependent infants
- Infants with neurologic or metabolic disorders that affect respiratory control
- Infants with chronic lung disease, especially those requiring O_2, CPAP, and/or mechanical ventilation

American Academy of Pediatrics: Apnea, SIDS and home monitoring, *Pediatrics* 111:914–917, 2003.

ACKNOWLEDGMENT

The editors gratefully acknowledge contributions by Drs. Mary Catherine Harris, Carlos Vega-Rich, and Peter Marro that were retained from the previous editions of *Pediatric Secrets*.

CHAPTER 13

NEPHROLOGY

Robert L. Seigle, MD, and Martin A. Nash, MD

ACID–BASE, FLUIDS, AND ELECTROLYTES

1. **In what situations can a child be hyponatremic but not hypotonic?**
   - **Increased extracellular osmotically active solutes:** When excessive glucose, mannitol, glycerol, or another osmotically active substances are added to or increased in the extracellular space, the osmotic gradient pulls water from the cells and dilutes the serum sodium concentration.
   - **Elevated plasma lipids and plasma proteins:** A measurement of 100 mL of serum actually contains about 93 mL of water and 7 mL (g) of plasma lipids and proteins. Increases in plasma lipids and protein decrease the amount of water (and sodium) in a fixed volume, so the serum sodium concentration as measured per volume is artifactually decreased.

     This is a classic question on rounds. In actuality, most labs now measure sodium in plasma water with an ion-specific electrode, so the question is more of historical and pedagogic interest.

2. **How is the cause of hyponatremia established?**
   Artifactual causes of hyponatremia should be ruled out. If the urine specific gravity is less than 1.003, causes of water intoxication (e.g., administration of inappropriate intravenous fluids, use of low-solute formulas or plain water in infants, excessive use of tap-water enemas, pathologic drinking behavior in psychiatric patients) should be sought by history. If none of these causes is likely, clinical evaluation on the basis of the patient's volume status and urinary sodium concentration will help categorize the disorder:

   If the patient is **hypovolemic**, evaluate urinary sodium concentration.
   If the urinary sodium concentration is less than 20 mEq/L, consider extrarenal losses:
   - Gastrointestinal problems (vomiting, diarrhea, drainage tubes, fistulas, gastrocystoplasty)
   - Skin problems (cystic fibrosis, heat stroke)
   - Third spacing (burns, pancreatitis, muscle trauma, effusions, ascites, peritonitis)
     If the urinary sodium concentration is more than 20 mEq/L, consider renal losses:
   - Diuretic induced
   - Osmotic diuresis
   - Salt-losing nephritis
   - Bicarbonaturia (renal tubular acidosis, metabolic alkalosis)
   - Mineralocorticoid deficiency
   - Pseudohypoaldosteronism

   If the patient is **euvolemic**, urine sodium concentration is usually more than 20 mEq/L, and the following should be considered:
   - Glucocorticoid or thyroid problem
   - Reset osmostat
   - Excessive antidiuretic hormone

If the patient is **hypervolemic**, evaluate urinary sodium concentration:

If the urinary sodium concentration is less than 20 mEq/L, consider edema-forming states:

■ Nephrosis
■ Congestive heart failure
■ Cirrhosis

If the urinary sodium concentration is more than 20 mEq/L, consider acute or chronic renal failure.

Avner ED: Clinical disorders of water metabolism: hyponatremia and hypernatremia, *Pediatr Ann* 24:23–30, 1995.

3. **Why are some children with congestive heart failure (CHF) hyponatremic while others are not?**

There are two stages to CHF: compensated and uncompensated. In the uncompensated state, there is decreased cardiac output with arterial underfilling. This results in activation of volume receptors in the atria, great vessels (carotid sinus), and other sites, leading to sympathetic nervous system stimulation and activation of the renin-angiotensin-aldosterone system to increase renal sodium reabsorption and to volume-mediated stimulation of antidiuretic hormone (ADH) release. The presence of ADH results in a reduced ability to excrete ingested or infused water, and the water retention produces hyponatremia.

The resulting sodium and water retention improves cardiac performance and the position on the Starling curve, leading to a new steady state in which the above mechanisms are no longer stimulated, and normal water excretion can return serum sodium concentration to normal.

In general, hyponatremia of any cause means ADH is stimulated. The clinical question is "why"? In the case of CHF, it is cardiac decompensation and a non–steady state with arterial underfilling.

4. **Describe the emergency treatment of symptomatic hyponatremia.**

Patients with central nervous system symptoms should receive urgent treatment with **hypertonic saline (3%)**; 1 mL/kg (which is equal to 0.513 mEq of sodium/mL) raises the serum Na by almost 1 mEq/L. Infusions of hypertonic saline at a rate of 3 mL/kg every 10 to 20 minutes are generally safe. Increasing the serum sodium by only 5 to 10 mEq/L is usually sufficient to stop hyponatremic seizures.

5. **How is the cause of hypernatremia established?**

A combination of history, clinical assessment of the patient's volume status, and urinary sodium concentration measurement is helpful for establishing the diagnostic categories.

If the patient is **hypovolemic**, evaluate urinary sodium concentration:

If the urinary sodium concentration is less than 20 mEq/L, consider extrarenal water losses:

■ Diarrhea
■ Excessive perspiration

If the urinary sodium concentration is more than 20 mEq/L, consider renal losses:

■ Renal dysplasia
■ Obstructive uropathy
■ Osmotic diuresis

If the patient is **euvolemic**, urinary sodium concentration is variable, and the following should be considered:

■ Extrarenal losses (insensible: dermal, respiratory)
■ Renal losses (central diabetes insipidus, nephrogenic diabetes insipidus)

If the patient is **hypervolemic**, urinary serum concentration is usually more than 20 mEq/L, and the following should be considered:

■ Improperly mixed formula in tube feeding
■ $NaCHO_3$ administration

- NaCl administration, poisoning
- Primary hyperaldosteronism (rare in children)

Avner ED: Clinical disorders of water metabolism: hyponatremia and hypernatremia, *Pediatr Ann* 24:23–30, 1995.

6. **Why can correcting hypernatremia too rapidly cause seizures?**
   Children with severe hyponatremia usually seize before treatment is started, whereas those with hypernatremia may develop seizures in response to therapy. In patients with hypernatremic dehydration, the increased extracellular tonicity draws fluid from the intracellular compartment, and cells shrink in size, including those in the brain. However, the brain can generate "idiogenic osmoles" to minimize the loss of fluids. These idiogenic osmoles are principally amino acids and other organic solutes that cause the brain to reabsorb some of that water. In fact, in chronic hypernatremia, brain size is back to almost normal. It takes about 24 hours to begin to generate or dissipate these idiogenic osmoles. If the correction of chronic (>24 hours' duration) hypernatremia is too rapid, water flows from the extracellular compartment back into the cerebral intracellular compartment, thereby causing cerebral edema. This can lead to seizures, cerebral hemorrhage, and even death. To prevent this situation, in patients with chronic hypernatremia, the serum Na should not be allowed to fall faster than 0.5 mEq/L per hour and ideally not more than 10 mEq/L in 24 hours.

   Schwaderer AL, Schwartz GJ: Treating hypernatremic dehydration, *Pediatr Rev* 28: 148–150, 2005.

7. **What treatment is available for nephrogenic diabetes insipidus (DI)?**
   Patients with this disease, by definition, do not respond to administration of vasopressin (unlike central DI). Therefore, desmopressin is not an option. The first step is to make certain that water is always available to avoid dehydration. Warn parents that these children can become dehydrated quickly during an episode of gastroenteritis, and medical intervention with intravenous fluid will be needed sooner than in an unaffected child. Decreasing the solute load for urinary excretion by modestly lowering salt and protein intake will decrease urine volume. If the volume of urine and frequency of urination is still intolerable, treatment with hydrochlorothiazide may be necessary. This drug is thought to decrease urine volume by establishing some degree of volume contraction, which stimulates proximal tubular reabsorption of sodium and water and decreases distal delivery and final urine volume. It may as well increase the number of aquaporin-2 channels. Because hydrochlorothiazide often produces hypokalemia, combined therapy with the potassium-sparing diuretic amiloride may be helpful.

8. **How does serum potassium concentration change with alterations in serum pH?**
   In patients with alkalosis, potassium moves into cells as hydrogen moves out of cells in response to the alkalinity. The opposite occurs in conditions of acidosis. For every 0.1 unit rise or fall in pH, there is a change in the opposite direction in the potassium concentration of between 0.4 and 0.6 mEq/L (i.e., lower pH leads to a higher potassium concentration). This is true in individuals and laboratory animals with acidosis as a result of mineral acids (e.g., HCl or NH_4Cl). The effects of organic acids on serum potassium are much less predictable.

9. **What are the clinical and physiologic consequences of progressive hypokalemia?**
   - Muscle weakness and paralysis, which can lead to hypoventilation and apnea
   - Constipation, ileus
   - Increased susceptibility for ventricular ectopic rhythms and fibrillation, especially in children receiving digitalis
   - Interference with the ability of the kidney to concentrate urine, leading to polyuria

10. **What should be the maximal rate and concentration of potassium infusions?**
Ideally, if potassium supplementation or replacement is needed, the concentration of potassium in the intravenous fluids should not exceed 40 mEq/L if given through a peripheral vein, or 80 mEq/L if given through a central vein. Infusion rates should not be more than 0.3 mEq K^+/kg per hour. Faster delivery can lead to local irritation of the veins, paresthesias, and/or weakness, and cardiac arrest because of changes in transmembrane potentials. For life-threatening conditions that result from hypokalemia (e.g., cardiac dysrhythmias, respiratory paralysis in a patient without alkalosis or acidosis), the rate may be increased up to 1 mEq K^+/kg per hour given centrally by an infusion pump. A continuous electrocardiogram monitor should be in place.

> Cronan KM, Norman ME: Renal and electrolyte emergencies. In: Fleisher GR, Ludwig S, editors: *Textbook of Pediatric Emergency Medicine*, ed 4, Baltimore, 2001, Lippincott Williams &Wilkins, pp 819–820.

11. **List the common causes of hypokalemia.**
   - Diuretics, occasionally laxatives
   - Metabolic alkalosis, especially in patients with pyloric stenosis
   - Severe diabetic ketoacidosis with dehydration
   - Diarrhea
   - Renal tubular acidosis, types I and II
   - Fanconi syndrome
   - Bartter syndrome, Gitelman syndrome
   - Hypermineralocorticoid states: Primary hyperaldosteronism, Cushing syndrome, adrenal tumors, rare forms of congenital adrenal hyperplasia, dexamethasone-suppressible hypertension
   - Pituitary tumors producing adrenocorticotropic hormone
   - Hyperreninemic states

12. **Which foods are high in potassium?**
See Table 13-1.

TABLE 13-1. FOODS HIGH IN POTASSIUM		
Food	Portion	Potassium (mg)
Raisins	2/3 cup	751
Baked potato (with skin)	1 medium	503
Cocoa	1 cup	480
Orange juice	8 oz	474
Banana	1 medium	451
French fries	3/5 cup	364
Carrot	1 raw	341

13. **List the causes of hyperkalemia in children.**
Increased intake: This is rarely a primary cause because the ability to dispose of a potassium load is so great. It is only important when renal excretion is compromised (renal failure with oliguria).
   Decreased renal excretion:
   - Acute oliguric renal failure: Acute glomerulonephritis or acute tubular necrosis
   - Oliguric end-stage renal failure
   - Hypoaldosteronism

Transcellular outward movement:

- Metabolic and acute respiratory acidosis
- Insulin deficiency and hyperglycemia in uncontrolled diabetes mellitus
- Increased tissue catabolism: Trauma, chemotherapy, hemolysis, rhabdomyolysis
- Exercise
- Medication related: Digoxin, β-blockers, succinylcholine, arginine
- Familial hyperkalemic periodic paralysis
- Medications: Potassium-sparing diuretics, angiotensin-converting enzyme (ACE) inhibitors
- Distal renal tubular acidosis, type IV
- Renal defect in potassium excretion (familial or obstructive)
  Pseudohyperkalemia (laboratory artifact):
- Thrombocytosis, leukocytosis, hemolysis
- Abnormal leaky red blood cell (RBC) membrane

McDonald RA: Disorders of potassium balance, *Pediatr Ann* 24:31–37, 1995.

14. **When are calcium infusions indicated in a patient with elevated serum potassium?**
    If the patient's **serum potassium level is higher than 8 mEq/L or cardiac dysrhythmia is present**. Calcium is the quickest way to treat an arrhythmia that is associated with hyperkalemia, but it has no effect on serum potassium concentrations. Hyperkalemia leads to an increase in the cell's membrane potential, thereby making cells more arrhythmogenic. Hypercalcemia raises the cell's threshold potential, restores the voltage difference between these two potentials, and decreases the likelihood of an arrhythmia. The effect of calcium infusion is transient, whereas potassium concentrations remain unchanged.

15. **What therapies are used for the emergency treatment of hyperkalemia?**
    - **Movement of potassium into cells** with sodium bicarbonate, 7.5% (1 mEq = 1 mL), 2 to 3 mL/kg, or glucose 50% plus insulin (regular), 1 unit for every 5 to 6 g of glucose, administered over 30 to 60 minutes; onset of action within 30 minutes; duration of action: 1 to 4 hours. Serum glucose should be monitored. Sodium bicarbonate is generally reserved for children who are also acidotic.
    - **Enhanced excretion of potassium** with Kayexalate, 1 g/kg; can be given in 10% glucose (1 g in 4 mL) or 25% sorbitol, every 4 to 6 hours; onset of action within hours; variable duration of action; route of administration: oral or rectal.
    - **Reversal of membrane effects** with 10% calcium gluconate, 0.5 to 1 mL/kg (up to 50 to 100 mg/kg), administered intravenously over 2 to 5 minutes; onset of action within minutes; duration of action: 30 to 60 minutes. The electrocardiogram (ECG) should be monitored, and treatment should be discontinued if the pulse rate rises above 100 beats/minute. This therapy should be reserved for the extreme situation in which immediate action is required to reduce ECG changes.
    - In newborn infants, inhaled albuterol has also been shown to lower serum potassium concentrations.

16. **Which children with acute renal failure are at the greatest risk for hyperkalemia?**
    The two most important determinants of potassium excretion are the rate of urine flow and aldosterone. Acute renal failure can be oliguric or nonoliguric. It is those with *oliguria* who are at the greatest risk for hyperkalemia because of low urine flow.

17. **What is the anion gap in serum?**
    The *anion gap* is the difference between the serum sodium concentration and the sum of chloride plus bicarbonate. It represents those anions that are not normally measured in clinical practice, such as sulfate, various organic anions, negatively charged albumin, and phosphate, which often is measured but is not included in the calculation of anion gap. The normal value is less than 15 mEq/L.

18. **What are the causes of an elevated anion gap acidosis?**
An increased anion gap reflects the addition of an acid with its anion that is not normally measured (i.e., not HCl). In methanol poisoning, it is formic acid with accumulation of formate causing the increased anion gap. In ethylene glycol ingestion (antifreeze), it is oxalate; in lactic acidosis, it is lactate. In diabetic ketoacidosis, it is β-hydroxybutyrate and acetoacetate. In salicylate poisoning, it is lactate and other organic anions.

For those who find mnemonics useful, the mnemonic **MUDPILES** is helpful to remember the causes of an elevated anion gap:
- **M**ethanol
- **U**remia (renal failure)
- **D**iabetic ketoacidosis, diarrhea of infancy
- **P**araldehyde, phenformin
- **I**ron, isoniazid, inborn errors of metabolism
- **L**actic acidosis (seen in clinical situations associated with hypoxia, severe cardiorespiratory depression, shock, and prolonged seizures)
- **E**thanol, ethylene glycol
- **S**alicylates

19. **Why is the determination of the anion gap useful?**
In the presence of metabolic acidosis, the calculation of the anion gap determines which of two diagnostic pathways is more likely. If the anion gap is increased, look for one of the causes in question 18. If it is normal, investigate for diarrhea or renal tubular acidosis.

20. **How limited is the respiratory response to metabolic alkalosis?**
Metabolic alkalosis occurs when a net gain of alkali or loss of acid leads to a rise in the serum bicarbonate concentration and pH. In metabolic alkalosis (as in metabolic acidosis), there is a measure of respiratory compensation in response to the change in pH. This response, which is accomplished by alveolar hypoventilation, is limited by the overriding need to maintain an adequate blood oxygen concentration. Usually the Pco_2 will not rise above 50 to 55 mm Hg, despite severe alkalosis.

21. **What is the differential diagnosis in a child presenting with symptoms of primary metabolic alkalosis?**
Metabolic alkalosis can be divided into two major categories on the basis of the urinary Cl^- concentration and the response to volume expansion with a saline infusion. The *saline-responsive metabolic alkaloses* usually involve a urine Cl^- concentration that is less than 10 mEq/L and significant volume depletion. Treatment with intravenously administered normal saline usually corrects the metabolic alkalosis; the classic example is pyloric stenosis. The *saline-resistant alkaloses* are associated with a high urine Cl^- and often hypertension. The administration of normal saline tends to aggravate rather than correct the metabolic alkalosis. In most cases, mineralocorticoid excess plays the central role in the generation of the acid-base disturbance.

Causes of saline-responsive metabolic alkalosis:
- Pyloric stenosis
- Vomiting
- Excessive upper gastrointestinal suctioning
- Congenital chloride diarrhea
- Laxative abuse
- Diuretic abuse
- Cystic fibrosis
- Chloride-deficient formulas in infants
- Posthypercapnia syndrome
- Poorly reabsorbable anion administration

- Posttreatment of organic acidemias (e.g., treatment of diabetic ketoacidosis with insulin → metabolism of acetoacetate resulting in the generation of bicarbonate)
  Causes of saline-resistant metabolic alkalosis:
- Primary hyperaldosteronism (extremely rare in children)
- Hyperreninemic hypertension
- Renal artery stenosis
- Heritable block in steroid hormone
- 17α-OH deficiency
- 11β-OH deficiency
- Licorice
- Liddle syndrome
- Bartter syndrome or Gitelman syndrome
- Severe potassium deficiency

22. **Why is the urine pH often acidic (pH 5.0 to 5.5) in a child with metabolic alkalosis from severe vomiting?**
    Prolonged vomiting results in metabolic alkalosis because of loss of hydrogen ions as well as volume depletion (dehydration). The volume depletion stimulates the release of aldosterone, resulting in increased distal reabsorption of sodium and increased excretion of hydrogen ions and potassium. The hydrogen ions lower the urine pH. To make matters worse, the resulting hypokalemia stimulates proximal tubular reabsorption of bicarbonate. All conspire to make the alkalosis worse. Only when volume is repleted, resulting in suppression of aldosterone, can the retained bicarbonate be excreted with sodium and the urine pH become alkaline (pH 6.5 or more), correcting the alkalosis.

    This is sometimes referred to as the "paradoxical aciduria of metabolic alkalosis," and your attending may use this term as well. If you are feeling courageous, you could respond that it is not paradoxical at all, once you understand the pathophysiology.

CLINICAL ISSUES

23. **How is enuresis categorized?**
    The terminology can be confusing. In an effort to standardize definitions, the 1998 International Children's Continence Society recommended the following:
    - **Enuresis:** A normal void occurring at a socially unacceptable time or place
    - **Nocturnal enuresis:** Voiding in bed during sleep that is socially unacceptable
    - **Primary nocturnal enuresis:** Monosymptomatic (no other urinary symptoms) bed-wetting in an individual who has never been dry at night for an uninterrupted period of 6 months
    - **Dysfunctional voiding:** Functional disturbances of voiding owing to overactivity of the pelvic floor during micturition (dysfunctional voiding is characterized by variable urinary stream, prolonged voiding, and incomplete bladder emptying, and it may be accompanied by daytime incontinence.)
    - **Diurnal enuresis:** Daytime enuresis characterized by normal voiding but at a socially unacceptable time or place; voiding is complete.

    Norgaard JP, van Gool JD, Hjalmas K, et al: Standardization and definitions in lower urinary tract dysfunction in children. International Children's Continence Society, *Br J Urol* 81(Suppl 3):1–16, 1998.

24. **How common is primary nocturnal enuresis in older children?**
    At the age of 5 years, about 20% of children (boys more than girls) wet the bed at least once monthly. Nightly wetting is not as common (<5%). By the age of 7 years, the overall rate is down to 10%, and by the age of 10 years, it is down to 5%. As a general rule, after age 7 years, nocturnal enuresis resolves at a rate of 15% per year so that by age 15 years, about 1% to 2% of teenagers still have nocturnal enuresis.

KEY POINTS: ENURESIS

1. This is a familial condition; 70% of enuretic children have a parent who has had the condition.

2. Nocturnal enuresis prevalence rates show a natural history of spontaneous resolution: 20% at 5 years, 10% at 7 years, and 5% at 10 years, with only a 1% to 2% persistence rate.

3. Isolated primary nocturnal enuresis rarely has identifiable organic pathology.

4. There is a high relapse rate when medications are stopped.

5. Enuresis alarms are the most therapeutically effective (especially in younger patients) and cost effective, but they require weeks of consistent use for full benefits.

25. **Why does nighttime bed-wetting persist in some children?**
Ninety-seven percent or more of the causes are nonpathologic, and a number of explanations have been theorized: maturational delay of neurodevelopmental processes, small bladder capacity, genetic influences, difficulties with waking, and decreased nighttime secretion of ADH. No data support the belief that wetting occurs during "deep sleep." Genetic influences are quite strong. If both parents were enuretic, a child's likelihood is about 75%; if one parent was involved, the likelihood is about 50%. Psychological problems are an unlikely cause of nocturnal enuresis, but they are more common if daytime symptoms are present.

Graham KM, Levy JB: Enuresis, *Pediatr Rev* 30:165–172, 2009.

26. **In what settings should a medical or surgical cause of enuresis be considered?**
Medical conditions include urinary tract infection (UTI), diabetes mellitus, diabetes insipidus, fecal impaction, and constipation. Suspicious symptoms include intermittent daytime wetness, polydipsia, polyuria, history of central nervous system trauma, and encopresis. *Surgical conditions* include ectopic ureter, neurogenic bladder, bladder calculus, and foreign body. These should be suspected if there is constant dampness, a dribbling urinary stream with abnormalities in gait, or obstructive sleep apnea. A thorough history and physical examination, along with urinalysis and urine culture (if indicated), is usually sufficient to eliminate the likelihood of any of these etiologies.

27. **What treatments are available for nocturnal enuresis?**
The therapeutic approach depends in large part on the age of the patient, the effect of the problem on the patient, and the parents' attitude. It is important to realize that 15% of patients per year will spontaneously improve.
- **Dry bed training:** Self-awakening routines, cleanliness training, bladder training, and rewards for dry nights; generally not effective as a sole intervention
- **Enuresis alarms:** Portable alarms (audio or vibratory) worn by the child at night and designed to awaken the child to the sensation of a full bladder; success rates as high as 70%; safe, but requires parental and child motivation
- **Desmopressin:** Synthetic analog of vasopressin that, at a renal level, increases distal tubular reabsorption of water, thus diminishing nighttime bladder volume; available in oral and nasal forms; up to 70% effective; high relapse rate after discontinuation (similar to placebo); possible adverse effects, including nasal irritation and hyponatremia; expensive
- **Imipramine:** Bladder effects include increasing capacity and decreasing detrusor excitability; high relapse rate; important central nervous system side effects in 10% (e.g., drowsiness, agitation, sleep disturbances)

■ **Oxybutynin:** Provides an anticholinergic, antispasmodic effect that reduces uninhibited detrusor muscle contractions; useful in patients with documented detrusor instability; 17% or less experience adverse reactions (e.g., dry mouth, flushing, drowsiness, constipation)

Neveus T: Diagnosis and management of nocturnal enuresis, *Curr Opin Pediatr* 199–202, 2009.

Silverstein DM: Enuresis in children: diagnosis and management, *Clin Pediatr* 43:317–221, 2004.

Nield LS, Kamat D: Enuresis: how to evaluate and treat, *Clin Pediatr* 43:409–415, 2004.

28. What are the causes of diurnal enuresis?

Organic causes account for less than 5% of cases. Of these, UTIs are probably the most common. An ectopic ureter should be suspected if dampness is constantly present; most children with diurnal enuresis have intermittent wetness. Rarely, a neurogenic bladder can cause this problem. Severe lower urinary tract obstruction can lead to bladder distention with overflow incontinence. Finally, pelvic masses (e.g., presacral teratoma, hydrocolpos, fecal impaction) that press on the bladder can lead to stress incontinence with running, coughing, or lifting.

Physiologic types of daytime wetting include the vaginal reflux of urine, giggle incontinence, and urgency incontinence. Reflux of urine into the vagina during micturition occurs frequently; after normal voiding, when the girl stands up and walks, the urine seeps out of the vagina and wets the underpants. Giggle incontinence is a sudden, involuntary, uncontrollable, and complete emptying of the bladder when giggling or laughing. Tickling or excitement may also lead to this problem. Urgency incontinence can be defined as an attack of intense bladder spasms that leads to abrupt voiding and wetting.

Psychogenic causes may be related to stress. Wetting can occur in any child who is significantly frightened. Chronic stress (e.g., the loss of a close relative, parental marital discord, hospitalization) can also lead to this kind of daytime wetting. The resistant child is one who is about 2½ years old and who refuses to be toilet trained. Seventy percent are males who are predominantly or totally wet. Often, this situation has occurred because of high-pressured attempts at toilet training. Most children with daytime wetness and nighttime dryness have a behavioral basis for the problem.

29. What is the most common genetic kidney disease?

Autosomal dominant polycystic kidney disease (ADPKD). The incidence is thought to be 1 in 800 to 1000. Each child of an affected parent has a 50% chance of acquiring the disease. Five percent of new cases arise due to spontaneous mutation. However, about one fourth of parents note no family history, indicating that a significant number of cases go undetected. ADPKD is characterized by fluid-filled cysts in the kidneys. Presentation may involve hypertension, gross hematuria after trauma, nephrolithiasis, pyogenic infection, or pain. ADPKD is a major cause of end-stage renal disease in children and adults.

Grantham JJ: Autosomal dominant polycystic kidney disease, *N Engl J Med* 359:1477–1485, 2008.

Polycystic Kidney Foundation: http://www.PKDcure.org.

PKD Alliance: http://www.arpkdchf.org.

30. How do you treat labial adhesions?

Labial adhesions are a relatively common gynecologic finding in girls between 4 months and 6 years of age. They may be complete or partial and are thought to result from local inflammation in a low-estrogen setting with resulting skin agglutination. Treatment consists of eliminating the underlying inflammation (if it is caused by an infection), sitz baths twice daily, maintenance of good perineal hygiene, and topical application of a 1% conjugated estrogen cream over the entire adhesion at bedtime for 3 weeks. The use of estrogen has an 80% to 90% cure rate and may be followed by the application of a petroleum jelly for 1 to 2 months nightly. It should be noted that the natural history of untreated asymptomatic labial adhesions is self-resolution: 50% resolve within 6 months, and nearly 100% resolve by 18 months. Surgical correction is almost never required.

Leung AKC, Robson WLM, Kao CP, et al: Treatment of labial fusion with topical estrogen therapy, *Clin Pediatr* 44:245–247, 2005.

GLOMERULONEPHRITIS

31. **During the evaluation of a patient with hematuria, what features suggest acute glomerulonephritis, chronic glomerulonephritis or nephritic syndrome?**
    Three presentations of glomerular involvement can occur:
    - **Acute glomerulonephritis:** Edema, proteinuria of 1^+ or greater, hypertension, oliguria, dysmorphic RBCs (small, misshapen RBC with blebs), or RBC casts on urinalysis
    - **Chronic glomerulonephritis:** Minimal acute symptoms; may have chronic fatigue, failure to thrive, or unexplained anemia with features of chronic renal failure, hypertension, abnormal urinalysis, and azotemia
    - **Nephrotic syndrome:** Proteinuria of greater than 40 mg/m^2 per hour, edema, hypoproteinemia, and hyperlipidemia

32. **If glomerulonephritis is suspected, what laboratory tests should be considered?**
    - Urinalysis
    - Blood urea nitrogen (BUN) and creatinine
    - Serum C3 and C4
    - Streptococcal serology
    - Throat culture; skin culture if lesions present
    - Serum albumin
    - Antinuclear antibody (ANA), anti-DNA antibodies (if systemic lupus erythematosus is suspected)
    - Hepatitis B and C serology (for patients living in endemic areas, those who have received transfusions, or those who engage in high-risk behavior)
    - Antineutrophil cytoplasmic antibody (ANCA) (if rapidly progressive glomerulonephritis or vasculitis is suspected)

33. **Which glomerulonephritides are associated with hypocomplementemia?**
    - **Postinfectious,** including poststreptococcal and other infectious antigens, such as subacute bacterial endocarditis. Formerly, shunt nephritis was a cause when the distal end of the shunt was placed in the atrium. This does not occur with ventriculoperitoneal shunt.
    - **Systemic lupus erythematosus**
    - **Membranoproliferative glomerulonephritis**

34. **Does the treatment of streptococcal skin or pharyngeal infections prevent poststreptococcal glomerulonephritis?**
    No study has ever demonstrated that the treatment of impetigo or pharyngitis prevents the glomerulonephritis in the index case. However, treatment lessens the likelihood of contagious spread to children who may be susceptible. Serum antistreptolysin (ASO) titers, which are elevated in patients with pharyngeal infections, are usually not elevated after skin infections. Therefore, to confirm the diagnosis of an antecedent skin infection, antihyaluronidase and anti-DNase B titers should be obtained.

35. **What is the usual time course for poststreptococcal glomerulonephritis?**
    About 7 to 14 days after a pharyngitis and as long as 6 weeks after a pyoderma with group A β-hemolytic streptococci, children typically have tea-colored urine and edema. The acute phase (e.g., hypertension, gross hematuria) can last as long as 3 weeks. Serum complement

levels may remain depressed for up to 8 weeks, but persistence beyond this point suggests another diagnosis. Chronic microscopic hematuria can persist for up to 2 years. In pediatric patients, full recovery is expected, and progression to chronic renal insufficiency is extremely rare.

36. **What percentage of children with poststreptococcal glomerulonephritis have elevated levels of serum ASO titers?**
About 80% to 85% of children with documented pharyngeal streptococcal infections develop elevated ASO titers. Streptolysin O is bound to lipids in the skin so that the percentage of individuals with streptococcal impetigo who develop positive ASO titers is much lower. For this reason, a normal ASO titer does not rule out recent ASO infection. Screening for other streptococcus-associated antigens, antihyaluronidase, and anti-DNAase B titers or the use of the Streptozyme test, which measures a variety of streptococcal antigens, will be positive in more than 95% of children with documented streptococcal infection.

37. **If pharyngitis and the brown urine occur on the same day or within 1 or 2 days, does this make poststreptococcal glomerulonephritis less likely?**
Yes. The occurrence of upper respiratory symptoms and gross hematuria at the same time would be more characteristic of Berger (or immunoglobulin A [IgA]) nephropathy.
As opposed to poststreptococcal glomerulonephritis, serum complement is normal in IgA nephropathy during the acute episode. These children tend to have recurrent episodes of gross hematuria associated with upper respiratory illnesses. On renal biopsy, there is the predominant deposition of IgA in the glomerular mesangium. Initially thought to be an example of "benign" hematuria, it is now apparent that 20% to 25% of patients will progress to end-stage renal disease over 25 years. There is no treatment that has been definitively shown to be beneficial in decreasing progression. Patients who excrete large amounts of protein have an increased risk for progression, and measures to decrease proteinuria (ACE inhibitors and angiotensin receptor blockers) are likely to be beneficial in this high-risk group.

HEMATURIA

38. **How common is hematuria in children?**
Microscopic hematuria (>5 RBCs/high-power field [HPF]) is common (0.5% to 2% of school-aged children) and often transient. In 70% to 80% of cases, no etiology is identified.

39. **What is the most identifiable cause of microscopic hematuria?**
Hypercalciuria, defined as elevated urinary calcium excretion without concomitant hypercalcemia. The likelihood changes depending on where you live. In areas of the southeastern United States—often called "the stone belt"—this is a common cause of isolated hematuria, with nearly one third of children with microscopic hematuria having hypercalciuria as the cause. In other parts of the United States, it is much less common. Overall, 3% to 6% of children will have idiopathic hypercalciuria.

Srivastava T, Schwaderer A: Diagnosis and management of hypercalciuria in children, *Curr Opin Pediatr* 21:214–219, 2009.

Bergstein J, Leiser J, Andreoli S: The clinical significance of asymptomatic gross and microscopic hematuria in children, *Arch Pediatr Adolesc Med* 159:353–355, 2005.

40. **What distinguishes lower from upper tract bleeding?**
As a general rule, brown, tea-colored, or cola-colored urine suggests *upper tract bleeding*, whereas bright red blood suggests *lower tract bleeding*. The darker urine has had more time to become oxidized within the urinary tract. However, exceptions occur. Rapid upper tract

bleeding may be red, and a dissolving clot within the bladder may produce brown urine. Establishing the source of microscopic hematuria can be difficult. *Glomerular bleeding* is said to produce RBCs that are small and dysmorphic with blebs or burr cells as opposed to the normal-sized RBCs seen in lower tract bleeding. Unfortunately, this change is best observed with phase-contrast microscopy, which is not readily available in most clinical settings. The presence of significant proteinuria also suggests upper tract (i.e., kidney) disease. The presence of even a single RBC or hemoglobin cast indicates a glomerular (or, rarely, tubular) etiology.

41. **If a healthy 10-year-old boy has bright red blood at the end of a previously clear urine stream, what is the likely diagnosis?**
In a preadolescent or early adolescent male, the occurrence of terminal hematuria often reflects engorged vessels around the entry of the prostatic duct into the urethra at the veru montanum. Although the etiology is unclear, it is a benign condition associated with hormonal changes at adolescence. It resolves spontaneously in weeks to months and does not require cystoscopy or other investigations.

42. **What is the "pink diaper" syndrome?**
This is a benign condition that is often misinterpreted as hematuria. A red-brown spot is noted in the diaper, which is caused by urate crystals.

43. **What evaluations should be considered during the evaluation of isolated hematuria?**
    - BUN and creatinine
    - Electrolytes
    - Urine calcium-to-creatinine ratio
    - Serologic evidence of recent streptococcal infection (unless hematuria has been present for several months)
    - Renal ultrasound: Evaluation for structural abnormalities (e.g., hydronephrosis, autosomal dominant or recessive polycystic kidney disease)
    - Hemoglobin electrophoresis: If sickle cell trait or disease is suspected
    - C3, C4. ANA is unnecessary in the asymptomatic child. It is sometimes positive in low titer, unrelated to the hematuria, but then requires further studies, creates much parental anxiety ("Oh, no, not lupus!"), and ends up being of no significance.
    - Urine culture: Unnecessary for recurrent gross hematuria or in an asymptomatic child with a 6-month history because there is a low likelihood of positivity

KEY POINTS: HEMATURIA

1. This is a very common condition; asymptomatic, microscopic hematuria is found in 0.5% to 2% of schoolchildren.

2. In most patients, the condition is benign, and evaluation yields no renal or urologic disease.

3. Hypercalciuria (>4 mg/kg per day) is found in some of these patients.

4. Patients with significant proteinuria along with hematuria are much more likely to have underlying pathology.

5. If the dipstick assessment is positive for blood but microscopic urinalysis is negative for RBCs, suspect hemolysis (positivity as a result of hemoglobin) or rhabdomyolysis (muscle breakdown with positivity as a result of myoglobin).

HYPERTENSION

44. How is hypertension defined in children?
The diagnosis of hypertension is made on the basis of comparison with the normative distribution blood pressure of healthy children of similar age, gender, and height. (This information is available in the 2004 article cited below as well as a more recent simplified approach.)

- **Hypertension:** Average systolic and or diastolic blood pressure is 95th percentile or higher on three or more occasions
- **Prehypertension:** 90th percentile or higher, but less than 95th percentile; as with adults, adolescents with blood pressure of 120/80 mm Hg or higher should be considered prehypertensive

Kaelber DC, Pickett F: Simple table to identify children and adolescents needing further evaluation of blood pressure, *Pediatrics* 123:e972–e974, 2009.

National High Blood Pressure Education Program Working Group on High Blood Pressure in Children and Adolescents: The fourth report on the diagnosis, evaluation, and treatment of high blood pressure in children and adolescents, *Pediatrics* 114:555–576, 2004.

KEY POINTS: HYPERTENSION

1. Common cause of artifactual elevation: Blood pressure cuff is too small

2. Essential (no detectable cause): Often a strong family history

3. Secondary (detectable lesion) hypertension: More likely with higher blood pressures and in younger children

4. Most cases of secondary hypertension in children caused by renal disease (renal anomalies, renal parenchymal disease, renal vascular abnormalities)

45. How do you determine the optimum cuff size for obtaining a blood pressure?
The length of the inflatable bladder inside the cuff (easily palpated) should almost completely encircle the arm and will overestimate the blood pressure if it is too short. Additionally, the height of the cuff should be the largest that comfortably fits from the axilla to the elbow. A cuff that is too small can produce falsely elevated blood pressure readings.

46. Which Korotkoff sound best represents diastolic blood pressure?
The Korotkoff sounds are produced by the flow of blood as the constricting blood pressure cuff is gradually released. There are five phases of Korotkoff sounds. The first appearance of a clear, tapping sound is called phase I and represents the systolic pressure. As the cuff continues to be released, soft murmurs can be auscultated; this is phase II. These are followed by louder murmurs during phase III, as the volume of blood passing through the constricted artery increases. The sounds become abruptly muffled in phase IV and disappear in phase V, which is usually within 10 mm Hg of phase IV.

In studies that compare intravascular blood pressure determinations with auscultatory readings, true diastolic pressure is most closely related to phase V (the disappearance of sound). However, in many young children, muffled sounds can be heard to zero and thus clearly do not always correlate with diastolic pressure. In these instances, it is best to record both the phase IV (the point at which sounds become muffled) and the phase V readings (e.g., 80/45/0).

47. **What is ambulatory blood pressure monitoring (ABPM) and is it useful in children?**

ABPM can mean either home monitoring of blood pressure, usually with an inflatable cuff and digital readout, or an automated process with continuous monitoring of blood pressure using an oscillometric method that obtains readings every 20 minutes during the day and less frequently at night. The digital device is useful, especially for monitoring the effects of therapy, but it is subject to selective filtering of results by the observer and gives a reading at only one point in time. The automated device is very useful in older children and especially adolescents, in whom blood pressure readings may be high only in an office setting ("white-coat hypertension") or in whom random determinations are only intermittently elevated. This device, which requires software for computerized analysis, can provide a great deal of information. It shows a complete record of blood pressure and pulse over a 24-hour period, the percentage of readings that are above the 95th percentile for age and body size, and whether or not there is a normal "dip" in pressure during sleep. The absence of such a dip is associated with true hypertension and the risk for end-organ damage. Although its use is currently somewhat cumbersome, it is likely that the automated device will find more frequent use in the future.

Swartz SJ, Srivaths PR, Croix B, Feig DI: Cost-effectiveness of ambulatory blood pressure monitoring in the initial evaluation of hypertension in children, *Pediatrics* 122:1177–1181, 2008.

KEY POINTS: CONSISTENT AND STRUCTURED WAYS TO AVOID MISDIAGNOSING HYPERTENSION

1. Properly sized cuff (age-dependent) with arm supported and raised to heart level

2. Quiet room, quiet patient

3. Repeated measurements over time and the use of averaged values

4. Get rid of the white coat

5. Sit at child level when taking the measurement

48. **When should hypertension be treated in the neonate?**

Hypertension is defined as a blood pressure higher than 90/60 mm Hg in term neonates and higher than 80/45 mm Hg in preterm infants. A sustained systolic blood pressure of more than 100 mm Hg in the neonate should be investigated and treated.

49. **What are the indications for the pharmacologic treatment of hypertension in older children?**

- Symptomatic hypertension
- Secondary hypertension
- Hypertensive target-organ damage (e.g., left ventricular hypertrophy on echocardiogram)
- Diabetes (types 1 and 2)
- Persistence despite nonpharmacologic measures

National High Blood Pressure Education Program Working Group on High Blood Pressure in Children and Adolescents: The fourth report on the diagnosis, evaluation, and treatment of high blood pressure in children and adolescents, *Pediatrics* 114:555–576, 2004.

50. **During the evaluation of a child with elevated blood pressure, what risk factors should be considered for identification and/or reduction?**

Important risk factors for hypertension in children include **family history** (if one parent has hypertension, the risk is about 25%; if both parents have hypertension, the risk is 45%), other genetic factors including **race** (blacks have twice the incidence of hypertension compared with whites, beginning in adolescence), **obesity**, history of **renal disease**, and **dietary factors** (mainly salt intake). More recently, a history of **prematurity** has been recognized as a risk factor.

Remembering that hypertension is a critical risk factor for cardiovascular disease, the important risk factors for this largest cause of mortality should also be addressed. These include diet and its effect on serum lipids, tobacco use, and lack of exercise.

51. **What are the most common causes of hypertension in various age groups?**
    See Table 13-2.

TABLE 13-2. INITIAL WORKUP FOR PEDIATRIC HYPERTENSION (IN ORDER OF PREVALENCE)	
Age Range	
First year of life	Secondary (99%) ■ Coarctation of the aorta ■ Renovascular* ■ Renal parenchymal disease ■ Miscellaneous causes[†] ■ Neoplasia (4%) ■ Endocrine (1%)
1-12 yr	Secondary (70%-85%) ■ Renal parenchymal disease ■ Coarctation of the aorta ■ Reflux nephropathy ■ Renovascular ■ Endocrine ■ Neoplasia ■ Miscellaneous Primary (essential) (15%-30%)
12-18 yr	Primary (essential) (85%-95%) Secondary (5%-15%): Same causes as 1-12 yr

*Renal artery/vein thrombosis, renal artery stenosis.
[†]Bronchopulmonary dysplasia (BPD), patent ductus arteriosus (PDA), intraventricular hemorrhage (IVH).
Data from Brady T, Siberry GK, Solomon B: Pediatric hypertension. Contemp Pediatr 25:49, 2008.

52. **What historical information suggests a secondary cause of hypertension?**
    See Table 13-3.

TABLE 13-3. SECONDARY CAUSES OF HYPERTENSION AS SUGGESTED BY HISTORY

History	Suggests
Known urinary tract infection; recurrent abdominal or flank pain with frequency, urgency, dysuria; secondary enuresis	Renal disease
Joint pains, rash, fever, edema	Renal disease, vasculitis
Complicated neonatal course, umbilical artery catheter	Renal artery stenosis
Renal trauma	Renal artery stenosis
Drug use (e.g., sympathomimetics, anabolic steroids, oral contraceptives, illicit drugs)	Drug-induced hypertension
Aberrant course or timing of secondary sexual characteristics; virilization	Adrenal disorder

53. **List the features on physical examination that suggest a secondary cause of hypertension.**
See Table 13-4.

TABLE 13-4. PHYSICAL FINDINGS THAT SUGGEST A POSSIBLE SECONDARY CAUSE OF HYPERTENSION

Physical Finding	Possible Secondary Cause
Blood Pressure	
>140/100 mm Hg at any age	Multiple secondary causes
Leg < arm blood pressure	Coarctation of the aorta
Adenotonsillar hypertrophy	Obstructive sleep apnea
Muscle weakness	Hyperaldosteronism
Joint swelling	Systemic lupus erythematosus, collagen vascular disease
Poor growth	Chronic renal disease
Short stature, features of Turner syndrome	Coarctation of the aorta
Multiple café-au-lait spots or neurofibromas	Renal artery stenosis, pheochromocytoma
Decreased or delayed pulse in leg	Coarctation of the aorta
Vascular Bruits	
Over large vessels	Arteritis
Over upper abdomen, flank	Renal artery stenosis
Flank or upper quadrant mass	Renal malformation, renal or adrenal tumor
Excessive virilization or secondary sex characteristics inappropriate for age	Adrenal disorder
Edema	Renal disease
Excessive sweating, increased resting heart rate	Pheochromocytoma

54. **What are the categories of antihypertensive medications used for outpatient management of hypertensive children?**
   - ACE inhibitors
   - Angiotensin receptor blockers (ARBs)
   - Calcium channel blockers
   - α-Blockers and β-blockers
   - Central α-agonists
   - Vasodilators
   - Diuretics

   Feld LG, Corey H: Hypertension in childhood, *Pediatr Rev*, 28:283–297, 2007.

55. **Why should patients with hypertension and/or those using diuretics avoid licorice?**
   True licorice contains glycyrrhizic acid, which has mineralocorticoid (i.e., sodium-retaining) properties. However, most American licorice contains only licorice flavoring and thus has no mineralocorticoid properties. Some chewing tobacco also contains licorice and has been associated with an excessive mineralocorticoid syndrome. Think of this if you are called to evaluate an edematous New York Yankees batboy.

PROTEINURIA AND NEPHROTIC SYNDROME

56. **How do the bedside methods for testing protein in random urine samples compare?**
   - **Dipstick assessment:** This relies on the reaction of protein (primarily albumin) with tetrabromophenol blue in a citrate buffer impregnated on the dipstick patch. Mild false-positive reactions can occur (1+ to 2+) when the patient's urine is alkaline or when the dipstick is allowed to sit in the urine for too long and the buffer strength is overcome. The results are reported qualitatively as 1+ to 3+, which corresponds to a range of 30 to 500 mg/dL.
   - **Sulfosalicylic acid:** This test precipitates protein in the urine and allows for a comparison with a group of previously prepared aqueous standards; it is reported in the same way as those standards. In contrast with the dipstick assessment, all proteins—not just albumin—are precipitated, as are iodinated contrast material and some antibodies. The finding of heavy proteinuria by sulfosalicylic acid testing with minimal proteinuria using the dipstick suggests the presence of large amounts of nonalbumin protein, most often as the result of multiple myeloma and the excretion of Bence Jones proteins. Look for this during a geriatrics—not a pediatrics—rotation.

57. **On a routine urinalysis, an asymptomatic 7-year-old boy has 1+ protein noted on dipstick assessment. How should this child be evaluated?**
   Assuming that the child is otherwise healthy and without any of the subtle signs of renal disease (e.g., short stature, pallor, hypertension), and assuming that this is isolated proteinuria, it is important to determine whether the proteinuria is intermittent or persistent. Intermittent (transient) proteinuria is entirely benign and does not require any workup. Persistent proteinuria may or may not be benign. The presence of persistent proteinuria can be determined by rechecking the urine at least three times over 2 to 3 weeks. If one of these tests is performed on a first-morning urine specimen (assuming the child voided before going to bed the night before), the patient can be evaluated for orthostatic proteinuria at the same time. Causes of transient proteinuria include fever, vigorous exercise, dehydration, stress, cold exposure, and seizures.

58. **Other than a timed urine collection, what is the best "spot" method for determining the degree of proteinuria?**

   Urinary protein-to-creatinine excretion ratio. Particularly in children, a 24-hour urine collection for protein is very difficult to obtain. Although both the dipstick and the sulfosalicylic testing methods estimate the concentration of protein in the urine, small amounts of protein in very concentrated urine will show up as more positive than the same amount of protein present in dilute urine. A number of studies have demonstrated that the urinary protein-to-creatinine ratio more closely approximates total 24-hour urinary protein excretion. Thus, on a random sample, a urine protein-to-creatinine ratio of less than 0.2 to 0.25 reflects a normal daily protein excretion, whereas values of more than 2 strongly suggest the presence of the nephrotic syndrome. This test has proved very effective both for the diagnosis of the nephrotic syndrome and for follow-up evaluations in children with prolonged and difficult-to-manage proteinuria. However, the test may overestimate protein excretion in individuals with abnormally low muscle mass (and hence lower creatinine excretion rates).

59. **How is the diagnosis of orthostatic proteinuria established?**

   By definition, individuals with orthostatic proteinuria have normal rates of protein excretion when lying recumbent but increased excretion rates when upright. Although all individuals excrete more protein when standing, some have an exaggerated response and may excrete as much as 1 g of urinary protein per day. Assuming the child emptied the bladder before going to bed, protein excretion when recumbent can be assessed semiquantitatively with a first-morning urine specimen immediately on arising using either a urine dipstick or a sulfosalicylic acid precipitation of the urine. More accurate assessment can be obtained using the urine protein-to-creatinine excretion ratio or as milligrams excreted per hour. In a reasonably concentrated first-morning urine specimen (urine specific gravity ≥ 1.018), a trace or negative value by dipstick assessment or sulfosalicylic acid precipitation is adequate to rule out proteinuria. At any urine specific gravity, a urine protein-to-creatinine ratio (mg/dL to mg/dL) of less than 0.25 is also considered normal. Remember, even individuals with renal disease may have increased protein excretion when standing and lower protein excretion rates when recumbent. The key to orthostatic proteinuria is that protein excretion is truly normal when recumbent and the individual is otherwise entirely healthy.

60. **What additional evaluation should be done for a patient with persistent proteinuria?**

   If the child's proteinuria is persistent and not orthostatic, protein excretion needs to be determined. Although the gold standard is the timed (24-hour) urine collection, this is often difficult to obtain in children. Because substantial amounts of urine are often lost, a 24-hour urinary creatinine excretion should be determined at the same time to assess for completeness. A standard definition of proteinuria was developed by the International Study for Kidney Disease in Children. Those researchers defined proteinuria as the excretion of more than 4 mg/m^2 of protein per hour (or 100 mg every 24 hours for a 30-kg child). More commonly, the urine protein-to-creatinine ratio is used.

   The evaluation of a child with persistent proteinuria includes many of the same tests required to evaluate glomerulonephritis, such as BUN and creatinine, electrolytes, and serum albumin, and often tests to document evidence of immunologic activation, such as C3, C4, ANA, and anti-DNA antibodies. Rarely, ANCA may be required. Finally, renal imaging studies and renal biopsy may be necessary for diagnosis.

61. **What is the natural history of orthostatic proteinuria?**

   Few prospective data exist about the long-term outcome of children and adolescents, but follow-up data for young adults for up to 50 years after diagnosis demonstrate a benign clinical course. Most agree that the prognosis is excellent, although the etiology remains unclear.

62. **What level constitutes "significant" proteinuria?**

Protein excretion of more than 4 mg/m^2 per hour on a timed urine collection is considered abnormal. Children with nephrosis excrete more than 40 mg/m^2 per hour. The upper limit of protein excretion in adults is 150 mg/day, but, for some reason, adolescents may excrete as much as 250 mg/day. A urine protein/urine creatinine ratio of >0.5 in children <2 years old and of >0.2 in older children is considered excessive.

63. **In a child with hematuria, can proteinuria be attributed simply to the protein that is contained in whole blood?**

Only in a child with grossly bloody urine. If the urine is normal in color (yellow or clear), any proteinuria above trace is abnormal.

64. **What disease should be considered if the quantification of total urinary protein is greatly in excess of the dipstick test for albumin?**

Dent disease is characterized by tubular proteinuria (so-called because it is due to defective reabsorption by the proximal tubule of filtered proteins), often associated with hypercalciuria, which may result in calcium stones, and slow but progressive chronic renal failure. The proteinuria is due to a defective chloride channel (CLCN5) in proximal tubular endosomes containing reabsorbed protein. The tubular proteinuria can be documented by measuring the excretion of β_2-microglobulin and retinal binding protein in urine.

65. **What constellation of clinical findings defines nephrotic syndrome?**

The nephrotic syndrome consists of **proteinuria, hypoalbuminemia, edema**, and **hyperlipidemia**. Of these, the proteinuria is primary, with the development of hypoalbuminemia, edema, and hyperlipidemia as secondary findings. It is not at all uncommon to find individuals with clear evidence of nephrotic-range proteinuria and mild to moderate hypoalbuminemia in whom evidence of hypolipidemia and peripheral edema are minimal.

66. **What distinguishes nephrosis from nephritis?**

The suffix "-itis" implies evidence of inflammation, which is seen on renal biopsy as the proliferation of the cellular elements within the glomerulus and often the presence of white blood cells. Clinically, these abnormalities produce a disruption of glomerular basement membrane structure and function that leads to hematuria and proteinuria. The proteinuria may be minimal to massive, depending on the type and severity of the **nephritis.** The finding of RBC casts in the urine is, with rare exceptions, diagnostic of glomerulonephritis.

Nephrosis is another term for the nephrotic syndrome. "Syndrome" implies a characteristic group of findings that may have diverse causes. As noted in the answer to the previous question, the nephrotic syndrome is caused by the renal loss of protein and the development of hypoalbuminemia, edema, and hyperlipidemia. This can be caused by a number of renal conditions, some of which demonstrate proliferative and inflammatory changes and some that do not demonstrate any evidence of nephritis (e.g., minimal change nephrotic syndrome). Thus, some but not all patients with (glomerulo)nephritis may have nephrosis, and some patients with the clinical syndrome called nephrosis may have evidence of nephritis on urinalysis (e.g., RBC casts) (Fig. 13-1) or on biopsy.

67. **Which childhood diseases appear primarily as glomerulonephritis or the nephrotic syndrome?**

Most of the conditions in Table 13-5 present symptoms of either a nephritic or a nephrotic picture; occasionally, a mixed picture will be noted.

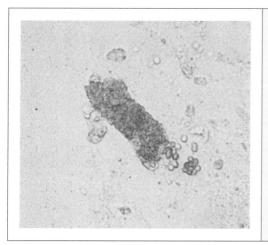

Figure 13-1. Red blood cell cast from a patient with streptococcal glomerulonephritis. These casts are almost always associated with glomerulonephritis or vasculitis and virtually exclude extrarenal disease. (From Zitelli BJ, Davis HW: Atlas of Pediatric Physical Diagnosis, 4th ed. St. Louis, Mosby, 2002, p 458.)

TABLE 13-5. CHILDHOOD DISEASES PRESENTING WITH SYMPTOMS OF GLOMERULONEPHRITIS OR NEPHROTIC SYNDROME

Glomerulonephritis	Nephrotic Syndrome
Postinfectious (both streptococcal as well as other bacteria, viruses, and parasites)	Minimal change nephrosis
Henoch-Schönlein nephritis	Focal segmental glomerulosclerosis
Immunoglobulin A nephropathy	Membranoproliferative
Membranoproliferative glomerulonephritis	Membranous nephropathy
Familial nephritis	Congenital nephrotic syndrome
Systemic lupus erythematosus	Systemic lupus erythematosus
Immune complex nephritis (infective endocarditis or "shunt nephritis")	Henoch-Schönlein nephritis
Rapidly progressive glomerulonephritis (Wegener granulomatosis or polyarteritis nodosa)	Immunoglobulin A nephropathy
Familial nephritis	

68. **At what level of albumin do children usually start to develop edema?**
When the serum albumin falls below 2.5 g/dL, edema usually begins to develop. When it falls below 1.8 g/dL, edema is almost always present, unless the child is receiving a diuretic.

69. **Why doesn't eating more protein restore the serum albumin concentration to normal in individuals with the nephrotic syndrome?**
The loss of urinary albumin is only part of the story. Under normal circumstances, very small amounts of albumin are filtered at the glomerulus. A very high percentage of what is filtered is then catabolized by the proximal tubular cells. Amino acids are reabsorbed from the tubular lumen back into the body and resynthesized into albumin within the liver. In patients with the nephrotic syndrome, significantly more albumin is filtered. Even with increased

catabolism and amino acid reabsorption at the renal tubular level, the rate of liver albumin synthesis is limited, and serum albumin levels fall. Feeding more protein would lead to increased protein absorption through the gastrointestinal tract, but the rate-limiting feature of insufficient liver synthesis cannot be overcome.

70. **What is the most common form of nephrotic syndrome seen in childhood?**
Minimal-change nephrotic syndrome (MCNS). Earlier names for this condition included *lipoid nephrosis* and *nil disease*. MCNS is a form of primary nephrotic syndrome and has a more favorable therapeutic response and prognosis. The etiology of MCNS is unknown, but it appears to be a condition of abnormal T-lymphocyte function. Other forms of primary nephrotic syndrome include conditions such as focal segmental glomerulosclerosis, membranous nephropathy, and membranoproliferative glomerulonephritis. Secondary forms of nephrotic syndrome may also occur as a consequence of infection, as a response to some medications, and as an autoimmune phenomenon.

71. **What is the most important historical factor to consider when assessing a patient for possible MCNS?**
Although the only definitive way to document the presence of MCNS is with a renal biopsy, most patients with MCNS show a constellation of signs and a response to treatment that are characteristic. The most important characteristic for a child with this condition is age on presentation. Between 75% and 80% of all children with nephrotic syndrome have MCNS, and about 80% of those present symptoms within the first 8 years of life. Appearance before the age of 1 year is unusual and should make one suspect various forms of congenital nephrotic syndrome or a secondary etiology such as congenital syphilis.

72. **What are the typical clinical features and therapeutic responses seen in patients with MCNS?**
Edema is generally present, blood pressure is normal, and gross hematuria is absent, but up to one third of these patients may have microscopic hematuria; however, RBC casts are not seen. In the absence of significant intravascular volume depletion, BUN, creatinine, and electrolytes are all within normal limits. Children who present symptoms in this manner should be started on daily prednisone; this is often called a *medical biopsy*.

The standard dose recommended for the initial episode is 2 mg/kg per day with a maximal dose of 80 mg/day. A single daily dose given in the morning is as effective as split doses and may lead to fewer steroid side effects. For the initial episode, daily steroids are continued for 4 to 6 weeks, regardless of how soon the patient responds. If the patient responds, then the daily prednisone is changed to alternate-day dosing at two thirds the previous dose for an additional 4 to 6 weeks every other day. Thereafter, the dose is either stopped completely or tapered over the next 2 months. Relapses are treated similarly, except the switch to alternate-day steroid is done when the urine dipstick assessment shows a negative or trace protein reaction for 3 to 4 days.

After the initiation of prednisone for an initial episode, 93% of patients or less will respond during the first month, with the mean time being 10 to 13 days. Response is indicated by the normalization of urinary protein excretion and diuresis. If therapy is prolonged for an additional month, another 4% will respond. About 3% of children with biopsy-proven MCNS will be steroid resistant despite 2 months of therapy.

73. **For whom should secondary MCNS therapies be considered?**
- For patients who do not respond to the initial course of prednisone
- For patients who become subsequent nonresponders to prednisone during relapses
- For patients who have frequent relapses
- For patients who develop significant side effects from steroids, primarily a decrease in the rate of growth in height

74. **Is there alternative therapy available for children who are experiencing growth retardation from steroid therapy for the nephrotic syndrome?**
    More than one third of children with steroid-responsive nephrotic syndrome will experience frequent relapses (more than four relapses per year), necessitating repeated courses of prednisone. Some of these children will have a fall-off in height growth (moving below their established height percentile). The ultimate prognosis remains excellent, but the therapy becomes a problem. Several agents have been used. Cyclophosphamide (2 to 3 mg/kg daily for 3 months) can often produce a prolonged remission, sometimes permanent, but most patients eventually relapse after a period free of steroids. The calcineurin inhibitors, cyclosporine and tacrolimus, have also been useful in maintaining remission without steroids, but relapse often recurs when the drugs are stopped. Mycophenolate mofetil is also used with success as a maintenance drug to avoid steroids.

75. **When are furosemide and albumin therapy indicated for patients with nephrotic syndrome?**
    Infusion of a 25% albumin solution in a dose of 0.5 to 1 g/kg of albumin over 1 to 2 hours, followed by a potent diuretic such as furosemide (1 to 2 mg/kg), can be used to induce diuresis in a child with nephrotic syndrome who is unresponsive to furosemide alone. This measure is only temporary because the rise in albumin will lead to increased protein excretion, thereby returning the serum level to the previous steady-state value. However, it is useful in a child with severe edema leading to incapacitating anasarca, cellulitis, skin breakdown, or respiratory embarrassment from pleural effusions. Albumin alone is useful for the child with a rising BUN caused by decreased renal perfusion; this situation is most often seen after vigorous diuretic therapy.

76. **What are the risks associated with the infusion of albumin with Lasix?**
    The administration of 25% albumin and furosemide is a serious therapy with important potential risks to the patient. The assumption in this treatment is that the fluid drawn back into the intravascular space by the albumin infusion will be excreted by the kidneys after the administration of furosemide. This may not be true when the nephrotic syndrome is associated with decreased renal function or in patients with pathology other than minimal change who have a normal or expanded intravascular volume. In that situation, the infusion may lead to intravascular volume overload, hypertension, and pulmonary edema. Pulse rate, respiratory rate, and blood pressure should be monitored frequently during the infusion and the rate slowed or stopped if signs of fluid overload develop.

77. **What is the mechanism of hypercoagulability associated with nephrotic syndrome?**
    Multiple factors contribute to the hypercoagulable state. *Blood viscosity* (in part as a result of hyperlipidemia) is increased. *Platelet adhesiveness* is increased. Nearly all *coagulation factors* and *clotting inhibitors* are altered. Fibrinogen levels are increased, and antithrombin III levels are decreased as a result of urinary losses. The overall tendency favors increased coagulation and decreased fibrinolysis.

78. **Which organisms are responsible for peritonitis in children with nephrotic syndrome?**
    Pneumococcus remains the most important cause, although gram-negative organisms, especially *Escherichia coli*, account for 25% to 50% of cases.

79. **What are the prognostic factors in children with nephrotic syndrome?**
    Prognosis in the nephrotic syndrome, as in most other renal diseases, is closely related to the level of proteinuria. The best prognosis is in MCNS when the proteinuria disappears completely with steroid therapy. Even a partial response, with a decrease in the rate of protein

excretion, appears to improve the prognosis. Proteinuria is not only a marker for the severity of the renal disease, it also can be injurious. In animal studies, it leads to the activation of cytokines, resulting in interstitial inflammation and fibrosis. Because of this observation, attempts are made to decrease the proteinuria through the administration of ACE inhibitors and angiotensin receptor blockers.

Hypertension can accelerate deterioration in severe renal disease. Therefore, the blood pressure should be monitored and hypertension treated.

80. **In which children with nephrotic syndrome should renal biopsy be considered?**
Children of any age who do not go into remission during their initial course of prednisone or who fail to respond to prednisone after relapses require a renal biopsy. Because older children are more likely to have other forms of nephrotic syndrome (e.g., focal segmental glomerulosclerosis, membranoproliferative glomerulonephritis), many pediatric nephrologists would biopsy those who present symptoms at the age of 8 years or older before beginning therapy. The presence of significant hypertension, renal insufficiency, RBC casts, multiple-organ involvement, partial lipodystrophy, or a low serum C3 level speaks against the finding of MCNS and requires a renal biopsy for definitive diagnosis.

RENAL FAILURE

81. **What clinical tools, including laboratory studies, are useful for distinguishing prerenal oliguria (e.g., volume depletion) from the oliguria of intrinsic acute renal failure (ARF)?**
Clinical assessment of hydration, volume, and perfusion status is critical because these are more likely to be impaired in a prerenal state. In patients with intrinsic ARF, these parameters are more likely to show normal or excess volume status, including possible evidence of edema or vascular congestion. If volume status assessment suggests a volume deficit, a fluid bolus with normal saline can be both diagnostic and therapeutic. Laboratory studies of some assistance are summarized in Table 13-6.

TABLE 13-6. LABORATORY STUDIES OF VALUE IN PRERENAL OLIGURIA AND ACUTE RENAL FAILURE

Parameter	Prerenal	Renal
U_{Na}—random mEq/L	<20	>40
FE_{Na}*	<1%	>1%
Urine osmolality (mOsm/L)	>500	<300

*$FE_{Na} = ([U_{Na} \times P_{Creat}]/[P_{Na} \times U_{Creat}]) \times 100\%$ (on a randomly collected, "spot" urine).

82. **What is the most common cause of ARF in young children in the United States?**
The answer traditionally has been **hemolytic uremic syndrome** (HUS), which in most cases is associated with gastrointestinal infection with Shiga toxin–producing *E. coli*, especially the O157:H7 serotype. However, when one considers all the cases of **acute tubular necrosis** in childhood that most commonly result from hypoxic, hypotensive, and/or hypovolemic

insults or drug-induced injury, it is difficult to place this broad category of ARF in second place. If you are asked on rounds and are in an argumentative mood, answer "acute tubular necrosis." (No one knows the true answer because statistics are not available for large populations.)

83. **What constitutes the triad of clinical findings of HUS?**
    - **Acute renal failure** that is usually—but not always—oligoanuric.
    - **Microangiopathic hemolytic anemia:** Examination of the smear is essential to identify RBC fragments, known as schistocytes. Anemia is nonimmune, Coombs negative.
    - **Thrombocytopenia** that may vary from mild to severe.

84. **What are the key elements in the pathophysiology of HUS?**
    Injury to endothelial cells is a primary event in pathogenesis. Arteriolar and capillary microthrombi and RBC fragmentation are also involved. Classification is based on whether the illness is triggered by a Shiga toxin, which in the United States is most commonly seen with *E. coli* O157:H7. This is the typical or classic form. Ninety percent of cases follow diarrhea.

85. **Does the use of antibiotic therapy in children with diarrhea caused by *E. coli* O157:H7 prevent HUS?**
    This is controversial. A 2000 study showed that children who received antibiotics (usually sulfa-containing or β-lactam antibiotics) during outbreaks have had a much higher rate (50% versus 7%) of HUS, but other larger studies have reported protection or no association. Most experts opt not to treat patients with *E. coli* O157:H7 with antibiotics because no benefit has been proved.

    American Academy of Pediatrics: *Escherichia coli* diarrhea. In: Pickering LK, Baker CJ, Long SS, McMillan JA, editors: *Red Book: 2009 Report of the Committee on Infectious Diseases*, ed 28, Elk Grove Village, IL, 2009, American Academy of Pediatrics, p 297.

    Safdar N, Said A, Gangnon RE, Maki DG: Risk of hemolytic-uremic syndrome after antibiotic treatment of *Escherichia coli* O157:H7 enteritis: a meta-analysis, *JAMA* 288:996–1001, 2002.

    Wong CS, Jelacic S, Habeeb RL, et al: The risk of hemolytic-uremic syndrome after antibiotic treatment of *Escherichia coli* O157:H7 infections, *N Engl J Med* 342:1930–1936, 2000.

86. **What is meant by the term "atypical hemolytic uremic syndrome?"**
    This term describes a group of children who present the classic features of HUS, as described previously, but who do not have infection by Shiga toxin as the cause. Unlike the Shiga toxin–associated HUS, these children are a heterogeneous group with diverse etiologies, including hereditary defects in complement regulatory genes, *Streptococcus pneumoniae*–related HUS, collagen vascular diseases (e.g., systemic lupus erythematosus), and medications (e.g., chemotherapeutic agents). Unlike typical HUS, which tends to occur in the summer months and primarily affects children between 6 months and 4 years of age, atypical HUS affects all ages in all seasons. The prognosis for atypical HUS is worse (as many as 50% may progress to end-stage renal disease compared with typical HUS, in which up to 85% recover renal function).

    Noris M, Remuzzi G: Atypical hemolytic-uremic syndrome, *N Engl J Med* 361:1676–1687, 2009.

87. **In a child with HUS, does the presence of a low level of the C3 component of complement have any special significance?**
    Yes, it does. These children often have a defect in one of the factors whose function is to put the brake on complement activation at the level of C3 in the alternate pathway, preventing the uncontrolled activation of terminal complement components C5 to C9 (the "membrane attack complex"). Defective factors include factor H, factor I, and membrane cofactor protein (MCP). These children are treated with infusions of fresh-frozen plasma and sometimes plasma exchange.

88. **What is the pathogenesis of renal osteodystrophy?**

    Renal osteodystrophy, which is also known as *renal metabolic bone disease* and *renal rickets*, is a condition that affects bone growth and development and that occurs in patients with chronic renal insufficiency. The pathogenesis is a combination of factors that lead to hypocalcemia. These include phosphate retention and hyperphosphatemia as a result of a decreased glomerular filtration rate and decreased production of 1,25-dihydroxyvitamin D by the kidney. This leads secondarily to the decreased absorption of calcium from the gastrointestinal tract and the decreased responsiveness of bone to parathyroid hormone. The hypocalcemia leads to an increased release of parathyroid hormone, which then increases bone resorption. Chronic disease leads to secondary hyperparathyroidism and bone marrow fibrosis, which is known as *osteitis fibrosis cystica*. Recognition of osteodystrophy, which often has its origins when the glomerular filtration rate is still about half of the normal rate, is important because early intervention with vitamin D and phosphate binders can prevent and/or heal the bone disease (although not necessarily enhance growth). Furthermore, in states of chronic acidosis, the skeleton acts as a buffer for the net acid retained. This results in the release of calcium, which contributes to osteopenia and bone disease.

89. **What are indications for dialysis in ARF?**

    Elevated BUN and creatinine. There are no established critical levels above which dialysis needs to be instituted. However, when the creatinine reaches 10 mg/dL or the BUN 100 mg/dL, the glomerular filtration rate is usually markedly reduced, which results in one or more of the following abnormalities:

    - Hyperkalemia, either rapidly rising or stable at a dangerously high level that is not controlled by Kayexalate-binding resin or other measures
    - Volume-dependent hypertension or signs of CHF not responsive to diuretics
    - Severe metabolic acidosis that cannot be treated with sodium bicarbonate
    - Signs or symptoms of uremia (e.g., fatigue, encephalopathy, anorexia, pruritus, cramps, bleeding, pericarditis)
    - Other severe electrolyte disturbances, including symptomatic hyponatremia, hypocalcemia, and hyperphosphatemia
    - Need for a blood transfusion in the presence of oligoanuria

90. **What are the main causes of chronic renal disease in children that result in renal transplantation?**
    - **Obstructive uropathy**
    - **Focal segmental glomerulosclerosis**
    - **Aplastic, hypoplastic, and dysplastic kidneys**

    Whyte DA, Fine RN: Chronic kidney disease in children, *Pediatr Rev* 29:335–340, 2008.

RENAL FUNCTION ASSESSMENT AND URINALYSIS

91. **What is the simplest way to estimate the glomerular filtration rate in the absence of a timed urine collection?**

    Use of the Schwartz formula requires only a serum creatinine level and the height of the child. No urine collection, timed or untimed, is necessary. The formula is as follows:

    Creatinine clearance $(mL/min/1.73\ m^2) = K \times height\ (cm)/serum\ creatinine\ (mg/dL)$

    K is 0.45 in infants younger than 1 year, 0.55 in infants older than 1 year and adolescent females, 0.33 in low-birthweight infants, and 0.7 in adolescent males.

92. **How can you be confident that a 24-hour urine collection (for anything) is complete?**
Because creatinine is produced in a continuous fashion and eliminated only through the kidneys, there is an expectation that a given amount, determined largely by muscle mass, will be excreted daily, independent of the level of renal function. Thus, the determination of total urine creatinine in a timed sample can give a reasonable estimate of whether the collection approximates that of 24 hours. The guidelines for expected creatinine excretion applicable to children and adolescents are as follows: for males, 15 to 25 mg/kg per day; for females, 10 to 20 mg/kg per day.

93. **When should routine urinalyses (UA) be performed in the pediatric age group?**
There has been some controversy regarding the use of the UA as a routine screening tool. It is a simple, inexpensive, and noninvasive study that is quite sensitive and specific, but the likelihood of this test uncovering significant, previously undiagnosed renal dysfunction is very low. Because of this, the likelihood of false-positive results is high, leading to unnecessary evaluations. The American Academy of Pediatrics in 2007 made the recommendation to discontinue routine urine dipsticks in healthy children as a screen for chronic kidney disease.

American Academy of Pediatrics: Committee on Practice and Ambulatory Medicine: Recommendations for preventive pediatric health care, *Pediatrics* 120:1376, 2007.

Sekhar DL, Wang L, Hoffenbeck CS, et al: A cost effectiveness analysis of screening urine dipsticks in well-child care, *Pediatrics* 125:660-663, 2010.

94. **How does Clinitest differ from typical urine dipstick testing for the evaluation of glucosuria?**
The **Clinitest tablet** detects reducing substances in the urine. These include reducing sugars (e.g., glucose, galactose, lactose, pentoses, fructose) and other compounds, including high amounts of amino acids, oxalate, ketones, and uric acid. It is also positive in the presence of many drugs, including high concentrations of ascorbic acid, penicillin, cephalosporins, nitrofurantoin, sulfonamides, and tetracycline. The **glucose oxidase square** on the dipstick is specific for glucose. The Clinitest may be helpful as an initial screening tool for a child who is suspected of having galactosemia, or it may be useful when testing the stool of a child who is suspected of having carbohydrate malabsorption or intolerance.

Liao JC, Churchill BM: Pediatric urine testing, *Pediatr Clin North Am* 48:1425–1440, 2001.

95. **What are the maximal and minimal urinary dilutional and concentrating capabilities of the renal system?**
Maximally dilute urine has a specific gravity of 1.001 and an osmolality of 50. Maximally concentrated urine has a specific gravity of about 1.032 and an osmolality of about 1200. Urine that is neither concentrated nor dilute (i.e., isosthenuric) has a specific gravity of about 1.010 and a corresponding osmolality of 300.

96. **What is the difference between urine specific gravity and urine osmolality?**
Both tests measure the concentration or dilution of the urine, and the relationship between the two is linear and direct, although osmolality is more physiologically correct. *Specific gravity* is determined by the density (and thus the weight and size) of solute in solution. *Osmolality*, on the other hand, depends on the number of particles (independent of their size) in solution and their effect on changing its freezing point. Therefore, when there are solutes with a relatively large molecular weight (e.g., albumin, glucose, contrast material) in the urine, specific gravity will disproportionately increase, and osmolality will be a better indicator of true urine concentration. A urine specific gravity of 1.040 is not achievable by the human kidney; in a child with nephrotic syndrome, levels that high do not represent supernormal concentrating capacity but rather artifactual effects of heavy proteinuria.

97. **What crystal, when seen in the urinary sediment, is always pathologic?**
The presence of a **cystine crystal**, which appears as a flat, simple, hexagon-shaped crystal, is never normal and is strong evidence for the amino acid transport disorder cystinuria. In classic cystinuria, the dibasic amino acids (cystine, ornithine, arginine, and lysine) are affected. The condition would be of little clinical significance except for the fact that cystine is very insoluble and results in nephrolithiasis.

SURGICAL ISSUES

98. **What are the risks associated with circumcision?**
The most common complications are bleeding and infection. With poor technique, injury or amputation of the glans can occur. Meatal stenosis as a consequence of meatal ulceration is another complication.

99. **Is circumcision now medically indicated?**
The debate continues. Data support that newborn circumcision protects males against UTIs in infancy and adulthood. Circumcision appears to decrease the transmission of certain sexually transmitted diseases (e.g., syphilis, chancroid, herpes simplex, human papillomavirus, human immunodeficiency virus). Other benefits can include improved lifetime genital hygiene, elimination of phimosis and local foreskin infections, and a lower incidence of penile cancer. There are many proponents both for and against circumcision. The decision at present, however, still rests primarily on nonmedical issues.

Brady MT: Newborn circumcision: Routine or not routine, that is the question. *Arch Pediatr Adolesc Med* 164:94-96, 2010.

Dickerman JD: Circumcision in the time of HIV: when is there enough evidence to revise the American Academy of Pediatrics' policy on circumcision? *Pediatrics* 119:1006–1007, 2007.

Tobian AAR, Serwadda D, Quinn TC, et al: Male circumcision for the prevention of HSV-2 and HPV infections and syphilis, *N Engl J Med* 360:1298–1309, 2009.

100. **What is the proper method of anesthesia for neonatal circumcision?**
Up to 85% of infant males in the United States undergo circumcision, and worldwide it remains the most commonly performed operation. Until recently, it was usually performed by most without anesthesia or analgesia. Although pacifiers, topical agents (3.0% lidocaine, EMLA cream), oral sucrose, and oral analgesics (e.g., acetaminophen) help alleviate some discomfort, the most effective means of minimizing pain are a ring block or a dorsal penile nerve block. The latter consists of injecting 0.3 to 0.4 mL of 1% lidocaine without epinephrine in both sides of the dorsal penile base.

Litman RS: Anesthesia and analgesia for newborn circumcision, *Obstet Gynecol Surg* 56:114–117, 2001.

101. **What distinguishes phimosis and paraphimosis?**
Phimosis is a narrowing of the distal foreskin, which prevents its retraction over the glans of the penis. In newborns, retraction is difficult because of normal adhesions that gradually self-resolve. Chronic inflammation or scarring can cause true phimosis with persistent narrowing and may require circumcision. **Paraphimosis** is incarceration of a retracted foreskin behind the glans. It occurs when the retracted foreskin is not repositioned. Progressive edema results, which, if uncorrected, can lead to ischemic breakdown. Local anesthesia, ice, and manual reduction usually correct the problem, but if these are unsuccessful, surgical reduction is necessary.

Huang CJ: Problems of the foreskin and glans penis, *Clin Pediatr Emerg Med* 10:56–59, 2009.

102. **What is hypospadias?**
Hypospadias occurs in 1 to 2 out of every 1000 live births and results from the failure or delay of the midline fusion of the urethral folds. It is often associated with a ventral band of fibrous tissue (chordee) that causes ventral curvature of the penis, especially with an erection, thereby making intercourse difficult or impossible. When assessing hypospadias, it is useful to describe where the urethral meatus appears (i.e., glandular, distal shaft, proximal shaft, or perineal) and also the degree and location of chordee. The treatment of hypospadias is surgical repair, usually as a one-step procedure. With the advent of microsurgical techniques, the optimal time for repair appears to be 6 to 12 months of age.

103. **How are the degrees of hypospadias classified?**
The mildest and most common form of hypospadias is distal hypospadias (Fig. 13-2A), which occurs in the subcoronal or glandular area in about 80% to 85% of cases. About 10% to 15% of cases occur in the penile shaft. Only 5% to 10% occur in the severe penoscrotal or perineal location (Fig. 13-2B).

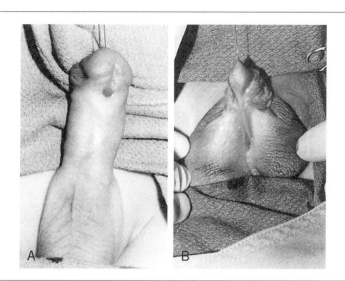

Figure 13-2. A, Distal hypospadias. **B**, Severe proximal hypospadias in the mid-scrotal area. (From Kay R: Hypospadias. In Resnick MI, Novick AC (eds): Urology Secrets, 3rd ed. Philadelphia, Hanley & Belfus, 2003, p 188.)

104. **What is the most common cause of urinary tract obstruction in the newborn?**
Posterior urethral valves, which are more commonly seen in male infants. The obstruction is frequently associated with high intravesicular pressures, which may damage the renal parenchyma if undetected. However, the adverse obstructive effects of the valves during intrauterine life may be associated with renal dysplasia. Thus, even with prompt recognition and treatment, renal insufficiency may progress.

105. **What is the natural history of hydroceles?**
Small hydroceles in infancy are benign and spontaneously resolve by 9 to 12 months of age. Large hydroceles rarely resolve and may cause vascular compromise and testicular atrophy; these should be resected. A communicating hydrocele (which changes in size) indicates a completely patent processus vaginalis and has the potential for hernia formation. This variety should also be repaired.

106. **When should undescended testicles be repaired?**
The optimal time for surgery on an undescended testicle is 12 months of age or shortly thereafter. Traditional teaching is that cryptorchidism usually resolves without intervention. Seventy-five percent of full-term infants and 90% of premature cryptorchid newborns will have full testicular descent by the age of 9 months, although recent data suggest that the rate of spontaneous descent is much lower. Spontaneous testis descent after 9 months is unlikely. During the second year of life, ultrastructural changes in the seminiferous tubules of the undescended testes begin to appear, but these may be halted by orchiopexy.

Wenzler DL, Bloom DA, Park JM: What is the rate of spontaneous testicular descent in infants with cryptorchidism? *J Urol* 171:849–851, 2004.

American Academy of Pediatrics: Timing of elective surgery on the genitalia of male children with particular reference to the risks, benefits, and psychological effects of surgery and anesthesia, *Pediatrics* 97:590–594, 1996.

107. **What is the most common genitourinary abnormality found on prenatal ultrasound?**
Hydronephrosis. This descriptive term indicates distention of the renal pelvis and calyces, which is often due to obstruction. However, it can also be seen with nonobstructing entities such as vesicoureteral reflux (VUR).

108. **What are the possible causes of prenatal hydronephrosis?**
- Ureteropelvic junction obstruction (most common)
- Posterior urethral valves
- VUR
- Prune belly syndrome
- Ectopic ureter or ureterocele
- Megaureter (obstructive and nonobstructive)
- Urethral atresia

109. **What is a reasonable approach to the management of prenatally detected hydronephrosis?**
See Figure 13-3.

110. **What physical findings should prompt a search for an underlying renal abnormality?**
- Abdominal mass
- Neonatal ascites
- High imperforate anus
- Oligohydramnios
- Perineal hypospadias
- Anuria-oliguria (especially in neonate)
- Exstrophy of the bladder
- Aniridia, hemihypertrophy (Wilms tumor)
- Ambiguous genitalia
- Poor urinary stream
- Prune belly syndrome
- Persistent wetness

TUBULAR DISORDERS

111. **Name the three main types of renal tubular acidoses (RTAs).**
This is a trick question, since type 3 no longer exists.
- Type 1, *Distal RTA*: Impairment in distal acidification
- Type 2, *Proximal RTA*: Impairment in proximal tubule bicarbonate reclamation

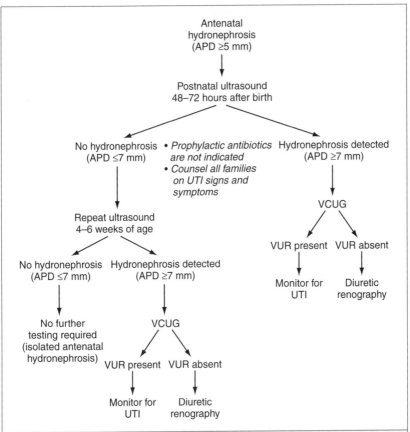

Figure 13-3. Algorithm for postnatal evaluation of antenatal hydronephrosis. APD, anterior-posterior diameter; UTI, urinary tract infection; VCUG, voiding cystourethrogram; VUR, vesicoureteral reflux. (From Becker AM: Postnatal evaluation of infants with an abnormal antenatal renal sonogram. Curr Opin Pediatr 21:209, 2009.)

- Type 4, *Distal hyperkalemic:* Occurs as a result of a lack of—or tubular insensitivity to—aldosterone
  All three types are associated with a hyperchloremic normal anion gap acidosis.

112. **Describe the clinical and laboratory manifestations of the various RTAs.**
RTAs of types 1 and 2 are associated with hypokalemia, whereas type 4 is characterized by hyperkalemia in addition to hyperchloremic acidosis. Hypercalciuria is typical of type 1 RTA and, in conjunction with hypocitraturia, often leads to nephrocalcinosis and renal calculi. Type 2 may be part of a more global defect of proximal tubule function, the Fanconi syndrome, which, in addition to bicarbonaturia, is characterized by aminoaciduria, glycosuria, phosphaturia (hypophosphatemia), and rickets. Type 4 RTA is most commonly observed in pediatric patients with obstructive uropathy, tubular unresponsiveness to aldosterone (pseudoaldosteronism) that is often transient during infancy, or decreased aldosterone secretion (hypoaldosteronism). Other signs and symptoms that are common with all forms of RTA are growth failure, polyuria, polydipsia, recurrent dehydration, and vomiting (Table 13-7).

TABLE 13-7. CLINICAL AND LABORATORY MANIFESTATIONS OF VARIOUS RENAL TUBULAR ACIDOSES

	Type 1 (Classic, Distal)	Type 2 (Proximal)	Type 4 (Aldosterone Deficiency)
Growth failure	+++	++	+++
Serum potassium	Normal or low	Normal or low	High
Nephrocalcinosis	Frequent	Rare	Rare
Low citrate excretion	+++	±	±
Fractional excretion of filtered HCO_3 at normal serum HCO_3 levels	<5%	5%-10%	<10%
Daily alkali treatment (mEq/kg)	1-3	5-20	1-3
Daily potassium requirement	Decreases with correction	Increases with correction	
Urine pH	>5.5	<5.5	<5.5
Presence of other tubular defects	Rare	Common	Rare

113. **What is the primary defect in type 1 RTA?**
An inability of the distal tubule to secrete hydrogen. Thus, in the presence of significant systemic acidosis, urine is not maximally acidified (pH <5.5). This defect in hydrogen secretion is associated with low rates of ammonium and titratable acid excretion.

114. **What is the main renal defect in type 2 RTA?**
The primary defect is a **decreased ability of the proximal tubule to reabsorb filtered HCO_3** at normal plasma HCO_3 concentrations—a "lowered tubular reabsorptive threshold." These patients typically have a chronic hyperchloremic metabolic acidosis, acid urine (pH <5.5), and a low fractional excretion (FE) of HCO_3 (<5%). When plasma HCO_3 levels are increased toward normal (and thus above the lowered tubular reabsorptive threshold), patients will lose HCO_3 in the urine (FE >15%), and the urine will be alkaline (pH >6.0).

115. **How is determining the urinary anion gap helpful for the evaluation of metabolic acidosis?**
Investigation of any child with a persistent metabolic acidosis must consider some form of RTA in the differential diagnosis. The urinary anion gap is a convenient and accurate screening test for RTA. It is an indirect estimate of urinary ammonium excretion (and thus urinary acid excretion) and is calculated by the following formula after determining urinary electrolyte concentrations:

$$Anion\ gap = Na^+ + K^- - Cl^-$$

If the anion gap is negative, it suggests a large chloride excretion and thus adequate ammonium excretion. The urinary anion gap is negative in hyperchloremic metabolic acidosis as a result of diarrhea, untreated proximal RTA, or prior administration of an acid load. If the anion gap is positive, it suggests an acidification defect, as is seen in patients with distal RTA. Results are not reliable if there are large amounts of unmeasured anions such as ketoacids, penicillin, or salicylates.

116. **How is RTA diagnosed in a patient with a hyperchloremic metabolic acidosis and a normal serum anion gap?**
See Figure 13-4.

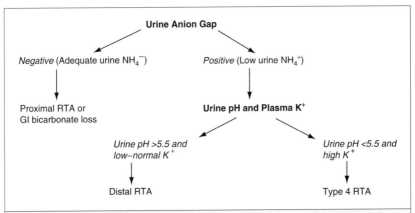

Figure 13-4. Diagnosis of renal tubular acidosis in patients with hyperchloremic metabolic acidosis and normal serum anion gap. (Adapted from Lash JP, Arruda JA: Laboratory evaluation of renal tubular acidosis. Clin Lab Med 13:117-129, 1993.)

117. **What is the recommended alkali therapy for the treatment of various forms of RTA?**
The goals of RTA therapy are to improve growth, correct metabolic bone disease, prevent nephrolithiasis and nephrocalcinosis, and control any underlying disease process.

Alkali therapy (sodium citrate or sodium bicarbonate): This is required for all forms of RTA, with the goal of a normal plasma HCO_3 level. Patients with distal RTA generally require only 2 to 3 mEq of alkali/kg/day. However, infants may also experience some increased urinary bicarbonate wasting and require up to 10 mEq/kg per day. Patients with proximal RTA require large quantities of alkali (5 to 20 mEq/kg/day). For type 4 RTA, patients usually need low-dose alkali therapy (1 to 3 mEq/kg/day) plus a potassium-restricted diet and mineralocorticoid therapy if there is hypoaldosteronism.

118. **What is the primary disease causing the Fanconi syndrome (the *renal* syndrome, not the *hematologic* one, both described by the same Swiss pediatrician, Guido Fanconi)?**
The *renal Fanconi* syndrome is the manifestation of multiple disorders of transport in the proximal tubule. It is characterized by the abnormal excretion of substances normally reabsorbed by the proximal tubule and for which there is no distal mechanism quantitatively sufficient to recapture the unabsorbed molecules. Thus, there is abnormal excretion of glucose, phosphate, amino acids, and bicarbonate. The phosphaturia produces hypophosphatemia; the bicarbonate loss causes metabolic acidosis. It is a surprise to many physicians to hear that cystinosis is the most common cause of the Fanconi syndrome. Other causes are Lowe oculocerebrorenal syndrome, galactosemia, hereditary fructose intolerance, glycogen storage disease, tyrosinemia, Wilson disease, and mitochondrial diseases.

119. **What is the clinical presentation of acute interstitial nephritis (AIN)?**
    AIN is caused by an immune-mediated inflammatory response that initially involves the renal interstitium and tubules, usually sparing the glomeruli and vasculature. AIN has a wide array of clinical presentations that range from isolated tubular disorders (e.g., Fanconi syndrome) to acute renal failure. Additional findings may suggest a hypersensitivity reaction (e.g., fever, rash, arthralgias).

120. **What drugs are known to be causes of AIN?**
    - Antibiotics (especially penicillin analogs, cephalosporins, sulfonamides, and rifampin)
    - Nonsteroidal anti-inflammatory drugs (NSAIDs)
    - Diuretics (especially thiazides and furosemide)

121. **What laboratory abnormalities are seen in patients with AIN?**
    - Urinary sediment: RBCs, leukocytes (eosinophils), leukocyte casts
    - Urinary protein excretion: Less than1 g/day; with NSAID use, may be more than 1 g/day
    - Fractional excretion of sodium: Usually more than 1
    - Proximal tubular defects: Glucosuria, bicarbonaturia, phosphaturia, aminoaciduria, proximal RTA
    - Distal tubular defects: Hyperkalemia, sodium wasting, distal RTA
    - Medullary defects: Sodium wasting, urinary concentrating defects

    Meyers CM: Acute interstitial nephritis. In: Greenberg A, editor: *Primer on Kidney Diseases. National Kidney Foundation*, San Diego, 1998, Academic Press, p 278.

122. **A young girl diagnosed with AIN has developed a painful red eye. Could there be a connection?**
    Yes, there most likely is a connection. There are several renal diseases associated with ocular inflammation. It is important to get the assistance of an ophthalmologist for definitive diagnosis and eye therapy. If this is anterior uveitis, there are several possible associations: sarcoidosis, Sjögren syndrome, and the syndrome of tubulointerstitial nephritis with uveitis (TINU). In the absence of pulmonary findings, the most likely diagnosis here is TINU. This is an interesting syndrome in which there may be a long delay in diagnosis because the uveitis may not appear for weeks to months after the onset of symptoms. There is usually persisting or intermittent fever with no etiology, associated with abdominal pain and considerable unexplained weight loss, often prompting a search for malignancy. The urine findings are minimal with low-grade proteinuria and mild pyuria. With time, the serum creatinine may increase. There may be a partial Fanconi syndrome (see earlier). Steroids are helpful for the uveitis and may help the interstitial nephritis, but this is not clear. Often the renal findings resolve, but the eye findings become a chronic problem.

URINARY TRACT INFECTIONS

123. **How helpful are dipstick testing and microscopic analysis of urine as screening tests for UTIs?**
    Recalling that sensitivity is the probability that test results will be positive among patients who have UTIs and specificity is the probability that test results will be negative among patients who do not have UTIs, the value of the components of the urinalysis individually and in combination as screening tools for the diagnosis of a UTI are summarized in Table 13-8.

TABLE 13-8. RAPID SCREENING TESTS FOR URINARY TRACT INFECTION IN CHILDREN: SENSITIVITY AND SPECIFICITY

Microscopy	Sensitivity (%) (range)	Specificity (%) (range)
≥5 WBC/HPF	67 (55, 88)	79 (77, 84)
Any bacteria/HPF	81 (16, 99)	83 (11, 100)
≥5 WBC or bacteria/HPF	99 (97, 100)	65 (67, 74)
Dipstick		
Any LE	83 (64, 89)	84 (71, 95)
Any nitrite only	50 (16, 72)	98 (95, 100)
Any nitrite or LE	88 (71, 100)	93 (76, 98)
≥ Moderate LE or nitrite	73 (62, 81)	99 (98, 99)
Both nitrite and LE	72 (14, 83)	96 (95, 100)
Dipstick + Microscopy		
Gram stain, any organism	93 (80, 98)	95 (87, 100)
Any positive on either LE, nitrite	99 (99, 100)	70 (60, 92)
≥5 WBC or bacteria/HPF	83 (74, 90)	87 (86, 88)

HPF = high-power field; LE = leukocyte esterase; WBC = white blood cells.
Data from Christensen AM, Shaw K: Urinary tract infection in childhood. In: Kaplan BS, Meyers KEC (eds): Pediatric Nephrology and Urology: The Requisites in Pediatrics. Philadelphia, Elsevier/Mosby, 2004, p 320.

124. **A child is urinating frequently and painfully, and culture revealed a UTI, but the original urinalysis had a negative nitrite study. Why?**
Members of the gram-negative, rod-shaped Enterobacteriaceae family can reduce dietary nitrate to nitrite. However, the bacteria need hours for this conversion. A first-morning void is more likely to be positive compared with the urinalysis of a child who has been urinating frequently with insufficient time to incubate in the bladder. A false-negative result is common with the nitrite test.

Patel HP: The abnormal urinalysis, *Pediatr Clin N Am* 53:325–337, 2006.

125. **Can the diagnosis of UTI be made on the basis of urinalysis alone?**
No. A urine culture is the only accurate means of diagnosing a UTI. Urinalysis can be valuable for selecting individuals for the prompt initiation of treatment while awaiting results of the urine culture. In older children (in whom UTI symptoms are more reliable indicators of infection), a negative nitrite test, a negative leukocyte esterase test, and the absence of UTI symptoms are highly correlated with the absence of infection. However, babies require a culture to exclude UTI.

KEY POINTS: URINARY TRACT INFECTION

1. *Escherichia coli* causes 90% of cases.

2. Antibiotic sensitivity testing is important because of the increasing incidence of ampicillin-resistant *E. coli*.

3. Infections may be caused by ascending bacteria from the urethral area.

4. Clean-bagged specimens are unreliable for diagnosis because of their high contamination rate.

5. Uncircumcised male infants have a 10-fold greater risk for infection than circumcised male infants.

126. **What bacterial counts constitute a positive urine culture?**
   - **Suprapubic aspiration:** At least 100 colony-forming units (CFU)/mL
   - **Catheterization:** At least 10,000 CFU/mL from midstream
   - **Midstream clean catch:** At least 100,000 CFU/mL of a single organism; 10,000 to 100,000 CFU/mL: suspicious and requires reculturing; less than 10,000 CFU/mL: usually indicates contamination
   - **Urine bag:** May be helpful if negative, but even at least 100,000 CFU/mL has an 85% false-positive result

127. **What factors can cause low colony counts despite significant urinary infection?**
   - High-volume urine flow
   - Recent antimicrobial therapy
   - Fastidious and slow-growing organisms (e.g., enterococci, *Staphylococcus saprophyticus*)
   - Low urine pH (<5.0) and specific gravity (<1.003)
   - Bacteriostatic agents in the urine
   - Complete obstruction of a ureter
   - Chronic or indolent infection
   - Use of inappropriate culture techniques

   Bock GH: Urinary tract infections. In: Hoekelman RA, Adam HM, Nelson HM, et al, editors: *Primary Pediatric Care*, ed 4, St. Louis, 2001, Mosby, p 1896.

128. **Why should urine specimens be refrigerated if they cannot be immediately processed?**
   The storage of urine specimens at room temperature is one of the most common causes of false-positive results. When left at room temperature, enteric organisms in specimens have a growth-doubling time of 12.5 minutes, and thus colony counts become an unreliable guide. If a urine specimen cannot be processed within 15 minutes, it should be refrigerated at less than 4°C to stop *in vitro* replication.

129. **What are the common presenting signs and symptoms of a UTI in an infant?**
   The presenting findings are nonspecific and can include fever, vomiting, diarrhea, irritability, hyperbilirubinemia, and poor feeding. These same findings are often seen in infants without UTIs—thus the importance of cultures in febrile infants.

130. **How common are UTIs in young febrile infants?**
   Quite common. In infants and toddlers between 2 and 24 months with unexplained fever (>38.3°C), the prevalence is about 7%, but it ranges between 2% and 9% depending on age

and sex. The younger the child, the more likely the presence of a UTI. Girls have twice as many infections (or more) as circumcised boys. White girls are twice as likely to have a UTI than black infants. In the first 3 months of life, uncircumcised males with fever have a 10-fold increased risk compared with circumcised boys. In infants younger than 2 months, 7.5% are likely to have UTIs, with boys having more than girls. Needless to say, the possibility of a UTI should always be considered in younger infants, particularly those without an identifiable source of infection.

Shaikh N, Morone ME, Bost JE, Farrell MH: Prevalence of urinary tract infection in childhood: a meta-analysis, *Pediatr Infect Dis J* 27:302–308, 2008.

131. Why are uncircumcised boys at greater risk for UTIs?

One theory is that the mucosal surface of the foreskin is more likely to harbor uropathogenic bacteria compared with the keratinized glans of the circumcised male owing to increased binding. Another is that there may be some partial obstruction of the meatus by the foreskin. There is an increased risk in boys whose foreskin is not able to be to be retracted to expose the meatus.

Hiraoka M, Tsukahara H, Ohshima Y, et al: Meatus tightly covered by the prepuce is associated with urinary infection, *Pediatr Int* 44:658, 2002.

Wiswell TE: The prepuce, urinary tract infections and consequences, *Pediatrics* 105:860–862, 2000.

132. What pathogens are associated with UTIs in children?

Between 80% and 90% of initial UTIs are caused by *E. coli*. Other organisms include *Proteus mirabilis*, *Klebsiella pneumoniae*, and *Pseudomonas*, *Enterobacter*, and some *Staphylococcus* species.

133. How is cystitis distinguished clinically from pyelonephritis?

Often with difficulty. Pyelonephritis tends to have more constitutional symptoms, such as fever, rigors, flank pain, and back pain, whereas cystitis has more bladder symptoms, such as enuresis, dysuria, frequency, and urgency. The presence of white blood cell casts or impaired urinary-concentrating ability is more indicative of pyelonephritis. Patients with pyelonephritis tend to have higher sedimentation rates, C-reactive proteins, and serum procalcitonin levels, but these results can also be seen in some patients with cystitis. Renal dimercaptosuccinic acid (DMSA) scintigraphy may be useful for identifying acute pyelonephritis. However, for most children, the treatments for cystitis and of pyelonephritis are essentially the same.

134. What should be the diagnostic approach regarding a possible UTI for a female infant aged 3 to 24 months with no known urinary tract abnormalities?

One algorithmic approach uses risk factors and likelihood ratios (a number <1 is less likely, >1 more likely) as well as urinalysis results to categorize the probability of UTI (Fig. 13-5). Diagnostic algorithms are also available for febrile males ages 3 to 24 months and for verbal children older than 24 months with urinary or abdominal symptoms.

135. Which patients with UTIs require hospitalization and parenteral antibiotics?

- Any infant younger than 2 months, because of an increased risk for urosepsis or other serious concomitant infections
- Any patient who is toxic, dehydrated, or unable to tolerate oral antibiotics

136. Should all pediatric patients with clinical pyelonephritis be hospitalized?

Traditionally, older patients with clinical evidence of pyelonephritis have been hospitalized for 24 to 48 hours for parenteral antibiotics and, if a good clinical response has occurred, discharged to home for additional oral antibiotic therapy. Data are emerging that the short- and long-term outcomes of patients (even as young as 2 months old) with uncomplicated pyelonephritis are the same for initial therapy with intravenous antibiotics

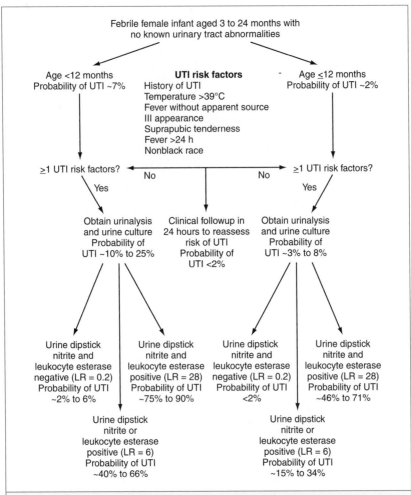

Figure 13-5. Diagnostic algorithm for febrile female infants aged 3 to 24 months suspected of having a urinary tract infection. LR = likelihood ratio. (From Shaikh N, Morone NE, Lopez J: Does this child have a urinary tract infection? *JAMA* 298:2902, 2007.)

and with oral, third-generation cephalosporins. Outpatient therapy clearly mandates the ability to tolerate oral antibiotics and that there are no concerns regarding compliance and careful and reliable follow-up.

137. **What is the expected resolution of fever after a child is started on an antibiotic for a UTI?**
In one study of 128 infants younger than 60 days with UTI treated with parenteral antibiotics, 85% became afebrile within 24 hours. Only 4% were febrile after 48 hours. In another study

involving 364 patients from ages 1 week to 18 years, 32% had fever beyond 48 hours (with older age being a risk factor for protracted fever).

Dayan RS, Hanson E, Bennett JE, et al: Clinical course of urinary tract infections in infants younger than 60 days of age, *Pediatr Emerg Care* 20:85–88, 2004.

Currie ML: *Arch Pediatr Adolesc Med* 157:1237–1240, 2003.

138. **What is the duration of antibiotic therapy for a UTI?**
Standard duration of therapy is 10 days (combined oral plus parenteral) for cystitis or pyelonephritis, although shorter courses are under study. Some experts lean toward 14 days of treatment for pyelonephritis. If the patient is not clinically improved within 2 to 3 days of starting therapy, the urine culture should be repeated and antibiotics adjusted, if indicated. Of note, follow-up cultures for a clinically improving patient are generally not indicated. In the two studies noted in question 137, none of the hospitalized patients who were treated according to available sensitivities from a positive culture had a persistent positive culture on repeat testing.

139. **In what cases are prophylactic antibiotics indicated for patients with UTIs?**
This is becoming very controversial. A 2007 study indicated that prophylaxis for recurrent UTI not only may not be protective, but may actually increase the likelihood of infections. Watchful waiting and rapid assessment when clinical concerns arise were the recommendations. Also, it is unclear whether preventing recurrent UTIs will prevent renal scarring. Consequently, prophylaxis for recurrent UTI in children with normal urinary tract anatomy is debated, particularly for younger infants. In some settings, however, prophylaxis is generally indicated:
■ Infants or children with their first UTI, who have finished their 10-day course of therapy and who are awaiting the completion of studies (e.g., voiding cystourethrogram [VCUG], renal ultrasound).
■ Patients with known urologic abnormalities that place them at high risk for recurrent UTIs (e.g., severe voiding disorders, high-grade VUR), although the utility of antibiotics in these situations is also being questioned.
A large trial, the Randomized Intervention for Children with Vesicoureteral Reflux study, is currently under way in an effort to provide some definitive answers regarding VUR.

Mattoo TK: Are prophylactic antibiotics indicated after a urinary tract infection? *Curr Opin Pediatr* 21:203–206, 2009.

Chesney RW, Carpenter MA, et al: Randomized Intervention for Children with Vesicoureteral Reflux (RIVUR): background commentary of RIVUR Investigators, *Pediatrics* 122(Suppl 5):233–239, 2008.

Conway PH, Cnaan A, Zaoutis T, et al: Recurrent urinary tract infection in children: risk factors and association with prophylactic antimicrobials, *JAMA* 298:179, 2007.

140. **Is cranberry juice helpful for the management of UTIs in children?**
The use of cranberry juice as a urine-acidifying agent and treatment for UTI has been popular for adults since the 1920s, and studies of adults have shown it to be helpful for diminishing the frequency of bacteriuria, possibly because of its antiadhesive properties against *E. coli*. Limited studies in children with chronic bacteriuria who require frequent catheterization have not shown positive benefits.

Schlager TA, Anderson S, Trudell J, Hendley JO: Effect of cranberry juice on bacteriuria in children with neurogenic bladder receiving intermittent catheterization, *J Pediatr* 135:698–702, 1999.

141. **Which patients with UTIs warrant imaging studies of the urinary tract?**
The 1999 American Academy of Pediatrics guidelines recommended renal ultrasonography and VCUG in children younger than 2 years with a UTI to detect anomalies or the presence of VUR. The value of these studies, particularly their role in preventing long-term renal sequelae, is under reexamination. Clinical trends include a more limited use of imaging studies with

emphasis on higher-risk patients and a reduction in the use of the VCUG. Guidelines in the United Kingdom rely on ultrasound and radionuclide studies rather than the VCUG. Patients at higher risk for having an abnormality identified include:

- Boys with a first UTI
- Infants younger than 1 year
- Recurrent UTI or bacteremia
- Infection with an unusual (non–*E. coli*) organism
- Abnormal renal function or abnormal urinary tract on antenatal screening
- Poor urinary stream
- Prolonged clinical course (symptoms >72 hours) or failure to respond to antibiotic therapy
- Palpable kidneys or abdominal mass

Marks SD, Gordon I, Tullus K: Imaging in childhood urinary tract infections: time to reduce investigations, *Pediatr Nephrol* 23:9, 2008.

Friedman AL: Acute UTI: what you need to know, *Contemp Pediatr* 25:68–76, 2008.

DeMuri GP, Wald ER: Imaging and antimicrobial prophylaxis following the diagnosis of urinary tract infection in children, *Pediatr Infect Dis J* 27:553–554, 2008.

Roberts K, Downs S, Hellerstein S, et al: Practice parameter: the diagnosis, treatment, and evaluation of the initial urinary tract infection in febrile infants and young children, *Pediatrics* 103:843–852, 1999.

142. **What imaging studies can be used for patients with UTIs who warrant evaluation?**
- VCUG or radionuclide cystogram, to evaluate for VUR (the most common abnormality found in children with UTIs)
- Renal ultrasound, to screen for urinary tract obstruction or other structural genitourinary abnormalities
- Renal cortical DMSA or MAG-3 (^{99m}Tc-mercaptoacetyltriglycine) scanning, recommended by some authorities to determine whether there is evidence of acute pyelonephritis or permanent renal scarring

143. **Is renal scarring a common occurrence in children with UTIs?**
Renal scars are relatively uncommon (<10% in children <2 years old) when DMSA scanning is done 6 months after a UTI if a patient has a normal urinary tract and no bladder dysfunction. Children with recurrent UTIs and concomitant VUR are at a higher risk for renal scarring. About 40% to 70% of children with grades II to IV reflux have renal scarring at the time of their initial renal scan. Much recent emphasis has focused on the importance of congenital abnormalities (e.g., hypoplasia, dysplasia) rather than ongoing VUR as contributors to chronic scarring observed after UTIs in children. The potential for the delayed appearance of renal scarring after normal initial studies remains controversial.

Orellana P, Baquedano, Rangarajan V, et al: Relationship between acute pyelonephritis, renal scarring, and vesicoureteral reflux: results of a coordinated research project, *Pediatr Nephrol* 19:1122–1126, 2004.

Wennerstrom M, Hansson S, Jodal U, Stokland E: Primary and acquired renal scarring in boys and girls with urinary tract infections, *J Pediatr* 136:30–34, 2000.

144. **Should children be screened for asymptomatic bacteriuria?**
Although 1% to 2% of girls older than 5 years have persistent bacteriuria, mass screening at present is not recommended for the following reasons:
- In girls with radiologically demonstrable anatomic abnormalities (0.2% to 0.5%), most renal injury appears to occur before the age of 5 years and may not progress.
- Older girls with asymptomatic bacteriuria and normal anatomy are unlikely to have sequelae if untreated.

The screening of infants and toddlers is technically more difficult, and the merits of screening are unclear. Infants and children at high risk should be considered for screening.

UROLITHIASIS AND NEPHROLITHIASIS

145. **Why are kidney stones increasing in frequency in children in the United States?**
The rise has been dramatic, with a nearly fivefold increase over the past two decades.
A leading theory is that increased salt intake, particularly by consumption of salty snacks and processed foods, and insufficient fluid intake have led to increased urinary calcium and oxalate concentrations with resultant stone formation. The rise of obesity is also paralleling the rise of urolithiasis in children.

VanDervoort K, Wiesen J, Frank R, et al: Urolithiasis in pediatric patients: a single center study of incidence, clinical presentation and outcome, *J Urol* 177:2300–2305, 2007.

146. **What are the clinical findings in pediatric urolithiasis?**
Patients present most commonly with flank pain, usually unilateral with nausea and vomiting. Although hematuria (>2 RBCs/HPF) is common, up to 15% may have no hematuria on testing. In about one third of cases, there is a family history of urolithiasis. Fever, dysuria, and costovertebral angle tenderness lower the likelihood of stones and make infection more likely.

Persaud AC, Stevenson MD, McMahon DR, Christopher NC: Pediatric urolithiasis: clinical predictors in the emergency department, *Pediatrics* 124:888–894, 2009.

147. **What is the composition of kidney stones in children?**
See Table 13-9.

TABLE 13-9. COMPOSITION OF KIDNEY STONES IN CHILDREN		
Stone Composition	**North America ($n = 340$)**	**Europe ($n = 315$)**
Calcium	58%	37%
Struvite	25%	54%
Cystine	6%	3%
Uric acid, urate	9%	2%
Others	2%	4%

Data from Polinsky MS, Kaiser BA, Baluarte HJ: Urolithiasis in childhood. Pediatr Clin North Am 34:683-710, 1987.

148. **What is the most common metabolic cause of pediatric urinary calculi?**
Hypercalciuria. The most common cause of this condition is familial idiopathic hypercalciuria. Multiple other causes include the following:
- Hypocitraturia
- Increased intestinal calcium absorption (vitamin D excess)
- Renal tubular dysfunction
- Endocrine abnormalities (hypothyroidism, adrenocorticoid excess, hyperparathyroidism)
- Bone metabolism disorders (immobilization, rickets, malignancies, juvenile rheumatoid arthritis)
- Drugs (certain diuretics, corticosteroids)
- Other (hypercalcemia, UTI, Williams syndrome)

Spivacow FR, Negri AL, del Valle EE, et al: Metabolic risk factors in children with kidney stone disease, *Pediatr Nephrol* 23:1129–1133, 2008.

Gillespie RS, Stapleton FB: Nephrolithiasis in children, *Pediatr Rev* 25:131–138, 2004.

149. **How is hypercalciuria defined in the infant and child?**
The strict definition of hypercalciuria in a child is more than 4 mg of urinary calcium per kilogram per 24 hours on an unrestricted diet that is normal for the child's age. Twenty-four-hour urine collections can be difficult in young children. Therefore, random urine collections have been used to screen for hypercalciuria. The urine calcium-to-creatinine ratio will vary with age. Morning nonfasting urine ratios that exceed the following correlate with quantitative hypercalciuria:
- Age >7 years: >0.24
- Age 5-7 years: >0.30
- Age 3-5 years: >0.41
- Age 1-2 years: >0.56
- Age <1 year: >0.81

150. **What laboratory studies are appropriate during the initial evaluation of children with renal stones?**
- Serum electrolytes, calcium, phosphorus, and creatinine
- 24-hour urine collection for sodium, calcium, creatinine, urate, citrate, uric acid, oxalate, and cystine
- Urine pH (by meter), urinalysis, and urine culture (if indicated)
- Stone analysis on any stone available
- In patients with hypercalciuria, hypercalcemia, or hypophosphatemia, obtain serum parathyroid hormone

Nicoletta JA, Lande MB: Medical evaluation and treatment of urolithiasis, *Pediatr Clin N Am* 53: 479–491, 2006.

151. **What percentage of pediatric patients with urolithiasis will not have hematuria?**
15%.

152. **How does the manipulation of urine pH affect renal calculi?**
Calcium oxalate stones, which are the most common type of renal calculi, are unaffected by the urine pH. These stones can be treated with thiazide diuretics, which increase renal calcium reabsorption and thereby decrease the urinary calcium excretion. Potassium citrate can be added if the urinary citrate excretion is low. Do not restrict calcium intake unless it is excessively high. Calcium phosphate stones may benefit from urinary acidification (in the absence of distal renal tubular acidosis, where lowering the urine pH is not possible). Uric acid stones form in acidic urine and also respond to alkalinization to a pH higher than 6.5. Additional therapy includes a reduction in purine intake and occasionally the use of allopurinol to block the formation of uric acid. High fluid intake plus urine alkalinization (pH >7) helps to block the formation of cystine stones. Penicillamine may also be required in some of these patients. Struvite or infection stones form in extremely alkaline urine. Urine acidification and antibiotics are the cornerstones of treatment for these stones.

153. **When is lithotripsy or surgery indicated for children with kidney stones?**
Most children with stones up to 5 mm will spontaneously pass them. Shock wave lithotripsy (SWL) is useful for children with pelvic or bladder stones that are radiopaque in whom fluoroscopy can be used to focus the shock waves. In general, SWL has a success rate of less than 50% with stones larger than 2 cm. Surgery (percutaneous nephrolithotomy) is generally reserved for children with stones that are causing urinary tract obstruction and for staghorn calculi in older patients that cannot be dissolved. Cystine stones are difficult to fragment by SWL. Ureteroscopy is suited for removal of distal urethral stones.

Durkee CT, Balcom A: Surgical management of urolithiasis, *Pediatr Clin N Am* 53:465–477, 2006.

Mandeville JA, Nelson CP: Pediatric urolithiasis, *Curr Opin Urol* 119:419–423, 2009.

VESICOURETERAL REFLUX

154. **How is VUR graded?**
Figure 13-6 demonstrates the five grades of VUR:
Grade I: Ureter only
Grade II: Ureter, pelvis, and calices; no dilation, normal caliceal fornices
Grade III: Mild dilation and/or tortuosity of the ureter and mild dilation of the renal pelvis; minor blunting of the fornices
Grade IV: Moderate dilation and/or tortuosity of the ureter and moderate dilation of the renal pelvis
Grade V: Significant blunting of most fornices; papillary impressions are no longer visible in most of the calices; gross dilation and tortuosity of the ureter; gross dilation of the renal pelvis and calices

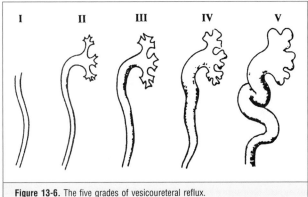

Figure 13-6. The five grades of vesicoureteral reflux.

Duckett JW, Bellinger MF: A plea for standardized grading of vesicoureteral reflux, *Eur Urol* 8:74–77, 1982.

155. **In addition to reflux, what other pathologic bladder findings may be noted on a VCUG?**
Diverticula may be seen, especially in the presence of outflow obstruction. A posterior urethral valve or urethral stricture can be detected during the voiding phase of the study. A ureterocele may be seen and appears as a filling defect in the bladder. Other features to note are the bladder capacity, residual volume after voiding, and thickening or trabeculation of the bladder from muscular hypertrophy.

156. **What is the normal bladder capacity in children?**
Volume (in ounces) = patient's age (in years) + 2. The normal adult bladder capacity is 12 to 16 ounces.

157. **What are the pros and cons of a VCUG versus a radionuclide cystogram (RNC) for the evaluation of reflux?**
   - Both studies require the catheterization of the bladder and the filling of the bladder with an imaging solution.
   - The RNC allows for continuous monitoring of the filling and emptying of the bladder compared with the intermittent fluoroscopy that occurs with the VCUG.
   - There is less radiation exposure with the RNC.

■ The VCUG provides greater anatomic detail of the urethra and bladder and can aid in the evaluation of bladder dysfunction better than the RNC.

■ The VCUG is more accurate for assessing and grading the degrees (I to V) of reflux.

■ In general, most authorities prefer the VCUG for the evaluation of a child with an initial UTI.

158. **How does the radiation exposure differ between RNC and VCUG?**
RNC has about 100 times less the absorbed radiation dose compared with a single radiograph VCUG. Many authorities recommend its use for the screening of siblings with reflux, for evaluating the child with myelomeningocele, and for the ongoing evaluation of significant reflux.

159. **What is the natural history of VUR?**
The likelihood that reflux will resolve spontaneously is influenced by the severity of the reflux at the time of initial diagnosis. About 80% to 90% of patients with grade I to II reflux, 45% with grade III reflux, and 25% with grade IV reflux will experience spontaneous resolution within 5 years. Grade V reflux always requires surgical intervention. The chances for resolution are better in children with unilateral—rather than bilateral—reflux.

KEY POINTS: VESICOURETERAL REFLUX

1. Spontaneous resolution more likely with grades I to III.

2. Thirty percent of these patients will have siblings with vesicoureteral reflux, but sequelae are rare.

3. About 30% of white children with urinary tract infections will have vesicoureteral reflux (less in certain racial groups).

4. Prophylactic antibiotics are intended to prevent pyelonephritis and to limit renal scarring and hypertension, but their utility in this regard is being questioned.

160. **How is VUR managed: medically or surgically?**
■ Grades I-II: These grades are usually managed medically if the family is reliable and will comply with outpatient regimens and follow-up studies.

■ Grades III-IV: If followed expectantly, these types of reflux will resolve slowly, at a rate of about 10% per year. Surgical intervention results in the elimination of this degree of reflux at least 95% of the time. Randomized studies have not shown any significant difference in long-term renal outcome (e.g., renal scarring, hypertension, reduced function) when comparing medical versus surgical treatment.

■ Grade V: Surgical intervention is indicated.

■ In recent years, the development of the STING procedure (subureteral injection of a hyaluronic acid complex, "Deflux") with cystoscopy has added a new, less invasive technique that has had a good rate of success in correcting reflux.

Lee RS, Retik AB: Does the Deflux procedure reduce the incidence of urinary tract infections in children with vesicoureteral reflux? *Nat Clin Pract Urol* 5:182–183, 2008.

Wheeler D, Vimalachandra D, Hodson EM, et al: Antibiotics and surgery for vesicoureteric reflux: a meta-analysis of randomized controlled trials, *Arch Dis Child* 88:688–694, 2003.

161. **Should asymptomatic siblings of a patient with VUR have urologic imaging done as a screen for reflux?**
The incidence of reflux is thought to be less than 1% in normal children, but some studies have demonstrated reflux in 33% to 45% of siblings of patients with reflux. Among identical

twins, the rate is 80%. Consequently, many authorities recommend screening siblings who are younger than 7 years with a radionuclide cystogram. Siblings older than 7 years who have a history of previous UTIs should also be screened for reflux. Although the incidence of reflux is higher in siblings, data are still lacking to prove that the screening and treatment of asymptomatic siblings decreases renal scarring.

ACKNOWLEDGMENT

The editors gratefully acknowledge contributions by Drs. Michael Norman, Thomas Kennedy, James Prebis, and Stephen J. Wassner that were retained from the first three editions of *Pediatric Secrets*.

CHAPTER 14

NEUROLOGY

Kent R. Kelley, MD

ANTIEPILEPTIC DRUGS

1. **Should treatment with antiepileptic drugs (AEDs) be started after the first afebrile seizure in a child?**
   Children with an isolated, uncomplicated seizure usually do not require AED therapy. Epidemiologic studies have shown that about one third of children with an uncomplicated single seizure, a normal neurologic examination, and normal electroencephalogram (EEG) will experience a second. "Delaying" treatment until after the second seizure does not adversely affect the long-term chance of epilepsy remission.

   AEDs are not without risks and side effects, both dose related and idiosyncratic. Other factors, including EEG results, antecedent neurologic history, family history, and imaging (in selective cases), influence the risk for recurrence and should be considered. Risk for recurrent seizures is sharply increased if the seizure was nocturnal, the neurologic status is not normal, there is a positive family history, if no immediate precipitating cause can be identified, and the EEG reveals epileptiform discharges.

   Guerrini R, Arzimanoglou A, Brouwer O: Rationale for treating epilepsy in children, *Epileptic Disord* 4: S9–S21, 2002.

   Hirtz D, Berg A, Bettis D, et al, Quality Standards Subcommittee of the American Academy of Neurology; Practice Committee of the Child Neurology Society: Practice parameter: treatment of the child with a first unprovoked seizure. Report of the Quality Standards Subcommittee of the American Academy of Neurology and the Practice Committee of the Child Neurology Society, *Neurology* 60:166–172, 2003.

   Holmes GL: Overtreatment in children with epilepsy, *Epilepsy Res* 52:35–42, 2002.

2. **What is the advantage of monotherapy chosen according to the epilepsy syndrome?**
   - Chronic toxicity is directly related to the number of drugs consumed.
   - As compared with monotherapy, intellectual and sensorium impairment is increased for any given AEDs (despite "normal" drug levels).
   - Drug interactions may paradoxically lead to loss of seizure control.
   - It is difficult to identify the cause of an adverse reaction.

   Menkes JH, Sankar R: Paroxysmal disorders. In Menkes JH, Sarnat HB, Maria BL, editors: *Child Neurology*, ed 7, Philadelphia, 2006, Lippincott Williams & Wilkins, pp 891–893.

3. **When should blood levels be obtained if seizures are poorly controlled or compliance is questionable?**
   Trough serum drug levels should be obtained to detect subtherapeutic or toxic concentrations. It is most helpful to check the serum level right before the dose, preferably in the morning before any medication is given. An inadequate serum concentration is the most common cause of persistent seizures, but drug toxicity, especially with phenytoin, may also manifest by deteriorating seizure control. There generally will be less variation in blood concentrations with tablets or capsules compared with liquid preparations; suspensions in particular result in notoriously inconsistent dosages.

Glauser TA, Pippenger CE: Controversies in blood-level monitoring: reexamining its role in the treatment of epilepsy, *Epilepsia* 41:S6–S15, 2000.

4. **Which AEDs are recommended for primary generalized tonic-clonic seizures in children?**

The "traditional" AEDs (phenobarbital, primidone, phenytoin) are no longer considered the drugs of choice for grand mal seizures for many age groups because of side effects, although phenobarbital remains the drug of choice for neonatal seizures. Studies have shown that most of the major anticonvulsants are comparable for reducing or eliminating seizure recurrences.

Class I evidence demonstrates that topiramate, lamotrigine, levetiracetam, valproate, and zonisamide are effective for the treatment of primary generalized tonic-clonic seizures. Carbamazepine and oxcarbazepine may cause an increased frequency of primary generalized seizures, especially absence and myoclonic types.

Shankar R: Initial treatment of epilepsy with antiepileptic drugs: pediatric issues, *Neurology* 63:S30–S39, 2004.

French JA, Kanner AM, Bautista J, et al: Therapeutics and Technology Assessment Subcommittee of the American Academy of Neurology; Quality Standards Subcommittee of the American Academy of Neurology; American Epilepsy Society: Efficacy and tolerability of the new antiepileptic drugs I: treatment of new onset epilepsy. Report of the Therapeutics and Technology Assessment Subcommittee and Quality Standards Subcommittee of the American Academy of Neurology and the American Epilepsy Society, *Neurology* 62:1252–1260, 2004.

Malphrus AD, Wilfong AA: Use of the newer antiepileptic drugs in pediatric epilepsies, *Curr Treat Options Neurol* 9:256-267, 2007.

5. **What is the drug of choice for absence epilepsy?**

Ethosuximide (Zarontin), **valproate** (divalproex sodium or Depakote), and **lamotrigine** (Lamictal) are all effective for eliminating or substantially reducing the number of absence attacks. Ethosuximide is traditionally the drug of choice, for several reasons:

- It works well for many patients. It not only stops the clinical attacks of absence, but it often normalizes the EEG by "erasing" the 3/second spike-wave discharges.
- It is well tolerated by most patients. Although rare cases of serious bone marrow, liver, or dermatologic disorders have occurred, routine or frequent blood tests are not considered obligatory by most physicians.
- It has a relatively long serum half-life (40 hours). Thus, once- or twice-daily dosing is appropriate and represents a real convenience to the patient.
- It is relatively inexpensive.

Disadvantages are that ethosuximide only protects against absence seizures. Children with coexisting generalized convulsions should be treated with valproate or lamotrigine. Disadvantages of valproate include the risks for idiosyncratic liver toxicity, weight gain, and teratogenicity. Lamotrigine should also be considered, with the relative risk for rash and generally favorable cognitive profile taken into account.

Glauser TA, Cnaan A, Shinnar S, et al: Ethosuximide, valproic acid, and lamotrigine in childhood absence epilepsy, *N Engl J Med* 362:790-799, 2010.

6. **Can AEDs paradoxically cause a worsening of seizures?**

A paradoxic worsening of seizure control by various AEDs has been noted for decades. Mechanisms may include nonspecific effects of drug intoxication. In addition, specific medications may exacerbate specific seizure types. For example, carbamazepine may worsen the absence, myoclonic, and astatic seizures seen in generalized epilepsy syndromes; phenytoin and vigabatrin may also worsen generalized seizures; and gabapentin and lamotrigine may worsen myoclonic seizures.

Perucca E, Gram L, Avanzini G, Dulac O: Antiepileptic drugs as a cause of worsening seizures, *Epilepsia* 39:5–17, 1998.

7. **What are the typical dose-related side effects of AEDs?**

   Dose-related side effects occur somewhat predictably and can be anticipated, particularly as the medication dose is initiated and escalated. Common dose-related side effects include sedation, headache, gastrointestinal irritation, unsteadiness, and dysarthria. Management commonly consists of reducing the dose by 25% to 50% and waiting about 2 weeks for tolerance to develop. In addition, behavioral and cognitive side effects can occur in some patients; these can be more subtle, and controversy exists regarding the relative effects of various AEDs.

   Loring DW, Meador KJ: Cognitive side effects of the antiepileptic drugs in children, *Neurology* 62: 872–877, 2004.

8. **What idiosyncratic drug reactions are associated with antiepileptic medications?**

   Idiosyncratic reactions occur unpredictably, are potentially fatal, and do not correlate with dose of medication.
   - **Carbamazepine:** Leukopenia, aplastic anemia, thrombocytopenia, hepatic dysfunction, rashes
   - **Ethosuximide:** Leukopenia, pancytopenia, rashes
   - **Phenobarbital:** Rashes, Stevens-Johnson syndrome, hepatic dysfunction
   - **Phenytoin:** Hepatic dysfunction, lymphadenopathy, movement disorder, Stevens-Johnson syndrome, fulminant hepatic failure
   - **Valproic acid:** Fulminant hepatic failure, hyperammonemia, pancreatitis, thrombocytopenia, rash, stupor

9. **Which children are most susceptible to valproic acid–induced acute hepatic failure?**

   The highest incidences occur in children younger than 2 years who are receiving polytherapy (1 in 540). In children younger than 2 years who are receiving valproic acid monotherapy, the rate is reduced to about 1 in 8000. The complication is unrelated to dosage and typically occurs during the first 3 months of therapy. Up to 40% of individuals who receive valproic acid will have dose-related elevations of liver enzymes, which are transient or resolve with dosage adjustments. However, liver function test monitoring is not helpful for predicting acute hepatic failure. It has been hypothesized that valproic acid may cause carnitine deficiency, hyperammonemia, and hepatotoxicity. Despite a lack of data from clinical trials, some clinicians recommend prophylactic carnitine supplementation.

   Bryant AE, Dreifuss FE: Valproic acid hepatic fatalities, *Neurology* 48:465–469, 1996.

10. **What are the warning signs and symptoms of hypersensitivity syndromes?**

    Symptoms often occur early, within the first months of treatment. Families need to be educated about the potential for drug reactions. Concerning symptoms include body temperature higher than 40°C, protracted vomiting, lethargy, exfoliation of the skin, mucosal (or palm or sole) lesions, facial edema, swelling of the tongue, confluent erythema, skin pain, palpable purpura, protracted bleeding from minor cuts, lymph node enlargement, and asthmatic symptoms. Multiple studies have shown that families fail to appreciate evolving symptoms of idiosyncratic reactions and continue to administer the offending agent. Examination may reveal lymphadenopathy, palpable purpura, blisters, and wheezing. Laboratory abnormalities may include eosinophilia, atypical lymphocytosis, and abnormal liver function enzymes. Routine surveillance of blood chemistries and complete blood counts (every 3 to 6 months) are standard practice, but they are unlikely to identify potentially life-threatening conditions.

    Browne TR, Holmes GL: Epilepsy, *N Engl J Med* 344:1145–1151, 2001.

    Stern RS: Improving the outcome of patients with toxic epidermal necrolysis and Stevens-Johnson syndrome, *Arch Dermatol* 136:410–411, 2000.

11. **What are the suggested dosing guidelines and therapeutic ranges of AEDs?**
See Table 14-1.

TABLE 14-1. GUIDELINES FOR DOSES OF ESTABLISHED ANTIEPILEPTIC DRUGS IN CHILDREN*			
Drug	Trade Name	Standard Maintenance Dose Range (mg/kg/day)	Target Plasma Drug Concentration Range (mg/mL)
Carbamazepine	Tegretol/Carbatrol	10-30	4-12
Ethosuximide	Zarontin	15-40	40-120
Gabapentin	Neurontin	30-45	5-15
Lamotrigine (monotherapy)	Lamictal	2-8	2-20
Levetiracetam	Keppra	10-20	Therapeutic range in children not yet established
Oxcarbazepine	Trileptal	20-40	5-50
Phenobarbital	Luminal	2-10	10-45
Phenytoin	Dilantin, Fosphenytoin	4-7	10-30
Tiagabine	Gabitril	1-2	5-70
Topiramate	Topamax	5-10	2-25
Valproate	Depakote	30-45	60-120
Zonisamide	Zonegran	4-12	10-40

*Therapeutic ranges are somewhat arbitrary. Levels above "normal" may be maintained to control seizures if side effects do not occur. Conversely, levels in the therapeutic range may have toxic effects. It is important to treat the patient and not the number.

12. **What is Diastat?**
Diazepam rectal gel (Diastat) has been approved for the treatment of status epilepticus and severe recurrent convulsive seizures in children. It is prescribed for home use by parents. Dosages (as they are for most medications in pediatric patients) are based on weight, and the medication is available in various premixed concentrations with syringe applicators.

13. **After what period can AEDs be safely discontinued?**
The withdrawal of antiepileptic drugs should be considered when the child is free of seizures for 2 years because well-controlled investigations have shown that the risk for relapse in children whose seizures have been in remission for 2 years is low. Although there is no uniform agreement about factors that are predictive of outcome, the highest remission rate appears to occur in those who are otherwise neurologically normal and in whom the EEG at the time of discontinuation lacks specific epileptiform features and displays a normal

background. The prognosis is the worst for children with symptomatic epilepsies, persistently abnormal EEGs, and abnormal neurologic examinations.

Greenwood RS, Tennison MB: When to start and stop anticonvulsant therapy in children, *Neurology* 56:1073–1077, 1999.

Smith R, Ball R: Discontinuing anticonvulsant medication in children, *Arch Dis Child* 87:259–260, 2002.

14. **When the decision is made to discontinue AEDs, should the tapering period be long or short?**
In practice, all AEDs should be tapered gradually rather than abruptly discontinued, although there is no actual withdrawal state produced by a "cold turkey" reduction of most AEDs (e.g., phenytoin, carbamazepine, valproate, ethosuximide). By contrast, a withdrawal syndrome of agitation, signs of autonomic overactivity, and seizures follow the sudden elimination of habitually consumed diazepam or short-acting barbiturates (e.g., secobarbital). The long elimination half-life of phenobarbital lessens the risk for withdrawal symptoms after abrupt discontinuation.

In a study of more than 100 children who had been seizure free for either 2 or 4 years, the risk for seizure recurrence during tapering and after discontinuation of the AED was no different if the period of taper was 6 weeks or 9 months. Rapid tapering appears to be an acceptable means of discontinuation.

Tennison M, Greenwood R, Lewis D, Thorn M: Discontinuing antiepileptic drugs in children with epilepsy: a comparison of a six-week and a nine-month taper period, *N Engl J Med* 330:1407–1410, 1994.

CEREBRAL PALSY

15. **What is cerebral palsy?**
Cerebral palsy (CP) describes a heterogeneous group of nonprogressive (static) motor and posture disorders of cerebral or cerebellar origin that typically manifest early in life. The primary impairment involves significant deficits in motor planning and control. Note that the definition does not imply etiology. Causes include cerebral malformations, metabolic and genetic causes, infection (both intrauterine and extrauterine), stroke, hypoxia-ischemia, and trauma. The process is nonprogressive, and the motor function that is affected results from the part of the brain that is involved. Although nonprogressive, clinical manifestations often change over time as the functional expression of the underlying brain is modified by normal brain development and maturation.

American Academy for Cerebral Palsy and Developmental Medicine: http://www.aacpdm.org.

United Cerebral Palsy Association: http://www.ucp.org.

16. **What are the Levine (POSTER) criteria for the diagnosis of CP?**
   - **P**osturing/abnormal movements
   - **O**ropharyngeal problems (e.g., tongue thrusts, swallowing abnormalities)
   - **S**trabismus
   - **T**one (hypertonia or hypotonia)
   - **E**volutional maldevelopment (primitive reflexes persist or protective/equilibrium reflexes fail to develop [e.g., lateral prop, parachute reflex])
   - **R**eflexes (increased deep tendon reflexes/persistent Babinski reflex)
   Abnormalities in four of these six categories strongly point to the diagnosis of CP.

Feldman HM: Developmental-behavioral pediatrics. In Zitelli BJ, Davis HW, editors: *Atlas of Pediatric Diagnosis*, ed 5, St. Louis, 2007, Mosby, p 82.

17. **What are the types of cerebral palsy?**

Clinical classification is based on the nature of the movement disorder and muscle tone and anatomic distribution. A single patient may have more than one type. Spastic cerebralpalsy is the most common, accounting for about two thirds of cases.

Spastic (or pyramidal) CP: Characterized by neurologic signs of upper motor neuron damage with increased "clasp knife" muscle tone, increased deep tendon reflexes, pathologic reflexes, and spastic weakness. Spastic CP is subclassified based on distribution:

- Hemiplegia: Primarily unilateral involvement, arm usually more than leg
- Quadriplegia: All limbs involved, with legs often more involved than arms
- Diplegia: Legs much more involved than arms, which may show no or only minimal impairment

Dyskinetic (nonspastic or extrapyramidal) CP: Characterized by prominent involuntary movements or fluctuating muscle tone with choreoathetosis the most common subtype. Distribution is usually symmetric among the four limbs.

Ataxic CP: Primarily cerebellar signs (including ataxia, dysmetria, past pointing, nystagmus)

Mixed types

Murphy N, Such-Neibar T: Cerebral palsy diagnosis and management: the state of the art, *Curr Probl Pediatr Adolesc Health Care* 33:146–169, 2003.

18. **What proportion of CP is related to birth asphyxia?**

In contrast with popular perception, large clinical epidemiologic and longitudinal studies indicate that perinatal asphyxia is an important—but relatively minor—cause. Estimates range from a low of 3% to a high of 21%. In most cases, the events leading to CP occur in the fetus before the onset of labor or in the newborn after delivery.

Nelson KB: Can we prevent cerebral palsy? *N Engl J Med* 349:1765–1769, 2003.

19. **How well do Apgar scores correlate with the development of CP?**

In a large study of 49,000 infants, a low Apgar score correlated poorly with the development of CP. Of term infants with scores of 0 to 3 at 1 or 5 minutes, 95% did not develop CP. Of those with scores of 0 to 3 at 10 minutes, 84% did not develop CP. If the 10-minute Apgar score improved to 4 or more, the rate for CP was less than 1%. A low Apgar score (0 to 3) at 20 minutes, however, had an observed CP rate of nearly 60%. Conversely, nearly 75% of patients with CP had 5-minute Apgar scores of 7 to 10.

Nelson KB, Ellenberg JH: Apgar scores as predictors of chronic neurologic disability, *Pediatrics* 68: 36–44, 1981.

Papile Lu-Ann: The Apgar score in the 21st century, *N Engl J Med* 344:519–520, 2001.

20. **Why is CP difficult to diagnose clinically during the first year of life?**

- Hypotonia is more common than hypertonia and spasticity in the first year, which makes the prediction of CP difficult.
- The early abundance of primitive reflexes (with variable persistence) may confuse the clinical picture.
- An infant has a limited variety of volitional movements for evaluation.
- Substantial myelination takes months to evolve and may delay the clinical picture of abnormal tone and increased deep tendon reflexes.
- Most infants who develop CP do not have identifiable risk factors; most cases are not related to labor and delivery events.

Shapiro BK, Capute AJ: Cerebral palsy. In McMillan JA, DeAngelis CD, Feigin RD, Warshaw JB, editors: *Oski's Pediatrics, Principles and Practice*, ed 3, Philadelphia, 1999, Lippincott Williams & Wilkins, pp 1910–1917.

KEY POINTS: CEREBRAL PALSY

1. Apgar scores correlate poorly with the ultimate diagnosis of cerebral palsy.

2. During the first year of life, hypotonia is more common than hypertonia in patients who are ultimately diagnosed with the disease.

3. Keep an eye on the eyes: As many as 75% of children with cerebral palsy have ophthalmologic problems (e.g., strabismus, refractive errors).

4. Spastic hemiplegia is the most common type of cerebral palsy that is associated with seizures.

5. Monitor regularly for hip subluxation, especially in patients with spastic diparesis, because earlier identification assists therapy.

21. **What behavioral symptoms during the first year should arouse suspicion about the possibility of CP?**
    - Excessive irritability, constant crying, and sleeping difficulties (severe colic is noted in up to 30% of babies who are eventually diagnosed with CP)
    - Early feeding difficulties with difficulties in coordinating suck and swallow, frequent spitting up, and poor weight gain
    - "Jittery" or "jumpy" behavior, especially at times other than when hungry
    - Easily startled behavior
    - Stiffness when handled, especially during dressing, diapering, and handwashing
    - Paradoxically "precocious" development, such as early rolling (actually a sudden, reflexive roll rather than a volitional one) or the stiff-legged "standing" with support of an infant with spastic diplegia

    Bennett FC: Diagnosing cerebral palsy—the earlier the better, *Contemp Pediatr* 16:65–76, 1999.

22. **What gross motor delays are diagnostically important in the infant with possible CP?**
    - Inability to bring the hands together in midline while in a supine position by the age of 4 months
    - Head lag persisting beyond 6 months
    - No volitional rolling by 6 months
    - Inability to independently sit straight by 8 months
    - No hands-and-knees crawling by 12 months

    Bennett FC: Diagnosing cerebral palsy—the earlier the better, *Contemp Pediatr* 16:65–76, 1999.

23. **What problems are commonly associated with CP?**
    - **Mental retardation:** Two thirds of total patients; most commonly observed in children with spastic quadriplegia
    - **Failure to thrive, growth retardation**
    - **Feeding problems** (including dysphagia, sialorrhea)
    - **Gastrointestinal problems** (gastroesophageal reflux, constipation)
    - **Learning disabilities**
    - **Ophthalmologic abnormalities** (strabismus, amblyopia, nystagmus, refractive errors)
    - **Hearing deficits**
    - **Communication disorders**

- **Epilepsy:** One half of total patients; most commonly observed in children with spastic hemiplegia
- **Behavioral and emotional problems** (especially attention-deficit hyperactivity disorder, depression, sleep problems)
- **Urinary problems** (incontinence, voiding dysfunction, urinary tract infections)
- **Spinal column changes** (kyphosis, scoliosis)
- **Respiratory problems** (upper airway obstruction, chronic aspiration)

Dodge NN: Cerebral palsy: medical aspects, *Pediatr Clin N Am* 55:1189–1207, 2008.

24. **What features in an infant suggest a progressive central nervous system (CNS) disorder rather than CP as the cause of a motor deficit?**
    - **Abnormally increasing head circumference:** Possible hydrocephalus, tumor, or neurodegenerative disorder
    - **Eye anomalies:** Cataracts, retinal pigmentary degeneration, optic atrophy (possible neurodegenerative disease), coloboma, chorioretinal lacuna, optic nerve hypoplasia (possible Aicardi syndrome or septo-optic dysplasia)
    - **Skin abnormalities:** Vitiligo, café-au-lait spots, nevus flammeus, port-wine stain (possible Sturge-Weber syndrome or neurofibromatosis)
    - **Hepatomegaly and/or splenomegaly** (possible storage disease)
    - **Decreased or absent deep tendon reflexes**
    - **Sensory abnormalities:** Diminished sense of pain, position, vibration, or light touch
    - **Developmental regression or failure to progress:** Rett syndrome or Leigh disease

    Taft LT: Cerebral palsy, *Pediatr Rev* 16:411–418, 1995.

25. **What therapies are used to treat the spasticity and dystonia of cerebral palsy?**
    - **Casting:** Serial "inhibitive" casting can reduce tone and allow improved gait and weight-bearing activities
    - **Nerve blocks, motor point blocks, botulinum toxin:** Injected to target spasticity in particular muscle groups
    - **Oral and intrathecal medications:** Including baclofen, dantrolene, carbidopa-levodopa, clonazepam
    - **Selective dorsal rhizotomy:** A neurosurgical procedure that interrupts the afferent component of the deep tendon (stretch) reflex
    - **Tendon-lengthening surgeries:** At ankle, knee, wrist, or elbow to prevent or delay joint contractures

    Pellegrino L: Cerebral palsy. In Batshaw ML, Pellegrino L, Roizen NJ, editors: *Children with Disabilities*, ed 6, Baltimore, 2007, Paul H. Brookes Publishing, pp 387–408.

    Bjornson K, Hays R, Graubert C, et al: Botulinum toxin for spasticity in children with cerebral palsy: a comprehensive evaluation, *Pediatrics* 120:49–58, 2007.

CEREBROSPINAL FLUID

26. **What is normal cerebrospinal fluid (CSF) pressure?**
    CSF pressure as measured during a lumbar puncture varies with age, positional technique, and combativeness of the patient. For truly accurate pressures, the child should be relaxed with legs extended. CSF can be seen in the manometer varying with respirations when the needle has been properly placed. As a general guide, upper limits of normal by age are as follows:
    - Neonate: 60 mm H_2O
    - 1 month to 4 years: 80 mm H_2O

- 4 to 12 years: 90 mm H_2O
- Adolescent to adult: 180 mm H_2O

Tureen JH: Meningitis. In Bergelson JM, Shah SS, Zaoutis TE, editors: *Pediatric Infectious Disease: The Requisites in Pediatrics*, Philadelphia, 2008, Mosby Elsevier, p 56.

27. **What are the normal CSF volumes in an infant, child, and adolescent?**
Estimates for the volume of the ventricular system are 40 to 50 mL in a term newborn, 65 to 100 mL in an older child, and 90 to 150 mL in a teenager or adult. The choroid plexus actively secretes a distillate of CSF at a rate of 0.3 to 0.4 mL/minute in children and adults, which equals about 20 mL/hour or 500 mL/day. This equates to an hourly CSF volume turnover rate of about 15%.

28. **What are the common causes of an elevated CSF protein?**
Elevated CSF protein (>30 mg/dL) is a nonspecific finding that is encountered in various neurologic disorders. Several common etiologies should be considered:
- **Infection:** Tuberculous meningitis, acute bacterial meningitis (pneumococcal, meningococcal, *Haemophilus influenzae*), syphilitic or viral meningitis, encephalitis
- **Inflammation:** Guillain-Barré syndrome (GBS), multiple sclerosis, peripheral neuropathy, postinfectious encephalopathy
- **Tumor** of the cerebral hemispheres or spinal cord
- **Vascular accidents,** such as cerebral hemorrhage (including subarachnoid hemorrhage, subdural hemorrhage, intracerebral hemorrhages) or stroke as a result of cranial arteritis, diabetes mellitus, or hypertension
- **Degenerative disorders** involving white-matter disease (e.g., Krabbe disease)
- **Metabolic disorders** (e.g., uremia)
- **Toxins** (e.g., lead)

29. **What CSF findings suggest metabolic disease as a cause of neurologic signs and symptoms?**
- **Elevated CSF protein concentration** is characteristic of metachromatic leukodystrophy and globoid cell encephalopathy.
- **Low CSF glucose concentration** is consistent with hypoglycemia caused by a defect of gluconeogenesis or a defect in the transport of glucose across the blood-brain barrier (GLUT-1 deficiency syndrome).
- **Low CSF folate concentration** suggests a defect involving folate metabolism.
- **Presence in the CSF of amino acids, specifically glycine, glutamate, and γ-aminobutyric acid (GABA),** may be diagnostic of nonketotic hyperglycinemia, pyridoxine-dependent epilepsy, or another defect in the GABA shunt.
- **Lactate** and **pyruvate** values are elevated in CSF disorders of cerebral energy metabolism, including pyruvate dehydrogenase deficiency, pyruvate carboxylase deficiency, numerous disturbances of the respiratory chain, and Menkes syndrome.
- **Low CSF lactate** value may be seen in the GLUT-1 deficiency syndrome.
- **Abnormal CSF biogenic amines** suggest several disorders that are associated with disturbed neurotransmission.

30. **As tests of meningeal irritation, what constitutes a positive Kernig or Brudzinski sign?**
Kernig sign, or the straight-leg-raising sign, consists of flexing the hip to 90 degrees and attempting to extend the knee. The limitation of knee extension as a result of painful resistance is a positive sign.

Brudzinski sign is a positive sign, and it is present if a reflex flexion of the thighs occurs when a patient's neck is passively flexed.

31. **How do the manifestations of increased intracranial pressure (ICP) differ in an infant compared with an older child?**
   - **Infant:** Increasing head circumference, delayed closure of the fontanel, suture separation, bulging fontanel, failure to thrive, macrocephaly, setting-sun sign, shrill cry
   - **Older child:** Headache (especially in the early morning, awakening the child from sleep, or association with vomiting), nausea, persistent vomiting, personality and mood changes, lethargy, anorexia, fatigue, somnolence, diplopia as a result of sixth-nerve palsy or third-nerve palsy with uncal herniation, papilledema

32. **What comprises the Cushing triad?**
   The *Cushing triad* consists of the development of **slow or irregular respirations, decreased heart rate,** and **elevated blood pressure** (particularly an increased systolic pressure with a widening pulse pressure) resulting from an increase in ICP. The Cushing triad may be observed in children with increased ICP or compression of the posterior fossa, which houses the medullary circulatory control center. It is a very late finding of increased ICP.

33. **How is hydrocephalus classified?**
   Communicating hydrocephalus is present if a tracer dye injected into one lateral ventricle appears in the lumbar CSF. This type of hydrocephalus is caused by an inability to normally reabsorb CSF by the arachnoid granulations, which can occur from meningeal scarring as a result of bacterial meningitis or intraventricular hemorrhage.

   Noncommunicating hydrocephalus refers to conditions causing intraventricular obstruction and alteration of the flow of dye into the lumbar CSF. Congenital malformations (especially aqueductal stenosis and Dandy-Walker syndrome with cystic dilation of the fourth ventricle) and mass lesions (e.g., tumors, arteriovenous malformations) can cause noncommunicating hydrocephalus.

   Hydrocephalus *ex vacuo* describes increases in volume without increased CSF pressure, which is seen in conditions of reduced cerebral tissue (e.g., malformation, atrophy).

34. **What is the normal growth rate of head circumference during the first year of life?**
   Head circumference at birth is about 34 cm for the term infant. The head circumference normally grows by 2 cm/month for the first 3 months of life, 1 cm/month for months 4 to 6, and 0.5 cm/month up to 1 year of life. The measurement of head circumference should be part of the examination of any child and should be plotted at every visit. The head circumference represents brain growth, but it is also influenced by hydrocephalus and subdural or epidural fluid collections.

35. **What are the complications of ventricular shunts?**
   Ventricular shunts drain CSF from the ventricles in patients whose normal outflow or absorption has been blocked. The fluid may be drained to a variety of different locations, including the peritoneum, kidney, or atrium. Shunts draining CSF have remarkably improved the outcome of children with hydrocephalus, but they are subject to obstruction, infection, or mechanical malfunction. Shunt malfunctions present signs of increased ICP. Children with shunt infections often have a low-grade fever as well as signs of increased ICP. Because it is impossible to know the compliance properties of the ventricular system, children with shunt malfunction or infection are at risk for sudden, catastrophic decompensation. Children suspected of having shunt malfunctions or infection require urgent attention, and they should be closely observed until the shunt has been fully evaluated.

   Piatt JH Jr, Garton HJL: Clinical diagnosis of ventriculoperitoneal shunt failure among children with hydrocephalus, *Pediatr Emerg Care* 24:201–210, 2008.

Duhaime A-C: Evaluation and management of shunt infections in children with hydrocephalus, *Clin Pediatr* 45:705–713, 2006.

36. **What are the characteristic features of pseudotumor cerebri?**
    Pseudotumor cerebri (also called *benign* or *idiopathic intracranial hypertension*) consists of an increased ICP in the absence of a demonstrable mass lesion and with a normal CSF formula. Characteristic features include the following:
    - Headache, fatigue, vomiting, anorexia, stiff neck, and diplopia from increased ICP
    - Normal neurologic examination except for papilledema or a third- or sixth-nerve palsy
    - Normal computed tomography (CT) scan, except sometimes for small ventricles
    - Normal CSF profile with the exception of an elevated opening pressure

37. **What causes pseudotumor cerebri?**
    Although there are multiple possible causes, more than 90% of cases are idiopathic. Among the reported causes are the following:
    - **Drugs:** Tetracycline, nalidixic acid, nitrofurantoin, corticosteroids, excess vitamin A
    - **Endocrine disorders:** Hyperthyroidism, Cushing syndrome, hypoparathyroidism
    - **Thrombosis** of the dural venous sinuses as a result of head trauma, otitis media, mastoiditis, or obstruction of jugular veins in the superior vena cava syndrome

38. **What treatment is recommended for severe cases of pseudotumor cerebri?**
    Patients with sustained visual field loss or severe refractory headache are candidates for treatment. Specific treatment depends on the presence of an identifiable precipitant, which should be removed when possible. For example, the cessation of the offending medication (e.g., tetracycline) or weight reduction in obese patients is recommended. Nonspecific treatment includes the administration of acetazolamide, furosemide, or hydrochlorothiazide and, sometimes, corticosteroids. In severe cases, surgical intervention is available through installation of a lumboperitoneal shunt or optic nerve sheath decompression.

    Matthews YY: Drugs used in childhood idiopathic or benign intracranial hypertension, *Arch Dis Child Educ Pract Ed* 93:19–25, 2008.

39. **Why is a stylet used during a lumbar puncture?**
    A stylet is typically used during a lumbar puncture to prevent epidermis (which might lodge in an open-ended needle) from being introduced into the subarachnoid space, where an epidermal tumor might form. There is debate about whether the stylet should be kept in place after the needle passes the subcutaneous space or removed at that point to allow a better assessment of CSF flow when the needle enters the subarachnoid space. After fluid has been collected, some experts advocate reinserting the stylet to minimize the potential to prevent attached arachnoid strands from causing prolonged CSF leakage through the dura, which may cause prolonged headaches.

    Ellenby MS, Tegtmeyer K, Lai S, Braner DAV: Videos in clinical medicine. Lumbar puncture, *N Engl J Med* 355:e12:2006.

    Baxter AL, Fisher RG, Burke BL, et al: Local anesthetic in stylet styles: factors associated with resident lumbar puncture success, *Pediatrics* 117:876–881, 2006.

    Strupp M, Brandt T, Muller A: Incidence of post-lumbar puncture syndrome reduced by reinserting the stylet: a randomized prospective study of 600 patients, *J Neurol* 245:589–592, 1998.

CLINICAL ISSUES

40. **What are the two key concepts in neurology?**
    - Localization of the lesion
    - Time course of the disorder: Paroxysmal, acute, subacute, or chronic

41. **What are general rules that govern localization of a potential neurologic problem?**
A problem can occur anywhere along the neuron axis: cerebrum, cerebellum, brainstem, spinal cord, nerve, neuromuscular junction, and muscle.
- **Cerebrum:** May present with seizures, mental status changes, headaches, unilateral signs (such as hemiparesis)
- **Cerebellum:** May involve ataxia, disturbances of speech, disorders of limb movement, nystagmus
- **Brainstem:** Combination of cranial nerve abnormalities and long-track signs (symmetrical weakness with or without sensory changes)
- **Spinal cord:** Defined level of impairment with motor and/or sensory changes below involved area and normal examination above
- **Neuropathy:** Distal more than proximal weakness with or without sensory changes
- **Muscle disease:** Proximal more than distal weakness with decreased deep tendon reflexes and normal sensation

Goldstein JL: Pediatric neurology in the emergency department: localization followed by differential diagnosis, *Clin Pediatr Emerg Med* 9:87, 2008.

42. **What distinguishes the pediatric neurologic examination?**
Observation. The most useful information is often acquired by watching the child move and play. The level of interaction, creativity, and degree of sustained attention can be observed and are all important components of the mental status examination. By observing eye movements, response to sounds, the child's reaction to visual stimuli introduced into the peripheral visual field, and the symmetry of facial movements, most of the cranial nerves can be tested. Persistent asymmetries of spontaneous motor activity (e.g., consistently reaching across midline for an object) are reliable signs of weakness. Inspection of the seated posture and gait of the child provides an assessment of the cerebellum and cerebellar outflow pathways.

43. **What are the advantages and disadvantages of various imaging procedures used in pediatric neurologic evaluation?**
- **Skull films** are useful for detection of fractures, lytic lesions, and widened sutures. They have poor sensitivity and specificity for intracranial pathology in the setting of trauma.
- **CT scan without contrast** is the best imaging technique for neurologic emergencies to screen a patient with significant head trauma for skull fractures, signs of herniation, or acute intracranial hemorrhage. It can also be used to screen for acute strokes and subarachnoid hemorrhages. Midline or ventricular shifts due to masses and cerebral edema or increased ICP can be noted. CT identifies bone clearly. This rapid study allows routine monitoring and is less expensive than magnetic resonance imaging (MRI). There is a small but defined risk associated with radiation from CT scans.
- **CT scan with contrast** uses radiodense contrast material to allow better identification of disruptions in the blood-brain barrier or of highly vascular structures, significantly improving detection of tumors, edema, focal inflammation, hemangiomas, and arteriovenous malformations.
- **MRI without contrast** is the preferred modality for most nonurgent examinations. It defines structures of brain more precisely than CT, especially within spinal cord, posterior fossa, and cisterns. It is more effective for subtle hemorrhages (especially subacute and chronic) and for tumors or masses. Different tissue-specific relaxation constants, called T1 and T2, and proton density allow for better definition of white and gray matter. It also provides an image in three dimensions. Its longer testing time may require sedation. Also, monitoring patients is more difficult in closed units. There are no known biologic

hazards from MRI, which measures the emission of radio waves released when protons return to a lower energy state after excitation within characteristic tissue environments. MRI is contraindicated in patients with metallic implants that are ferromagnetic.

- **MRI with contrast** is helpful in defining brain metastases and distinguishing postoperative scarring from other pathology.
- **Magnetic resonance angiography (MRA)** is a special type of MRI that displays larger arteries and veins without the use of contrast. It is less invasive than traditional arteriograms, and it is useful in defining arterial stenosis and identifying intracranial hemangiomas, arteriovenous malformations, and vascular aneurysms.
- **MR spectroscopy (MRS)** allows for *in vivo* examination of some chemical constituents of the brain including choline (NAA), a neuronal marker, and lactate (a marker of energy metabolism).
- **Functional MRI (fMRI)** allows for *in vivo* anatomic localization of the motor strip and components of expressive and receptive language.
- **Positron emission tomography (PET)** detects localized functional abnormalities using short half-life isotopes of carbon, nitrogen, oxygen, and fluorine. Labeled glucose ligands are useful in the evaluation of epileptic foci before surgery. These are areas of reduced cerebral glucose metabolism during interictal periods.
- **Single-photon emission computed tomography (SPECT)** uses gamma-ray emission of lipophilic isotopes in the measurement of cerebral blood flow and is also used in the study of refractory epilepsies.

Menkes JH, Moser FG, Maria BL: Neurologic examination of the child and infant. In Menkes JH, Sarnat HB, Maria BL, editors: *Child Neurology*, ed 7, Philadelphia, 2006, Lippincott Williams & Wilkins, pp 18–27.

44. **A child presents with progressive left leg weakness and diplopia, especially when looking toward the left. Where is the lesion?**
The above history, in combination with an examination showing upper motor neuron nerve dysfunction, long tract signs, brisk reflexes, upgoing toe (Babinski sign), and a contralateral third-nerve palsy (down and out), localizes the lesion to the **right pyramidal tract before the decussation** (crossing over) and involves a lesion of the **right third-nerve nucleus**. The progressive course suggests a slow-growing lesion, such as a pontine glioma.

45. **A dilated and unreactive pupil indicates the compression of what structure?**
The third cranial nerve. This may be the result of compression anywhere along the course of the nerve. Uncal herniation is a medial displacement of the uncus of the temporal lobe and may cause this sign.

46. **Pinpoint pupils and respiratory changes indicate the compression of what structure?**
Progressive central herniation of the brain downward through the foramen magnum causes compression of the **pons** and can produce this finding.

47. **How does the presentation of stroke differ between infants and older children?**
Infants usually have a seizure, whereas older children have acute hemiplegia.

Calder K, Kokorowski P, Tran T, Henderson S: Emergency department presentation of stroke, *Pediatr Emerg Care* 19:320–328, 2003.

Children's Hemiplegia and Stroke Association: http://www.chasa.org.

Pediatric Stroke Network: http://www.pediatricstrokenetwork.org.

48. **What is the differential diagnosis of stroke in children?**
Cerebrovascular disease, or stroke, can be the result of primary vascular disease, bleeding disorder (hemorrhagic stroke), or a variety of secondary problems that lead to thrombotic or embolic occlusions (most commonly of the middle cerebral artery). Diagnostic possibilities include the following:
- **Cardioembolic:** Cyanotic congenital heart disease, atrial myxoma, endocarditis, rheumatic or other valvular heart disease
- **Hematologic:** Hemoglobinopathies (especially sickle cell disease), hypercoagulable states (antithrombin III deficiency, protein C or S deficiency), hyperviscosity (leukemia, hyperproteinemia, thrombocytosis), coagulation disorders (lupus-associated antibodies, hemophilia, thrombocytopenia, factor V abnormalities, hyperhomocysteinemia)
- **Circulatory:** Vasculitis (infectious or inflammatory), occlusive (homocystinuria, arteriosclerosis, fibromuscular dysplasia of the internal carotid artery, posttraumatic carotid scarring), carotid or vertebral artery dissection, moyamoya disease, atrioventricular malformation with steal syndrome, anomalous circulation, posttraumatic air embolism, arterial aneurysm, hemiplegic migraine
- **Metabolic:** Mitochondrial disease

Pappachan J, Kirkham FJ: Cerebrovascular disease and stroke, *Arch Dis Child* 93:890–898, 2008.

Carlin TM, Chanmugam A: Stroke in children, *Emerg Med Clin North Am* 20:671–685, 2002.

49. **What is the derivation of "moyamoya" in moyamoya disease?**
Moyamoya, which is Japanese for "puff of smoke," refers to the cerebral angiographic appearance of patients with this primary vascular disease that results in stenosis of the internal carotid artery. It also occurs in a wide variety of conditions, such as neurofibromatosis type 1, sickle cell disease, Down syndrome, and tuberous sclerosis, in addition to the idiopathic condition that is endemic in Japan. Because it is a chronic condition, fine vascular collaterals can develop, and it is these collaterals that create the "puff of smoke" appearance on angiography.

Scott RM, Smith ER: Moyamoya disease and moyamoya syndrome, *N Engl J Med* 360:1226–1237, 2009.

50. **A child who develops weakness, incontinence, and ataxia 10 days after a bout of influenza likely has what diagnosis?**
Acute disseminated encephalomyelitis is thought to be a postinfectious or parainfectious process that is targeted against central myelin. Any portion of the white matter may be affected. Multiple lesions with a perivenular lymphocytic and mononuclear cell infiltration and demyelination are seen on pathologic examination. Acute disseminated encephalomyelitis has been associated with mumps, measles, rubella, varicella-zoster, influenza, parainfluenza, mononucleosis, and immunization. An associated transverse myelitis may be acute (developing over hours) or subacute (developing over 1 to 2 weeks), with both motor and sensory tract involvement. Bladder and bowel dysfunction is often early and severe. CSF examination shows mild increase of pressure and up to 250 cells/mm^3, with a lymphocyte predominance. The MRI shows an increased T2 signal intensity. Prognosis, particularly with the use of intravenous corticosteroids, is good.

51. **In patients with acute injury to the brain, what two types of edema may occur?**
- **Vasogenic edema** results from increased permeability of the capillary endothelium with resulting exudation. It is more marked in cerebral white matter and occurs as a result of inflammation (meningitis and abscess), focal processes (hemorrhage, infarct, or tumor), vessel pathology, or lead or hypertensive encephalopathy.
- **Cytotoxic edema** results from the rapid swelling of cells, especially astrocytes, and also from neurons and endothelial cells as a result of dysfunction of the membranes and ionic

pumps from energy failure, which may lead to cellular death. Hypoxia caused by cardiac arrest, hypoxic-ischemic encephalopathy (HIE), various toxins, severe infections, status epilepticus, infarct, or increased ICP is also a possible cause.

52. **What are the treatments for increased ICP?**
   - **Hyperventilation:** The usual goal is to lower the P_{CO_2} to 25 to 30 mm. This causes vasoconstriction, which decreases the intracranial vascular volume.
   - **Fluid restriction, osmotic diuretics,** and **hypertonic mannitol solution** all work to shrink brain water content, provided there is an intact blood-brain barrier.
   - **Head elevation** in a midline position to 30 degrees maximizes venous return.
   - **External ventricular drains** are sometimes placed, both to monitor pressure and to allow for a minimal amount of CSF withdrawal.
   - **Normalization of physiologic parameters:** It is important to avoid significant hypotension, hypoxia, hypoglycemia, and hyperthermia.

53. **How is brain death defined?**
   Brain death is defined by an irreversible absence of cortical and midbrain activity. There must be an absence of a reversible etiology (i.e., toxic-metabolic, medication, hypothermia, hypotension, or surgically remediable causes). Spinal cord, peripheral nerve, or reflex muscular activity may persist despite brain death. Decorticate or decerebrate posturing, however, is inconsistent with brain death. The examination must remain unchanged over time. Other countries have defined brain death as the absence of brainstem function alone, but in the United States, the absence of cortical function also must be demonstrated. The clinical hallmark of brain death is deep, unremitting, unresponsive coma.

   Banasiak KJ, Lister G: Brain death in children, *Curr Opin Pediatr* 15:288–293, 2003.

   Wijdicks EFM: The diagnosis of brain death, *N Engl J Med* 344:1215–1221, 2001.

54. **How is the diagnosis of brain death made?**
   Patients with suspected brain death should be observed over 12 to 24 hours for the following:
   - Unresponsive coma and the absence of eye opening, extraocular movements, vocalizations, or other cerebral-generated activity
   - The complete absence of brainstem function, including nonresponsive, midposition, or fully dilated pupils; no spontaneous or reflexive eye movements on oculovestibular testing ("doll's eyes" and calorics); no bulbar muscle function (i.e., corneal, gag, cough, sucking, and rooting reflexes); and no respirations on apnea testing
   Supportive testing, if needed, to document brain death can include absent cerebral cortical activity as evidenced by a properly recorded "flat," "isoelectric," or electrocerebral silence (determined by EEG), the absence of blood flow to the hemispheres by cerebral arteriography or radionuclide study, or the presence of ICP that exceeds mean blood pressure for several hours.

   Banasiak KJ, Lister G: Brain death in children, *Curr Opin Pediatr* 15:288–293, 2003.

   Wijdicks EFM: The diagnosis of brain death, *N Engl J Med* 344:1215–1221, 2001.

55. **How do the criteria for the determination of brain death vary by age?**
   The Task Force on Brain Death in Children recommends that no determination of brain death be made in neonates younger than 7 days old. In infants who are 7 days to 2 months old, two examinations and EEGs separated by at least 48 hours are recommended. In infants 2 months to 1 year old, two examinations and EEGs separated by at least 24 hours are recommended. A repeat examination and EEG are not required if cerebral blood flow study shows absence of flow. In children older than 1 year, if the etiology is irreversible, laboratory testing is not required, and a 12-hour period of observation is recommended. If there is a

potentially reversible condition (e.g., HIE), at least a 24-hour period of observation is recommended. In practice, there is variability in adherence to these guidelines.

Mathur M, Petersen L, Stadtler M, et al: Variability in pediatric brain death determination and documentation in southern California, *Pediatrics* 121:988–993, 2008.

Report of special task force of the American Academy of Pediatrics Task Force on Brain Death in Children: Guidelines for the determination of brain death in children, *Pediatrics* 80:298–300, 1987.

56. **Compare the persistent vegetative state with the minimally conscious state.**
   ■ The **persistent vegetative state** is "a form of eyes-open permanent unconsciousness in which the patient has periods of wakefulness and physiological sleep/wake cycles, but at no time is the patient aware of himself or herself or the environment." If this state persists for more than 3 months in children, the long-term outlook is grim.
   ■ The **minimally conscious state** occurs on emergence from this vegetative state, and a patient must demonstrate a reproducible action in one or more of four types of behavior: (1) simple command following; (2) gestural or verbal "yes/no" responses; (3) intelligible verbalization; or (4) purposeful behaviors.

   Giacino JT, Ashwal S, Childs N, et al: The minimally conscious state: definition and diagnostic criteria, *Neurology* 58:349–353, 2002.

   American Academy of Neurology: Position of the American Academy of Neurology on certain aspects of the care and management of the persistent vegetative state patient. Adopted by the Executive Board, American Academy of Neurology, April 21, 1988, Cincinnati, Ohio, *Neurology* 39:125–126, 1989.

57. **What is the differential diagnosis of an intracranial bruit?**
   An intracranial bruit can be found in normal children and may be augmented by contralateral carotid compression. Disorders that may be associated with an intracranial bruit include vascular malformations and conditions characterized by increased cerebral blood flow:
   ■ Fever
   ■ Cerebral angioma
   ■ Intracerebral tumors
   ■ Thyrotoxicosis
   ■ Cerebral aneurysm
   ■ Any cause of increased ICP
   ■ Anemia
   ■ Cerebral arteriovenous malformations
   ■ Meningitis
   ■ Cardiac murmurs

   Mace JW, Peters ER, Mathies AW Jr: Cranial bruits in purulent meningitis in childhood, *N Engl J Med* 278:1420–1422, 1968.

58. **In a previously normal child who develops acute ataxia, what are the two most common diagnoses?**
   1. **Drug ingestion,** especially antiepileptic drugs, heavy metals, alcohol, and antihistamines.
   2. **Acute postinfectious cerebellitis,** most commonly after varicella: This is a diagnosis of exclusion if drug screening, CT or MRI, CSF evaluation, and other tests are negative.

59. **What are the causes of toe walking?**
   ■ CP (spastic diplegia)
   ■ Muscular dystrophy
   ■ Spinal dysraphism
   ■ Hereditary or acquired polyneuropathies
   ■ Intraspinal and filum terminale tumor
   ■ Equinovarus deformity

- Isolated congenital shortening of the Achilles tendon
- Variation of normal in early stages of walking
- Normal development pattern in some toddlers

Sala DA, Shulman LH, Kennedy RF, et al: Idiopathic toe-walking: a review, *Dev Med Child Neurol* 41:846–848, 1999.

60. **What is the Babinski response?**
Stimulation of the lateral aspect of the sole of the foot to the distal metatarsals may elicit a plantar response (extension); this indicates a lack of cortical inhibition and aids in the diagnosis of central hypotonia. It is abnormal outside of the neonatal period, when a flexor response develops, and can be a sign of disturbed pyramidal tract function. The stimulus elicits a number of sensory pathways with competing functions (including grip and withdrawal) and is somewhat dependent on the state of the infant and the examiner's technique. Its value as a localizing sign in the neonate is more controversial, but a consistent asymmetry is abnormal.

61. **A 7-year-old child with progressive ataxia, kyphoscoliosis, nystagmus, pes cavus (high arch), and an abnormal electrocardiogram (ECG) likely has what diagnosis?**
Friedreich ataxia. This heredodegenerative disease is an autosomal recessive disorder with childhood onset of gait ataxia, absent tendon reflexes, and extensor plantar responses. The spinal cord shows degeneration and sclerosis of the spinocerebellar tracts, the posterior column, and the corticospinal tracts. The condition is rare. The gene for Friedreich ataxia has been mapped to chromosome 9q13, contains a trinucleotide repeating sequence (GAA), and encodes for a protein called frataxin. A deficiency of frataxin leads to the accumulation of iron in the mitochondria and to oxidative stress, which leads to cell death.

Alper G, Narayanan V: Friedreich's ataxia, *Pediatr Neurol* 28:335–341, 2003.

62. **What clinical features help to distinguish peripheral from central vertigo?**
Peripheral vertigo implies dysfunction of the labyrinth or vestibular nerve, whereas central vertigo is associated with abnormalities of the brainstem or temporal lobe.
Peripheral
- Hearing loss, tinnitus, and otalgia may be associated.
- Past pointing and falling in the direction of unilateral disease occur.
- In bilateral disease, ataxia occurs with the eyes closed.
- Vestibular and positional nystagmus are present.
Central
- Cerebellar and cranial nerve dysfunction are frequently associated.
- No hearing loss is present.
- An alteration of consciousness may be associated.

Fenichel GM: *Clinical Pediatric Neurology: A Signs and Symptoms Approach*, ed 6, Philadelphia, 2009, Elsevier, p 365.

63. **In what settings is hyperacusis noted?**
Hyperacusis, or increased sensitivity to sound, is found in patients with injury to the facial nerve (CN VII), which innervates the stapedius muscle, or in those with injury to the trigeminal nerve (CN V), which innervates the tensor tympani muscle. Exaggerated startle response to sound or vibration occurs in patients with lysosomal storage diseases (e.g., sphingolipidoses such as Tay-Sachs disease, GM_1 gangliosidosis, and Sandhoff disease), Williams syndrome, hyperkalemia, tetanus, and strychnine poisoning.

64. **What is the most common cause of asymmetrical crying facies?**
In this entity, one side of the lower lip depresses during crying (on the normal side), and the other does not. Often misdiagnosed as a facial nerve palsy resulting from forceps delivery, the most common cause is **congenital absence of the depressor anguli oris muscle** of the lower lip. Its occasional association with heart defects warrants ECG and chest radiograph in these patients.

65. **What are the common causes of peripheral seventh-nerve palsy?**
Facial weakness caused by a lesion of the facial nerve (cranial nerve VII) is common. The facial weakness involves both the upper and lower face and affects both emotional and volitional facial movements. Any part of the nerve can be disturbed: the nucleus itself, the axon as it passes through the pons, or the peripheral portion of the nerve. Common etiologies include the following:
- Trauma
- Developmental hypoplasia or aplasia, including the Möbius anomaly
- Bell palsy (usually idiopathic, but may follow nonspecific viral infections)
- Infections, including Ramsay Hunt syndrome (herpes zoster invasion of the geniculate ganglion producing herpetic vesicles behind the ear and painful paralysis of the facial nerve); Lyme disease; local invasion from suppurative mastoiditis or otitis media; mumps, varicella, Epstein-Barr virus, cytomegalovirus, rubella, human immunodeficiency virus, or enterovirus neuritis; sequelae of bacterial meningitis; and parotid gland infection, inflammation, or tumor
- Guillain-Barré syndrome
- Tumor of the brainstem or cerebellar pontine angle tumors
- Inflammatory disorders such as sarcoidosis

66. **How is a *peripheral* seventh-nerve palsy distinguished from a *central* seventh-nerve palsy?**
The patient with a suspected palsy is asked to wrinkle the forehead, raise the eyebrows, and close the eyes tightly. In *peripheral* seventh-nerve palsy, no forehead furrows are noted, and the affected eye does not open as wide as the unaffected eye. In *central* seventh-nerve palsy, forehead furrowing and relatively good eye opening occur because the cells of the facial nucleus that innervate the upper face receive fibers from both cerebral hemispheres. Lower facial muscles are innervated from only the single contralateral cerebral hemisphere.

Gilden DH: Bell's palsy, *N Engl J Med* 351:1323–1331, 2004.

67. **During recovery from Bell palsy, why do the eyes water at mealtime?**
These are *crocodile tears*. The facial nerve supplies autonomic motor function to the lacrimal and salivary glands. Because of aberrant reinnervation during the course of healing from a facial nerve palsy, tasting a meal can trigger tearing rather than salivation. Folklore has it that crocodiles feel compassion for their victims and weep while munching.

68. **When are "doll's eyes" movements considered normal or abnormal?**
The *oculovestibular reflex* (also called *oculocephalic, proprioceptive head-turning reflex*, or *doll's eyes reflex*) is used most commonly as a test of brainstem function. The patient's eyelids are held open while the head is briskly rotated from side to side. A positive response is contraversive conjugate eye deviation (i.e., as the head rotates to the right, both eyes deviate to the left). Doll's eyes movements are interpreted as follows:
- In healthy awake newborn infants (who cannot inhibit or override the reflex with willful eye movements), the reflex is easy to elicit and is a normal finding. It can be used to test the range of the extraocular movements of infants during the first weeks of life.

- In healthy, awake, mature individuals, normal vision overrides the reflex, which is thus normally absent, and so the eyes follow the head turning.
- In a patient in a coma with preserved brainstem function, the depressed cortex does not override the reflex, and doll's eyes movements occur in rapid head rotation. Indeed, the purpose of eliciting this reflex in the comatose patient is to demonstrate that the brainstem still functions normally.
- In a patient in a coma with brainstem damage, the neural circuits that carry out the reflex are impaired, and the reflex is abolished.

69. **How are cold calorics done?**
As a test of brainstem function in an obtunded or comatose individual, 5 mL of ice-cold water is placed in the external ear canal (after ensuring the integrity of the tympanic membrane), with the head elevated at 30 degrees. A normal response occurs with deviation of the eyes to the side in which the water was placed. No response indicates severe dysfunction of the brainstem and the medial longitudinal fasciculus.

70. **What causes pinpoint pupils?**
Pupillary size represents a dynamic balance between the constricting influence of the third nerve (representing the parasympathetic autonomic nervous system) and the dilating influence of the ciliary nerve (which conducts fibers of the sympathetic nervous system). Pinpoint pupils indicate that the constricting influence of the third cranial nerve is not balanced by opposing sympathetic dilation. Etiologies could include the following:
- **Structural lesion in the pons** through which the sympathetic pathways descend
- **Metabolic disorders**
- **Opiates,** such as heroin or morphine
- **Other agents,** including propoxyphene, organophosphates, carbamate insecticides, barbiturates, clonidine, meprobamate, pilocarpine eyedrops, and mushroom or nutmeg poisoning

71. **What is the differential diagnosis of ptosis?**
Ptosis is the downward displacement of the upper eyelid as a result of dysfunction of the muscles that elevate the eyelid. A drooping eyelid may represent pseudoptosis caused by swelling of the eyelid as a result of local edema or active blepharospasm. True ptosis results from weakness of the eyelid muscles or interruption of its nerve supply. Etiologies include the following:
- **Muscular:** Congenital ptosis, which may occur alone or in the setting of Turner or Smith-Lemli-Opitz syndrome, myasthenia gravis (associated with marked daytime fluctuation), botulism, or some muscular dystrophies
- **Neurologic:** Horner syndrome, which results from the interruption of the sympathetic supply to Müller smooth eyelid muscle, and third-nerve palsy, which innervates the levator palpebral muscle; brainstem or orbital tumor (concerning if blurred vision also present)

72. **What does the Marcus Gunn pupil detect?**
An **afferent pupillary defect**. The pupils are normally equal in size (except for patients with physiologic anisocoria) as a result of the consensual light reflex: light entering either eye produces the same-strength "signal" for the constriction of both the stimulated and nonstimulated pupil. Some diseases of the maculae or optic nerves affect one side more than the other. For example, a meningioma may develop on one optic nerve sheath. As a result of unilateral or asymmetrical optic nerve dysfunction, a Marcus Gunn pupil may result.

73. **How is the swinging flashlight test done to detect a Marcus Gunn pupil?**
    - The patient is examined in a dim room, and fixation is directed to a distant target. This permits maximal pupillary dilation because of a lack of direct light and accommodation reflexes.
    - Light presented to the "good" eye produces the equal constriction of both pupils. A flashlight is swung briskly over the bridge of the nose to the eye with the "defective" optic nerve. The abnormal pupil remains momentarily constricted from the lingering effects of the consensual light response. However, the impaired eye with its reduced pupillomotor signal soon escapes the consensual reflex and actually dilates, despite being directly stimulated with light. The pupil that paradoxically dilates to direct light stimulation displays the afferent defect.

EPILEPSY

74. **What is epilepsy?**
    Epilepsy describes a syndrome of recurrent, unprovoked seizures, typically two or more, not the result of fever or a systemic medical condition. It is derived from the Greek verb *epilepsia* meaning "to seize upon" or "to take hold of." The early Greeks referred to it as the sacred disease, but Hippocrates debunked this notion and argued from clinical evidence that it arose from the brain. Epilepsy is not an entity or even a syndrome but rather a symptom complex arising from disordered brain function that itself may be the result of a variety of pathologic processes.

    American Epilepsy Society: http://www.aesnet.org.

    Chang BS, Lowenstein DH: Epilepsy, *N Engl J Med* 349:1257–1266, 2003.

    Epilepsy Foundation: http://www.epilepsyfoundation.org.

75. **What is the long-term outcome for children with epilepsy?**
    There are many different causes of epilepsy, and, in large part, the outcome relates to the underlying etiology. Children with idiopathic or genetically determined epilepsy have the best prognosis, whereas children with antecedent neurologic abnormalities fare less well. Nearly 75% of children will enter into a sustained remission 3 to 5 years after the onset of their epilepsy. There is no evidence that antiepileptic medications as they are currently used in clinical practice are neuroprotective or that they alter the long-term outcome of patients. Although there is a favorable prognosis for the remission of seizures, children with epilepsy are at an increased risk for having other long-term challenges, including difficulties achieving social, educational, and vocational goals. Treatment with antiepileptic medications is one important part of the management of the child, but other critical aspects of the physician–patient interaction, including educating, counseling, and advocacy, are equally important.

76. **How often are EEGs abnormal in healthy children?**
    About 10% of "normal" children have mild, nonspecific abnormalities in background activity. About 2% to 3% of healthy children have unexpected incidental epileptiform (i.e., spikes or sharp wave) patterns. Some may have heritable, familial EEG abnormalities without a clinical seizure disorder (e.g., centrotemporal spikes seen in benign seizure-susceptibility syndromes such as rolandic epilepsy).

77. **Should an EEG be done on all children who have a first afebrile seizure?**
    This is a major controversial issue. Of new-onset seizures in children, about one third do not involve fever. The American Academy of Neurology has recommended that all children with a first seizure without fever undergo an EEG in an effort to better classify the

epilepsy syndrome. Others argue that the quantity of expected information from obtaining EEGs for all cases is too low to affect treatment recommendations in most patients. They suggest that a selective approach to EEG use should be pursued, particularly for children with a seizure of focal onset, for children younger than 1 year, and for any child with unexplained cognitive or motor dysfunction or abnormalities on neurologic examination.

Gilbert DL, Buncher CR: An EEG should not be routinely obtained after first unprovoked seizure in childhood, *Neurology* 54:635–641, 2000.

Hirtz D, Ashwal S, Berg A, et al: Practice parameter: evaluating a first nonfebrile seizure in children. Report of the Quality Standards Subcommittee of the American Academy of Neurology, the Child Neurology Society, and the American Epilepsy Society, *Neurology* 55:616–623, 2000.

78. **In a patient with a suspected seizure disorder, but a normal EEG, how can the sensitivity of the EEG be increased?**
    - Repeat the EEG
    - Obtain following sleep deprivation
    - Use hyperventilation and photic stimulation (e.g., strobe lights)
    - Obtain a prolonged EEG (1 to 3 days) with or without video

79. **Which types of epilepsy are characterized by specific EEG findings?**
    - **Rolandic epilepsy:** Midtemporal spikes (only during sleep in 30%)
    - **Benign epilepsy with occipital focus:** Continuous unilateral or bilateral occipital high-voltage spike waves
    - **Absence epilepsy:** Characteristic 3-Hz spike-wave pattern
    - **Juvenile myoclonic epilepsy:** Spike and polyspike-wave patterns
    - **Infantile spasms:** Hypsarrhythmia, a markedly disorganized pattern
    - **Lennox-Gastaut syndrome:** Slow spike-wave forms at less than 3-Hz frequency
    - **Landau-Kleffner syndrome:** Spike-wave discharges that persist during sleep

80. **Which disorders commonly mimic epilepsy?**
    Many conditions are characterized by the sudden onset of abnormal consciousness, awareness, reactivity, behavior, posture, tone, sensation, or autonomic function. Syncope, breath-holding spells, migraine, hypoglycemia, narcolepsy, cataplexy, sleep apnea, gastroesophageal reflux, and parasomnias (night terrors, sleep walking, sleep talking, nocturnal enuresis) feature an abrupt or "paroxysmal" alteration of brain function and suggest the possibility of epilepsy. Perhaps one of the most difficult attacks to distinguish is the "nonepileptic" seizure (also called a *pseudoepileptic* or *hysterical seizure*).

81. **What are the two key questions for the classification of the epilepsy syndrome?**
    1. **Where does the seizure begin?** If the seizure appears to begin in part of the brain, it is partial or localization-related. Partial seizures (formerly called *focal seizures*) are divided into simple and complex types.
    2. **Is brain development normal?** If the seizure arises from a developmentally normal brain, it is a primary or idiopathic epilepsy; arising from an abnormal brain makes it a secondary or symptomatic epilepsy. *Cryptogenic* is the term used to describe seizures in a child who has not had normal neurologic development and in whom the etiology cannot be found.

82. **What are the categories of seizures in children?**
    The syndrome classification as codified by the International League against Epilepsy distinguishes seizure on the basis of type rather than etiology (Table 14-2). Combinations of seizure types may occur in an individual patient.

TABLE 14-2. INTERNATIONAL LEAGUE AGAINST EPILEPSY SEIZURE CLASSIFICATION

Partial (Focal, Local) Seizures	Generalized Seizures

Simple partial seizures
 ■ With motor signs: Focal motor, jacksonian, versive, postural, phonatory
 ■ With somatosensory or special sensory symptoms (simple hallucinations, e.g., tingling, light flashes, buzzing): somatosensory, visual, auditory, olfactory, gustatory, vertiginous
 ■ With autonomic symptoms and signs
 ■ With psychic symptoms (disturbances of higher cerebral functions): Dysphasic, dysmnesic, cognitive, affective, illusions, structured hallucinations
 Unclassified Epileptic Seizures
 ■ Complex partial seizures (with impairment of consciousness)
 ■ Simple partial onset followed by impairment of consciousness
   ■ With no other features
   ■ With simple partial features
   ■ With automatisms
 ■ Partial seizures evolving to secondarily generalized tonic-clonic seizures
	■ Absence seizures, with impairment of consciousness, with clonic, atonic, tonic, or autonomic components, or with automatisms occurring alone or in combination
	 ■ Atypical absences, more pronounced changes of tone than in absence seizures; onset and/or cessation not abrupt
	 ■ Monoclonic seizures (single or multiple)
	 ■ Clonic seizures
	 ■ Tonic seizures
	 ■ Tonic-clonic seizures
	 ■ Atonic seizures

Adapted from Vedanarayanan VV: Diagnosis of epilepsy in children. Pediatr Ann 28:218-224, 1999.

83. **What are the causes of symptomatic seizures?**
Symptomatic seizures are those that are caused by an identifiable injury to the brain, as opposed to idiopathic or cryptogenic epilepsy. The seizures are a sign of underlying disease or pathology that must be managed, if possible, independently of the seizure (Table 14-3).

84. **If a previously normal child has an afebrile, generalized tonic-clonic seizure, what should parents be told about the risk for recurrence?**
Studies indicate that the recurrence rate is between 25% and 50%. The EEG is an important predictor of recurrence. A subsequent normal EEG reduces the 5-year recurrence risk to 25%. Occurrence of the seizure during sleep increases the risk to 50%. Half of recurrences will occur during the first 6 months after the first seizure; two thirds will occurs

TABLE 14-3. CAUSES OF SYMPTOMATIC SEIZURES

Fever
- Simple febrile seizures
- Complicated febrile seizures

Trauma
- Impact seizures
- Early posttraumatic seizures
- Late posttraumatic seizures

Hypoxia
- Complicated breath-holding spells
- Hypoxic seizures

Metabolic
- Acquired metabolic disorders
- Neurologic effects of systemic disease
- Inborn errors of metabolism

Toxins
- Drugs
- Drug withdrawal
- Biologic toxins

Stroke
- Ischemic stroke
- Embolic stroke
- Hemorrhagic stroke

Intracranial Hemorrhage
- Subdural hemorrhage
- Subarachnoid hemorrhage
- Intracerebral hemorrhage

Adapted from Evans OB: Symptomatic seizures. Pediatr Ann 28:231-237, 1999.

within 1 year, and 90% or more will have occurred within 2 years. The child's age at the time of the first seizure and the duration of the seizure do not affect the recurrence risk.

Shinnar S, Berg AT, Moshe SL, et al: The risk of seizure recurrence after a first unprovoked afebrile seizure in childhood: an extended follow-up, *Pediatrics* 98:216–225, 1996.

85. **Should all children with a new-onset afebrile generalized seizure have a CT or MRI evaluation?**
Although most adults with new-onset seizures should have a head imaging study (preferably MRI), the relatively high frequency of idiopathic seizure disorders in children often obviates a scan in those with generalized seizures, nonfocal EEGs, and normal neurologic examinations. Consider obtaining a cranial imaging study in the following situations:
- Any seizure with focal components (other than mere eye deviation)
- Newborns and young infants with seizures
- Status epilepticus at any age
- Focal slowing or focal paroxysmal activity on EEG

Hirtz D, Berg A, Bettis D, et al: Quality Standards Subcommittee of the American Academy of Neurology; Practice Committee of the Child Neurology Society: Practice parameter: treatment of the child with a first unprovoked seizure. Report of the Quality Standards Subcommittee of the American Academy of Neurology and the Practice Committee of the Child Neurology Society, *Neurology* 60:166–175, 2003.

Hsieh DT, Chang T, Tsuchida TN, et al: New-onset afebrile seizures in infants: role of neuroimaging, *Neurology* 74-150-156, 2010.

86. **What are the most common inherited seizure or epilepsy syndromes?**
- Febrile convulsions
- Rolandic epilepsy, childhood absence epilepsy
- Juvenile myoclonic epilepsy (of Janz)

87. **What are the clinical features of rolandic epilepsy?**
Rolandic epilepsy is an idiopathic localization-related epilepsy that represents 10% to 15% of all childhood seizure disorders.
- It begins in school-aged children (4 to 13 years old) who are otherwise healthy and neurologically normal.
- Seizures are idiopathic or familial (autosomal dominant inheritance with age-dependent penetrance).
- Seizures may be simple or complex and partial or generalized. Classically, there is a history of one-sided facial paresthesias and twitching and drooling that may be followed by hemiclonic movements or hemitonic posturing. Consciousness is typically preserved. The seizures are primarily nocturnal and may secondarily generalize.
- Often referred to as *benign* because the individual is developmentally normal, seizures are usually rare and nocturnal, and they most often resolve after puberty.

88. **What are the types of absence seizures?**
Typical absence
- EEG: 3-Hz spike wave
- Observations: Abrupt onset and ending (typically 5 to 10 seconds)
- Simple subtype: Unresponsiveness with no other associated features except minor movements (e.g., lip smacking or eyelid twitching)
- Complex subtype: Unresponsiveness with more prolonged mild atonic, myoclonic, or tonic features or automatisms
Atypical absence (most common in Lennox-Gastaut syndrome)
- EEG: 2-Hz (or slower) spike wave
- Observations: Gradual onset and ending; frequency is more cyclic; unresponsive with more prolonged and pronounced atonic, tonic, myoclonic, or tonic activity

89. **In a child who is suspected of having absence seizures, how can a seizure be elicited during an examination?**
Hyperventilation for at least 3 minutes is a useful provocative maneuver to precipitate an absence seizure. Young patients may be coaxed into overbreathing by making a game of it. Hold a tissue paper in front of the child's mouth, and then instruct the patient to keep breathing fast enough to keep the tissue aloft.

90. **What percentage of patients with absence seizures also have occasional grand mal seizures?**
About 30% to 50%.

91. **What is the prognosis for children with absence epilepsy?**
The prognosis for patients with childhood absence epilepsy has been studied prospectively, and nearly 90% of patients who have normal intelligence, normal neurologic examination, normal EEG background activity, no family history of convulsive epilepsy, and no history of tonic-clonic convulsions will become free of seizures. Conversely, the complete absence of favorable factors is associated with a poor prognosis for the cessation of seizures. It may be that absence seizures are expressed on a spectrum from typical childhood absence epilepsy that is genetic in origin to the Lennox-Gastaut syndrome, which is symptomatic of brain injury.

92. **A teenager, like his father, develops brief, bilateral, intermittent jerking of his arms. What seizure disorder is he likely to have?**
Juvenile myoclonic epilepsy, which is also called *myoclonic epilepsy of Janz*, is a familial form of primary idiopathic generalized epilepsy that typically involves "fast" 3- to 5-Hz

spike-wave discharges on EEG ("impulsive petit mal") and autosomal dominant inheritance. The distinctive clinical features of this type of epilepsy include morning myoclonic jerks, generalized tonic-clonic seizures upon awakening, normal intelligence, a family history of similar seizures, and onset between the ages of 8 and 20 years.

93. **What are myoclonic seizures?**
    These seizures are characterized by rapid, bilateral, symmetrical muscle contractions of short duration—"quick jerks." They may be isolated, or they may occur repetitively. Myoclonic seizures may be the sole manifestation of epilepsy, or, more commonly, they may be associated with absence attacks or tonic-clonic attacks.

KEY POINTS: EPILEPSY

1. Definition: Repeated, unprovoked seizures

2. Classified as localization related (focal partial onset) and generalized

3. Most important classification questions: Where does the seizure begin? Is brain development normal?

4. Epilepsy syndromes further subdivided as idiopathic (presumed genetic), symptomatic (known etiology), and cryptogenic

5. Proper classification of epilepsy syndromes guidance of treatment options and prognosis

94. **What distinguishes atonic and akinetic seizures?**
    Atonic seizure involves the sudden and usually complete loss of tone in the limb, neck, and trunk muscles. Muscle control is lost without warning, and the child may be seriously injured. This situation is often aggravated by the occurrence of one or more myoclonic jerks immediately before muscle tone is lost so that the fall is associated with an element of propulsion. Atonic seizures are particularly common in children with static encephalopathies, and they may prove refractory to therapy. In **akinetic seizures,** movement is arrested without a significant loss of muscle tone; this is rare.

95. **What is the classic triad of infantile spasms?**
    Spasms, hypsarrhythmia, and developmental regression. Infantile spasms are known as West syndrome, and the condition is named for the physician who first described the condition in his own son in 1841.

96. **What characterizes hypsarrhythmia?**
    The term means "mountainous slowing," and it describes the classic interictal EEG of infantile spasms that is characterized by extremely high-voltage, slow, and disorganized brain waves with multifocal spike activity. Hypsarrhythmia may either precede or follow the onset of infantile spasms. This EEG configuration may appear first or most obviously in non–rapid eye movement sleep and confirms the clinical diagnosis of infantile spasms.

97. **How commonly is a cause identified in infantile spasms?**
    A cause can be identified in up to 90% of children with infantile spasms, particularly in those who are symptomatic at the time of the initial seizure. Of identifiable causes, three fourths are prenatal or perinatal, and one fourth are postnatal. All patients with infantile spasms should have detailed neuroimaging and metabolic and genetic studies. Causes, including some possible specific examples, include the following:

- **Prenatal and perinatal:** Neurocutaneous disorders (tuberous sclerosis), brain injury (hypoxic-ischemic encephalopathy), intrauterine infection (cytomegalovirus), brain malformations (lissencephaly, agenesis of the corpus callosum), inborn metabolic errors (nonketotic hyperglycinemia, phenylketonuria, maple syrup urine disease, pyridoxine dependency)
- **Postnatal:** Infectious (herpes encephalitis), hypoxic-ischemic encephalopathy, head trauma

98. **What is the prognosis for infants with infantile spasms?**
Prognosis in large part depends on the clinical state at the time of the first seizure. In the cryptogenic or idiopathic group (10% to 15%, which are those without an underlying disorder identifiable), development, neurologic examination, and imaging studies are usually normal at the onset. With adrenocorticotropic hormone (ACTH) treatment, up to 40% will have a complete or near-complete recovery with normal cognitive development. In the symptomatic group (85% to 90%, which comprises those with a specific etiology), neurologic deficits, developmental delays, or cranial abnormalities are typically present before the first seizure. In this group, complete or near-complete recovery is achieved by only 5% to 15%. Twenty-five to 50% will develop Lennox-Gastaut syndrome.

Kivity S, Lerman P, Ariel R, et al: Long-term cognitive outcomes of a cohort of children with cryptogenic infantile spasms treated with high-dose adrenocorticotropic hormone, *Epilepsia* 45:255–262, 2004.

99. **What is the treatment of choice for infantile spasms?**
Currently in the United States, most children with infantile spasms are treated with ACTH as the first treatment option; most patients will respond to this medication. Vigabatrin, particularly in infants with tuberous sclerosis and those younger than 3 months, has been found in some studies to be useful. However, Vigabatrin is not approved for use in the United States in part because of possible side effects with retinal toxicity with constriction of peripheral visual fields as well as cerebral white matter changes.

Desguerre I, Nabbout R, Dulac O: The management of infantile spasms, *Arch Dis Child* 93:462–463, 2008.

Mackay MT, Weiss SK, Adams-Webber T, et al, American Academy of Neurology; Child Neurology Society: Practice parameter: medical treatment of infantile spasms, *Neurology* 62:1668–1681, 2004.

100. **What are the side effects that are associated with ACTH?**
The potential side effects of ACTH are prodigious. The treatment is associated with about 5% mortality in some series as a result of massive gastric hemorrhage from ulceration of the mucosa, sepsis as a result of immunologic compromise, or cardiac failure caused by a dilated cardiomyopathy. Echocardiography can reveal changes in advance of the clinical hypertension and may be a useful screening tool for the latter complication. The routine testing of the stool for occult blood, the regular monitoring of blood pressure, the screening of the urine for glucose, and the institution of a low-salt diet are other appropriate precautions. In addition to these short-term side effects of ACTH, there are other complications that are related to prolonged use, as are seen with other steroid treatments.

101. **What is the most likely diagnosis in a child of Ashkenazi descent with stimulus-sensitive seizures, cognitive deterioration, and a cherry-red spot?**
The classic lysosomal lipid storage disorder presenting symptoms of a progressive encephalopathy during infancy is **Tay-Sachs disease**. The infantile forms of GM_2 gangliosidosis includes Tay-Sachs disease, which is caused by a deficiency of hexosaminidase A, and Sandhoff disease, which is caused by a deficiency of

hexosaminidase A and B. Tay-Sachs is an autosomal recessive disorder that is localized to chromosome 15, with an incidence of 1 in 3900 in the Ashkenazi Jewish population of Eastern or Central European descent. The enzymatic defect leads to intraneuronal accumulation of GM_2 ganglioside. Normal development is seen until 4 to 6 months of age, when hypotonia and a loss of motor skills occur, with the subsequent development of spasticity, blindness, and macrocephaly. The classic cherry-red spot is present in the ocular fundi of more than 90% of patients.

102. **A patient with seizures, microcephaly, and a low CSF glucose but a normal serum glucose has what likely condition?**
The **GLUT-1 deficiency syndrome,** which was previously referred to as the *glucose transporter protein deficiency syndrome*, was first described in 1991. The clinical phenotype is variable, but the child usually presents symptoms during the first years of life with seizures and delays of motor and mental development. The head circumference decelerates during the first years of life. The diagnosis should be suspected if CSF reveals low glucose (and lactate) concentrations without evidence of inflammation and blood sugars are normal.

103. **What is the clinical triad of the Lennox-Gastaut syndrome?**
Lennox-Gastaut syndrome is characterized by **mental retardation, seizures** of various types, and disorganized **slow spike-wave activity** on an EEG. The seizures usually begin during the first 3 years of life and are characteristically severe and refractory to anticonvulsant drugs. Prognosis is poor, with more than 80% of children continuing to have seizures into adulthood.

Crumrine PK: Lennox-Gastaut syndrome, *J Child Neurol* 17:S70-S75, 2002.

104. **A 5-year-old with a history of normal language development who develops seizures and inattention to speech with severe regression of language skills has what likely condition?**
Landau-Kleffner syndrome. First described in 1957, this is a condition of acquired epileptic aphasia with nocturnal EEG abnormalities, reduction in language function, and problems with attention. Despite the use of various AEDs and/or ACTH, recovery is often delayed, and communication problems persistent.

Robinson F: Landau-Kleffner syndrome: current issues, *Neurology* 19:53–56, 2003.

105. **How is status epilepticus defined?**
- Because of uncertainty regarding at precisely what time morbidity ensues in the course of a prolonged seizure, there is a variance in definitional length regarding status epilepticus. In general, more than 20 to 30 minutes of continuous or sequential seizure activity has previously defined status epilepticus.
- Recurrent seizures without full recovery of consciousness between seizures.

106. **Why is status epilepticus so dangerous?**
With the onset of a seizure, catecholamine release and sympathetic discharge result in increased heart rate and blood pressure. Cerebral flow increases dramatically to compensate for the increased metabolic needs of the brain. With persistence of the seizure, compensatory mechanisms begin to fail. Respiratory acidosis and metabolic acidosis develop. Systemic blood pressure falls. Intracranial pressure increases. The inability to meet the increased oxygen demands of the brain results in an intracranial change to anaerobic metabolism with acidosis, increased CSF lactate, and cerebral edema. The prolonged electrical discharges by themselves may also cause neuronal damage.

Hanhan UA, Fiallos MR, Orlowski JP: Status epilepticus, *Pediatr Clin N Am* 48:683–695, 2001.

107. **How should a child who presents with status epilepticus be managed?**
- **0 to 5 minutes:** Confirm the diagnosis. Maintain the airway by head positioning or oropharyngeal airway. Administer nasal oxygen. Suction as needed. Obtain and frequently monitor vital signs using pulse oximetry and ECG. Establish an intravenous line. Obtain venous blood for laboratory determinations (e.g., glucose, serum chemistries, hematology studies, toxicology screen, culture, anticonvulsant levels if patient is a known epileptic). Administer antipyretics as indicated.
- **5 to 15 minutes:** If hypoglycemic (or if a rapid reagent strip for glucose testing is not available), administer 2 mL/kg of $D_{25}W$ or 5 mL/kg of $D_{10}W$. In an infant with no known seizure disorder, give 100 mg of pyridoxine intravenously. Monitor oxygenation by pulse oximetry and vital signs. Administer lorazepam, 0.1 mg/kg (up to 4 mg) intravenously at 2 mg/minute. If intravenous access cannot be established, give diazepam, 0.5 mg/kg rectally.
- **10 to 20 minutes:** Repeat lorazepam in 5 to 10 minutes if seizure persists. Intramuscular therapy is not recommended.
- **15 to 35 minutes:** If seizures persist, administer fosphenytoin (preferred for children) intravenously at 20 mg phenytoin equivalents (PE)/kg loading dose at 150 mg PE/minute or 3 mg PE/kg per minute. If phenytoin is used, the dose is 15 to 20 mg/kg at 0.5 to 1 mg/kg per minute intravenously while monitoring ECG and blood pressure. The infusion should be slowed if dysrhythmia or QT-interval widening develops. For neonates younger than 1 month, administer a loading dose of phenobarbital, 20 mg/kg intravenously as the second-line medication.
- **30 to 50 minutes:** If seizures persist for 15 minutes after the use of phenytoin, administer additional doses of fosphenytoin/phenytoin, 10 mg/kg to a maximum of 30 mg/kg total. If seizures persist, give phenobarbital (20 mg/kg) intravenously at a rate of 1 mg/kg/minute (maximum: 60 mg/minute). With the use of phenobarbital after benzodiazepines, the risk for respiratory depression is increased, and the likely need for intubation increases and should be anticipated. If phenobarbital fails to stop the seizure, other measures (e.g., general anesthesia) are usually necessary. Other third line medications for refractory SE, including levetiracetam and valproate, are currently utilized in some centers prior to the use of phenobarbital.

Abend NS, Huh JW, Helfaer MA, Dlugos DJ: Anticonvulsant medications in the pediatric emergency room and intensive care unit, *Pediatr Emerg Care* 24:705-718, 2008.

Goldstein J: Status epilepticus in the pediatric emergency department, *Clin Ed Emerg Med* 9:96–100, 2008.

Yoong M, Chin RFM, Scott RC: Management of convulsive status epilepticus in children, *Arch Dis Child Educ Pract Ed* 94:1–9, 2009.

108. **What is the most common cause of refractory seizures?**
An inadequate serum concentration of antiepileptic medication is the most common cause of persistent seizures, but other causes should be considered:
- **Drug toxicity,** especially with phenytoin, may manifest by deteriorating seizure control.
- **Metabolic abnormalities,** particularly in patients with inborn errors of metabolism, may be seen.
- **Medications** may have a paradoxic reaction and exacerbate certain types of seizures, particularly in children with mixed seizure disorders. For example, carbamazepine or phenytoin may control generalized tonic-clonic seizures in patients with juvenile myoclonic epilepsy, but they may aggravate myoclonic and absence seizures.
- **Incorrect identification** of the epilepsy syndrome may be a cause. Partial seizures may masquerade as a generalized form of epilepsy in the very young child (bilateral symmetrical tonic posturing may be seen in partial seizures). Conversely, generalized forms of epilepsy may first appear as partial seizures (severe infantile myoclonic epilepsy). Treatment based on an epilepsy syndrome rather than ictal semiology usually improves control in these circumstances.

109. **What is the role of the ketogenic diet for the treatment of seizures?**

The *ketogenic diet* is effective for the treatment of all seizure types, particularly in children with myoclonic forms of epilepsy. The diet involves supplying most calories through fats, with concurrent limitation of carbohydrates and protein. The mechanism of seizure control is unclear, but it is perhaps related to a switch in the cerebral metabolism from the use of glucose to the use of β-hydroxybutyrate. After 24 hours of fasting, the child is placed on a high-fat diet in which the ratio of fats to carbohydrates and protein combined is 3:1 to 4:1. Anticonvulsant drugs may be reduced or eliminated entirely if the diet is effective. The regimen must be followed closely, and parents must understand the demands of close adherence to the diet. A skilled dietitian is instrumental for providing variety and palatability to the diet. It is important to recall that the diet may have adverse effects, including serious, potentially life-threatening complications such as hypoproteinemia, lipemia, and hemolytic anemia.

Freeman JM, Kossoff EH, Hartman AL: The ketogenic diet: one decade later, *Pediatrics* 119:535-543, 2007.

Kossoff EH, Zupec-Kania BA, Rho JM: Ketogenic diets: an update for child neurologists, *J Child Neuro* 24:979-988, 2009.

110. **What is the role of the vagal nerve stimulator in seizure control?**

The *vagal nerve stimulator* is a surgically implanted device that intermittently stimulates the left vagus nerve. Why this decreases seizure frequency is not well understood. It is a palliative—not curative—procedure that has been performed in adults and in some children with intractable complex partial seizures or generalized tonic seizures who were thought not to be candidates for definitive surgical cure. The vagal nerve stimulator has been placed in children as young as 2 to 3 years old, but most of the experience is in older children.

Buchhalter JR, Jarrar RG: Therapeutics in pediatric epilepsy. Part 2: epilepsy surgery and vagus nerve stimulation, *Mayo Clin Proc* 78:371–378, 2003.

Wheless JW, Maggio V: Vagus nerve stimulation therapy in patients younger than 18 years, *Neurology* 59(6 Suppl 4):S21–S25, 2002.

111. **What should a teenager with epilepsy be told about the potential of obtaining a driver's license?**

State requirements vary regarding individuals with epilepsy and the right to drive. The most common requirement is a specified seizure-free period and submission of a physician's evaluation of the patient's ability to drive safely. Many states require the periodic submission of medical reports while the license is active. In addition, many states allow exceptions under which a license may be issued for a shorter seizure-free period (e.g., if a seizure occurred in isolation as a result of medication change or intercurrent illness), or they may issue licenses with restrictions (e.g., daytime driving only). A summary of requirements for each state is available from the Epilepsy Foundation.

Epilepsy Foundation: http://www.epilepsyfoundation.org.

112. **When should a child be referred for epilepsy surgery evaluation?**

Although many epilepsy syndromes in childhood have spontaneous remission, 20% of incident epilepsy is intractable, and 5% of patients with intractable epilepsy may benefit from epilepsy surgery. Indications for surgery are intractable disabling seizures and/or deteriorating development. In general, outcome is determined by the completeness of the evaluation and the congruence of the data, the completeness of the resection, and the etiology of the seizures.

Lee JYK, Adelson PD: Neurosurgical management of pediatric epilepsy, *Pediatr Clin N Am* 51:441–456, 2004.

Nordli DR, Kelley KR: Selection and evaluation of children for epilepsy surgery, *Pediatr Neurosurg* 34:1–12, 2001.

FEBRILE SEIZURES

113. How are febrile seizures defined?

Febrile seizures are defined as a convulsion caused by a fever that is without evidence of CNS pathology or acute electrolyte imbalance that occurs in children between the ages of 1 month and 7 years (most commonly between the ages of 6 months and 5 years, with a peak at the end of the second year of life). Children with a history of epilepsy who have an exacerbation of seizures with fever are excluded. Febrile seizures occur in 2% to 5% of children. There is often a positive family history of febrile convulsions.

114. What is the likelihood of recurrence of a febrile seizure?

The likelihood of recurrence increases with younger age of onset, with a recurrence rate about 1 in 2 if the patient is younger than 1 year when the initial seizure occurs and 1 in 5 if the patient is older than 3 years during the initial seizure. About half of recurrences are within 6 months of the first seizure; three fourths occur within 1 year, and 90% occur within 2 years. Other risk factors for recurrence are a lower temperature (close to 38°C) at the time of seizure, less than 1 hour's duration of fever before the seizure, and a family history of febrile seizures. Overall, the recurrence rate in the pediatric population is about 30%.

Sadleir LG, Scheffer IE: Febrile seizures, *BMJ* 334:307–311, 2007.

115. What features make a febrile seizure complex rather than simple?

- **Simple febrile seizure:** Relatively brief (<15 minutes long) and occurs as a solitary event (one attack in 24 hours) in the setting of fever not caused by CNS infection
- **Complex (also called atypical or complicated) febrile seizure:** Focal features either at the onset or during the seizure, extended in duration (>15 minutes long), or occurring more than once in 1 day

116. Why are complex febrile seizures more worrisome than simple febrile seizures?

They suggest a more serious problem. For example, a focal seizure raises concern of a localized or lateralized functional disturbance of the CNS. An unusually long seizure (>15 minutes) also raises the suspicion of primary CNS infectious, structural, or metabolic disease. Repeated seizures within a 24-hour period likewise imply a potentially more serious disorder or impending status epilepticus.

117. When should a lumbar puncture be performed as part of the evaluation of a young child with a simple febrile seizure?

This is often a difficult question when a well-appearing infant or toddler is examined after a febrile seizure, and approaches vary by clinician and textbook. The American Academy of Pediatrics conservatively recommends that, after a seizure with fever in children 6 to 12 months of age, a lumbar puncture should be *strongly considered* because signs and symptoms associated with meningitis may be minimal or absent in this age group. In children between 12 and 18 months old, a lumbar puncture should be *considered* because signs and symptoms can be subtle. In children older than 18 months, when meningeal signs are typically present in meningitis, a lumbar puncture can be deferred if such signs are not present. In younger patients who have received prior antibiotic therapy, a lumbar puncture should be strongly considered because treatment can mask the signs and symptoms of meningitis. Other features that might prompt a lumbar puncture in children younger than 2 years include a prior history of irritability, decreased feeding or lethargy, a complex seizure, or a prolonged postictal period of altered consciousness. It should be noted that a simple, brief, nonfocal seizure as the sole manifestation of bacterial meningitis in febrile children is unusual. In one retrospective study of 503 patients with meningitis, none was noted to have bacterial meningitis manifesting solely as a simple seizure. Rates of bacterial meningitis are declining in the era of the pneumococcal conjugate vaccine. One recent large cohort study found no patients between 6 and 18 months presenting with a simple febrile seizure to have bacterial meningitis and called for reconsideration of the American Academy of Pediatrics recommendations.

Kimia AA, Capraro AJ, Hummel D, et al: Utility of lumbar puncture for first simple febrile seizure among children 6 to 18 months of age, *Pediatrics* 123:6–12, 2009.

American Academy of Pediatrics: Provisional Committee on Quality Improvement: Practice parameter: the neurodiagnostic evaluation of the child with a first simple febrile seizure, *Pediatrics* 97:769–775, 1996.

Green SM, Rothrock SG, Clem KJ, et al: Can seizures be the sole manifestation of meningitis in febrile children? *Pediatrics* 92:527–534, 1993.

118. **How common is bacterial meningitis as a cause of febrile status epilepticus?**
About 1 in 5. Consequently, when febrile status epilepticus occurs, antibiotics should be administered until stabilization of the patient permits a lumbar puncture.

Chin RFM, Neville BG, Scott RC: Meningitis is a common cause of convulsive status epilepticus with fever, *Arch Dis Child* 90:66–69, 2005.

119. **Do prolonged febrile seizures result in an increased peripheral white blood cell count?**
A common clinical question in children is whether a leukocytosis, if found, can be explained on the basis of a prolonged seizure as a stress reaction. In a study of 203 children with seizures and fever, 61% had a normal peripheral white blood cell count. No association was found between blood leukocytosis and febrile seizure duration in children.

van Stuijvenberg M, Moll HA, Steyerberg EW, et al: The duration of febrile seizures and peripheral leukocytosis, *J Pediatr* 133:557–558, 1998.

120. **What ancillary testing should be considered in a patient with a complex febrile seizure?**
Most children with their first complex febrile seizure should undergo a CSF examination to rule out intracranial infection. Children with focal motor seizures or postictal lateralized deficits (motor paresis, unilateral sensory or visual loss, sustained eye deviation, or aphasia) should be considered for neuroimaging to check for a structural abnormality. However, if the patient is neurologically normal, data suggest an emergent CT may not be necessary. The immediate performance of an EEG offers limited insight into the patient's disease. Prominent generalized postictal slowing is not unexpected. Definite focal slowing suggests a possible structural abnormality. For a simple febrile seizure, an EEG is not indicated because it is not predictive of either the risk for recurrence of febrile seizures or the development of epilepsy.

Teng D, Dayan P, Tyler S, et al: Risk of intracranial pathologic conditions requiring emergency intervention after a first complex febrile seizure episode among children, *Pediatrics* 117:304–308, 2006.

DiMario FJ: Children presenting with complex febrile seizures do not routinely need computed tomography scanning in the emergency department, *Pediatrics* 117:528–530, 2006.

121. **What is the risk for epilepsy after a febrile seizure?**
The risk depends on several variables. In otherwise normal children with a simple febrile seizure, the risk for later epilepsy is about 2%. The risk for epilepsy is higher if any of the following is present:
■ There is a close family history of nonfebrile seizures.
■ Prior neurologic or developmental abnormalities exist.
■ The patient had an atypical or complex febrile seizure, defined as focal seizures, seizures lasting at least 15 minutes, and/or multiple attacks within 24 hours.
One risk factor increases the risk to 3%. If all three risk factors are present, the likelihood of later epilepsy increases to 5% to 10%.

Waruiru C, Appleton R: Febrile seizures: an update, *Arch Dis Child* 89:751–756, 2004.

KEY POINTS: FEBRILE SEIZURES

1. Simple: Brief and lasting <15 minutes

2. Complex: Focal, >15 minutes long or recurrence within 1 day

3. Risk for recurrent febrile seizure increases if positive family history or seizure occurs at <1 year of age and/or body temperature of <40°C

4. Risk for developing future nonfebrile seizures is low (only 2% by age 7 years)

5. Normal long-term intellect and behavior compared with controls

6. Increased risk for developing epilepsy if complex febrile seizure, prior neurologic abnormality, or family history of seizure disorder

---

122. **What is the long-term outcome for children with febrile seizures?**
In a previously normal child, the risk for death, neurologic damage, or persistent cognitive impairment from a single febrile seizure is near zero. These potential complications are more likely with complex febrile seizures, but the risk is still exceedingly low. Impaired cognition in the latter group is more likely if afebrile seizures subsequently develop. Febrile status epilepticus has a very low mortality with proper treatment in recent years, and the development of mesial temporal sclerosis is less than 1 in 70,000.

Chang YC, Guo NW, Wang ST, et al: Working memory of school-aged children with a history of febrile convulsions: a population study, *Neurology* 57:37–42, 2001.

Verity CM, Greenwood R, Golding J: Long-term intellectual and behavioral outcomes of children with febrile convulsions, *N Engl J Med* 338:1723–1728, 1998.

123. **After a febrile seizure, should a child be treated with prophylactic antiepileptics?**
For most children, a simple febrile seizure is an unwanted but transient disruption of their health, and treatment is not necessary. Treatment, with phenobarbital or valproic acid, may be considered in the very young child if febrile seizures recur frequently and in children with preexisting neurologic abnormalities or with complex febrile seizures. In general, however, the side effects of continuous prophylaxis outweigh the relatively minor risks of recurrence. Long-term prophylaxis does not improve the prognosis in terms of subsequent epilepsy or motor or cognitive ability.

Offringa M, Moyer VA: Evidence based management of seizures associated with fever, *BMJ* 323: 1111–1114, 2001.

Baumann RJ, Duffner PK: Treatment of children with simple febrile seizures: the AAP practice parameter. American Academy of Pediatrics, *Pediatr Neurol* 23:11–17, 2000.

124. **Is the aggressive use of antipyretic therapy at the start of a febrile illness effective in reducing the likelihood of a febrile seizure?**
Despite being recommended frequently by pediatricians, aggressive antipyretic use (as well as oral and rectal phenobarbital and oral diazepam) have not been shown to be effective in preventing recurrence of a febrile seizure. Rectal diazepam can reduce the risk, but side effects (drowsiness and ataxia) can interfere with the clinical evaluation of a possible serious febrile illness.

Menkes JH, Sankar R, Maria BL: editors: Paroxysmal disorders. In Menkes JH, Sarnat HB, editors: *Child Neurology*, ed 7, Philadelphia, 2006, Lippincott Williams & Wilkins, pp 920–992.

HEADACHE

125. **What are the emergency priorities when evaluating a child with a severe headache?**
As with all common presenting symptoms, the main priority is to rule out diagnostic possibilities that may be life-threatening:
    - Malignant hypertension
    - Increased intracranial pressure (e.g., mass lesion, acute hydrocephalus)
    - Intracranial infections (e.g., meningitis, encephalitis)
    - Subarachnoid hemorrhage
    - Stroke
    - Acute angle closure glaucoma (may appear as a headache, but rare in children)

126. **When should neuroimaging be considered in a child with headache?**
    - Abnormal neurologic signs
    - Headache increasing in frequency and severity
    - Headache occurring in early morning or awakening child from sleep
    - Headache made worse by straining or by sneezing or coughing (may be a sign of increased ICP)
    - Headache associated with severe vomiting without nausea
    - Headache worsened or helped significantly by a change in position
    - Fall off in linear growth rate
    - Recent school failure or significant behavioral changes
    - New-onset seizures, especially if seizure has a focal onset (see previous discussion)
    - Migraine headache and seizure occurring in the same episode, with vascular symptoms preceding the seizure (20% to 50% risk for tumor or arteriovenous malformation)
    - Cluster headaches in any child or teenager

    Lewis DW, Ashwal S, Dahl G, et al, Quality Standards Subcommittee of the American Academy of Neurology; Practice Committee of the Child Neurology Society: Practice parameter: evaluation of children and adolescents with recurrent headaches. Report of the Quality Standards Subcommittee of the American Academy of Neurology and the Practice Committee of the Child Neurology Society, *Neurology* 59:490–498, 2002.

    Schor NF: Brain imaging and prophylactic therapy in children with migraine: recommendations versus reality, *J Pediatr* 143:776–779, 2003.

KEY POINTS: CLASSIC HEADACHE OF INCREASED INTRACRANIAL PRESSURE

1. Awakens patient from sleep at night

2. Pain present upon awakening in the morning

3. Vomiting without associated nausea

4. Made worse by straining, sneezing, or coughing

5. Intensity of pain changes with changes in body position

6. Pain lessens during the day

127. **What are the three primary headache disorders in children?**
These are recurrent headaches not attributable to underlying physical disease.
    - **Migraine:** Most common type in children (4% in childhood and more common in teenage girls and young women)

- **Tension type:** Features different from migraine—bilateral, nonpulsating, not aggravated by activity; school problems with stress and absences and family dysfunction are frequently noted
- **Cluster:** Uncommon in childhood; consist of severe unilateral orbital or supraorbital pain with conjunctival injection and tearing

128. **What is the origin of the word *migraine*?**
Ancient Greek physicians recognized a specific type of recurring head pain that was unilateral. The modern word *migraine* is a French modification of the Greek term *hemikrania*.

129. **What are the clinical features of migraine headaches in children?**
Migraine is a periodic disorder with symptom-free periods characterized by headaches with a throbbing nature, unilateral in older children and commonly bilateral in younger children, lasting 1 to 72 hours, pulsating with moderate or severe intensity, aggravated by routine physical activity and exercise, and associated with nausea and/or photophobia and phonophobia. There may be a history of recurrent vomiting or motion sickness. There is often a family history of migraine, and the genetics may be multifactorial.
- **Migraine with aura:** Previously called *classic migraine*, this is less common in children. The aura is a prodrome of variable focal neurologic features such as visual scotoma, sensory symptoms (numbness, tingling), sluggishness, and difficulty concentrating or motor features (weakness, dysphasia).
- **Migraine without aura:** Previously called common migraine, these are the more frequent type in childhood.

Headache Classification Subcommittee of the International Headache Society: The international classification of headache disorders, *Cephalalgia* 24(Suppl 1):1–160, 2004.

130. **Which physical findings are important during the initial evaluation of possible migraine headache?**
- Height and weight should be normal for age. Pituitary tumor, craniopharyngioma, and partial ornithine transcarbamylase deficiency may all result in growth failure and mimic migraine headache. Head circumference should be normal, ruling out hydrocephalus.
- Skin should be checked for abnormalities. Throbbing headaches are common in neurofibromatosis and systemic lupus erythematosus, both of which have easily recognizable skin manifestations.
- Blood pressure should be normal.
- Check for sinus tenderness or pain with head movement (implying cervical spine disease). The patient should be examined for carious teeth, misaligned bite, or disordered chewing and jaw opening (temporomandibular joint dysfunction).
- Auscultation should reveal no cranial bruits (if present, these suggest possible arteriovenous malformation or mass lesion).
- The neurologic examination should be normal.

131. **When do children begin to have migraine headaches?**
About 20% suffer their first headache before the age of 10 years.

132. **Which foods have been associated with the development of migraine headaches?**
Tyramine-rich foods (cheese, red wine), foods with monosodium glutamate (Asian food), nitrate-rich foods (smoked and lunch meats, salami), alcoholic beverages, caffeinated beverages, chocolate, citrus fruits, and sulfites (food coloring).

133. **What is familial hemiplegic migraine?**
Familial hemiplegic migraine is an autosomal dominant disorder that is clinically characterized by transient hemiparesis and aphasia followed by migraine headache. About 20% are affected by progressive cerebellar ataxia. Mutations in CACNA1A (which encodes a neuronal calcium channel) on chromosome 19 are found in half of affected families.

Wessman M, Kaunisto MA, Kallela M, et al: The molecular genetics of migraine, *Ann Med* 36: 462–473, 2004.

134. **What is the likely diagnosis for a 10-year-old girl with a history of headaches and a family history of migraines who has had 10 minutes of a spinning sensation and double vision followed by an occipital headache and has a normal neurologic examination in the office?**
Basilar-type migraine, which occurs in 3% to 19% of childhood migraines. Symptoms related to balance, gait, and visual disturbance are followed by headache, which, unlike most migraines, is occipital.

Lewis DW: Pediatric migraine, *Pediatr Rev* 28:43–53, 2007.

135. **How do the triptans work to treat an acute migraine headache?**
Triptans are serotonin receptor subtype-selective drugs which were thought initially to work primarily through their vasoconstrictive effects on arterial smooth muscle in cranial blood vessels. However, there are questions whether the primary mechanism is central or peripheral. Triptans act on peripheral nerve endings, preventing the release of proinflammatory and vasoactive peptides, including substance P and calcitonin gene–related peptide (GCRP). Also unclear is the apparent selectivity of triptans for migraine pain but not other kinds of somatic pain.

Ahn AH, Basbaum AI: Where do triptans act in the treatment of migraine? *Pain* 115:1–4, 2005.

136. **What nonpharmacologic therapies are available for the prevention of migraine?**
- Migraine elimination diet
- Normalization of sleep habits
- Discontinuance of possible triggering medications (e.g., analgesic overuse, bronchodilators, oral contraceptives)
- Biofeedback
- Relaxation therapy
- Family counseling (if family stress is a trigger)
- Self-hypnosis

Damen L, Bruijn J, Verhagen AP, et al: Prophylactic treatment of migraine in children. Part 1. A systematic review of nonpharmacological trials, *Cephalalgia* 26:373–383, 2006.

137. **What categories of medication are available for the prevention of migraine in children?**
As with many therapies used for children, most studies involve adults with extrapolation to children for whom the mediations may not work as well. These medications are regularly used by clinicians but not yet approved by the U.S. Food and Drug Administration for children. Keys to therapy are gradually increasing the dose until effectiveness is or is not established or adverse effects intervene.
- Antidepressants (especially tricyclics)
- Antihistamine (especially cyproheptadine with antiserotonergic effects)
- Antihypertensives (including β-blockers and calcium channel blockers)

■ Anticonvulsants (including divalproate sodium and topiramate)
■ Nonpharmaceuticals (including riboflavin, coenzyme Q, and butterbur extract)

Damen L, Bruijn JK, Verhagen AP, et al: Prophylactic treatment of migraine in children. Part 2. A systematic review of pharmacological trials, *Cephalalgia* 26:373–383, 2006.

138. **Who should be started on prophylactic medication for migraine headaches?**
There are no precise criteria, but generally prophylactic treatment should be considered if any of the following are present:
■ Headaches with aura occur frequently.
■ Headaches with aura are poorly responsive to abortive medication.
■ School attendance is significantly affected.
■ Headaches, although infrequent, last for several days.

139. **How long are the prophylactic medications continued?**
The optimal duration of therapy remains unclear, but many authorities suggest a treatment duration of 3 to 6 months followed by an attempt at weaning. Less than 50% will require the reinitiation of medication.

140. **What distinguishes tension-type headaches from migraines?**
Unlike migraines, these headaches are bilateral with a pressing and tightening quality (as opposed to the pulsatile quality of migraines) and usually of mild or moderate intensity. They are not associated with nausea or vomiting and typically not worsened by light or sound. Pericranial muscle tenderness is common.
Psychological stress is associated with and can aggravate tension-type headaches. Activation of hyperexcitable peripheral afferent neurons from head and neck muscles, as well as abnormalities in central pain processing and pain sensitivity, likely contribute to the problem.

Loder E, Rizzoli R: Tension-type headache, *BMJ* 336:88–92, 2008.

MOVEMENT DISORDERS

141. **What are the various types of pathologic hyperkinetic movements?**
■ **Tremors:** Rhythmic oscillatory movements, both supination-pronation and flexion-extension, seen in resting state or with activity
■ **Chorea:** Quick dancing movements of proximal and distal muscles with irregular unpredictable random jerks
■ **Athetosis:** Irregular, slow, distal writhing movements
■ **Stereotypy:** Repetitive, purposeless motions (e.g., body rocking, head rolling) that resemble voluntary movements often associated with akathisia (sensory and motor restlessness)
■ **Dystonia:** Slow, twisting, sustained movements; may result in abnormal postures and progress to contractures
■ **Ballismus:** Abrupt, random, violent, flinging movements, often proximal and unilateral
■ **Myoclonus:** Abrupt, brief, jerky contractions of one or more muscles, often stimulus sensitive
■ **Tics:** Rapid, sudden, repetitive movements or vocalizations

142. **What techniques can be used to elicit abnormal movements (particularly chorea)?**
Methods of provocative testing include the maintenance of posture in extension against gravity, hyperpronation (or "spooning," especially above the head), tongue protrusion ("trombone tongue"), squeezing the finger of the examiner ("milk-maid's grip"), pouring liquid, and drawing a spiral.

143. **What disorders are commonly associated with the various hyperkinetic movements?**
    - **Tremors, resting:** Primary juvenile Parkinson disease, secondary Parkinson disease
    - **Tremors, kinetic:** Essential (familial) tremor, cerebellar disorders, brainstem tumors, hyperthyroidism, Wilson disease, electrolyte disturbance (e.g., glucose, calcium, magnesium), heavy-metal intoxication (e.g., lead, mercury), multiple sclerosis
    - **Chorea:** Sydenham chorea (associated with rheumatic fever), Huntington disease, hyperthyroidism, infectious mononucleosis, pregnancy, anticonvulsants, neuroleptic drugs, closed head injury, systemic lupus erythematosus, carbon monoxide poisoning, Wilson disease, hypocalcemia, polycythemia, parainfectious and infectious encephalopathies (e.g., rubeola, syphilis)
    - **Athetosis:** CP, other static encephalopathies, Lesch-Nyhan syndrome, kernicterus
    - **Stereotypy:** Autism, Rett syndrome, neuroleptic drugs (i.e., tardive dyskinesia), schizophrenia
    - **Dystonia:** Idiopathic primary dystonias (e.g., torsion dystonia), Sandifer syndrome, spasmus nutans, neuroleptic drugs, static encephalopathy, perinatal asphyxia, familial dystonia (sometimes dopa-responsive)
    - **Ballismus:** Encephalitis, closed head injury
    - **Myoclonus:** Sleep myoclonus, benign myoclonus of infancy, postanoxic encephalopathy, uremic encephalopathy, hyperthyroidism, urea cycle defects, side effects of tricyclic therapy, slow virus infections, Wilson disease, myoclonus-opsoclonus, neuroblastoma, epileptic encephalopathies, mitochondrial disease, prion disease, Tay-Sachs disease, startle disease, sialidosis

144. **What constitutes a tic?**
    Tics are brief, sudden, repetitive, stereotyped, involuntary, and purposeless movements or vocalizations. They most commonly involve muscles of the head, neck, and respiratory tract. Their frequency can be increased by anxiety, stress, excitement, and fatigue. They are decreased during sleep and relaxation, during activities involving high concentration, and, at times, through voluntary action. In some cases, premonitory feelings (e.g., irritation, tickle, temperature change) can precipitate the motor or vocal response.

145. **What is the range of clinical tics?**
    - **Motor (simple clonic):** Eye blinking, eye jerking, head twitching, shoulder shrugging
    - **Motor (simple dystonic):** Bruxism, abdominal tensing, shoulder rotation
    - **Motor (complex):** Grunting, barking, sniffing, snorting, throat clearing, spitting
    - **Vocal (complex):** Coprolalia (obscene words), echolalia (repeating another's words), palilalia (rapidly repeating one's own words)

146. **What makes a tic tick?**
    Transient and chronic tic disorders usually do not have an identifiable cause. However, dyskinesias such as tics can be found in association with a number of other conditions:
    - **Chromosomal abnormalities:** Down syndrome, fragile X syndrome
    - **Developmental syndromes:** Autism, pervasive developmental disorder, Rett syndrome
    - **Drugs:** Anticonvulsants, stimulants (e.g., amphetamines, cocaine, methylphenidate, pemoline)
    - **Infections:** Encephalitis, postrubella syndrome

147. **How should simple tics be treated?**
    Simple motor tics are common and occur in more than 5% to 21% of school-aged children. Simple tics generally do not require pharmacologic intervention and can be treated expectantly by developing relaxation techniques, minimizing stresses that exacerbate the problem, avoiding punishment for tics, and decreasing fixation on the problem. Most simple tics self-resolve in 2 to 12 months. Moderate or severe tics, especially when significant patient distress is involved, may warrant pharmacologic treatment.

148. **What comorbidities occur in children with tics?**

The prevalence of tic disorder is higher in younger children and in males and is associated with school dysfunction, obsessive-compulsive disorder, and attention-deficit/hyperactivity disorder. In addition, separation anxiety, overanxious disorder, simple phobia, social phobia, agoraphobia, mania, major depression, and oppositional defiant disorder were found to be significantly more common in children with tics.

149. **When do tics warrant pharmacologic intervention?**

Tics that have a significant disabling impact on a child's educational, social, or psychological well-being (particularly if they have been present for >1 year) may require intervention. When the complexity of tics increases or the diagnosis of Tourette syndrome is suspected, pharmacotherapy should also be considered. Most theories point to a hyperdopaminergic state of the basal ganglia as the most likely etiology for unregulated movements. Pharmacologic management includes α_2-agonists (e.g., clonidine, guanfacine) or the administration of atypical neuroleptics (e.g., risperidone, haloperidol) and/or the cessation of any stimulant drugs that can cause dopamine release. Because of the high associated incidence of obsessive-compulsive disorder and attention-deficit/hyperactivity disorder, other medications may be needed, and consultation with a pediatric psychiatrist or neurologist is often warranted.

150. **What are the diagnostic criteria for Tourette syndrome?**

In 1885, Gilles de la Tourette described a syndrome of motor tics and vocal tics with behavioral disturbances and a chronic and variable course. *Diagnostic and Statistical Manual of Mental Disorders* (DSM IV) criteria for Tourette syndrome require the following:
- Multiple motor tics
- One or more vocal tics
- Onset before the age of 21 years
- Waxing and waning course
- Presence of tics for more than 1 year (usually on a daily basis)
- No identifiable medical etiology

151. **What is coprolalia?**

Coprolalia is an irresistible urge to utter profanities, occurring as a phonic tic. Only 20% to 40% of patients with Tourette syndrome have this phenomenon, and it is not essential for the diagnosis.

152. **What behavioral problems are associated with Tourette syndrome?**
- Obsessive-compulsive disorder
- Attention-deficit/hyperactivity disorder
- Severe conduct disorders
- Learning disabilities (particularly math)
- Sleep abnormalities
- Depression, anxiety, and emotional lability

Tourette Syndrome Association: http://www.tsa-usa.org.

153. **Why is the diagnosis of Tourette syndrome commonly delayed?**
- Tendency to associate unusual symptoms with attention-getting or psychological problems
- Incorrect belief that all children with Tourette syndrome must have severe tics
- Attribution of vocal tics to upper respiratory infections, allergies, or sinus or bronchial problems
- Diagnosis of eye blinking or ocular tics as ophthalmologic problems
- Mistaken belief that coprolalia is an essential diagnostic feature

Singer HS: Tic disorders, *Pediatr Ann* 22:22–29, 1993.

154. **What is the cause of tardive dyskinesia?**
Tardive dyskinesia is a hyperkinetic disorder of abnormal movements, most commonly involving the face (e.g., lip smacking or pursing, chewing, grimacing, tongue protruding). Tardive dyskinesia occurs during treatment with neuroleptics (e.g., chlorpromazine, haloperidol, metoclopramide) or within 6 months of their discontinuance. This disorder is thought to be a result of dopaminergic dysfunction of the basal ganglia because these drugs act as dopamine-receptor blockers.

155. **For a patient taking neuroleptic medication, how long must therapy last before symptoms of tardive dyskinesia can develop?**
About 3 months of continuous or intermittent treatment with neuroleptics is needed before the risk for tardive dyskinesia increases.

156. **What is neuroleptic malignant syndrome?**
Neuroleptic malignant syndrome is a syndrome of movement (rigidity, tremor, chorea, and dystonia), autonomic dysfunction (fever, hypertension, tachycardia, diaphoresis, irregular respiratory pattern, urinary retention), alteration of consciousness, and rhabdomyolysis with an elevation of creatinine kinase. It occurs within weeks of starting neuroleptics, and there is a 20% associated mortality rate in adults.

157. **Which movement disorder in children presents with "dancing eyes and dancing feet"?**
Opsoclonus-myoclonus (infantile polymyoclonus syndrome or acute myoclonic encephalopathy of infants) is a rare but distinctive movement disorder in children that is seen during the first 1 to 3 years of life. Opsoclonus is characterized by wild, chaotic, fluttering, irregular, rapid, conjugate bursts of eye movements (saccadomania). Myoclonus is sudden, shocklike muscular twitches of the face, limbs, or trunk. The anatomic site of pathology is the cerebellar outflow tracts. The etiology may be direct viral invasion, postinfectious encephalopathy, or neuroblastoma.

NEONATAL SEIZURES

158. **How are neonatal seizures classified?**
Although there is no universally accepted standard classification system, one based on clinical criteria is commonly used. It divides neonatal seizures into four types:
- Subtle
- Tonic (partial or generalized)
- Clonic (partial or multifocal)
- Myoclonic (partial, multifocal, or generalized)

All seizure types are recognized as paroxysmal alterations in behavioral, motor, or autonomic function. Not all clinically observed phenomena, however, are accompanied by associated epileptic surface-EEG activity, and this electroclinical disassociation is increased after AED treatment. Partial clonic, tonic, and myoclonic seizures have been shown to have the most consistent EEG ictal correlate.

159. **What is the most common type of clinical seizure during the neonatal period?**
The so-called **subtle seizure**. Rather than arising as an abrupt dramatic "convulsion" with obvious forceful twitching or posturing of the muscles, the subtle seizure appears as an unnatural, repetitive, stereotyped choreography, featuring oral-buccal-lingual movements, eye blinking, nystagmus, lip smacking, or complex integrated limb movements (swimming, pedaling, or rowing) and other fragments of activity drawn from the limited repertoire of normal infant activity. These neonates frequently have HIE and moderately to markedly abnormal EEGs, and they are at significantly greater risk for mental retardation, CP, and epilepsy.

160. **What are the causes of neonatal seizures?**
 ■ Hypoxic-ischemic encephalopathy caused by asphyxia
 ■ Infection
 ■ Toxins (e.g., inadvertent fetal injection with local anesthetic; cocaine, including withdrawal)
 ■ Metabolic abnormalities (e.g., hypoglycemia, hypocalcemia, hypomagnesemia, pyridoxine deficiency, inborn errors)
 ■ CNS malformations
 ■ Cerebrovascular lesions (e.g., intraventricular, periventricular hemorrhage, subarachnoid hemorrhage, infarction, arterial cerebral occlusion)
 ■ Benign familial neonatal-infantile seizures (e.g., a sodium channelopathy)

 Zupanc ML: Neonatal seizures, *Pediatr Clin North Am* 51:961–978, 2004.

161. **In premature and full-term infants, how do the causes of seizures vary with regard to relative frequency and time of onset?**
 See Table 14-4.

TABLE 14-4. VARIANCE IN RELATIVE FREQUENCY AND TIME OF ONSET OF CAUSES OF SEIZURES

Etiology	Postnatal Time of Onset		Relative Frequency	
	0-3 days	>3 days	Premature	Full-Term
Hypoxic-ischemic	+		+++	+++
Intracranial hemorrhage*	+	+	++	+
Hypoglycemia	+		+	+
Hypocalcemia	+	+	+	+
Intracranial infection†	+	+	++	+
Developmental defects	+	+	++	++
Drug withdrawal	+	+	+	+

*Hemorrhages are principally germinal matrix-intraventricular in the premature infant and subarachnoid or subdural in the term infant.
†Early seizures occur usually after intrauterine nonbacterial infections (e.g., toxoplasmosis, cytomegalovirus infection), and later seizures usually occur with herpes simplex encephalitis or bacterial meningitis.
Adapted from Volpe JJ (ed): Neurology of the Newborn, 3rd ed. Philadelphia, WB Saunders, 1995, p 184.

162. **What is an acceptable workup in a newborn with seizures?**
 The workup should include a careful prenatal and natal history as well as a complete physical examination. Laboratory studies should include blood for glucose, electrolytes, calcium, phosphorus, and magnesium. A lumbar puncture should be performed to rule out meningitis. Neuroimaging studies (cranial ultrasound, CT scan, or MRI) are mandatory. Additional studies, where warranted, include blood levels for ammonia, lactate, and pyruvate; additional CSF studies (e.g., lactate, pyruvate, glycine, CSF neurotransmitters if metabolic disease is suspected); and urine studies for organic and amino acid analysis for possible inborn errors of metabolism. Serial use of EEG polygraphy can document persistent seizures, especially the persistence of electrographic seizures without clinical seizures after initial treatment.

163. **In what settings should an inborn error of metabolism be suspected as a cause of neonatal seizures?**
    - The onset of seizures is beyond day 1 of life (the exception is pyridoxine deficiency).
    - The infant becomes symptomatic after the introduction of enteral or parenteral nutrition.
    - The seizures are intractable and do not respond to conventional AEDs.

    Characteristic EEG patterns may be seen in maple syrup urine disease, propionic acidemia, and pyridoxine deficiency.

    Scher MS: Neonatal seizures. In Polin RA, Yoder MC, editors: *Workbook in Practical Neonatology*, ed 4, Philadelphia, 2007, Saunders Elsevier, p 363.

164. **How are seizures differentiated from tremors in the neonate?**
    See Table 14-5.

TABLE 14-5. TREMORS VERSUS SEIZURES		
Clinical Feature	Tremors	Seizures
Abnormality of gaze or eye movement	0	+
Movements are exquisitely stimulus sensitive	+	0
Predominant movement	Tremor	Clonic jerking
Movements cease with passive flexion	+	0
Autonomic changes	0	+

Adapted from Volpe JJ (ed): Neurology of the Newborn, 3rd ed. Philadelphia, WB Saunders, 1995, p 182.

165. **What are the treatment options for neonatal seizures?**
    Neonatal seizures may be treated with phenobarbital. Studies of the pharmacokinetics of phenobarbital in neonates have indicated that it is most appropriate to load with a full 20 mg/kg rather than smaller fractions. If seizures persist, additional increments of phenobarbital to total loading doses of 40 mg/kg can be given. Continued seizures may be treated with a loading dose of 20 mg/kg of phenytoin (or phenytoin equivalents in the case of fosphenytoin). The usual maintenance dose for phenobarbital is between 3 and 6 mg/kg per day and between 4 and 8 mg/kg per day for phenytoin. Efficacy from either of these two agents is low, with only one third of patients showing an immediate complete response. Even after apparently successful intravenous treatment with phenobarbital and phenytoin with the resolution of clinical seizures, electrographic seizures may continue unabated. The significance of this finding is unclear, and the need to suppress electrographic seizures without clinical accompaniments is controversial.

    Levene M: The clinical conundrum of neonatal seizures, *Arch Dis Child Fetal Neonatal Ed* 86:F75–F77, 2002.

    Rennie JM, Boylan GB: Neonatal seizures and their treatment, *Curr Opin Neurol* 16:177–181, 2003.

166. **What is the treatment for refractory seizures in the neonate?**
    Frequent and recurrent seizures are not uncommon in newborns and are especially common in the setting of asphyxia. If seizures are refractory to full dosing of phenobarbital and phenytoin, the addition of drugs in the benzodiazepine family (e.g., diazepam, lorazepam) or of paraldehyde is generally effective. It is important to ensure that no underlying biochemical disturbance is present before the serum levels of anticonvulsants are raised to

maximal concentrations. Although pyridoxine-dependent seizures are rare, a trial dose of pyridoxine should be administered intravenously to infants with recurrent seizures of uncertain etiology. If possible, simultaneous EEG recording should be performed to document the cessation of seizure activity and the normalization of the EEG within minutes of pyridoxine treatment. Infants with pyridoxine-dependent epilepsy may have profound autonomic dysfunction (apnea, bradycardia, and hypotension) in response to initial pyridoxine administration and should be monitored carefully.

167. **Of what prognostic value is the interictal EEG in a neonate with seizures?**
This study can have significant prognostic value. Severe interictal EEG abnormalities (e.g., burst suppression, marked voltage suppression, flat or isoelectric) are highly predictive (90%) of a fatal outcome or severe neurologic sequelae. Conversely, a normal interictal EEG in a term infant with seizures confers a very low (10%) likelihood of significant neurologic impairment. Moderate abnormalities (e.g., voltage asymmetries, immature patterns) have a mixed outcome.

Laroia N, Guillet R, Burchfiel J, McBride MC: EEG background as predictor of electrographic seizures in high risk neonates, *Epilepsia* 39:545–551, 1998.

168. **After an infant has recovered from a seizure, how long should medication be continued?**
Maintenance therapy typically involves the use of phenobarbital because it is difficult to achieve therapeutic levels of phenytoin with oral administration in infancy, and other medications (e.g., carbamazepine) are less well studied. Although phenobarbital is generally well tolerated, it may have deleterious effects on behavior, attention span, and possibly brain development. It does not prevent the later development of epilepsy.
Many authorities recommend discontinuing therapy if the neurologic examination has normalized. In addition, if the neurologic examination is abnormal but an EEG by the age of 3 months reveals no seizure activity, consideration can also be given to stopping phenobarbital.

169. **In patients with neonatal seizures, how does the cause affect the prognosis?**
See Table 14-6.

NEUROCUTANEOUS SYNDROMES

170. **What are the three most common neurocutaneous syndromes?**
- Neurofibromatosis
- Tuberous sclerosis complex
- Sturge-Weber syndrome

171. **What are the inheritance patterns of the various neurocutaneous syndromes?**
- **Neurofibromatosis:** Autosomal dominant
- **Tuberous sclerosis complex:** Autosomal dominant
- **von Hippel-Lindau syndrome:** Autosomal dominant
- **Incontinentia pigmenti:** X-linked dominant
- **Sturge-Weber syndrome:** Sporadic
- **Klippel-Trénaunay-Weber syndrome:** Sporadic

172. **What is the derivation of the term *phakomatosis*?**
The term *phakomatosis* is derived from the Greek *phakos*, meaning "lentil" or "lens-shaped," and it refers to patchy, circumscribed dermatologic lesions that are the hallmark of this group of disorders. In addition to dermatologic features, these syndromes have hamartomatous involvement of multiple tissues, especially the CNS and the eye. More commonly, the term *neurocutaneous syndrome* is used.

TABLE 14-6. RELATIONSHIP BETWEEN CAUSE AND PROGNOSIS OF NEONATAL SEIZURE

Etiology	Favorable Outcome*	Mixed Outcome	Unfavorable Outcome*
Toxic-metabolic	Simple late-onset hypocalcemia Hypomagnesemia Hyponatremia Mepivacaine toxicity	Hypoglycemia Early-onset complicated hypocalcemia Pyridoxine dependency	Some aminoacidurias
Asphyxia	—	Mild hypoxic-ischemic encephalopathy	Severe hypoxic-ischemic encephalopathy
Hemorrhage	Uncomplicated subarachnoid hemorrhage	Subdural hematoma Intraventricular hemorrhage (grades I and II)	Intraventricular hemorrhage (grades III and IV)
Infection	—	Aseptic meningoencephalitis; some bacterial meningitides	Herpes simplex encephalitis; some bacterial meningitides
Structural	—	Simple traumatic contusion	Malformations of the central nervous system

*Favorable prognosis implies at least an 85% to 90% chance of survival and subsequent normal development. Unfavorable prognosis implies a high likelihood (85% to 90%) of death or serious handicap in survivors.
From Scher MS: Neonatal seizures. In Polin RA, Yoder MC (eds): Workbook in Practical Neonatology, 4th ed. Philadelphia, Saunders Elsevier, 2007, p 370.

---

173. **What are the diagnostic criteria for neurofibromatosis-1 (NF1)?**
Two or more of the following:
■ Café-au-lait spots (six or more that are >0.5 cm in diameter before puberty; six or more that are >1.5 cm in diameter after puberty)
■ Skinfold freckling (axillary or inguinal region)
■ Neurofibromas (two or more) of any type, or at least one plexiform neurofibroma
■ Iris hamartomas, also called *Lisch nodules* (two or more)
■ Characteristic osseous lesion (i.e., sphenoid dysplasia, thinning of the cortex of the long bones with or without pseudoarthrosis)
■ First-degree relative with NF1 diagnosed by the above criteria

Williams VC, Lucas J, Babcock MA, et al: Neurofibromatosis type 1 revisited, *Pediatrics* 123:124–133, 2009.

174. **How does NF1 differ from NF2?**
NF1, which is also known as *classic von Recklinghausen disease*, is much more common (1 in every 3000 to 4000 births) than NF2 and accounts for up to 90% of cases of neurofibromatosis. NF2 (1 in every 50,000 births) is characterized by bilateral acoustic neuromas, intracranial and intraspinal tumors, and affected first-degree relatives. NF1 has been linked to alterations on chromosome 17, whereas NF2 is linked to alterations on chromosome 22. Dermatologic findings and peripheral neuromas are rare in NF2. Other rarer subtypes of neurofibromatoses (e.g., segmental distribution) have been described.

Asthagiri AR, Parry DM, Butman JA, et al: Neurofibromatosis type 2, *Lancet* 373:1974–1986, 2009.

175. **How common are café-au-lait spots at birth?**
Up to 2% of black infants will have three café-au-lait spots at birth, whereas one café-au-lait spot occurs in only 0.3% of white infants. White infants with multiple café-au-lait spots at birth are more likely than black infants to develop neurofibromatosis. In older children, a single café-au-lait spot that is more than 5 mm in diameter can be found in 10% of white and 25% of black children.

Hurwitz S: Neurofibromatosis. In Hurwitz S, editor: *Clinical Pediatric Dermatology*, ed 2, Philadelphia, 1993, WB Saunders, pp 624–629.

176. **If a 2-year-old child has seven café-au-lait spots that are larger than 5 mm in diameter, what is the likelihood that neurofibromatosis will develop, and how will it evolve?**
Up to 75% of these children, if followed sequentially, will develop one of the varieties of neurofibromatosis, most commonly type 1. In a study of nearly 1900 patients, 46% with sporadic NF1 did not meet criteria by the age of 1 year. By the age of 8 years, however, 97% met the criteria, and by the age of 20 years, 100% did. The typical order of appearance of features is café-au-lait spots, axillary freckling, Lisch nodules, and neurofibromas. Yearly evaluation of patients with suspicious findings should include a careful skin examination, ophthalmologic evaluation, and blood pressure measurement.

DeBella K, Szudek J, Friedman JM: Use of the National Institutes of Health criteria for the diagnosis of neurofibromatosis 1 in children, *Pediatrics* 105:608–614, 2000.

Korf BR: Diagnostic outcome in children with multiple café-au-lait spots, *Pediatrics* 90:924–927, 1992.

177. **What are Lisch nodules?**
Pigmented iris hamartomas (Fig. 14-1). Although these are not usually present at birth in patients with NF1, up to 90% will develop multiple Lisch nodules by the age

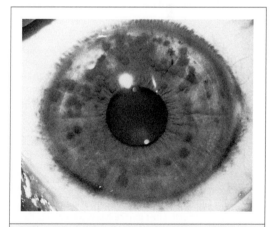

Figure 14-1. Lisch nodules. (From Zitelli BJ, Davis HW: Atlas of Pediatric Physical Diagnosis, 5th ed. Philadelphia, Mosby, 2007, p 568.)

of 6 years. Hamartomas are focal malformations that are microscopically composed of multiple tissue types, and these can resemble neoplasms. However, unlike neoplasms, they grow at similar rates as normal components and are unlikely to pathologically compress adjacent tissue.

178. **How common is a positive family history in cases of NF1?**
Because of the high spontaneous mutation rate for this autosomal dominant disease, only about 50% of newly diagnosed cases are associated with a positive family history.

179. **What are the primary diagnostic criteria for tuberous sclerosis complex (TSC)?**
TSC is characterized by hamartomatous growths that occur in multiple tissues. The National Institutes of Health Consensus Conference in 1998 revised the diagnostic criteria for TSC on the basis of major or minor features. Definite TSC consisted of two major features or one major and two minor features; probable and possible TSC had fewer features (Table 14-7). No single finding was considered pathognomonic for TSC. Two gene site abnormalities, TSC1 (chromosome 9) and TSC2 (chromosome 16), have been identified. Genetic testing is now available.

TABLE 14-7. DIAGNOSTIC FEATURES FOR TUBEROUS SCLEROSIS COMPLEX

Major Features	Minor Features
Facial angiofibromas	Dental enamel pits
Nontraumatic ungual or periungual fibroma	Bone cysts
Hypomelanotic macules (>3)	Hamartomatous rectal polyps
Shagreen patch	Gingival fibromas
Multiple retinal nodular hamartomas	Cerebral white matter migration tracts
Cortical tuber	
Subependymal nodule or giant cell astrocytoma	
Cardiac rhabdomyoma, single or multiple	

Crino PB, Nathanson KL, Henske EP: The tuberous sclerosis complex, *N Engl J Med* 355: 1345–1356, 2006.

180. **What is the classic triad of TSC?**
1. Seizures
2. Mental retardation
3. Facial angiofibroma (adenoma sebaceum)
However, less than one third of patients will develop these classic features.

181. **What is the most common presenting symptom of TSC?**
Seizures. About 85% of patients have seizures, and infantile spasms are the most common. Tonic and atonic seizures are also seen. Complex partial seizures are frequently seen in conjunction with other seizure types. Mental retardation is especially common with the onset of seizures before the age of 2 years. Autism and other behavioral disturbances are also frequently seen in children with TSC.

Curatolo P, Bombardieri R, Jozwiak S: Tuberous sclerosis, *Lancet* 372:657–668, 2008.

182. **What are skin findings in patients with tuberous sclerosis?**
See Table 14-8.

TABLE 14-8. SKIN FINDINGS IN TUBEROUS SCLEROSIS

Age at Onset	Skin Findings	Incidence (%)
Birth or later	Hypopigmented macules	80
2-5 yr	Angiofibromas	70
2-5 yr	Shagreen patches	35
Puberty	Periungual and gingival fibromas	20-50
Birth or later	Café-au-lait spots	25

183. **Why is the term *adenoma sebaceum* a misnomer when used to describe patients with tuberous sclerosis?**
On biopsy, these papules are actually angiofibromas. They have no connection to sebaceous units or adenomas. This rash occurs in about 75% of patients with tuberous sclerosis, usually developing on the nose and central face between the ages of 5 and 13 years. It is red, papular, and monomorphous, and it is often mistaken for acne (Fig. 14-2). The diagnosis of tuberous sclerosis should be entertained in children who develop a rash that is suggestive of acne well before puberty.

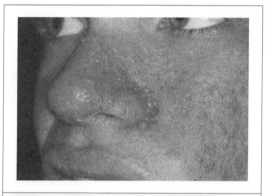

Figure 14-2. Adenoma sebaceum in patient with tuberous sclerosis. (From Sahn EE: Dermatology Pearls. Philadelphia, Hanley and Belfus, 1999, p 86.)

184. **What is the "tuber" of tuberous sclerosis?**
These 1- to 2-cm lesions consist of small stellate neurons and astroglial elements that are thought to be primitive cell lines resulting from abnormal differentiation. They may be located in various cortical regions. They are firm to the touch, like a small potato or tuber.

185. **What is the tissue type of a shagreen patch?**
A shagreen patch is an area of cutaneous thickening with a pebbled surface that, on biopsy, is a **connective tissue nevus**. The term *shagreen* derives from a type of leather that is embossed by knobs during the course of processing.

186. **Which types of facial port-wine stains are most strongly associated with ophthalmic or CNS complications?**
Port-wine stains can occur as isolated cutaneous birthmarks or, particularly in the areas underlying the birthmark, in association with structural abnormalities in the following areas:

(1) the choroidal vessels of the eye, thereby leading to glaucoma; (2) the leptomeningeal vessels of the brain, thus leading to seizures (Sturge-Weber syndrome); and (3) hemangiomas in the spinal cord (Cobb syndrome). Glaucoma or seizures are most often associated with port-wine stains in children demonstrating the following:

- Involvement of the eyelids
- Bilateral distribution of the birthmark
- Unilateral involvement of all three branches (V_1, V_2, V_3) of the trigeminal nerve
- Ophthalmologic assessment and radiologic studies (CT or MRI) are indicated for children exhibiting these findings.

Thomas-Sohl KA, Vaslow DF, Maria BL: Sturge-Weber syndrome: a review, *Pediatr Neurol* 30: 303–310, 2004.

Tallman B, Tan OT, Morelli JG, et al: Location of port-wine stains and the likelihood of ophthalmic and/ or central nervous system complications, *Pediatrics* 87:323–327, 1991.

187. **What are the three stages of incontinentia pigmenti?**
Incontinentia pigmenti is an X-linked dominant disorder that is associated with seizures and mental retardation. The condition is presumed to be lethal to boys in utero because nearly 100% of cases are female.
- **Stage 1—Vesicular stage:** Lines of blisters are present on the trunk and extremities of the newborn that disappear in weeks or months. They may resemble herpetic vesicles. Microscopic examination of the vesicular fluid demonstrates eosinophils.
- **Stage 2—Verrucous stage:** Lesions develop in the patient at about 3 to 7 months of age that are brown and hyperkeratotic, resembling warts; these disappear over 1 to 2 years.
- **Stage 3—Pigmented stage:** Whorled, swirling (marble cake–like), macular, hyperpigmented lines develop. These may fade over time, leaving only remnant hypopigmentation in late adolescence or adulthood (which is sometimes considered a fourth stage).

188. **What is the likely diagnosis for a 7-year-old who is noted to have recurrent nosebleeds, cutaneous telangiectasias on his lips, and an intracranial arteriovenous malformation on MRI?**
Hereditary hemorrhagic telangiectasia, which has also been known as *Osler-Weber-Rendu disease*. This condition may affect up to 1 in 5000 in the United States. The condition consists of nosebleeds; skin lesions; visceral manifestations due to arteriovenous malformations in the lung, liver, gastrointestinal tract, and CNS; and a positive family history. Genetic mutations involve transforming growth factor-β, which causes abnormalities in blood vessel formation.

Mei-Zahav M, Letarte M, Faughnan ME, et al: Symptomatic children with hereditary hemorrhagic telangiectasia: a pediatric center experience, *Arch Pediatr Adolesc Med* 160:596–601, 2006.

NEUROMUSCULAR DISORDERS

189. **How can the anatomic site responsible for muscle weakness be determined clinically?**
See Table 14-9.

190. **What are the causes of acute generalized weakness?**
- **Infectious and postinfectious conditions:** Acute infectious myositis, GBS, enteroviral infection
- **Metabolic disorders:** Acute intermittent porphyria, hereditary tyrosinemia

TABLE 14-9. CLINICAL DETERMINATION OF ANATOMIC SITE RESPONSIBLE FOR MUSCLE WEAKNESS

	Upper Motor Neuron	Anterior Horn Cell	Neuromuscular Junction	Peripheral Nerve	Muscle
Tone	Increased (may be decreased acutely)	Decreased	Normal, variable	Decreased	Decreased
Distribution	Pattern (e.g., hemiparesis, paraparesis) Distal > proximal	Variable, asymmetrical	Fluctuating, cranial nerve involvement	Nerve distribution	Proximal > distal
Reflexes	Increased (may be decreased early)	Decreased to absent	Normal (unless severely involved)	Decreased to absent	Decreased
Babinski	Extensor	Flexor	Flexor	Flexor	Flexor
Other	Cognitive dysfunction, atrophy only very late	Fasciculations, atrophy, no sensory involvement	Fluctuating course	Sensory nerve involvement, atrophy, rare fasciculations	No sensory deficits; may be tenderness and signs of inflammation

Adapted from Packer RJ, Berman PH: Neurologic emergencies. In Fleisher GR, Ludwig S (eds): Textbook of Pediatric Emergency Medicine, 3rd ed. Baltimore, Williams & Wilkins, 1993, p 584.

- **Neuromuscular blockade:** Botulism, tick paralysis
- **Periodic paralysis:** Familial (hyperkalemic, hypokalemic, normokalemic)

Fenichel GM: *Clinical Pediatric Neurology: Signs and Symptoms Approach*, ed 5, Philadelphia, 2009, Elsevier, p 197.

191. **If a child presents with weakness, what aspects of the history and physical examination suggest a myopathic process?**

History
- Gradual rather than sudden onset
- Proximal weakness (e.g., climbing stairs, running) rather than distal weakness (more characteristic of neuropathy) predominates
- Absence of sensory abnormalities, such as "pins-and-needles" sensations
- No bowel and bladder abnormalities

Physical examination
- Proximal weakness is greater than distal weakness (except in myotonic dystrophy)
- Positive Gower sign (patient arises from a sitting position by pushing the trunk erect by bracing the arms against anterior thigh as a result of weakness of the pelvic girdle and the lower extremities)
- Neck flexion weaker than neck extension
- During the early stages, reflexes normal or only slightly decreased
- Normal sensory examination
- Muscle wasting but no fasciculations
- Muscle hypertrophy seen in some dystrophies

Weiner HL, Urion DK, Levitt LP: *Pediatric Neurology for the House Officer*, Baltimore, 1988, Williams & Wilkins, pp 136–138.

192. **How does electromyography help to differentiate between myopathic and neurogenic disorders?**

Electromyography measures the electrical activity of resting and voluntary muscle activity. Normally, the action potentials are of standardized duration and amplitude, with two to four distinguishable phases. In **myopathic** conditions, the durations and amplitudes are shorter than expected; in **neuropathies,** they are longer. In both conditions, extra phases (i.e., polyphasic units) are usually noted.

193. **How is pseudoparalysis distinguished from true neuromuscular disease?**

Pseudoparalysis (hysterical paralysis) or weakness may be seen in conversion reactions (i.e., emotional conflicts presenting as symptoms). In conversion reactions, sensation, deep tendon reflexes, and Babinski response are normal; movement may also be noted during sleep. *Hoover sign* is also helpful in cases of unilateral paralysis. With the patient lying supine on the table, the examiner places a hand under the heel of the unaffected limb and asks the patient to raise the plegic limb. In pseudoparalysis, no pressure is felt under the heel on the unaffected side.

194. **Why is it important to localize the cause of hypotonia?**

Localization of the level of the lesion is critical for determining the nature of the pathologic process. In the absence of an acute encephalopathy, the differential diagnosis of hypotonia is best approached by asking the question, "Does the patient have normal strength despite the hypotonia, or is the patient weak and hypotonic?" The combination of weakness and hypotonia usually points to an abnormality of the anterior horn cell or the peripheral neuromuscular apparatus, whereas hypotonia with normal strength is more characteristic of brain or spinal cord disturbances.

KEY POINTS: HYPOTONIA

1. Localization of lesion is critical for determining pathologic process.

2. Most important question: Is strength normal or abnormal?

3. Hypotonia *with weakness*: Think abnormality in anterior horn cell or peripheral neuromuscular apparatus.

4. Hypotonia *without weakness*: Think brain or spinal cord disturbance.

195. **How can you detect myotonia clinically?**
Myotonia is a painless tonic spasm of muscle that follows voluntary contraction, involuntary failure of relaxation, or delayed muscle relaxation after a contraction. It can be elicited by grip (e.g., handshake), forced eyelid closure (or delayed eye opening in crying infants), lid lag after upward gaze, or percussion over various sites (e.g., thenar eminence, tongue).

196. **How do the presentations of the two forms of myotonic dystrophy differ?**
The presentation of **congenital** myotonic dystrophy is during the immediate newborn period. Symptoms include hypotonia, facial diplegia with "tenting" of the upper lip, and, frequently, severe respiratory distress as a result of intercostal and diaphragmatic weakness, especially in the right hemidiaphragm. Feeding problems as a result of poor suck and gastrointestinal dysmotility are also present. The **juvenile** presentation of this condition is during the first decade of life. This form is characterized by progressive weakness and atrophy of the facial and sternocleidomastoid muscles and shoulder girdle, impaired hearing and speech, and excessive daytime sleepiness. Clinical myotonia is more likely, and there may be mental retardation.

197. **In a newborn with weakness and hypotonia, what obstetric and delivery features suggest a diagnosis of congenital myotonic dystrophy?**
A history of spontaneous abortions, polyhydramnios, decreased fetal movements, delays in second-stage labor, retained placenta, and postpartum hemorrhage all raise the concern for congenital myotonic dystrophy. Because the mother is nearly always affected in congenital myotonic dystrophy (although previously diagnosed in only half the cases), a careful clinical and electromyographic evaluation of the mother is essential.

198. **Why is myotonic dystrophy an example of the phenomenon of "anticipation"?**
Genetic studies have shown that the defect in myotonic dystrophy is an expansion of a trinucleotide (CTG) in a gene on the long arm of chromosome 19 that codes for a protein kinase. The gene product was named myotonin-protein kinase, and it is thought to be involved in sodium- and chloride-channel function. In successive generations, this repeating sequence has a tendency to increase, sometimes into the thousands (normal is <40 CTG repeats), and the extent of repetition correlates with the severity of the disease. Thus, each succeeding generation is likely to get more extensive manifestations and earlier presentations of the disease (i.e., the phenomenon of anticipation).

199. **How does the pathophysiology of infant botulism differ from that of food-borne and wound botulism?**
■ **Infant botulism** results from the ingestion of *Clostridium botulinum* spores that germinate, multiply, and produce toxin in the infant's intestine. The source of the spores is often unknown, but it has been linked to honey in some cases, and spores have been found in corn syrups. Therefore, these foods are not advised for infants younger than 1 year old.

- **Food-borne botulism** involves cases in which preformed toxin is already present in the food. Improper canning and anaerobic storage permit spore germination, growth, and toxin formation, which result in symptoms if the toxin is not destroyed by proper heating.
- **Wound botulism** occurs if spores enter a deep wound and germinate.

200. **What is the earliest indication for intubation in an infant with botulism?**
Intubation is indicated if there is a loss of protective airway reflexes. This occurs before respiratory compromise or failure because diaphragmatic function is not impaired until 90% to 95% of the synaptic receptors are occupied. An infant with hypercarbia or hypoxia is at very high risk for imminent respiratory failure.

Schreiner MS, Field E, Ruddy R: Infant botulism: a review of 12 years' experience at the Children's Hospital of Philadelphia, *Pediatrics* 87:159–165, 1991.

201. **In an infant with severe weakness and suspected botulism, why is the use of aminoglycosides relatively contraindicated?**
The botulism toxin acts by irreversibly blocking acetylcholine release from the presynaptic nerve terminals. Aminoglycosides, tetracyclines, clindamycin, and trimethoprim also interfere with acetylcholine release; therefore, they have the potential to act synergistically with the botulinum toxin to worsen or prolong neuromuscular paralysis.

202. **What are the two most common symptoms in children with juvenile myasthenia gravis?**
Ptosis and **diplopia.** Myasthenia gravis is characterized by a highly variable clinical course of fluctuating weakness (characteristically with increasing contractions) that initially involves muscles that are innervated by the cranial nerves. It is caused by a defect in neuromuscular transmission that is caused by an autoimmune antibody-mediated attack on the acetylcholine receptors.

203. **What are the risks to a neonate who is born to a mother with myasthenia gravis?**
Passively acquired neonatal myasthenia develops in about 10% of infants born to myasthenic mothers because of the transplacental transfer of antibody directed against acetylcholine receptors (AChR) in striated muscle. Signs and symptoms of weakness typically arise within the first hours or days of life. Pathologic muscle fatigability commonly causes feeding difficulty, generalized weakness, hypotonia, and respiratory depression. Ptosis and impaired eye movements occur in only 15% of cases. The weakness virtually always resolves as the body burden of anti-AChR immunoglobulins diminishes. Symptoms typically persist for about 2 weeks but may require several months to disappear completely. General supportive treatment is usually adequate, but oral or intramuscular neostigmine may help to diminish symptoms.

204. **How does the pathophysiology of juvenile versus congenital myasthenia gravis differ?**
Juvenile (and adult) myasthenia gravis is caused by circulating antibodies to the AChR of the postsynaptic neuromuscular junction. Occurrence is rare before the age of 2 years.
Congenital myasthenia gravis is a nonimmunologic process. It is caused by morphologic or physiologic features affecting the presynaptic and postsynaptic junctions, including defects in ACh synthesis, end-plate acetylcholinesterase deficiency, and end-plate AChR deficiency. Neonatal myasthenia gravis refers to the transient weakness that occurs in infants of mothers with myasthenia gravis.

205. **How is the edrophonium (Tensilon) test done?**
Edrophonium is a rapid-acting anticholinesterase drug of short duration that improves symptoms of myasthenia gravis by inhibiting the breakdown of ACh and increasing its concentration in the neuromuscular junction. A test dose of 0.015 mg/kg is given intravenously; if it is tolerated, the full dose of 0.15 mg/kg (up to 10 mg) is given. If measurable improvement in ocular muscle or extremity strength occurs, myasthenia gravis is likely. Because edrophonium may precipitate a cholinergic crisis (e.g., bradycardia, hypotension, vomiting, bronchospasm), atropine and resuscitation equipment should be available.

206. **Does a negative antibody test exclude the diagnosis of juvenile myasthenia gravis?**
No. Up to 90% of children with juvenile myasthenia have measurable anti-AChR antibodies, but, in the other 10%, continued clinical suspicion is necessary because their symptoms are usually milder (e.g., ocular muscle weakness, minimal generalized weakness). In these children, other tests (e.g., edrophonium, electrophysiologic studies, single-fiber electromyography) may be needed to make the diagnosis.

207. **What are the four characteristic features of damage to the anterior horn cells?**
Weakness, fasciculations, atrophy, and hyporeflexia.

208. **What processes can damage the anterior horn cells?**
- **Degenerative** (spinal muscular atrophy): Werdnig-Hoffman, Kugelberg-Welander
- **Metabolic:** Tay-Sachs disease (hexosaminidase deficiency), Pompe disease, Batten disease (ceroid-lipofuscinosis), hyperglycinemia, neonatal adrenoleukodystrophy
- **Infectious:** Poliovirus, Coxsackie virus, echoviruses

209. **What is the primary genetic abnormality in infants and children with spinal muscular atrophy (SMA)?**
Disruption of the **survival motor neuron 1 (*SMN1*) gene**. SMAs are a group of diseases that affect the motor neuron, resulting in widespread muscular denervation and atrophy. Carrier frequency is estimated between 1 in 50 to 80. SMAs are the second most common hereditary neuromuscular disease after Duchenne muscular dystrophy. How changes in the SMN protein result in the disease process and phenotypic variability is unclear.

Lunn MR, Wang CH: Spinal muscular atrophy, *Lancet* 371:2120–2133, 2008.

Spinal Muscular Atrophy Association: http://www.smafoundation.org.

210. **How are the inherited progressive spinal muscular atrophies distinguished?**
See Table 14-10.

211. **What are muscular dystrophies?**
A muscular dystrophy is an inheritable myopathy that affects limbs or facial muscles and that is progressive, with pathologic evidence of degeneration or regeneration without any abnormal storage material.

Muscular Dystrophy Association: http://www.mdausa.org.

212. **What is the clinical importance of dystrophin?**
Dystrophin is a muscle protein that is presumed to be involved in anchoring the contractile apparatus of striated and cardiac muscle to the cell membrane. As a result of a gene mutation, this protein is completely missing in patients with Duchenne muscular dystrophy. On the other hand, muscle tissue from patients with Becker muscular dystrophy contains reduced amounts of dystrophin or, occasionally, a protein of abnormal size.

TABLE 14-10. PROGRESSIVE SPINAL MUSCULAR ATROPHIES (SMAs)

Disorder	Inheritance	Age of Onset	Clinical Features
Acute infantile SMA (Werdnig-Hoffmann disease, SMA type 1)	Autosomal recessive	In utero to 6 mo	Frog-leg posture; areflexia; tongue atrophy and fasciculations, progressive swallowing, and respiratory problems; survival <4 yr
Intermediate SMA (chronic Werdnig-Hoffmann disease, SMA type 2)	Autosomal recessive; rarely autosomal dominant	3 mo to 15 yr	Proximal weakness; most sit unsupported; decreased or absent reflexes; high incidence of scoliosis, contractures; survival may be up to 30 yr
Kugelberg-Welander disease (SMA type 3)	Autosomal recessive; rarely autosomal dominant	5-15 yr	May be part of the spectrum of SMA 2; hip girdle weakness; calf hypertrophy; decreased or absent reflexes; may be ambulatory until fourth decade

SMA = spinal muscular atrophy.
Adapted from Parke JT: Disorders of the anterior horn cell. In McMillan JA, DeAngelis CD, Feigin RD, Warshaw JB (eds): Oski's Pediatrics: Principles and Practice, 3rd ed. Philadelphia, JB Lippincott, 1999, p 1959.

213. **How are Duchenne and Becker muscular dystrophies distinguished?**
See Table 14-11.

214. **Is corticosteroid therapy effective for the treatment of Duchenne muscular dystrophy?**
Several studies have documented an improvement in strength with an optimal dose of prednisone of 0.75 mg/kg per day. The strengthening effect lasts for up to 3 years while the steroid is continued. Appropriate timing and duration of treatment have not been established, and side effects (weight gain and increased susceptibility to infection) may outweigh the benefits in many cases.

Manzur AY, Kinali M, Muntoni F: Update on the management of Duchenne muscular dystrophy, *Arch Dis Child* 93:986–990, 2008.

215. **What is the most likely diagnosis in a child with progressive walking difficulties evolving over several days?**
Guillain-Barré syndrome (GBS) is an acute demyelinating neuropathy that is characterized by ascending, acute, progressive peripheral and cranial nerve dysfunction and paresthesias. In younger children (<6 years), it may be heralded by pain. It is frequently preceded by a viral respiratory or gastrointestinal illness and rarely by surgery or immunizations. The disease is characterized by the presence of multifocal areas of the inflammatory

TABLE 14-11. DUCHENNE VERSUS BECKER MUSCULAR DYSTROPHY

	Genetics	Diagnosis	Manifestations
Duchenne	1 in 3500 male births X-linked Several different deletions, point mutations in dystrophin gene result in a completely nonfunctional protein New mutations occur Carrier females may have mild weakness or cardiomyopathy	Whole-blood DNA may reveal a deletion in about 65%; otherwise, electromyogram and muscle biopsy studies are definitive	Clinically evident at 3-5 years of age Regular, stereotyped course of progressive proximal weakness Calf hypertrophy Loss of ambulation by 9-12 years Worsening scoliosis and contractures Eventual dilated cardiomyopathy and/or respiratory failure Life expectancy of 16-19 years
Becker	1 in 20,000 male births X-linked Various mutations in dystrophin gene result in reduced amount of or partially functional protein	More benign clinical course Reduced dystrophin levels in muscle cells (by immunostaining) or abnormal dystrophin	Clinically evident during early second decade Milder, slower course as compared with Duchenne Calf pseudohypertrophy Pes cavus Cardiac and central nervous system involvement unusual Ambulatory until 18 years or beyond Life expectancy twice as long as compared with Duchenne

Adapted from Tsao VY, Mendell JR: The childhood muscular dystrophies: making order out of chaos. Semin Neurol 19:9-23, 1999.

demyelination of nerve roots and peripheral nerves. As a result of the loss of the healthy myelin covering, the conduction of nerve impulses (action potentials) may be blocked or dispersed. The resulting clinical effects are predominantly motor (i.e., the evolution of flaccid, areflexic paralysis). There is a variable degree of motor weakness. Some individuals have mild brief weakness, whereas fulminant paralysis occurs in others. Autonomic signs (e.g., tachycardia, hypertension) and sensory symptoms (e.g., painful dysesthesias) are not uncommon, but they are overshadowed by the motor signs. More than half of these patients develop facial involvement, and mechanical ventilation may be required. The *Miller Fisher variant* is characterized by gait ataxia, areflexia, and ophthalmoparesis.

Guillain-Barré syndrome: http://www.gbsfi.com.

Winer JB: Guillain-Barré syndrome, *BMJ* 337:227–231, 2008.

216. **What CSF findings are characteristic of GBS?**
The classic CSF finding is the **albuminocytologic** dissociation. Most common infections or inflammatory processes generate an elevation of white blood cell count and protein. The CSF profile in GBS includes a normal cell count with elevated protein, usually in the range of 50 to 100 mg/dL; however, at the onset of disease, the CSF protein concentration may be normal.

217. **Outline the management of acute GBS.**
Early clinical monitoring is focused on the development of bulbar or respiratory insufficiency. Bulbar weakness manifests as unilateral or bilateral facial weakness, diplopia, hoarseness, drooling, depressed gag reflex, or dysphagia. Frank respiratory insufficiency may be preceded by air hunger, dyspnea, or a soft muffled voice (hypophonia). The autonomic nervous system is occasionally involved, and this is signified by the presence of labile blood pressure and body temperature. The management of GBS includes the following:
- Observation in an intensive care unit is critical, with frequent monitoring of vital signs.
- The early institution of plasmapheresis or intravenous immunoglobulin shortens the clinical course and lessens long-term morbidity; corticosteroid therapy is thought to be ineffective.
- If bulbar signs are present, the patient should receive nothing orally, and the mouth is suctioned frequently. Hydration is maintained intravenously, and nutritional support is provided by nasogastric feedings.
- The vital capacity (VC) is measured frequently. In children, the normal VC may be calculated as VC = 200 mL × age in years. If the VC falls below 25% of normal, endotracheal intubation is performed. Careful pulmonary toilet is conducted to minimize atelectasis, aspiration, and pneumonia.
- Meticulous nursing care includes careful patient positioning to prevent pressure sores, compression of peripheral nerves, and venous thrombosis.
- Physical therapy is conducted to prevent the development of contractures by passive range-of-movement exercises and splinting to maintain physiologic hand and limb postures until muscle strength returns.

Vucic S, Kiernan MC, Cornblath DR: Guillain-Barré syndrome: an update, *J Clin Neurol* 16:733–741, 2009.

Burns TM: Guillain-Barré syndrome, *Semin Neurol* 28:152–167, 2008.

218. **What is the prognosis for children with GBS?**
Children appear to recover more quickly and more fully than adults. Fewer than 10% have significant residual deficits. In rare cases, the neuropathy may recur as a chronic inflammatory demyelinating polyneuropathy.

219. **How do syndromes of ascending paralysis compare in the clinical presentation?**
See Table 14-12.

220. **How does multiple sclerosis appear during childhood?**
Multiple sclerosis is extremely rare in childhood (0.2% to 2.0% of all cases). Studies of affected children demonstrate a variable predominance of boys during early childhood and females during adolescence. Ataxia, muscle weakness, and transient visual or sensory

TABLE 14-12. FEATURES OF FOUR SIMILAR SYNDROMES OF ASCENDING PARALYSIS

Feature	Tick Paralysis	Guillain-Barré Syndrome	Spinal Cord Lesion	Poliomyelitis
Ataxia	Present	Absent	Absent	Absent
Rate of progression	Hours to days	Days to weeks	Gradual or abrupt	Days to weeks
Muscle-stretch reflexes	Absent	Absent	Variable	Absent
Babinski sign	Absent	Absent	Present	Absent
Sensory loss	None	Mild	Present	None
Meningeal signs	Absent	Rare	Absent	Present
Fever	Absent	Rare	Absent	Present
Cerebrospinal Fluid				
Protein level	Normal	High	Normal or high	High
White cell count (per mm^3)	<10	<10	Variable	>10
Time to recovery	<24 hr after tick removal	Weeks to months	Variable, depending on cause	Months to years or no recovery (permanent paresis)

Adapted from Felz MW, Smith CD, Swift TR: A six-year-old girl with tick paralysis. N Engl J Med 342:90-94, 2000.

symptoms are relatively common presentations. CSF examination may demonstrate mild ($<$25 cells/mm^3) mononuclear pleocytosis with an increasing probability of oligoclonal bands with each recurrence. MRI is the single most useful diagnostic test: the presence of multiple, periventricular white matter plaques (bright areas on T2 images) confirms the diagnosis.

Renoux C: Natural history of multiple sclerosis with childhood onset, *N Engl J Med* 356:2603–2613, 2007.

SPINAL CORD DISORDERS

221. **Which spinal segments do each of the common reflexes test?**
See Table 14-13.

TABLE 14-13. SPINAL SEGMENTS AND COMMON REFLEXES

Deep Tendon Reflex	Superficial Reflex	Peripheral Nerve	Segmental Organization
	Pupillary	Optic/oculomotor	CN II-III
Jaw jerk		Trigeminal	CN V
	Corneal	Trigeminal/facial	CN V-VII
	Gag	Glossopharyngeal/vagal	CN IX-X
Biceps		Musculocutaneous	C5-C6
Brachioradialis		Radial	C5-C6
Triceps		Radial	C6-C8
Finger flexion		Median/ulnar	C7-T1
Abdominal reflex		Thoracic	T8-T12
	Umbilical	Thoracic	T8-T12
	Cremasteric	Genitofemoral	L1-L2
Adductor		Femoral/obturator	L2-L4
Quadriceps		Femoral	L2-L4
	Plantar reflex	Sciatic	S1-S2
	Anal wink	Pudendal	S3-S5

222. **How common are asymptomatic spinal anomalies in normal children?**
Up to 5% of children have spina bifida occulta, an incomplete fusion of the posterior vertebral arches, which is usually noted as an incidental radiographic finding. The defect most commonly involves the lower lumbar lamina of L5 and S1.

223. **Which sacral dimples and coccygeal pits in a newborn are concerning for an occult spinal dysraphism (OSD)?**
These occur in up to 4% of newborns. Certain features are more likely to be associated with an OSD and warrant a screening ultrasound.
- Location above the gluteal crease (typically $>$2.5 cm from the anus)
- Deep dimples (if base cannot be visualized, do not probe because of risk for introducing an infection if a direct communication with the spinal canal is present)
- Larger size ($>$0.5 cm)
- Pits with cutaneous markers (lipoma, hypertrichosis, hemangioma)

Williams H: Spinal sinuses, dimples, pits and patches: what lies beneath? *Arch Dis Child Educ Pract Ed* 91:3p75–3p80, 2006.

KEY POINTS: NEONATAL SACRAL FINDINGS SUGGESTIVE OF OCCULT SPINAL DYSRAPHISM

1. Location above the gluteal crease (typically >2.5 cm from the anus)

2. Deep dimples

3. Larger dimple size (>0.5 cm)

4. Sacral pits with cutaneous markers (lipoma, hypertrichosis, hemangioma)

224. **What is the recurrence rate of open neural tube defects?**

Open neural tube defects (myelomeningocele or spina bifida and anencephaly) usually have multifactorial causes, but in some cases, they may be the result of mendelian recessive inheritance. The general recurrence rate is 2.5% for mothers of affected children, sisters of the mother of an affected child, and female children born to individuals with spina bifida. Daily folic acid intake of 400 mcg reduces the risk of spina bifida by as much as 70%. Serum and amniotic α-fetoprotein can detect open neural tube defects, and ultrasound is also a useful tool.

Spina Bifida Association of America: http://www.sbaa.org.

225. **What are the two main features of the Chiari malformations?**

Cerebellar elongation and **protrusion of the foramen magnum into the cervical spinal cord**. Anatomic anomalies of the hindbrain and skeletal structure result in different positioning of the various structures relative to the upper cervical canal and foramen magnum with different clinical features.

226. **What are the types of Chiari malformations?**

Type I is clinically the least severe and is generally asymptomatic during childhood. The presentation of a Chiari I malformation may be insidious. Epilepsy is found in a small minority of these patients. There may be paroxysmal vertigo, drop attacks, vague dizziness, and headache, which may be increased by the Valsalva maneuver. Occipital headache precipitated by exertion may progress to torticollis, downgaze nystagmus, periodic nystagmus, and oscillopsia. MRI findings in patients with Chiari I malformations include malformations of the base of the skull and of the upper cervical spine, including hydromyelia, syringomyelia, and syrinx.

Type II is the most common of those diagnosed during childhood. Medulla and cerebellum, together with part or the entire fourth ventricle, are displaced into the spinal canal. A variety of cerebellar, brainstem, and cortical defects can occur. This type is strongly associated with noncommunicating hydrocephalus and lumbosacral myelomeningocele.

Type III comprises any of the features of types I and II, but the entire cerebellum is herniated throughout the foramen magnum, with a cervical spina bifida cystica. Hydrocephalus is a common feature.

Sarnat HB: Neuroembryology, genetic programming and malformations of the nervous system. In Menkes JH, Sarnat HB, Maria BL, editors: *Child Neurology*, ed 7, Philadelphia, 2006, Lippincott Williams & Wilkins, pp 299–301.

KEY POINTS: EARLY CLUES TO SPINAL CORD COMPRESSION

1. Scoliosis producing sustained poor posture

2. Back or abdominal pain beginning abruptly during sleep

3. Increased sensitivity of spinal column to local pressure or percussion

4. Bowel or bladder dysfunction

5. Diminished sensation in the anogenital region and lower limbs

227. **What is the full anatomic expression of myelomeningocele?**
Children with myelomeningocele have a complex, multifaceted, congenital disorder of structure that represents a dysraphic state (i.e., a defective closure of the embryonic neural groove). In its full expression, it is typified anatomically by the following:
- The presence of unfused or excessively separated vertebral arches of the bony spine (spina bifida)
- Cystic dilation of the meninges that surround the spinal cord (meningocele)
- Cystic dilation of the spinal cord itself (myelocele)
- Hydrocephalus and the spectrum of congenital cerebral abnormalities

228. **What is the likelihood that a patient with myelomeningocele will have hydrocephalus?**
Hydrocephalus is seen in 95% of children with thoracic or high lumbar myelomeningocele. The incidence decreases progressively with more caudal spinal defects to a minimum of 60% if the myelomeningocele is located in the sacrum.

229. **What is the usual cause of stridor in a child with myelomeningocele?**
The stridor is usually caused by **dysfunction of the vagus nerve,** which innervates the muscles of the vocal cords. In their resting position, the edges of the cords meet in the midline; during speech, they move apart. Hence, in bilateral vagal nerve palsies, the free edges of the vocal cords are closely opposed and obstruct air flow, thereby resulting in stridor. In symptomatic patients, the motor nucleus of the vagus nerve may be congenitally hypoplastic or aplastic. More commonly, the vagal dysfunction is believed to arise from a mechanical traction injury caused by hydrocephalus, which produces progressive herniation and inferior displacement of the abnormal hindbrain. Shunting the hydrocephalus may alleviate the traction and improve the stridor. Sometimes the later recurrence of stridor indicates the reaccumulation of hydrocephalus as a result of ventriculoperitoneal shunt failure.

230. **What are the principal options for managing urinary incontinence in patients with myelomeningocele?**
About 80% of patients have a neurogenic bladder, which most commonly manifests as a small, poorly compliant bladder and an open and fixed sphincter. Options include the following:
- Clean intermittent catheterization, which results in more complete emptying than simple Credé maneuvers

- Artificial urinary sphincter to increase outlet resistance
- Surgical urinary diversion (e.g., suprapubic vesicostomy), which is uncommonly used
- Augmentation cystoplasty to increase bladder capacity in combination with the use of oxybutynin (a smooth muscle antispasmodic)

    Blum RW, Pfaffinger K: Myelodysplasia in childhood and adolescence, *Pediatr Rev* 15:480–488, 1994.

231. **How frequently is myelomeningocele associated with mental retardation?**
    Only 15% to 20% of patients have associated mental retardation. Hydrocephalus *per se* does not cause the mental retardation that is associated with this syndrome. (Recall that children with appropriately treated congenital hydrocephalus caused by simple aqueductal stenosis usually have normal psychomotor development.) Only severe hydrocephalus with a very thick cortical mantle predicts lower intelligence. Mental retardation is usually attributed to acquired secondary CNS infection or subtle microscopic anomalies of neuronal migration and differentiation, which may coexist with the macroscopically visible malformation of the hindbrain.

232. **In an infant born with myelomeningocele, how does the initial evaluation predict long-term ambulation potential?**
    The level of motor function—and not the level of the defect—is most predictive of ambulation.
    - **Thoracic:** No hip flexion is noted. Almost no younger children will ambulate, and only about one third of adolescents will ambulate with the aid of extensive braces and crutches.
    - **High lumbar (L1, L2):** The patient is able to flex the hips, but there is no knee extension. About one third of children and adolescents will ambulate, but only with extensive assistive devices.
    - **Mid-lumbar (L3):** The patient is able to flex the hips and extend the knee. The percentage of those able to ambulate is midway between those with high and low lumbar lesions.
    - **Low lumbar (L4, L5):** The patient is able to flex the knee and dorsiflex the ankle. Nearly half of younger children and nearly all adolescents will ambulate, with varying degrees of braces or crutches.
    - **Sacral (S1-S4):** The patient is able to plantar flex the ankles and move the toes. Nearly all children and adolescents will ambulate, with minimal or no assistive devices.

ACKNOWLEDGMENT

The editors and the author gratefully acknowledge contributions by Drs. Douglas R. Nordli, Jr., Peter Bingham, and Robert R. Clancy that were retained from the first three editions of *Pediatric Secrets*.

CHAPTER 15

ONCOLOGY

Richard Aplenc, MD, MCSE, Emily G. Lipsitz, MD,
and Peter C. Adamson, MD

CHEMOTHERAPY AND RADIATION THERAPY

1. **What was the first cytotoxic chemotherapeutic agent used for the treatment of children with leukemia?**
   In 1948, Sidney Farber reported success using aminopterin (4-aminopteroyl-glutamic acid) in 16 children with acute leukemia. Aminopterin was a precursor to the antifolate drug methotrexate, which is commonly used today.

   Farber S, Diamond LK, Mercer RD, et al: Temporary remissions in acute leukemia in children produced by folic acid antagonist, 4-amino-pteroylglutamic acid (aminopterin), *N Engl J Med* 238:787–793, 1948.

2. **Name the common cytotoxic chemotherapeutic drug classes.**
   Chemotherapeutic drugs are usually classified by their primary site and mechanism of action or source. The most common are the **alkylators, antimetabolites, antitumor antibiotics,** and **plant toxins**.

3. **We can thank the guinea pig for a major (albeit serendipitous) breakthrough in the treatment of childhood acute lymphoblastic leukemia (ALL). What role did our rodent friend the *Cavy* play?**
   In 1953, investigators discovered that whole guinea pig serum could bring about regression of certain transplanted lymphosarcomas in inbred mice. By 1961, it was determined that the fraction of guinea pig serum responsible for its antileukemic effect contained significant asparaginase activity. Most leukemic lymphoblasts were then found to be asparagine autotrophs, requiring exogenous asparagine for survival. A bacterial source (*Escherichia coli*) of asparaginase was identified, and pharmaceutical production of L-asparaginase began, increasing the complete remission rate for children with ALL from about 80% to more than 95%.

4. **Which chemotherapeutic agents are cell cycle dependent? In which phase are they most active?**
   See Figure 15-1.

5. **What is the difference between adjuvant and neoadjuvant chemotherapy?**
   Adjuvant chemotherapy is administered *after* the primary treatment of a tumor (surgical resection or radiation therapy), when there is no remaining gross tumor that can be assessed for response to the chemotherapy.
   Neoadjuvant chemotherapy is administered *before* the delivery of definitive local treatment and then continues afterward in the adjuvant setting. For children with solid tumors, several cycles of neoadjuvant chemotherapy are often administered to improve the chances of achieving complete surgical resection and improved local control of a primary tumor.

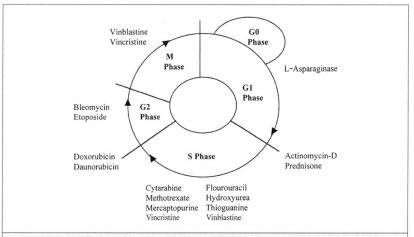

Figure 15-1. Phases in which cell cycle–dependent chemotherapy agents are most active. G0 = resting phase (nonproliferation), G1 = gap1 (pre-DNA synthesis with diploid RNA and protein synthesis), S = DNA synthesis, G2 = gap2 (post-DNA synthesis), M = mitosis. (From Weiner MA, Cairo MS: Pediatric Hematology/Oncology Secrets. Philadelphia, Hanley & Belfus, 2000, p 96.)

6. **Why are most chemotherapeutic drug dosages based on body surface area (BSA)?**
   In theory, BSA correlates better than body weight with cardiac output and hence hepatic and renal perfusion. Because most drug clearance occurs by hepatic and renal mechanisms, anticancer drugs that have a very narrow therapeutic index are usually dosed in a manner that is normalized to BSA. The exception is made for infants, who have a very high BSA-to-body weight ratio; infants receive chemotherapy based on body weight. BSA can be estimated using height and weight. One estimate can be obtained with the following formula:

$$BSA\ (m^2) = \sqrt{[(weight \times height)/3600]}$$

7. **Which chemotherapeutic agents can be administered intrathecally to either treat or prevent meningeal malignancy?**
   Methotrexate, cytarabine, and hydrocortisone are commonly administered intrathecally to treat or prevent meningeal leukemia and lymphoma. Thiotepa and a novel formulation of BCNU are also used for nonhematologic malignancies with meningeal involvement.
   Most systemically administered anticancer drugs have limited penetration into the cerebrospinal fluid (CSF). Intrathecal chemotherapy has the advantage of delivering high drug concentration to the CSF while minimizing systemic toxicities.

8. **What is the difference between pharmacokinetics and pharmacodynamics?**
   Pharmacokinetics refers to the effect of the body on the drug. It is the study of how drugs are absorbed, distributed, metabolized, and eliminated from the body. Common parameters include elimination half-life, peak concentration, clearance, and area under the concentration-time curve.
   Pharmacodynamics refers to the effect of the drug on the body. A pharmacodynamic effect can be a toxicity measurement (decrease in blood counts) or an anticancer measurement (decrease in the size of a tumor) after chemotherapy.

9. **What are the phases of clinical trials?**
   ■ **Phase I:** *The dose determination phase*. This phase is designed primarily to recommend a dose for further testing in children, usually the maximal tolerated dose. Pharmacokinetic studies are performed during phase I trials to help learn whether children handle a drug differently than adults. Phase 1 trials typically enroll 18 to 30 children.
   ■ **Phase II:** *The efficacy phase*. Usually a group of children with the same diagnosis are studied, and the percentage of patients in whom the drug causes a tumor to decrease in size is determined. Phase II trials enroll 30 to 150 children, depending on how many different tumor types are being studied.
   ■ **Phase III:** *The comparative phase*. This phase studies whether a new drug (or a new combination of drugs) that was found to be efficacious in a phase II trial can improve therapy relative to the best current therapy. Phase III trials are randomized and can enroll hundreds to thousands of children.

   Balis FM, Fox E, Widemann BC, Adamson PC: Clinical drug development for childhood cancers, *Clin Pharmacol Ther* 85:127–129, 2009.

10. **What is the major dose-limiting toxicity for the alkylating agents?**
   Myelosuppression. Alkylating agents are chemically reactive compounds that covalently add an alkyl group; this is most important with regard to macromolecules involved in DNA synthesis, damaging templates, and inhibiting synthesis. Agents include the nitrogen mustards, oxazaphosphorines (including cyclophosphamide and ifosfamide), busulfan, and cisplatin.

11. **What are the common side effects of methotrexate?**
   Myelosuppression and **mucositis.** In high doses, the drug can be nephrotoxic and cause dermatitis, hepatitis, and mucositis. Most important, toxicity is primarily a function of duration of exposure. Because methotrexate can collect within fluid compartments (e.g., pleural or peritoneal effusions), it should be avoided in patients with significant third-space fluid collections.

12. **If one had to choose a single laboratory test to obtain before administering high-dose methotrexate, which one should it be?**
   Determination of serum creatinine is essential before administering high-dose methotrexate. The kidneys eliminate more than 90% of methotrexate. In the presence of abnormal renal function, high-dose methotrexate carries a high risk for severe or fatal toxicity.

   Widemann BC, Adamson PC: Understanding and managing methotrexate nephrotoxicity, *Oncologist* 11:694–703, 2006.

13. **In what way do the side-effect profiles of cisplatin and carboplatin differ?**
   Carboplatin causes significant myelosuppression, primarily thrombocytopenia. *Cisplatin* causes only mild myelosuppression but is associated with significant nephrotoxicity, ototoxicity, and neurotoxicity.

14. **What factors are associated with an increased risk for developing anthracycline-induced cardiotoxicity?**
   Total cumulative dose, mediastinal radiotherapy, young age, and female gender are associated with an increased risk for developing anthracycline (doxorubicin, daunorubicin)-induced cardiotoxicity. Cumulative anthracycline dose has long been associated with an increased risk, with the incidence of clinically apparent congestive heart failure rising significantly with doxorubicin doses exceeding 450 mg/m^2. Late cardiotoxicity appears to be more common in children than in adults because the heart is to unable to grow in proportion to the child, resulting in a small, poorly compliant left ventricle. Thus, younger children,

particularly children younger than 5 years, are at higher risk. There is also some evidence that girls have a higher incidence of abnormal cardiac findings at any given cumulative dose than boys.

Barry E, Alvarez JA, Scully RE, et al: Anthracycline-induced cardiotoxicity: course, pathophysiology, prevention and management, *Expert Opin Pharmacother* 8:1039–1058, 2007.

15. **What is a vesicant?**
A *vesicant* is an agent that produces a vesicle; in oncology, it is a chemotherapeutic drug that can cause a severe burn if the drug infiltrates around the intravenous catheter. The anthracyclines (doxorubicin, daunorubicin), dactinomycin, and the vinca alkaloids (vincristine, vinblastine) are all vesicants. These drugs must be administered either through a central venous catheter or through a newly placed, free-flowing intravenous catheter that does not cross over a joint space.

16. **Which classes of chemotherapeutic agents have most commonly been implicated in causing secondary leukemias?**
The alkylating agents (e.g., cyclophosphamide) and topoisomerase II inhibitors (etoposide) increase the risk for developing secondary leukemia. Etoposide-induced leukemias tend to occur earlier, usually within 2 to 3 years of exposure.

17. **Why is intrathecal chemotherapy dosed based on patient age, whereas systemic (oral, intravenous) dosing is based on weight or body surface area?**
The brains of children grow disproportionately more quickly than their bodies (hence the tendency of infants who have recently learned to sit to readily tip over). The CSF increases in parallel with central nervous system (CNS) growth, such that by the age of 3 years, CSF volume is 80% that of adult CSF volume. Scaling intrathecal doses to body size would undertreat younger children, whereas scaling doses in adolescent patients, whose CNS size has plateaued relative to body size, would unnecessarily expose them to potentially more toxic drug concentrations.

18. **What are the most effective antiemetics for the prevention and treatment of chemotherapy-induced vomiting?**
The serotonin receptor antagonists ondansetron and granisetron are the most effective agents for chemotherapy-associated emesis. They work less well for delayed emesis, for which combinations of antihistamines and phenothiazines may be used. Dexamethasone is a useful adjunct when administering highly emetogenic chemotherapy.

Dupuis LL, Nathan PC: Options for the prevention and management of acute chemotherapy-induced nausea and vomiting in children, *Pediatr Drugs* 5:597–613, 2003.

19. **What drug, made famous in Frank Capra's 1944 film about two sweet old ladies, is now used in the treatment of one form of leukemia?**
The remedy used by the ladies in *Arsenic and Old Lace* is making an encore performance. In the early 1990s, investigators in China reported that arsenic, an ancient remedy, was found to be highly effective in the treatment of patients with acute promyelocytic leukemia. Arsenic appears to trigger an apoptotic response in promyeloblasts, but its precise mechanism of action is still under investigation.

20. **Who develops the "somnolence syndrome"?**
Transient symptoms attributed to temporary demyelination have been observed 6 to 8 weeks after completion of CNS radiation, most commonly for CNS prophylaxis for ALL. Children who develop the somnolence syndrome have lethargy, headache, and anorexia that last for about 2 weeks. Computed tomography and CSF studies show no consistent abnormality,

but an electroencephalogram often reveals a slow-wave activity consistent with diffuse cerebral disturbance. The use of steroids during irradiation appears to minimize the occurrence of the syndrome.

21. **What are the differences between conventional external radiation, intensity-modulated radiation therapy (IMRT), and proton-beam radiation?**
Both conventional radiation and IMRT use photon or electron beams to deliver radiation to the patient. IMRT uses many radiation fields, with each field having a unique radiation intensity profile that varies as a function of position within the field. This differs from conventional radiation, in which each field has a constant, or fixed intensity profile across the field area and thus allows for dose reduction to normal tissues or critical structures. Because of the physical properties of protons and their ability to deposit energy over a short distance, proton therapy may have the advantage of reducing radiation dose to nontarget normal tissues while allowing higher doses to be delivered to the tumor.

22. **What is radiation recall?**
Radiation recall is a delayed effect that results from the interaction of certain chemotherapeutic agents (doxorubicin, daunorubicin, or actinomycin-D) with radiation. After radiation therapy, an erythematous rash in the previous radiation field develops. The rash is geographic, usually precisely following the outline of the radiation field. Many of these occur months after the radiation treatment.

23. **What is a "fraction" of radiation?**
Radiation therapy is coordinated so that a patient receives a maximally tolerated total amount of radiation dose. However, exposure to large amounts of radiation in one instance does not necessarily result in optimal cellular destruction, and it may have significant side effects. As a result, radiation is "fractionated" into smaller doses. Patients may receive up to dozens of individual fractions to achieve total radiation doses. For solid tumors, radiation is delivered over 2 to 6 weeks.

24. **A 10-year-old girl is being treated for acute myelogenous leukemia (AML) with a combination of high-dose cytarabine and daunorubicin. Five days after the initiation of therapy, she develops the onset of nystagmus, ataxia, and dysmetria. A computed tomography scan of the brain reveals no focal abnormalities. What is the most likely cause of her symptoms?**
High-dose cytarabine (ara-C) can result in an **acute cerebellar syndrome** leading to nystagmus, ataxia, dysmetria, and dysdiadochokinesia. Imaging at the onset of symptoms is typically normal. In most cases, neurologic symptoms resolve within a week, but as many as 30% of patients do not regain full cerebellar function. The risk for developing cerebellar syndrome is related to the dose and schedule of cytarabine, with the highest risk being observed with administration of high doses over 6 or more days.

25. **What are the long-term sequelae of chemotherapy and irradiation?**
A variety of problems can ensue, depending on the age of the patient and the types of treatment. Four areas of prime concern include **cognitive deficits** (particularly in children <5 years old), **cardiac disease** (especially with the intensive use of anthracyclines), **endocrinopathies** (especially hypopituitarism, thyroid abnormalities, and gonadal end-organ failure), and **second malignancies.**

Friedman DL, Meadows AT: Late effects of childhood cancer therapy, *Pediatr Clin North Am* 49:1083–1106, 2002.

Oberfield SE, Sklar CA: Endocrine sequelae in survivors of childhood cancer, *Adolesc Med* 13: 161–169, 2002.

CLINICAL ISSUES

26. **A patient has a central venous catheter and develops a fever. What should be done?**
    The risk for bacteremia is increased in patients with central venous catheters. As such, any patient with an indwelling central venous catheter and a fever (temperature usually ≥38.5°C) should have a blood culture obtained from each lumen of the catheter and intravenous antibiotics administered until evidence of a negative blood culture is provided.

27. **A patient is neutropenic and has a fever. What should be done?**
    Because neutropenic patients are at risk for invasive bacterial infections, patients who are neutropenic (absolute neutrophil count <500/mm³ or <1000/mm³ and falling) should have blood cultures obtained and should receive broad-spectrum antibiotics. Antibiotic coverage should include both gram-negative and gram-positive organisms, including antibiotics that are active against *Pseudomonas aeruginosa*. Broad-spectrum antibiotics are continued until neutrophil counts show definitive signs of recovery.

28. **A patient remains febrile and neutropenic despite appropriate antibiotics for several days. Is there cause for concern?**
    Although it is not uncommon for a neutropenic patient to remain febrile for many days despite administration of broad-spectrum antibacterial agents, persistent fever is associated with an increased likelihood of invasive fungal infection. Because the ability to recover fungi in routine blood cultures is limited, the approach to such patients is to empirically add antifungal coverage after a period of persistent fever. Depending on the underlying disease and treatment, antifungal agents are generally added after 3 to 7 days of persistent fever. Choices of empirical antifungal therapy have expanded over recent years and now include liposomal formulations of amphotericin B, azoles (e.g., voriconazole), and echinocandins (e.g., caspofungin).

29. **Describe three different types of infection that are associated with central venous catheters, and how the treatment approaches to these infections differ.**
    For external catheters (Hickman, Broviac), an **exit site infection,** manifested as inflammation and occasionally exudate limited to where the catheter emerges through the skin, can usually be managed with a combination of local care and systemic antibiotics. Patients with indwelling catheters are at increased risk for **blood infections.** Many bacterial blood infections associated with central lines can be cleared with intravenous antibiotics administered through the central catheter, rotating lumens for multiline catheters. The potentially most serious bacterial infection is a **tunnel infection,** manifested by inflammation and tenderness along the entire subcutaneous tract of the catheter. These infections mandate prompt removal of the catheter and administration of intravenous antibiotics.

30. **How should a patient who has oral candidiasis or esophageal candidiasis be treated?**
    Candida species of yeast are a common cause of oral or esophageal infections in immunocompromised hosts. Topical antifungals (e.g., nystatin) may be tried in cases of simple oral candidiasis, and these can be added to regimens to treat esophageal candidiasis. However, systemic therapy is usually indicated in cases of esophageal candidiasis. Fluconazole is the first-line agent that can be used against candidal mucosal infections.

31. **After receiving broad-spectrum antibiotic therapy for 4 days for fever and neutropenia, a patient develops a new fever that is associated with abdominal cramps and bloody diarrhea. What is the most likely diagnosis?**
    The patient most likely has ***Clostridium difficile* colitis** brought on by treatment with broad-spectrum antibiotics. The diagnosis should be confirmed by detection of the *C. difficile* toxins

in the stool, and either metronidazole (preferred) or oral vancomycin should be initiated promptly.

32. **Why do patients on chemotherapy receive trimethoprim-sulfamethoxazole?**
Trimethoprim-sulfamethoxazole is used to prevent *Pneumocystis carinii* pneumonia. Prophylaxis can be achieved with 2 to 3 days of consecutive-day dosing per week.

33. **What paraneoplastic syndromes can occur in childhood?**
Paraneoplastic signs or symptoms are those that are unrelated to a malignancy but that can herald cancer. They occur more commonly in adults than children. However, unexplained high calcium, watery diarrhea, polymyositis, dermatomyositis, unexplained high hemoglobins, hypertension, precocious puberty, and opsoclonus or myoclonus can be associated with childhood malignancies.

    de Graaf JH, Tamminga RY, Kamps WA: Paraneoplastic manifestations in children, *Eur J Pediatr* 153:784–791, 1994.

34. **What is the triad of tumor lysis syndrome?**
Hyperuricemia, hyperkalemia, and **hyperphosphatemia.** These metabolic complications occur as a result of the rapid lysis of a large tumor burden, especially in Burkitt lymphoma and T-cell leukemia and lymphoma. Secondary renal failure and symptomatic hypocalcemia can also occur.

35. **What factors can contribute to renal failure in tumor lysis syndrome?**
    - **Uric acid nephropathy:** The degradation of nucleic acids leads to increases in serum uric acid, which is soluble at physiologic pH but can precipitate in the acid milieu of the collecting tubules.
    - **Calcium-phosphate crystallization:** Lymphoblasts (which contain four times the phosphate of lymphocytes) release phosphate, and, if the calcium-phosphate product exceeds 60, crystals can form in the renal microvasculature.
    - **Tumor burden:** The tumor itself may contribute to preexisting renal problems by parenchymal involvement, obstructive uropathy, and venous stasis.

36. **What two pharmacologic agents can be used to prevent or treat hyperuricemia caused by tumor lysis syndrome?**
Allopurinol inhibits the enzyme xanthine oxidase, a key enzyme required for the formation of uric acid. Its administration blocks further uric acid *production*. **Rasburicase** is a recombinant enzyme that catalyses the conversion of uric acid to allantoin, which is more soluble than uric acid, and more readily *excreted* by the kidney.

37. **Why is bicarbonate often used in the initial management of tumor lysis syndrome?**
The mainstay of tumor lysis therapy is aggressive hydration with initial alkalinization (with diuresis when necessary). Uric acid is relatively insoluble in the acidic pH of the urine, but this solubility increases with increased urine pH. Bicarbonate increases the pH and solubility of uric acid. After the uric acid normalizes and allopurinol is being administered, alkalinization is stopped.

38. **A child with newly diagnosed leukemia experiences a rapid decline in hemoglobin soon after administration of rasburicase. What is the basis for this drug-related adverse event?**
Rasburicase is contraindicated in patients with glucose-6-phosphate dehydrogenase (G6PD) deficiency because of the risk for hemolysis and development of methemoglobinemia.

39. **A child undergoing induction chemotherapy for leukemia develops right lower quadrant pain and tenderness. What diagnosis should be considered?**
Typhlitis. Although patients with cancer or those receiving chemotherapy may develop appendicitis, typhlitis is a severe necrotizing infection of the ileocolonic junction that occurs in neutropenic patients.

40. **Is it true that the newest form of asparaginase, PEG-asparaginase, was affectionately named after its inventor?**
Although a Peggy may certainly have been involved in its development, PEG stands for polyethylene glycol. By conjugating the native enzyme L-asparaginase to this large polymer, the half-life of the drug is greatly extended, and the exposed antigenic sites that can result in allergic reactions are diminished. Thus, instead of requiring up to nine intramuscular injections every other day, children with ALL can now be treated with a single injection.

41. **What is the difference between a Broviac and a Port-A-Cath?**
Children who require repeated blood draws or intravenous medications often have a semipermanent central venous catheter placed.
- A **Broviac catheter** is tunneled through the subcutaneous tissues of the chest and emerges as a thin plastic tube, usually at the level of the second or third rib.
- A **Port-A-Cath** contains a subcutaneous reservoir and is implanted under the skin of the chest. It is not visible, but it must be accessed by inserting a small needle through the skin and into the reservoir.

   Gallieni M, Pittiruti M, Biffi R: Vascular access in oncology patients, *CA Cancer J Clin* 58:323–346, 2008.

42. **What is the differential diagnosis of an anterior mediastinal mass?**
The five "Ts" can be used to remember the differential diagnosis of an anterior mediastinal mass: teratoma (germ-cell tumor), thymoma, thyroid tumor, T-cell leukemia, and terrible lymphoma.

43. **What is superior mediastinal syndrome? How is it managed?**
Superior mediastinal syndrome, also called superior vena cava syndrome results from the presence of an anterior mediastinal mass that compresses the trachea and the superior vena cava. Patients have a cough and dyspnea, particularly when supine, and they have swelling of the head and upper extremities as a result of venous compression. Patients with a large mediastinal mass must not be anesthetized because of the risk for complete airway obstruction and vascular collapse. The optimal management of a mediastinal mass is prompt diagnosis and the initiation of appropriate treatment. Irradiation of the mass may provide emergent relief while the diagnosis is being made.

44. **Which tumors most commonly cause superior mediastinal syndrome?**
In childhood, the most common primary cause is non-Hodgkin lymphoma. Less frequent causes are Hodgkin disease, neuroblastoma, and sarcomas. Nonmalignant infectious causes are unusual but can include histoplasmosis or tuberculosis. The most frequent cause in children, however, is iatrogenic, resulting from vascular thrombosis after surgeries for congenital heart disease, shunting procedures for hydrocephalus, or central catheterization for venous access.

45. **Why is a generous mediastinal shadow on the radiograph much more worrisome in a teenager than an infant?**
Among infants, the incidence of Hodgkin disease is extremely low. The thymus normally has a distinctive shape with flaring at the base and indentations from the ribcage ("sail sign"), which can usually be delineated on plain film. In teenagers, thymic enlargement has a higher likelihood of malignancy, particularly Hodgkin disease, which is usually accompanied by

lymphadenopathy in other areas of the mediastinum, particularly the paratracheal, tracheobronchial, and hilar regions.

46. **Which neoplasms are associated with hemihypertrophy?**
Wilms tumor, hepatoblastoma, and **adrenal cortical carcinoma** are associated with hemihypertrophy either as part of Beckwith-Wiedemann syndrome or in isolation. Between 1% and 3% of Wilms tumor patients have hemihypertrophy.

47. **Which cancers are often associated with splenomegaly?**
Acute leukemia, chronic myeloid leukemia, chronic myelomonocytic leukemia, Hodgkin disease, and non-Hodgkin lymphoma. Solid tumors rarely metastasize to the spleen to the point of causing splenomegaly.

48. **What are the predictors of malignancy in the pediatric patient with peripheral lymphadenopathy?**
A common clinical problem is determining which patients with enlarged lymph nodes require biopsy for diagnosis. In a study of 60 patients, risk for malignancy increased with increasing size (>1 cm), increasing number of adenopathy sites, and increasing ages (≥8 years old). Supraclavicular location, abnormal chest radiograph, and fixed nodes were also significantly predictive of malignancy.

Nield LS, Kamat D: Lymphadenopathy in children: when and how to evaluate, *Clin Pediatr* 43:25–33, 2004.

Soldes OS, Younger JG, Hirschl RB: Predictors of malignancy in childhood peripheral lymphadenopathy, *J Pediatr Surg* 34:1447–1452, 1999.

49. **What are the common indications for transfusion support for children with cancer?**
Although there are no absolute criteria, in most centers, packed red blood cells are given when a patient has a hemoglobin level of less than 8.0 g/dL. Platelets are empirically administered for a platelet count of less than 10,000 to 20,000/mm^3 in an otherwise well patient; a higher threshold may be used if there is active bleeding, disseminated intravascular coagulation (DIC), or a planned procedure. Granulocyte transfusions may be effective in neutropenic patients with a refractory infection caused by a gram-negative organism. Transfusions with plasma may be used for the treatment of coagulopathies.

50. **Why are blood products irradiated and leukocytes depleted?**
Irradiation of blood products prevents transfusion-associated graft-versus-host disease (GVHD), which occurs when small numbers of T cells in the blood product are transferred into an immunocompromised patient. Leukocyte depletion removes other white blood cells that would increase the risk for febrile transfusion reactions, alloimmunization, and the transmission of cytomegalovirus.

51. **What are the most common symptoms experienced by oncology patients receiving end-of-life care?**
Fatigue, pain, and **dyspnea.** Parents report that these symptoms are managed effectively in less than one third of children. As compared with adults, twice as many children die in hospitals during the final stages of disease, and half of them are on a ventilator. Insufficient attention to palliative care is a large problem.

Hewitt M, Goldman A, Collins GS, et al: Opioid use in palliative care of children and young people with cancer, *J Pediatr* 152:39–44, 2008.

Himelstein BP, Hilden JM, Boldt AM, et al: Pediatric palliative care, *N Engl J Med* 350:1752–1762, 2004.

Wolfe J, Grier HE, Klar N, et al: Symptoms and suffering at the end of life in children with cancer, *N Engl J Med* 342:326–333, 2000.

EPIDEMIOLOGY

52. What are the frequencies of relative incidence of the childhood cancers in the United States?
- Leukemias: 27%
- CNS tumors: 21%
- Lymphomas: 11%
- Neuroblastoma: 7%
- Wilms tumor: 6%
- Soft tissue tumors: 6%
- Bone tumors: 5%
- Retinoblastoma: 3%
- Other tumors: 14%

Gurney JG, Severson RK, Davis S, et al: Incidence of cancer in children in the United States. Sex-, race-, and 1-year age-specific rates by histologic type, *Cancer* 75:2186–2195, 1995.

53. How do the types of malignancies compare between infants and adolescents?
See Figures 15-2 and 15-3.

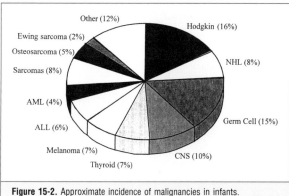

Figure 15-2. Approximate incidence of malignancies in infants.

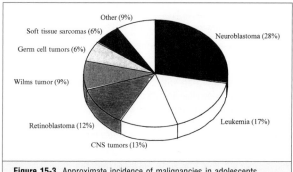

Figure 15-3. Approximate incidence of malignancies in adolescents.

54. **Is cancer the most common cause of death in children younger than 15 years?**
Cancer ranks a distant second, accounting for 10% of deaths in children younger than 15 years. Accidents account for nearly 45% of deaths among this age group; congenital anomalies rank third, at 8%, and homicide ranks fourth, at 5%.

55. **Although in psychic lore a "seer" can look into the future, for cancer researchers SEER has a different connotation. What is it?**
SEER stands for surveillance, epidemiology, and end-results database. SEER collects cancer incidence, prevalence, and survival data in specific geographic areas in the United States. These areas represent about 26% of the U.S. population. SEER data are freely available to qualified investigators and can be used to study epidemiology trends in cancer incidence, prevalence, and survival.

   http://seer.cancer.gov/.

56. **What are the relative risks for children to develop leukemia?**
See Table 15-1.

TABLE 15-1. RELATIVE RISK FOR CHILDREN TO DEVELOP LEUKEMIA	
Population at Risk	Estimated Risk
U.S. white children	1 in 2800
Siblings of a child with leukemia	1 in 700
Identical twin of a child with leukemia	1 in 5
Children with:	
Down syndrome	1 in 75
Fanconi syndrome	1 in 12
Bloom syndrome	1 in 8
Ataxia-telangiectasia	1 in 8
Exposures:	
Atom bomb within 100 m	1 in 60
Ionizing radiation	?
Benzene	1 in 960
Alkylating agents	1 in 2000?

Data from Mahoney DH Jr: Neoplastic diseases. In McMillan JA, DeAngelis CD, Felgin RD, Warshaw JB (eds): Oski's Pediatrics, Principles and Practice, 3rd ed. Philadelphia, JB Lippincott, 1999, p 1494.

57. **Is cell phone use associated with an increased risk for brain tumors?**
Currently, the available epidemiologic data do not support an association between cellular phone use and brain tumors. Theses studies are complicated by many factors, including recall bias (patients with brain tumors recalling cell phone exposure differently than subjects without brain tumors), difficulties in estimating actual radiofrequency exposure, and incomplete follow-up of study subjects.

   Patrick K, Griswold WG, Raab F, Intille SS: Health and the mobile phone, *Am J Prevent Med* 35: 177–181, 2008.

58. **Which cancers have a significant racial predilection?**
Wilms tumor has a higher incidence among black female infants. **Ewing tumor** is about 30 times more common in whites than in blacks. **Hodgkin disease** is rare in those of East Asian descent.

59. **What cancers are most commonly associated with a second neoplasm?**
See Table 15-2.

TABLE 15-2. CANCERS MOST COMMONLY ASSOCIATED WITH A SECOND NEOPLASM	
Primary Tumors	**Secondary Tumors**
Retinoblastoma	Osteosarcoma
	Pinealoblastoma
Hodgkin disease	Acute nonlymphoblastic leukemia
	Non-Hodgkin lymphoma
	Sarcoma (in radiation field)
	Thyroid carcinoma
	Breast carcinoma (in radiation field)
Acute lymphoblastic leukemia	Brain tumors
	Non-Hodgkin lymphoma
Sarcomas	Sarcomas

60. **What is the most well-documented risk factor for hepatoblastoma?**
Multiple studies have demonstrated that **low birthweight** (<1000 g) is a risk factor for hepatoblastoma. Presently, it is not known whether this is due to other factors associated with low birthweight, such as hyperalimentation use, or the low birthweight itself.

61. **Are there any known transplacental carcinogens?**
Diethylstilbestrol, which was used to prevent spontaneous abortion, has been associated with an increased risk for vaginal cancer in the female offspring. It has also been reported that there is a 10-fold increased risk for monoblastic leukemia in the infants of mothers who smoke marijuana. It has been suggested that sedatives and a number of nonhormonal drugs are transplacental carcinogens, but this is not proved. It also has not been proved that cigarette smoke and the use of oral contraceptives are transplacental carcinogens.

62. **Is prenatal ultrasound associated with a risk for leukemia later in childhood?**
No. In vitro, ultrasound has been shown to cause cell membrane changes, and thus concern has been expressed regarding potential effects on embryogenesis and prenatal and postnatal development. However, in a study of all deaths from leukemia in Swedish children over a 16-year period, no association with prenatal ultrasound was found. Of note, the only known association of prenatal ultrasound with alterations in development has been a preference for left-handedness.

Kieler H, Ahlsten G, Haglund B, et al: Routine ultrasound screening in pregnancy and aspects of the children's subsequent neurological development, *Obstet Gynecol* 91:750–756, 1998.

Naumburg E, Bellocco R, Cnattingius S, et al: Prenatal ultrasound examinations and risk of childhood leukaemia: case-control study, *BMJ* 320:282–283, 2000.

63. **Do children living near electrical power lines have an increased risk for developing cancer?**
Although a few small studies have suggested an association between power lines and an increased risk for ALL, the largest and best-designed study as reported by Linet did not find evidence to support this hypothesis. Since that time, additional studies have not demonstrated a significant risk.

Draper G, Vincent T, Kroll ME, Swanson J: Childhood cancer in relation to distance from high-voltage power line in England and Wales: a case-control study, *BMJ* 330:1290–1293, 2005.

Linet MS, Hatch EE, Kleinerman RA, et al: Residential exposure to magnetic fields and acute lymphoblastic leukemia in children, *N Engl J Med* 337:1–7, 1997.

LEUKEMIA

64. **What are the most common clinical findings in the initial presentation of ALL?**
   - **Hepatosplenomegaly:** 70% (10% to 15% of children have marked enlargement of the liver or spleen to a level below the umbilicus)
   - **Fever:** 40% to 60%
   - **Lymphadenopathy:** 25% to 50% with moderate or marked enlargement
   - **Bleeding:** 25% to 50% with petechiae or purpura
   - **Bone and joint pain:** 25% to 40%
   - **Fatigue:** 30%
   - **Anorexia:** 20% to 35%

KEY POINTS: ACUTE LYMPHOBLASTIC LEUKEMIA

1. Most common childhood malignancy

2. Increased risk: Patients with Down syndrome, congenital immunodeficiency syndrome, exposure to ionizing radiation; sibling of patient with acute lymphoblastic leukemia

3. Chemotherapy phases: Induction (to achieve remission), delayed intensification, maintenance

4. Survival (if in standard risk group) >80% at 5 years after completion of therapy

5. Most common sites of relapse: Bone marrow, central nervous system, testis

65. **What are the typical hematologic findings noted during the presentation of ALL?**
   Leukocyte count (mm³)
   - <10,000: 45% to 55%
   - 10,000 to 50,000: 30% to 35%
   - >50,000: 20%

   Hemoglobin (g/dL)
   - <7.5: 45%
   - 7.5 to 10.0: 30%
   - >10: 25%

   Platelet count (mm³)
   - <20,000: 25%
   - 20,000 to 99,000: 50%
   - >100,000: 25%

66. **What studies of tumor cells are useful for determining a patient's prognosis?**
The cytogenetics and DNA index (ratio of DNA content in abnormal cells compared to normal reference cells) are determinants of the number and structure of chromosomes and chromosomal material in tumor cells. More than 50 chromosomes or a DNA index of more than 1.16 is favorable. Certain chromosomal translocations are unfavorable. Immunophenotyping is also useful and involves the determination of B- or T-cell lineage, with maturity or immaturity of cells.

   Pui C-H, Relling MV, Downing JR: Acute lymphoblastic leukemia, *N Engl J Med* 350: 1535–1548, 2004.

67. **Why do children with ALL who are younger than 1 year have poorer prognoses?**
Most infants with ALL in this age group often have a full complement of unfavorable features: high white blood cell count, CNS leukemia, bulky extramedullary disease, and t(4;11) (a translocation associated with poor response to therapy). By contrast, the prognosis for infants with AML is not necessarily less favorable than that of older children.

68. **Why do boys with ALL fare more poorly than girls?**
In boys, after a full course of chemotherapy with remission, testicular involvement is a common site of relapse, occurring in up to 10% of cases. In older boys and teenage boys, there is a higher incidence of T-cell disease than in girls. T-cell disease is associated with adverse prognostic factors (high white blood cell count, hepatosplenomegaly, and mediastinal masses) and alone carries a poorer prognosis. In girls, ovarian relapse is very rare, although it is difficult to diagnose after bone marrow relapse.

69. **Is ethnicity related to treatment outcome in patients with acute leukemia?**
Ethnicity appears to be related to outcome in both ALL and AML in children. In both leukemias, African American ethnicity is associated with a poorer outcome. Although the reasons are not known, these differences may be the result of either host or leukemia characteristics.

KEY POINTS: HIGHER-RISK GROUPS WITH POORER PROGNOSIS OF PATIENTS WITH ACUTE LYMPHOBLASTIC LEUKEMIA

1. Age: <1 year and >10 years

2. White blood cell count: >50,000/mm^3

3. Chromosomal translocation abnormalities, specifically t(8;14), t(9;22), and t(4;11)

4. Hypoploidy (<45 chromosomes)

5. Malignant cells, with mature B-cell or T-cell immunophenotyping

6. Central nervous system involvement

7. Black and Hispanic patients

8. Males

70. **In the United States, what are the four most common types of pediatric leukemia, and about how many children are diagnosed each year with each type?**
    ALL, with about 2500 new diagnoses yearly; **AML,** with about 500 new diagnoses yearly; **chronic myelogenous leukemia** (CML), with about 100 new diagnoses yearly; and **juvenile myelomonocytic leukemia** (JMML), with about 50 new diagnoses yearly.

71. **In addition to leukemia, what other diagnoses should be considered when evaluating a child who shows symptoms of pancytopenia?**
    - Aplastic anemia
    - Viral-induced suppression
    - Drug-induced suppression
    - Metastatic disease to the bone marrow
    - Hemophagocytic syndromes
    - Disseminated histoplasmosis
    - Transfusion-associated graft-versus-host disease (GVHD)

72. **Although many prognostic factors have come and gone for childhood ALL, which two have remained significant for the past 40 years?**
    The two most consistent prognostic factors are age and elevation of presenting white blood cell count. Children younger than 1 year or older than 10 years old have a worse prognosis, as do those with a presenting white blood cell count of $50,000/mm^3$ or greater. Prognostic factors are important because, although 95% of ALL patients achieve remission (<5% lymphoblasts in bone marrow), 25% relapse. Identifying patients at higher risk is important so that more aggressive or novel therapy can be considered.

73. **Other than age at diagnosis and white blood cell count, what factor has the greatest prognostic impact on long-term survival?**
    A better prognosis is seen in patients who have a **brisk initial response to therapy**. This has been defined differently in separate studies. The Children's Cancer Group found an improved prognosis in patients with less than 5% blasts in the bone marrow after 14 days of chemotherapy. The Berlin-Frankfurt-Münster group found a similar prognosis in patients who had less than $1000 blasts/mm^3$ in the peripheral blood after 7 days of prednisone.

74. **What is MRD and how is it used?**
    MRD stands for *minimal residual disease*, which is typically detected by flow cytometry at several time points during therapy. In ALL, MRD detects patients who have a normal appearing bone marrow by light microscopy, but in fact have an increased risk for relapse owing to low-level, persistent disease. MRD use in AML is not as well defined as in ALL.

75. **What is the acute risk for a very elevated blast count noted at the time of the initial diagnosis of leukemia?**
    An elevated blast count at diagnosis may cause **CNS leukostasis and stroke.** The risk is higher in patients with AML because myeloblasts are larger and may have procoagulant activity that increases the risk for stroke or hemorrhage. Leukocytapheresis is sometimes used to reduce the blast count before initiating therapy, but its impact on improving outcome remains unproved.

76. **What are the most common sites of extramedullary relapse of ALL?**
    The most common is the **meninges,** and this is followed by **testicular relapse.** Testicular disease is accompanied by painless testicular swelling (usually unilateral). The diagnosis must be confirmed by biopsy. Patients with testicular disease require irradiation in addition to intensive retreatment with chemotherapy.

77. **What are the long-term side effects of cranial radiation administered for the prevention of CNS leukemia?**
A number of endocrinologic complications can occur, including growth hormone deficiency, hypothyroidism, hypogonadism, impaired fertility, and premature ovarian failure. Children are also at risk for deficits in attention, memory, and intelligence quotient. Less commonly, leukoencephalopathy may occur. Finally, children receiving cranial radiation are at risk for developing a second malignant neoplasm.

78. **Which distinct form of AML uses an analog of a common vitamin as a core component of its treatment?**
Treatment of acute promyelocytic leukemia (APL), or AML FAB subtype M3, includes oral administration of the **vitamin A analog all-*trans*-retinoic acid (ATRA).** ATRA can differentiate a malignant promyeloblast into a mature functioning neutrophil. Inclusion of ATRA in current treatment protocols has dramatically increased cure rates for patients with APL.

79. **What is a chloroma?**
A *chloroma* is a tumor that is formed by a coalescence of AML blasts. It may appear in bones, skin, soft tissue, or other sites. Its name is derived from its green appearance on its cut surface.

Downing JR, Burnett A: Acute myeloid leukemia, *N Engl J Med* 341:1051–1062, 1999.

80. **What is the significance of the Philadelphia chromosome?**
The **Philadelphia chromosome,** discovered in Philadelphia in 1960 by Nowell and Hungerford, was the first clonal cytogenetic abnormality (a balanced translocation between chromosomes 9 and 22) described in leukemia. The result is a new fusion gene that codes for a tyrosine kinase with increased enzymatic activity. The Philadelphia chromosome is seen in more than 90% of patients with CML but also in 5% or less of children with ALL (20% of adult ALL) and in 2% or less of children with AML. Different isoforms of the fusion gene may be present in ALL. ALL in a child with the Philadelphia chromosome has a much poorer prognosis.

Arico M, Valsecchi MG, Camitta B, et al: Outcome of treatment in children with Philadelphia chromosome-positive acute lymphoblastic leukemia, *N Engl J Med* 342:998-1006, 2000.

81. **What is the appropriate treatment for CML?**
Currently, there is debate about the most appropriate treatment for CML. Many physicians use the tyrosine kinase inhibitor (TKI) imatinib as first-line therapy and then use second-generation TKIs (dasatinib, nilotinib) for patients who are imatinib intolerant or refractory. Other physicians will use imatinib as first-line therapy and then move to allogeneic stem cell transplantation (SCT) for imatinib-intolerant or imatinib-resistant patients. A minority of physicians continue to use SCT as primary therapy for pediatric patients with CML.

CML treatment decisions are difficult because the TKI are generally very well tolerated with very few long-term side effects, unlike SCT, which has a measurable mortality rate and substantial long-term complications. However, TKIs are not considered curative, whereas a successful SCT will cure a patient with CML.

82. **If you saw a car with the license plate, "FLT3 ITD," what would the most likely interest of its driver be?**
Studying childhood AML would likely occupy most of this driver's free time. FLT3 or "FMS-like tyrosine kinase 3" is a tyrosine kinase located on chromosome 13. Internal tandem duplications (ITD) of the juxtamembrane region of FLT3 protein are associated with an increased risk for relapse in AML. In pediatric AML, this increased risk for relapse is particularly evident for patients who have a high allelic ratio, or an increased number of the ITDs.

LYMPHOMA

83. **What is the malignant cell of Hodgkin disease?**
The **Reed-Sternberg cell.** Its normal cell of origin remains unclear, with the predominance of evidence indicating a B or T lymphocyte. However, the cells alone are not pathognomonic of Hodgkin disease and may be seen in infectious mononucleosis, non-Hodgkin lymphoma, carcinomas, and sarcomas.

84. **How is Hodgkin disease staged?**
Hodgkin lymphoma, like non-Hodgkin lymphoma, is classified according to the stage of disease and histology, as in the Ann Arbor System. It is also staged according to whether there are symptoms. Patients with no symptoms are referred to as having *A disease.* Patients with documented fever, involuntary weight loss of more than 10%, or night sweats are considered to have *B disease.* Intractable pruritus may also be a symptom, but it is not among the B symptoms used for staging.
    Stage is determined both clinically and pathologically. Location of lymph node regions is the critical factor: I (single region), II (regions on the same side of the diaphragm), III (regions on both sides of the diaphragm), or IV (diffuse disease). Clinical staging refers to staging that is done without histologic proof. Pathologic staging refers to biopsy-proven disease in a given region and usually involves a staging laparotomy and splenectomy to determine the extent of disease.

85. **What are B symptoms?**
Fever, night sweats, and **weight loss.** Their presence carries a poorer prognosis for patients with Hodgkin disease.

86. **What is the histologic classification of Hodgkin disease?**
See Table 15-3.

TABLE 15-3. THE RYE, NEW YORK, HISTOLOGIC CLASSIFICATION*

Type	Lymphocytes	Reed-Sternberg Cells	Other	Incidence (%)
Lymphocyte predominant	Many	Few	Histiocytes	10-15
Nodular sclerosing	Many	Few or many	Bands of refractile fibrosis	40-70
Mixed cellularity	Many	Few or many	Eosinophils, histiocytes	20-30
Lymphocyte depletion	Few	Many	No refractile fibrosis	<5

*Based on the relative number of lymphocytes and Reed-Sternberg cells.

87. **What is the prognosis for the various stages of Hodgkin disease?**
The prognosis for children with Hodgkin disease is excellent in that most are cured. For stages I and IIA, the 5-year relapse-free survival rate is higher than 80% for patients treated with radiation only, and it may be higher than 90% for patients treated with radiation and

chemotherapy. For stage IIB, prognosis is not as good, especially if there is a massive mediastinal tumor, but 5-year survival is still higher than 80%. The same survival figures pertain to stage IIIA disease, but treatment generally is more extensive than that for a limited stage II disease. For stage IV disease, the 5-year relapse-free survival rate is 70% to 90%.

88. **The classification of lymphomas has evolved over time, but an international effort has brought consistency to diagnosing these diverse cancers. Describe the World Health Organization (WHO) classification system for non-Hodgkin lymphomas.**
The current WHO system classifies pediatric lymphomas as **common, uncommon,** and **rare.** The common classification is further divided into B-cell lymphoma (precursor B-cell lymphoblastic lymphoma or leukemia, Burkitt lymphoma, diffuse large-B cell lymphoma, and mediastinal [thymic] large-B cell lymphoma) and T-cell lymphoma (precursor T-cell lymphoblastic lymphoma or leukemia, anaplastic large cell lymphoma, and peripheral T-cell lymphoma, unspecified). The uncommon lymphomas include follicular lymphoma, hepatosplenic T-cell lymphoma, and extranodal marginal B-cell lymphoma of mucosa-associated lymphoid tissue (MALT) lymphoma. The rare lymphomas include mycosis fungoides, subcutaneous panniculitis-like T-cell lymphoma, adult T-cell human T-cell lymphotropic virus type 1–associated lymphoma, primary cutaneous CD30-positive T-cell lymphoproliferative disorders, and extranodal natural killer or T-cell lymphoma.

89. **What differentiates B- and T-cell precursor leukemia from lymphoma?**
The **bone marrow blast percentage** is used to differentiate B- and T-cell precursor leukemia from lymphoma. If the bone marrow blast percentage is greater than or equal to 25%, the diagnosis of leukemia is given. If the blast percentage is less than 25% and the patient has other sites of malignant disease, the diagnosis of lymphoma is given.

90. **What are the common types of lymphoma in children?**
As compared with adults, aggressive, **high-grade lymphomas** occur more frequently in children. The three most common types are Burkitt lymphoma, lymphoblastic lymphoma, and large cell lymphoma.

91. **How does anaplastic large cell lymphoma typically present?**
Patients typically present in adolescence with nodal involvement and may have involvement of extranodal sites including the skin and soft tissues. About 25% of patients may have bone marrow involvement, and 75% will have a t(2;5)(p23;q35) translocation that will involve the *ALK* gene.

92. **What is an eosinophilic granuloma?**
Eosinophilic granuloma is a lytic tumor of bone that is accompanied by pain and sometimes swelling. Its histology is identical to that of Langerhans cell histiocytosis, with which it is now classified. Biopsy of an isolated eosinophilic granuloma is often curative, although lesions may also regress spontaneously.

93. **What are the features of Langerhans cell histiocytosis (LCH)?**
LCH is a multifaceted disorder and replaces the diseases grouped under the term *histiocytosis X.* The presenting symptoms of LCH may be isolated bone lesions (eosinophilic granuloma), bone lesions together with exophthalmos and diabetes insipidus (Hand-Schüller-Christian disease), or with disseminated disease (Letterer-Siwe disease). Other features include skin rashes that resemble seborrheic dermatitis, chronic otitis externa, lymphadenopathy, hepatosplenomegaly, pancytopenia, neurologic deficits, and pulmonary disease. Mild forms of the disease tend to wax and wane even without treatment, whereas disseminated disease is often resistant to therapy.

NERVOUS SYSTEM TUMORS

94. **How are CNS tumors classified?**
    Most are typically classified on the basis of histology:
    - **Glioma:** Arises from supportive tissue (astrocytes)
    - **Ependymoma:** Arises from the ependymal cells that line the ventricles
    - **Germ cell tumor:** Arises from totipotent germ cells
    - **Rhabdoid:** Arises from an unknown cell type
    - **Craniopharyngioma:** Arise from embryonic precursors to anterior pituitary gland

---

KEY POINTS: CENTRAL NERVOUS SYSTEM TUMORS

1. Second most common neoplasm of childhood, after leukemia

2. Older children (>1 year): Most tumors are infratentorial (cerebellar or brainstem)

3. Younger children (<1 year): Most tumors are supratentorial

4. Gold standard for diagnosis: Magnetic resonance imaging with and without gadolinium enhancement

5. Back pain, extremity weakness, and/or bowel and bladder dysfunction suggestive of spinal cord lesions or metastases

---

95. **Where is the most common area for each tumor to occur?**
    - **Glioma:** Cerebellum and optic pathway (more commonly benign and low grade); cerebrum or brainstem (more commonly malignant and higher grade)
    - **Ependymoma:** Fourth ventricle; less commonly the spinal cord
    - **Germ cell tumor:** Pineal or supracellar region
    - **Primitive neuroectodermal tumor (PNET) medulloblastoma:** Midline of the cerebellum
    - **Rhabdoid:** Posterior fossa
    - **Craniopharyngioma:** Choroid plexus

96. **What are the most common supratentorial brain tumors? What are their symptoms?**
    Supratentorial tumors include tumors of the cerebrum, basal ganglia, thalamus, and hypothalamus. They can be gliomas, ependymomas, PNETs, germ cell tumors, choroid plexus tumors, or craniopharyngiomas. These tumors can show signs of increased intracranial pressure, such as headache and vomiting. In addition, these tumors may be accompanied by focal deficits, such as memory loss, weakness, and visual changes.

    Hawley DP, Walker DA: A symptomatic journey to the centre of the brain, *Arch Dis Child Educ Pract Ed* 95:59-64, 2010.

97. **What are the most common infratentorial tumors? What are their symptoms?**
    Infratentorial tumors include tumors of the cerebellum and brainstem. They can be astrocytomas, medulloblastomas, ependymomas, or gliomas. If infratentorial tumors block CSF outflow, headache and vomiting may be the presenting signs; they can also become apparent with localizing signs such as cranial nerve palsies or ataxia.

98. **Which common parameters should be closely monitored in a child after resection of a brain tumor?**
    It is important to closely monitor **urine output** and **serum sodium** in children undergoing CNS surgery. Resection of a hypothalamic glioma, germ cell tumor, or craniopharyngioma

can directly disrupt the function of the pituitary gland and lead to diabetes insipidus. Alternatively, some patients may develop a cerebral salt-wasting syndrome after resection.

99. **Which cranial nerve abnormality is most common in children showing signs of increased intracranial pressure as the result of a posterior fossa tumor?**
Inability to abduct one or both eyes **(cranial nerve VI palsy)** may result from an elevation in intracranial pressure and can be a false localizing sign for the primary brain tumor.

100. **What are the three Es of the diencephalic syndrome?**
Diencephalic syndrome is the constellation of symptoms that result from the presence of a hypothalamic tumor: **euphoria, emaciation,** and **emesis.**

101. **What is Parinaud syndrome?**
Parinaud syndrome is the result of increased intracranial pressure at the dorsal midbrain, causing downgaze, papillary dilation, and nystagmus.

102. **In addition to imaging studies, what should be included in the evaluation of a possible CNS germ cell tumor?**
Both serum and cerebrospinal **tumor α-fetoprotein** and **human chorionic gonadotropin** should be obtained. Significant elevation of these markers is diagnostic of CNS germ cell tumor in a patient with an intracranial mass.

103. **What are the key evaluations for a child with a newly diagnosed medulloblastoma?**
Medulloblastomas may spread contiguously to the cerebellar peduncle, to the floor of the fourth ventricle, into the cervical spine, or above the tentorium. In addition, medulloblastomas may disseminate through the CSF. Every patient should thus be evaluated with diagnostic imaging (magnetic resonance imaging) of the spinal cord and of the whole brain. Examination of CSF should be performed after resection of the primary tumor.

Pizer B, Clifford S: Medulloblastoma: new insights into biology and treatment, *Arch Dis Child Educ Pract Ed* 98:137–144, 2008.

104. **What is a "dropped met"?**
Most brain tumors do not metastasize; they are fatal because of local invasion. A *dropped metastasis* occurs when a primary brain tumor spreads through CSF pathways, thereby resulting in meningeal deposits along the spinal cord. These metastases have "dropped" from their original site down to the spinal cord or cauda equina.

105. **What are the differences among a glioma, an astrocytoma, and glioblastoma multiforme?**
- A **glioma** (from the Greek word *glia* for glue and the suffix *-oma* for tumor) is a neoplasm that is derived from one of the various types of cells that form the interstitial tissue of the central nervous system, such as astrocytes, oligodendria, and ependymal cells. Of the gliomas, astrocytomas of variable malignancy are the most prevalent.
- **Astrocytomas** are subdivided into categories (grades) on the basis of the degree of tumor anaplasia and the presence or absence of necrosis. The juvenile pilocytic and subependymal astrocytoma are low-grade gliomas. Anaplastic astrocytoma (grade 3) grow more rapidly than the more differentiated astrocytomas.
- **Glioblastoma multiforme** is the highest-grade astrocytoma (grade 4).

Ullrich NJ, Pomeroy SL: Pediatric brain tumors, *Neurol Clin* 21:897–913, 2003.

106. **What is the most common malignancy associated with neurofibromatosis type 1 (NF1)?**
Optic pathway glioma. These low-grade astrocytomas occur in 15% to 20% of patients with NF1. Fortunately, only about half of them become symptomatic, and therefore treatment is not always indicated. Because greater than 70% of patients with optic pathway glioma have NF1, a new diagnosis of this optic glioma mandates an evaluation for this common autosomal dominant genetic disease.

107. **Why is the prognosis for children with brainstem gliomas so poor?**
A basic tenet of CNS tumors is that a gross total resection is necessary to achieve the greatest chance of long-term cure. Brainstem tumors most commonly are fully intrinsic to the pons and unresectable. Although radiation can improve symptoms, there currently is no known curative therapy for most children with brainstem gliomas.

108. **Cancer therapy uses many different modalities of treatment. Patients with high-risk neuroblastoma require treatment with virtually all known therapeutic modalities to maximize the likelihood of cure. Can you name the modalities?**
Children with stage IV neuroblastoma therapy are currently managed by using almost all known therapeutic modalities for cancer therapy. Therapy often requires administration of multiagent chemotherapy, surgical resection, stem cell transplantation, radiation therapy, differentiation therapy with 13-*cis*-retinoic acid (Accutane), and most recently, immunotherapy.

109. **Why can neuroblastoma arise in a spectrum of locations in children?**
Neuroblastomas are tumors of the neural crest tissue. Abnormal migration of neural crest cells, which are destined for the adrenal medulla or the para-aortic sympathetic ganglia, forms pockets of immature neuroma. Thus, tumors arise anywhere along the neuraxis and in the adrenal glands.

KEY POINTS: NEUROBLASTOMA

1. Most common pediatric extracranial solid tumor

2. Most common malignant tumor among infants

3. Majority of children <4 years old

4. Poorer prognosis: >1 year old, metastatic disease, Myc-N amplification

5. Most metastatic at diagnosis

6. Paraneoplastic syndromes: VIP syndrome (diarrhea as a result of increased vasoactive intestinal peptide), opsoclonus-myoclonus ("dancing eyes, dancing feet"), and catecholamine excess (with flushing, sweating, headache, hypertension)

110. **What are the most common presentations of neuroblastoma?**
Children with disseminated neuroblastoma are irritable and ill, and they often have exquisite bone pain, proptosis, and periorbital ecchymoses. Seventy percent of neuroblastomas arise in the abdomen; half of these arise in the adrenal gland, and the other half arise in the parasympathetic ganglia and are distributed throughout the retroperitoneum and the paravertebral area in the chest and neck. The tumor produces and excretes catecholamines,

which can on occasion cause systemic symptoms such as sweating, hypertension, diarrhea, and irritability. Children with localized neuroblastoma may have symptoms referable to a mass.

Maris JM: Recent advances in neuroblastoma, *N Engl J Med* 362: 2202-2211, 2010.

111. **What is Horner syndrome?**
Ptosis, miosis (with unequal pupils), and **anhidrosis.** The syndrome can occur from congenital brachial plexus injury, but acquired Horner syndrome requires evaluation for cervical, intrathoracic, or intracranial pathology, particularly neuroblastoma.

112. **Where does neuroblastoma tend to metastasize?**
Neuroblastoma spreads to the **liver, the bone,** the **bone marrow,** and, less commonly, the **skin.**

113. **What is meant by "dancing eyes, dancing feet"?**
"Dancing eyes, dancing feet" is a descriptive term for opsoclonus-myoclonus, a condition in which children with neuroblastoma develop horizontal nystagmus and involuntary lower extremity muscle spasm. These symptoms are thought to arise from a nonspecific antibody reaction to neuroblastoma that cross-reacts with the motor end plate. These symptoms do not always improve, despite appropriate neuroblastoma therapy.

114. **What urinary test aids in the diagnosis of neuroblastoma?**
Urinary concentrations of catecholamines and metabolites, including dopamine, homovanillic acid, and vanillylmandelic acid, are often increased (>3 standard deviations above the mean per milligram creatinine for age) in children with neuroblastoma.

115. **Which molecular abnormality is associated with a more aggressive form of neuroblastoma?**
Myc-N amplification is often seen in patients with stage IV neuroblastoma. The presence of myc-N amplification renders a patient at higher risk for recurrence regardless of staging.

116. **What does the S stand for in stage IVS neuroblastoma?**
Stage IVS is a "special" type of neuroblastoma that is found only in children younger than 1 year. Along with a primary tumor, these infants may have bone marrow, liver, and skin disease as well. Even without therapy, these cancers spontaneously regress and disappear over time. Treatment is only indicated if the patient is symptomatic from the underlying disease (e.g., large abdominal mass, liver disease).

117. **What nuclear medicine agent has been useful in both the diagnosis and treatment of neuroblastoma?**
^{131}I-metaiodobenzylguanidine (^{131}I-MIBG) was developed by Wieland and colleagues at the University of Michigan in the 1970s for use as an antihypertensive agent. It is structurally similar to norepinephrine and found to concentrate within the neurosecretory granules of catecholamine producing cells. In the 1980s, studies confirmed the usefulness of I-MIBG in localizing neuroblastoma; 90% of neuroblastomas have uptake of I-MIBG in both primary and metastatic sites. In the late 1980s, studies investigating the use of I-MIBG as a therapeutic modality came about and are ongoing.

118. **How can the site of spinal cord compression be clinically localized?**
Spinal tenderness on percussion correlates with localization in up to 80% of patients. In addition, **neurologic evaluation** of strength, sensory level changes, reflexes, and anal tone can help to pinpoint the location in the spinal cord, the conus medullaris (the terminal neural portion of the spinal cord), or the cauda equina. Progression is rapid with spinal cord compression but may be rapid or variable with compression of the conus medullaris or the cauda equina. The levels of the spine most frequently affected are summarized in Table 15-4.

TABLE 15-4. FREQUENCY OF INVOLVEMENT OF CERVICAL, THORACIC, AND LUMBOSACRAL SPINE FROM TUMOR COMPRESSION	
Spinal Level	Involvement (%)
Cervical	10
Thoracic	70
Lumbar	20

Data from Gates RA, Fink RM: Oncology Nursing Secrets, 2nd ed. Philadelphia, Hanley & Belfus, 2001, p 470.

119. **What is leukokoria?**
    Leukokoria, or white pupil, can be obvious, or it can be a subtle asymmetry on pupillary red reflex evaluation. Although other diagnoses can accompany leukokoria, the most significant one is retinoblastoma.

120. **What is the heredity of retinoblastoma?**
    Although most cases are sporadic, retinoblastoma can be inherited as an autosomal dominant trait with nearly complete penetrance. Of all cases, 60% are nonhereditary and unilateral, 15% are hereditary and unilateral, and 25% are hereditary and bilateral. Families of patients with retinoblastoma should have genetic counseling.

121. **What is the "two-hit" hypothesis of cancer, particularly retinoblastoma?**
    Alfred Knudson's "two-hit" hypothesis is a basic tenet of malignant transformation. In 1971, Knudson calculated the genetic probabilities of developing retinoblastoma and hypothesized that patients with bilateral disease first inherited a germline mutation and then underwent a second somatic mutation to develop the disease. Patients with unilateral or sporadic disease developed two somatic mutations during early childhood. The identification of the genes associated with the first of the "two hits" correctly predicted the presence of tumor suppressor genes.

    Knudson A: Two genetic hits (more or less) to cancer, *Nat Rev Cancer* 1:157–162, 2001.

122. **In what age group does retinoblastoma usually occur?**
    Retinoblastoma most often occurs in younger children, with 80% of cases diagnosed before the age of 5 years. Retinoblastoma is usually confined to the eye, with more than 80% of children being cured with current therapy.

    Shields CL, Shields JA: Basic understanding of current classification and management of retinoblastoma, *Curr Opin Ophthalmol* 17:228–234, 2006.

123. **Patients with retinoblastoma are at increased risk for other tumors. How significant a risk is this?**
    Patients with the hereditary type of retinoblastoma have a markedly increased frequency of second malignant neoplasms. The cumulative incidence is about 26% ± 10% in nonirradiated patients and 58% ± 10% in irradiated patients by 50 years after diagnosis of retinoblastoma. Most of the second malignant neoplasms are osteosarcomas, soft tissue sarcomas, and melanomas.

OTHER SOLID NON–CENTRAL NERVOUS SYSTEM TUMORS

124. **What are the peak ages of incidence of the most common solid tumors of childhood?**
Neuroblastoma and Wilms tumor are tumors of early childhood. Ewing sarcoma and osteosarcoma are more prevalent during adolescence. Rhabdomyosarcoma occurs throughout childhood and the teenage years.

125. **What are "blastemal" tumors?**
Many pediatric solid tumors are thought to arise from a primitive blastemal cell. A *blastema* is a mass of embryonic cells from which an organ or a body part develops. Thus, these cells are undifferentiated and, if mutated, may develop into tumors such as neuroblastoma, pleuropulmonary blastoma, hepatoblastoma, or Wilms tumor, to name a few.

126. **What is a Wilms tumor?**
A primary malignant renal tumor of large histologic diversity. The age at which a child is most commonly diagnosed with Wilms tumor is summarized in Figure 15-4.

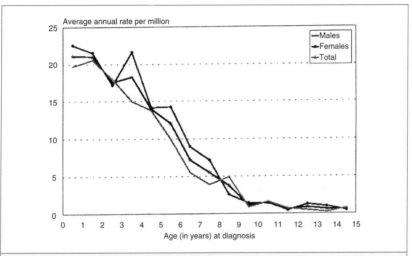

Figure 15-4. Age at diagnosis of Wilms tumor. (From Weiner MA, Cairo MS: Pediatric Hematology/Oncology Secrets. Philadelphia, Hanley & Belfus, 2000, p 157.)

127. **What are the three histologic components of a Wilms tumor?**
Wilms tumors are considered triphasic, consisting of a **blastemal** (immature) component, an **epithelial** (tubular) component, and a **stromal** (muscular) component.

128. **How is Wilms tumor distinguished radiographically from neuroblastoma?**
- **Wilms tumor:** Computed tomography images will show intrinsic distortion of the kidney parenchyma and the collecting system. Only 10% of children with Wilms tumor have calcifications.
- **Neuroblastoma:** This is almost always extrarenal and causes displacement—not distortion—of the renal parenchyma and collecting system. Calcifications are seen in more than 50% of children with abdominal neuroblastoma.

129. **Where does Wilms tumor tend to metastasize?**
Locally, Wilms tumor can grow through the renal capsule, invade the renal veins, extend into the vena cava, and even progress into the chambers of the heart. The lungs, regional lymph nodes, and liver are the most common sites of metastasis.

130. **What is a stage V Wilms tumor?**
Bilateral Wilms tumor is known as a stage V tumor. Each tumor is staged independently; prognosis with bilateral disease is not necessarily poor.

131. **What is WAGR syndrome?**
The constellation of **Wilms tumor, aniridia, genitourinary abnormalities**, and **mental retardation.**

132. **"Small, round, blue cell tumor" is often used in the description of which childhood tumors?**
Neuroblastoma, rhabdomyosarcoma, Ewing sarcoma, lymphoblastic leukemia, and **lymphoma**. All appear as small, round, blue cells on low-power microscopic examination. High-power microscopic examination, usually in combination with a panel of immunohistochemical stains and molecular diagnostics, is required for definitive diagnosis.

133. **What factors influence the prognosis of a patient with Wilms tumor?**
Overall, Wilms tumor carries a good prognosis. Factors that influence the prognosis include tumor stage and histology as well as chromosomal abnormalities such as loss of heterozygosity (LOH). LOH for markers on the distal arm of chromosome 16 has been found in about 20% of Wilms tumors, whereas loss of the short arm of chromosome 1 has been found in about 10% of cases. LOH of either locus portends an adverse prognosis, independent of tumor stage and histology.

134. **Where are the most common locations of Ewing sarcoma?**
The **pelvis, leg, upper arm**, and **rib.** These tumors arise in extraskeletal (soft tissue) locations and can locally invade the bone.

135. **What molecular abnormality is commonly seen in Ewing sarcoma?**
The **t(11:22) translocation** is pathognomonic of Ewing sarcoma. This translocation results in the fusion gene *EWS-FLI1*, which is thought to disrupt transcriptional regulatory pathways. About 85% of Ewing sarcomas carry this translocation.

136. **What are the two most common sites of metastases for patients with Ewing sarcoma?**
Ewing sarcoma often metastasizes to the **lungs** and somewhat less frequently to other **bones.** In general, lymph nodes are not involved, which suggests that dissemination of this tumor is primarily hematogenous.

137. **What is osteosarcoma?**
A **malignant spindle cell tumor** in which the cells produce neoplastic osteoid. It is the most common primary malignancy of bone in children.

138. **Osteosarcoma generally arises in which part of the bone?**
The **metaphyses of long bones** of the extremities. Between 60% and 80% of tumors are located in the metaphyses of the knee (i.e., the proximal tibia or the distal femur).

139. **Do all patients with osteosarcoma require surgical resection of the primary tumor?**
Surgical resection of the primary tumor is a requirement for curative treatment of osteosarcoma. In contrast to Ewing sarcoma, osteosarcoma is a relatively radiation-resistant tumor, and thus surgical resection after neoadjuvant chemotherapy is a mainstay of treatment.

140. **For patients with localized osteosarcoma, what factor is most predictive of a favorable outcome?**
Patients with more than 95% necrosis of the primary tumor (as determined by pathologic examination) after neoadjuvant chemotherapy have a better prognosis than those with lesser amounts of necrosis.

141. **What do Ewing sarcoma and osteosarcoma have in common?**
Both are treated with neoadjuvant chemotherapy, which is an initial 2- to 3-month period of chemotherapy, followed by local control with surgery. For select cases of Ewing sarcoma, radiation therapy is also used. Both tumors can develop distant metastases in the lungs and in other bones, and both tumors are cancers of adolescence. Although both Ewing sarcoma and osteosarcoma appear to be soft tissue tumors arising in bone, only osteosarcoma is truly a tumor of bone, whereas Ewing sarcoma is a primitive neuroectodermal tumor.

142. **In what solid tumor has the surgical resection of pulmonary metastases been shown to result in long-term cure?**
Although many pediatric sarcomas metastasize to the lungs, only surgical resection of pulmonary metastases from osteosarcoma has been definitively shown to contribute to cure, and only, in general, when the metastases are few in number. The role of the surgical resection of pulmonary metastases arising from other sarcomas (e.g., rhabdomyosarcoma, Ewing sarcoma) is less clear and is only undertaken in select circumstances.

143. **What is a limb salvage procedure?**
In an attempt to save as much natural tissue as possible, patients with soft tissue sarcomas often undergo a "limb salvage" surgery, in which cancerous tumor is removed from the bone without amputation. Because of the proximity of osteosarcomas to the knee joint, this often results in the removal of the joint as well. Patients who undergo a limb salvage procedure will require a prosthesis or crutches to ambulate.

144. **What is a rhabdomyosarcoma?**
A soft tissue tumor that arises from cells that give rise to striated skeletal muscle. It is the most common soft tissue tumor of childhood.

145. **Where do rhabdomyosarcomas usually arise?**
The four most common areas are as follows: (1) the head and neck; (2) the genitourinary region; (3) the extremities; and (4) the orbit. The survival rate for those with tumors in other areas is dependent on the amount, if any, of tumor left after resection and the presence or absence of metastatic disease.

146. **What sites of disease are associated with the best outcomes for children with rhabdomyosarcoma?**
Favorable locations include the orbit, the head and neck (except for parameningeal tumors), the vagina, and the biliary tract. Unfavorable locations include the bladder, the prostate, and the parameninges.

Crist WM, Anderson JR, Meza JL, et al: Intergroup rhabdomyosarcoma study-IV: results for patients with nonmetastatic disease, *J Clin Oncol* 15:3091–3102, 2001.

147. **What are the two major histologic subtypes of rhabdomyosarcoma?**
Alveolar rhabdomyosarcoma, a name derived from its superficial appearance histologically to lung tissue, tends to occur in older children and adolescents. Most of these tumors carry the t(2;13) translocation, and they carry a higher risk for recurrence. *Embryonal rhabdomyosarcomas* tend to occur in younger children, and they are the predominant histology associated with favorable site tumors.

148. **Which germ cell tumor is usually seen in young children?**
Most germ cell tumors that appear in young children are **benign teratomas** occurring in the sacrococcygeal region. In general, patients with mature teratomas are managed by surgical resection, with care taken for sacrococcygeal tumors to be sure that the entire coccyx is removed.

149. **Virilization may be associated with which childhood cancer?**
Tumors that cause virilism are most commonly those that produce large quantities of dehydroepiandrosterone, a 17-ketosteroid. Tumors that produce testosterone may also cause virilization. Most commonly, these are benign tumors of the adrenal gland; rarely are they malignant. However, the distinction between carcinoma and benign adenoma is frequently difficult. Occasionally, males with primary hepatic neoplasms may become virilized because of the production of androgens by the tumor.

150. **How great is the risk for malignant transformation in undescended testes?**
The risk for malignancy may be **5 to 10 times higher** in the undescended testis than in a normal testis. The risk in the contralateral testis may also be increased. Orchidopexy decreases, but does not eliminate, the risk for subsequent malignant transformation.

151. **What are the most common primary liver tumors of childhood?**
Hepatoblastoma and **hepatocellular carcinoma.** Hepatoblastomas usually develop in infants and young children, whereas hepatocellular carcinomas develop throughout childhood. Infection with hepatitis B and C virus are the greatest risk factors for the occurrence of hepatocellular carcinoma.

152. **Which tumor marker is most likely to be elevated in children with hepatic tumors?**
Most patients with either hepatoblastoma or hepatocellular carcinoma have an elevated concentration of **α-fetoprotein** that parallels disease activity. Lack of a significant decrease of α-fetoprotein with treatment may signify a poor response to therapy. Occasionally, hepatoblastomas produce β-human chorionic gonadotropin and can result in isosexual precocity.

153. **Lance Armstrong's treatment for metastatic testicular germ cell tumor had an important modification from standard therapy. What was it and why did this seven-time winner of the *Tour de France* find this important?**
Lance Armstrong had a testicular germ cell tumor with metastases to the brain. The therapy for germ cell tumors is typically a combination of cisplatin, etoposide, and bleomycin. Bleomycin is a glycopeptide antibiotic that can result in pulmonary fibrosis and impaired lung function. Fortunately, a number of other agents have excellent activity in the treatment of germ cell tumors, including ifosfamide and etoposide, and thus Mr. Armstrong was effectively treated without administration of bleomycin. In general, gonadal germ cell tumors, even when metastatic, have a good prognosis.

STEM CELL TRANSPLANTATION

154. **Identify the three types of stem cell transplantation.**
    - **Allogenic:** The transfer of bone marrow, peripheral blood stem cells, or umbilical cord blood from a donor to another individual
    - **Autologous:** The use of a person's own bone marrow or peripheral blood stem cells
    - **Syngeneic:** The transfer of bone marrow, peripheral blood stem cells, or umbilical cord blood from a genetically identical donor (i.e., identical twins)

155. **When a stem cell transplant physician refers to a "conditioning" regimen, is the doctor embarking on a plan to improve the hairstyle of the patient?**
    Not quite. *Conditioning* refers to the process of bone marrow ablation and immune suppression needed for the successful engraftment of the donor marrow. The two most commonly used conditioning regimens are cyclophosphamide with total-body irradiation (Cy/TBI) and busulfan with cyclophosphamide (BuCy). Many physicians prefer Bu/Cy because the regimen does not have the long-term endocrine and cognitive side effects (particularly seen in small children) that Cy/TBI has. However, for some cancers, the addition of radiation to the conditioning regimen may provide additional anticancer effect.

156. **What are the major side effects from total-body irradiation used in conditioning?**
    In the short term, total-body irradiation may cause **interstitial pneumonitis** and **nephritis.** Over the long term, total-body irradiation may lead to cataracts, growth retardation, hypothyroidism, other endocrine dysfunction, infertility, and secondary malignancies. The long-term effects of total-body irradiation on pulmonary, cardiac, and neuropsychiatric function continue to be studied.

157. **Do all transplant patients require complete ablation of their recipient bone marrow?**
    No. Stem cell transplants that do not ablate the recipient bone marrow are called nonmyeloablative transplants. Such transplants require vigorous immune suppression to maintain the donor graft as well as a disease that does not require intensive chemotherapy or full donor engraftment for success. Thus, patients with leukemias that respond well to a graft-versus-leukemia effect may benefit from the decreased morbidity and mortality of a reduced-intensity preparative regimen.

158. **What is the chance of siblings having the same human leukocyte antigen (HLA) type?**
    The HLAs, which are located on chromosome 6, approximate simple mendelian inheritance, with two siblings having a 1 in 4 chance of having the same typing. A 1% crossover of material may also occur during meiosis. The larger the family, the more likely a match becomes, as shown by the formula $[1 - (0.75)^n]$, with n being the number of siblings. Thus, a child with five brothers and sisters has a 76% chance of having a sibling with an HLA match.

159. **What is the chance of finding an HLA-matched unrelated donor?**
    Although in theory the number of possibilities would equal or even exceed the world's population, thereby making a match astonishingly unlikely, HLA types cluster in individuals of similar genetic and racial backgrounds. In one estimate of persons of European ancestry, about 200,000 individuals would need to be screened to reach a 50% chance of finding a match.

Gahrton G: Bone marrow transplantation with unrelated volunteer donors, *Eur J Cancer* 27:1537–1539, 1991.

160. **How are tumor cells purged from a marrow or peripheral blood stem cell specimen?**
    - Immunologic methods using monoclonal antibodies
    - *Ex vivo* use of chemotherapy
    - Selective binding of tumor cells to lectins
    - Treatment of marrow with antisense complementary DNA
    - Selective culture of normal cells
    - Selection of normal hematopoietic progenitor cells (e.g., CD34 cells)

161. **What are the different sources of stem cells for transplantation?**
    Stem cells may be obtained either from the **peripheral blood,** the **bone marrow** itself, or the **umbilical cord blood** of a newborn. Peripheral blood stem cells are collected by leukocytapheresis, whereas bone marrow stem cells are collected by multiple bone marrow aspirates. Cord blood is harvested from the placenta at the time of delivery. Stored placental or cord blood is a useful source for patients without a related histocompatible donor because of less GVHD.

    Copelan EA: Hematopoietic stem-cell transplantation, *N Engl J Med* 354:1813–1826, 2006.

162. **What are the advantages and disadvantages of umbilical cord blood as the source for a stem cell transplantation?**
    Advantages
    - No risk to mother or infant
    - Available on demand after cryopreservation
    - Can target minority families
    - Donors not lost as a result of age, illness, or relocation

    Disadvantages
    - Limited number of stem cells in collection
    - Possible lack of availability of additional donor cells if graft failure or relapse occurs
    - Undiagnosed medical condition may be present in newborns

163. **Worldwide, what is the most common indication for stem cell transplantation?**
    β-Thalassemia.

164. **Which prophylactic measures should be taken after stem cell transplantation?**
    Patients may receive antibiotics for gut decontamination. An oral antifungal agent such as fluconazole is also frequently administered. Patients should receive *P. carinii* prophylaxis and replacement of immunoglobulins with intravenous immunoglobulin. Acyclovir may also be administered.

165. **What are the major features of graft-versus-host disease (GVHD)?**
    Acute GVHD typically begins with a fever that is followed by a salmon-colored rash on the palms and soles. The rash may be pruritic and may desquamate. Hepatitis (with jaundice and transaminase elevation) and gastroenteritis (with diarrhea, weight loss, and abdominal pain) may also occur.

166. **How is GVHD managed?**
    Doses of methotrexate, cyclosporine, or tacrolimus during the immediate posttransplantation period may be given in an attempt to prevent the development of acute GVHD. T-cell depletion of the bone marrow graft also decreases the incidence of GVHD. For the treatment of acute GVHD, steroids, cyclosporine, or tacrolimus may be used alone or in combination, depending on the extent of donor-recipient mismatch and the severity of GVHD.

    Carpenter PA, MacMillan ML: Management of acute graft-versus-host disease in children, *Pediatr Clin North Am* 57:273–295, 2010.

167. **What are the risk factors for GVHD?**
There are multiple risk factors for GVHD. First and foremost is the relatedness of the donor to the recipient. An unrelated donor transplant will have a higher risk for GVHD than a matched related donor transplant. Second, the number of T cells received is a risk factor with higher T-cell numbers associated with a higher GVHD risk. Donor age and parity status are also risk factors, with older donors and multiparous donors having higher GVHD risks.

168. **How are acute GVHDs of the skin, gut, and liver graded?**
See Table 15-5.

TABLE 15-5.	GRADING OF ACUTE GRAFT-VERSUS-HOST DISEASE OF SKIN, GUT, AND LIVER			
	Grade I	Grade II	Grade III	Grade IV
Skin (area involved)	<25%	25-50%	>50%	Desquamation or blood loss
Gut (diarrhea)	<0.5 L/day	0.5-1.0 L/day	1.0-1.5 L/day	Ileus, bloody diarrhea
Liver (bilirubin)	<3 mg/dL	3-6 mg/dL	6-15 mg/dL	>15 mg/dL or ↑ ALT or AST

ALT=alanine transaminase; AST=aspartate transaminase.

169. **What is graft-versus-leukemia (GVL)?**
Graft-versus-leukemia occurs when the donor marrow recognizes antigens on the leukemic blast cell as foreign and initiates immune-mediated clearance of the malignant cell. GVL is most easily obtained in patients who have been transplanted for CML, although patients with AML and ALL may also experience a GVL effect (AML usually more than ALL). Thus, GVL constitutes an important part of the antileukemic effect of transplantation, particularly for CML and AML. Current research is directed at separating a graft-versus-host effect from a GVL effect.

170. **What is the most likely diagnosis for a patient who experiences weight gain, right upper quadrant pain, and hepatomegaly 10 days after stem cell infusion?**
The patient most likely has **veno-occlusive disease (VOD),** also known as **sinusoidal obstruction syndrome (SOS).** VOD/SOS is due to damage to the hepatic endothelial cells that then leads to activation of the clotting cascade within the hepatic sinusoids and subsequent reversal of blood flow through the liver. Severe VOD/SOS may be characterized by more than 10% weight gain, respiratory failure, hepatorenal syndrome, and mental status changes. The treatment of VOD centers on maintaining adequate intravascular volume without compromising respiratory function and administration of defibrotide.

ACKNOWLEDGMENT

The editors gratefully acknowledge contributions by Drs. Peter Langmuir and Jeffrey Skolnik that were retained from prior editions of *Pediatric Secrets*.

CHAPTER 16

ORTHOPEDICS

Benjamin D. Roye, MD, MPH

CLINICAL ISSUES

1. **What causes a Sprengel deformity?**
   Sprengel deformity (congenital elevation of the scapula) results from the failure of normal scapular descent during fetal life, thereby resulting in an elevated, hypoplastic scapula. The affected side of the neck appears shorter and broader and may give the appearance of torticollis. A fibrocartilaginous band or omovertebral bone may bridge the space between the medial upper scapula and the spinous process of a cervical vertebra. Abduction of the ipsilateral arm is usually limited, but this limitation may not be clinically significant. Sprengel deformity may be associated with congenital scoliosis and renal anomalies.

2. **What is torticollis?**
   Also called a "cock-robin" deformity, *torticollis* is a combined head tilt in one direction with rotation in the opposite direction. This deformity may be fixed or flexible.

3. **What is the differential diagnosis for torticollis?**
   - **Osseous:** Atlanto-occipital anomalies, unilateral absence of C1, Klippel-Feil syndrome (fusion of cervical vertebrae), atlantoaxial rotatory displacement, basilar impression
   - **Nonosseous:** Congenital muscular torticollis, Sandifer syndrome (severe gastroesophageal reflux), ocular dysfunction (strabismus, oculogyric crisis), infections (cervical adenitis, retropharyngeal abscess), central nervous system tumors, syringomyelia, Arnold-Chiari malformation, abnormal skin webs (pterygium colli)

4. **Are stretching exercises helpful for congenital muscular torticollis?**
   Yes. Studies have shown that management with manual stretching—particularly when initiated at an early age—significantly reduces the need for surgical correction.

   Cheng JC, Wong MW, Tang SP, et al: Clinical determinants of the outcome of manual stretching in the treatment of congenital muscular torticollis in infants: a prospective study of eight hundred and twenty-one cases, *J Bone Joint Surg Am* 83:679–687, 2001.

5. **What is infantile cortical hyperostosis?**
   Caffey disease (or syndrome), which usually occurs before 6 months of age, is a condition of unknown etiology that consists of tender, nonsuppurative, cortical swellings of the shafts of bone, most commonly the mandible and clavicle. It remits spontaneously, but exacerbations may persist for several years. In severe cases, corticosteroids may be helpful. Infantile cortical hyperostosis is a rare condition. The presence of periosteal reaction, especially if asymmetrical, should raise the suspicion of battered child syndrome (child abuse).

6. **What is rickets?**
   Rickets is the failure of osteoid to calcify in a growing child, most commonly caused by a lack of vitamin D. The adult equivalent is osteomalacia.

7. **Why is rickets reappearing?**
   There has been an increase in exclusive breastfeeding for prolonged periods without vitamin D supplementation. Human milk is low in vitamin D, and the American Academy of Pediatrics recommends vitamin supplementation for breastfed infants. Additionally, reduced maternal sunlight exposure for cultural, societal, or personal reasons has become more common. Immigrant groups who have increasingly migrated to more temperate regions have more children with this condition; reasons remain unclear for the increased incidence among these groups.

   Misra M, Pacaud D, Petryk A, et al: Vitamin D deficiency in children and its management: review of current knowledge and recommendations, *Pediatrics* 122:398–417, 2008.

8. **What are the physical signs that are suggestive of rickets?**
   The anatomic abnormalities of rickets result primarily from the inability to normally mineralize osteoid; the bones become weak and subsequently distorted. Signs of rickets include the following:
   - Short stature (often <3rd percentile)
   - Femoral and tibial bowing
   - Delayed suture and fontanel closure, widening of suture lines
   - Pectus carinatum or "pigeon breast" (anterior protrusion of the sternum)
   - Frontal thickening and bossing of the forehead
   - Defective tooth enamel, extensive caries
   - Harrison groove (a rim of rib indentation at the insertion of the diaphragm)
   - Widened physes at wrists and ankles
   - "Rachitic rosary" (enlarged costochondral junctions)

9. **Which bones are known to develop aseptic necrosis?**
   The **osteochondroses** are a group of disorders in which aseptic necrosis of epiphyses occurs with subsequent fragmentation and repair (Table 16-1). The exact cause is unknown. The patient usually has pain at the affected site.

TABLE 16-1. TYPICAL AGE OF ONSET OF OSTEOCHONDROSES

Location	Eponym	Typical Age of Onset (yr)
Tarsal navicular bone	Köhler disease	6
Capitellum of distal humerus	Panner disease	9-11
Carpal lunate	Kienböck disease	16-20
Distal lunar epiphysis	Burns disease	13-20
Head of femur	Legg-Calvé-Perthes disease	3-5

10. **What are skeletal dysplasias?**
    Skeletal dysplasias, also known as *osteochondrodysplasias*, are a group of disorders characterized by an intrinsic abnormality in the growth and remodeling of cartilage and bone. These generalized disturbances in the development of the skeleton affect the skull, spine, and extremities to varying degrees. Children with these conditions frequently have disproportionate short stature (dwarfism) and dysmorphic facial features. The most common viable form of dwarfism is achondroplasia.

11. **What is the principal genetic abnormality in achondroplasia?**
    A mutation in the gene for **fibroblast growth factor receptor 3** (*FGFR3*). More than 95% of patients have the same point mutation, and more than 80% are new mutations. The functional change affects many tissues, but in particular the cartilaginous growth plate.

    Horton WA, Hall JG, Hecht JT: Achondroplasia, *Lancet* 370:162–172, 2007.

12. **What are the inheritance patterns and clinical features of osteogenesis imperfecta?**
These constitute a group of heterogenous genetically transmitted diseases in which different mutations result in different degrees of clinical features and skeletal fragility (Table 16-2). Incidence overall is about 1 in 20,000.

Osteogenesis Imperfecta Foundation: http://www.oif.org.

TABLE 16-2. TYPES OF OSTEOGENESIS IMPERFECTA		
Type	Inheritance	Clinical Features
I	Autosomal dominant	Bone fragility, blue sclerae, onset of fractures after birth (most at preschool age)
A		*Without* dentinogenesis imperfecta
B		*With* dentinogenesis imperfecta
II	Autosomal recessive	Lethal in perinatal period, dark blue sclerae, concertina femurs, beaded ribs
III	Autosomal recessive	Fractures at birth, progressive deformity, normal sclerae and hearing

13. **McCune-Albright syndrome is associated with what skeletal abnormalities?**
Polyostotic fibrous dysplasia (i.e., fibrous tissue replacing bones). The fibrous dysplasia occurs most commonly in the long bones and the pelvis and may result in deformity and/or increased thickness of bone. Fibrous dysplasia associated with precocious puberty and café-au-lait spots is known as *McCune-Albright syndrome*.

14. **What are the causes of in-toeing gait (pigeon-toeing)?**
In-toeing can be due to problems in the foot, tibia, or hip:
Foot:
- Metatarsus adductus
- Talipes equinovarus (clubfoot)
Leg:
- Tibial torsion (internal)
Hip:
- Femoral anteversion (medial femoral torsion)
- Paralysis (polio, myelomeningocele)
- Spasticity (cerebral palsy)
- Maldirected acetabulum

Tunnessen WW Jr: *Signs and Symptoms in Pediatrics*, ed 3, Philadelphia, 1999, Lippincott Williams & Wilkins. pp 693–695.

15. **Is in-toeing a problem?**
Most cases of in-toeing are not a pathologic problem. There is a normal range of foot placement during gait that can range from slightly internally rotated to slightly externally rotated. Many children will improve their walking as they get older; most children do not have a mature gait pattern until about age 7 years. Many elite runners turn their feet in when running because they are faster this way—most parents love this piece of information.

16. **When, if ever, does in-toeing need to be treated?**
In-toeing rarely requires treatment other than reassurance to the family that their child's walking will improve with time. Femoral anteversion and tibial torsion almost never require treatment in the neurologically normal child. Traditional treatments such as the infamous boots and bars and orthopedic shoes do nothing to change the natural history of these problems. Metatarsus adductus often spontaneously resolves in the first 2 years of life, but feet that are rigid (i.e., the foot cannot easily be manipulated into a normal position) or severe cases may require casting, straight laced shoes, or in extreme cases, surgery.

17. **A 15-year-old with tibial pain (worse at night and relieved by nonsteroidal anti-inflammatory drugs) has a small lytic area surrounded by reactive bone formation on radiograph. What is the likely diagnosis?**
Osteoid osteoma, a benign bone-forming tumor, is typically seen in older children and adolescents and exhibits a male predominance (male-to-female ratio, 2:1). Most children complain of localized pain, usually in the femur and tibia; however, arms and vertebrae may also be involved. Radiographs may demonstrate an osteolytic area surrounded by densely sclerotic reactive bone, and bone scans reveal "hot spots." Computed tomography (CT) scans will show a "nidus" in the middle of the lesion that is pathognomonic for this diagnosis. The site is usually less than 1 cm in diameter and arises at the junction of old and new cortex. Pathologically, the lesion is highly vascularized fibrous tissue with an osteoid matrix and poorly calcified bone spicules surrounded by a dense zone of sclerotic bone. Treatment is surgical excision.

18. **What is the clinical significance of limb-length discrepancy?**
A significant portion of the population has mild limb-length discrepancy. Limb-length discrepancies of less than 2 cm in a skeletally mature individual usually require no treatment. In addition to quantifying leg discrepancy in a skeletally immature child, it is important to estimate what the limb-length discrepancy will be at skeletal maturity. This can be done by periodically measuring the discrepancy radiographically and using charts, such as the Green and Anderson "growth-remaining graph," the Moseley "straight-line graph," or the Paley "multiplier method" to calculate anticipated leg-length discrepancy at skeletal maturity. Assessment of skeletal age is based on the bone age from an anteroposterior hand and wrist radiograph.

19. **What are the possible causes of a limb-length discrepancy?**
   - **Congenital anomalies:** Congenital short femur, proximal femoral focal deficiency, congenital absence of fibula, posteromedial bowing of tibia, tibial hypoplasia, congenital hemihypertrophy
   - **Tumors:** Neurofibromatosis, fibrous dysplasia, enchondromatosis, hereditary multiple exostosis, Klippel-Trénaunay-Weber syndrome
   - **Trauma**: Physeal injuries, fracture
   - **Infection:** Septic arthritis, osteomyelitis (the infection can damage the growth plates)
   - **Inflammatory**: Juvenile rheumatoid arthritis

20. **What are the long-term effects of uncorrected limb-length discrepancy?**
Limp and low back pain are the most common sequelae of a leg-length discrepancy because the pelvic tilt places increased stress on the lumbosacral spine. Other complications include an equinus contracture of the ankle and late degenerative arthritis of the hip.

21. **What are the general management principles for a limb-length discrepancy?**
   - 0–2 cm: No treatment
   - 2–5 cm: Shoe lift, epiphysiodesis (surgical fixation across the growth plate to slow growth of the longer extremity)

- 5–20 cm: Limb lengthening
- >20 cm: Prosthetic fitting

There is flexibility in these guidelines to account for factors such as environment, motivation, intelligence, compliance, emotional stability, patient and parent wishes, predicted final height, and associated pathology in the limbs. As surgical morbidity has decreased, limb-lengthening procedures are being increasingly used for lesser discrepancies.

Friend L, Widmann RF: Advances in the management of limb length discrepancy and lower limb deformity, *Curr Opin Pediatr* 20:46–51, 2008.

22. **A 2-year-old who is refusing to use her right arm after being lifted by her parent over a curb by her outstretched arm likely has what problem?**
    Also known as a "pulled elbow," a **nursemaid elbow** is a subluxation of the radial head under the orbicular ligament resulting from axial traction applied to the extended arm of a young child. The child is typically unwilling to move the affected limb (pseudoparalysis), and there is tenderness directly over their radial head. Radiographs are normal, so the diagnosis must be made by history and physical examination. The subluxated radial head is reduced by supinating the extended forearm followed by fully flexing the elbow. An audible and palpable click is often present. After successful reduction, the child will begin to use the arm spontaneously (usually after a few minutes of crying). If symptoms persist, the child should be reassessed for a possible occult fracture of the radial head or distal humerus.

Meckler GD, Spiro DM: Technical tip: radial head subluxation, *Pediatr Rev* 29:e42–e43, 2008.

23. **What signs and symptoms suggest a serious cause of back pain in a child that warrants further evaluation?**
    - **Symptoms:** Age younger than 5 years; pain interfering with daily activities in school, play, or athletics; pain lasting longer than 4 weeks; night pain (often associated with tumor); pain radiating down the leg, fever, or other systemic symptoms (especially weight loss); limp or altered gait; bowel or bladder habit changes
    - **Signs:** Postural changes; clawing of the toes, gait changes, bowel and bladder habit changes, other neurologic abnormalities; reproducible point tenderness; pain with hyperextension of the back, bruising

Davis PJC, Williams HJ: The investigation and management of back pain in children, *Arch dis Child Educ Pract Ed* 93:73–83, 2008.

24. **What is the differential diagnosis of back pain in children?**
    - **Infectious:** Diskitis, vertebral osteomyelitis, vertebral tuberculosis
    - **Developmental:** Spondylolysis, spondylolisthesis, Scheuermann kyphosis, scoliosis
    - **Traumatic:** Herniated disk, muscle strain, fractures, vertebral apophyseal fracture
    - **Inflammatory:** Juvenile rheumatoid arthritis, ankylosing spondylitis
    - **Neoplastic:** Eosinophilic granuloma, osteoid osteoma or osteoblastoma, aneurysmal bone cyst, leukemia, lymphoma, Ewing sarcoma, osteosarcoma
    - **Visceral:** Urinary tract infection, hydronephrosis, ovarian cysts, inflammatory bowel disease

25. **Do school backpacks contribute to back pain?**
    Probably, but this is controversial. Some experts suggest that the limits of maximal loads lifted by children should be 10% to 15% of body weight. In some studies, more than one third of students carried more than 30% of their body weight at least once during the school week. Loads greater than 20% body weight result in contact pressures above the ischemic threshold of skin.

Macias BR, Murthy G, Chambers H, Hargens AR: Asymmetric loads and pain associated with backpack carrying by children, *J Pediatr Orthop* 5:512–517, 2008.

26. **What constitutes an orthopedic emergency?**
There are few true emergencies in orthopedics that require immediate attention, but conditions that fall into this category include open fractures, impending compartment syndrome, femoral neck fractures (including unstable slips of the proximal femoral physis or slipped capital femoral epiphysis [SCFE]), dislocation of major joints (i.e., knee, hip, spine), septic arthritis, and cauda equina syndrome.

KEY POINTS: PEDIATRIC ORTHOPEDIC EMERGENCIES—NO DELAY!

1. Open fracture

2. Impending compartment syndrome

3. Dislocation of major joints

4. Septic arthritis

5. Arterial injury

FOOT DISORDERS

27. **Do infants and children need shoes?**
Barefoot is the natural state of the foot. Humans evolved without shoes, and individuals who spend most of their lives unshod have stronger feet and fewer foot deformities than those who wear shoes. Before they begin walking, infants do not need foot coverings other than to keep their feet warm. After the child begins to walk, shoes will offer protection from the cold and from sharp objects. The American Academy of Pediatrics recommends soft, light, flexible shoes for new walkers—not bulky, heavy supportive shoes.

28. **What advice should be given to a parent about buying shoes for a toddler?**
The best shoe is one that simulates the bare foot:
- The shoe should easily flex.
- The bottom of the shoe should be flat. Heels should be avoided because they tend to force the foot forward and cramp the toes.
- The shoe should be foot shaped and generously fitted. The toe box should be wide and high to properly accommodate the toddler's pudgy feet.

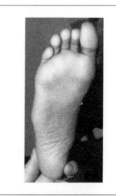

Figure 16-1. Metatarsus adductus. (From Jay RM: Foot and Ankle Pearls. Philadelphia, Hanley & Belfus, 2002, p 52.)

29. **What is the most common congenital foot abnormality?**
Metatarsus adductus. In patients with this condition, the forefoot is turned toward the midline as a result of adduction of the metatarsal bones at the tarsometatarsal joints. The hindfoot (heel) is normal (Fig. 16-1). Most cases are mild and flexible, with the foot easily

straightened by passive stretching. A simple test to determine whether the kidney-shaped curvature is within normal limits is to draw a line that bisects the heel. When extended, this line normally falls between the second and third toe space. If it falls more laterally, metatarsus adductus is present. In utero positioning is the suspected cause of the condition in many cases. It is seen more frequently in first-born children, presumably because primigravida mothers have stronger muscle tone in their uterine and abdominal walls.

30. **How is metatarsus adductus treated?**
If the foot can be passively abducted beyond neutral, the prognosis is excellent for a spontaneous correction without any therapeutic intervention. In feet that are stiffer, a program of passive stretching is in order. The parents are taught to hold the heel in a neutral position and manually abduct the forefoot using the thumb placed over the cuboid as a fulcrum. This exaggerated position should be held for a few seconds and the stretching repeated 10 times each session. These sessions should occur with bathing and diaper changing. If this fails to improve, foot bracing and/or casting can be of help.

31. **How is clubfoot distinguished from severe metatarsus adductus?**
Clubfoot, or *talipes equinovarus,* is distinguished pathologically by a combination of forefoot and hindfoot abnormalities, which results in a fixed (rigid) equinus and varus deformity of the hindfoot. Metatarsus adductus is often a component of clubfeet, but in isolated metatarsus adductus, the hindfoot (heel) is *normal*. If the ankle can be dorsiflexed to neutral or beyond, metatarsus is the most likely diagnosis.

32. **How are clubfeet treated?**
Most clubfeet respond well to serial casting using the Ponseti method. The casts should be applied soon after birth, and they are changed weekly. Over the course of three to eight casts, significant improvement in the shape of the foot can be expected. About 80% of the feet that are corrected with casting will require an Achilles tenotomy to correct the equinus deformity. Those feet that are not adequately corrected with casting require a more extensive surgical release.

33. **What is a calcaneovalgus foot?**
This common deformity, a sort of anti-clubfoot, is the result of an *in utero* "packaging defect" and is considered a normal variant. The deformity is the exact opposite of the clubfoot: the foot lies in an acutely dorsiflexed position, with the top of the foot in contact with the anterolateral surface of the leg. The heel is in severe valgus, and the forefoot is markedly abducted. Overall, the foot is flexible, and both the heel and the forefoot can be corrected into a neutral position. Spontaneous correction is the norm. However, having parents passively stretch the foot is often beneficial (and makes the parents feel better and proactive).

34. **What foot abnormality results in the appearance of a "Persian slipper" foot?**
Also called "rocker-bottom foot," this abnormality is due to **congenital vertical talus**. Lateral radiographs reveal a vertically oriented talus with dislocation of the talonavicular joint. On examination, the forefoot is markedly dorsiflexed, and the heel is rigid and points downward, giving the sole the characteristic convex or boat-shaped appearance. Serial casting and subsequent surgical reversion are the usual treatments. The syndrome most commonly associated with this deformity is trisomy 18.

35. **What should be suspected when pes cavus is noted on examination?**
Pes cavus, or high-arched feet (often associated with claw toes), can result from contractures or disturbed muscle balance (Fig. 16-2). A neurologic etiology should always be considered and looked for. The differential diagnosis includes a normal familial variant, Charcot-Marie-Tooth disease, spina bifida, cauda equina, peroneal muscle atrophy, Friedreich ataxia, Hurler syndrome, and polio.

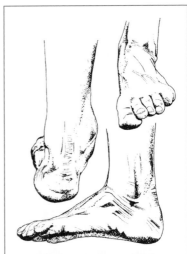

Figure 16-2. Pes cavus. (From Mellion MB, Walsh WM, Shelton GL: The Team Physician's Handbook, 2nd ed. Philadelphia, Hanley & Belfus, 1997, p 603.)

36. **Should children with flexible flat feet be given corrective shoes?**
Only very rarely. Flexible flat feet (pes planovalgus) is a common finding in infants and children (up to nearly 50%) and about 15% of adults. During weight-bearing activity, the ligaments supporting the medial longitudinal arch stretch and the arch becomes flattened. The heel may also go into an increased valgus (outward) position. There are no radiographic parameters that define a flexible flat foot; it is thought to be a normal variant that results from ligamentous laxity. Children typically do not complain of pain, and an arch can be created easily by removing weight from the feet, having the child stand on the toes, or by dorsiflexing the great toe. This condition is distinguished from pathologic flat feet in which lack of weight bearing does not lessen the flatness and rigidity is present on physical examination. This condition occurs in less than 1% of children. Prospective studies have shown that corrective shoes or orthotic insets are not necessary in young children with asymptomatic flexible flat feet because the arch can spontaneously develop during the first 8 years of life.

Pfeiffer M, Kotz R, Ledl T, et al: Prevalence of flat foot in preschool-aged children, *Pediatrics* 118:634–639, 2006.

Wenger DR, Mauldin D, Speck G, et al: Corrective shoes and inserts as treatment for flexible flat feet in infants and children, *J Bone Joint Surg* 71:800–810, 1989.

37. **When should I worry about a child with flat feet?**
Flat feet become concerning if they are rigid (as opposed to flexible) or painful, or if they cause a disability (such as decreased walking or running endurance). If any of these conditions occur, the child should be evaluated by a specialist for possible treatment, including physical therapy (to stretch the Achilles tendon and to strengthen the foot and ankle muscles), orthotics, or in rare cases, surgery.

38. **How does the cause of foot pain vary by age?**
   - **0 to 6 years:** Ill-fitting shoes, foreign body, occult fracture, osteomyelitis, juvenile rheumatoid arthritis (if other joints are involved), rheumatic fever (hypermobile flat foot)
   - **6 to 12 years:** Ill-fitting shoes, foreign body, accessory navicular bone, occult fracture, tarsal coalition (peroneal spastic flat foot), ingrown toenail, hypermobile flat foot
   - **12 to 19 years:** Ill-fitting shoes, foreign body, ingrown toenail, pes cavus, hypermobile flat foot with tight Achilles tendon, ankle sprains, stress fracture

Gross RH: Foot pain in children, *Pediatr Clin North Am* 33:1395–1409, 1986.

39. **A 10-year-old boy with recurrent ankle sprains and painful flat feet should be evaluated for what possible diagnosis?**
Tarsal coalition. Fusion of various tarsal bones through fibrous or bony bridges can result in a stiff foot that inverts with difficulty. When inversion of the foot is done during an examination, tenderness occurs on the lateral aspect of the foot, and peroneal tendons become very prominent. Thus, this condition is also referred to as *peroneal spastic flat foot*. Unless the condition is very severe and warrants surgery, corrective shoes are usually adequate treatment. Other possible causes of a rigid flat foot include rheumatoid arthritis, septic arthritis, posttraumatic arthritis, neuromuscular conditions, and congenital vertical talus.

FRACTURES

40. **What are the fracture patterns unique to children?**
Children can suffer from **physeal (growth plate) fractures, buckle fractures, greenstick fractures,** and **plastic deformation injuries.** Most fractures in children incorporate one or more of these patterns.

41. **What is a buckle fracture?**
Children's bones are softer and more plastic than adult bones. Their bones can bend without actually breaking. A buckle (or torus) fracture occurs when a bone is bent (usually as a result of a fall) and compressive forces cause the cortex to actually buckle out, causing a bump in the bone. This is analogous to what happens to the sheet metal in a car involved in a collision. Although this is a fracture, the bone is still in one piece and stable, which is why these fractures are often diagnosed 1 or 2 weeks after injury, much to the surprise and chagrin of the parents who had been ignoring their child's complaints.

42. **What is a greenstick fracture?**
A *greenstick* is an incomplete fracture of a long bone. It is called this because the fracture pattern is similar to what happens when you try to snap a still living branch (or green stick) in half: the branch will break on one side but not all the way through. Similarly, in a greenstick fracture, only one cortex fractures while the other cortex remains intact, although usually bent.

43. **What does plastic deformation mean?**
The softness, or plasticity, of a child's bones allows them to bend without breaking. When you take a metal rod and bend it just a little, it tends to spring back to its original position. However, if you bend it more, it may spring back, but not all the way, leaving you with a bent rod. The same thing happens in children's bones. Depending on how much force and energy are imparted into the bone as a result of an injury, the bone will first bend, then buckle, then break. So a little bit of force will bend the bone, leaving the child with a bent forearm (far and away the most common location for this pattern of injury). A little more force may cause the cortex to buckle, and even more force will cause a fracture line to extend across the bone. It is important to realize that plastically deformed bones do not remodel because there is no healing response as there is when the bone is actually cracked. Therefore, patients with plastically deformed bones usually require them to be straightened (in the operating room or under sedation). This maneuver often results in a complete fracture occurring, which may require internal fixation with rods, wires, or plates.

44. **Where are the most frequent sites of fractures among children?**
- Clavicle
- Distal radius
- Distal ulna

45. **What is an open fracture?**

In an *open fracture*, the fracture site communicates with the external environment, usually as a result of the bone piercing the skin. Often, the bone pokes out, then falls back beneath the skin, so any laceration of a fracture site must be presumed to be an open fracture until proved otherwise. Open fractures have higher incidence of infection and a higher degree of soft tissue damage when compared with closed fractures.

46. **What is a toddler fracture?**

A *toddler fracture* is a fracture of the tibia in a child 9 months to 3 years old as a result of low-energy rotational forces. Typically, these fractures have a spiral appearance and are not displaced. The fibula is rarely fractured. The child will limp or more commonly refuse to bear weight. If the child is comfortable at rest, no immobilization is required, but some children (and families) will be more comfortable in a cast or splint for about 2 to 3 weeks.

47. **How are growth-plate fractures classified?**

The Salter-Harris classification of growth-plate (physis) injuries (Fig. 16-3) was devised in 1963:

- **Type I:** Epiphysis and metaphysis separate; usually no displacement occurs as a result of the strong periosteum; radiograph may be normal; tenderness over the physis may be the only sign; normal growth after 2 to 3 weeks of cast immobilization
- **Type II:** Fragment of metaphysis splits with epiphysis; usually closed reduction; casting is for 3 to 6 weeks (longer for lower extremity than upper extremity); growth is usually not affected, except distal femur and tibia
- **Type III:** Partial plate fracture involving a physeal and epiphyseal fracture to the joint surface; occurs when growth plate is partially fused; closed reduction more difficult to achieve
- **Type IV:** Extensive fracture involving epiphysis, physis, metaphysis, and joint surface; high risk for growth disruption unless proper reduction (usually done operatively) is obtained
- **Type V:** Crush injury to the physis; high risk for growth disruption

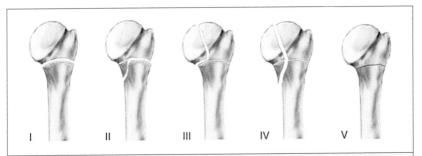

Figure 16-3. Salter-Harris classification. (From Dormans JP [ed]: Pediatric Orthopaedics and Sports Medicine: The Requisites in Pediatrics. Philadelphia, Mosby, 2004, p 22.)

48. **What are the sequelae of growth-plate fractures?**

Most growth-plate fractures heal without incidence. If there is an injury to the growth plate, a growth disturbance may occur, caused by the formation of a bony bridge or bar at the site of physeal damage. If there is damage to the entire physis, premature physeal closure occurs, with resulting longitudinal growth arrest. Asymmetrical closure leads to angular deformity of the limb. Fractures of the distal femoral physis are particularly prone to premature closure.

49. **What is the most common cause of a pathologic fracture?**
Also called *secondary fractures,* these are fractures through a bone weakened by a pathologic process. The most common such fracture is through **unicameral bone cysts** (simple bone cysts). These cysts usually occur in the metaphysis of a long bone, most frequently the humerus. They occur predominantly in males, are usually asymptomatic (unless a fracture occurs), are centrally located in the bone, and are often quite large.

50. **In a patient with a suspected fracture, what are the key points on physical examination?**
Assess "the five Ps" in the affected extremity:
■ **P**ain and point tenderness
■ **P**ulse (distal to the fracture), to evaluate vascular integrity
■ **P**allor, to evaluate vascular integrity
■ **P**aresthesia (distal to the fracture), to assess for sensory nerve injury
■ **P**aralysis (distal to the fracture), to assess for motor nerve injury
    Examine for pain above and below the suspected injury site because multiple fractures can occur in the same limb. The involved extremity should also be carefully examined for deformity, swelling, crepitus, discoloration, and open wounds. A primary concern in any evaluation is a distal neurovascular compromise, which may require immediate surgical intervention. Although the neurologic examination can be challenging in the setting of pain, especially in the younger child who is not cooperative, it is very important to do as thorough an examination as possible.

51. **What are the signs of compartment syndrome?**
The five Ps noted in the preceding question are seen in impending or established compartment syndrome in which swelling is causing distal ischemia. However, the most important symptom is pain, especially pain that does not respond to pain medication and pain with passive range of motion of the digits (fingers or toes) distal to the fracture. If one waits for numbness and paralysis to make the diagnosis of compartment syndrome, it is too late—permanent damage has likely been done. Compartment syndrome is often unrecognized in unconscious patients, so a high index of suspicion must be maintained in patients with severe injuries and an altered mental status. In addition, a frightened young child or infant may be very difficult to examine. If there is any concern about compartment syndrome, the compartment pressures must be measured.

52. **What is the treatment of compartment syndrome?**
Compartment syndrome is a true orthopedic emergency. Increased pressure in a compartment is relieved by incising the skin and fascia encompassing the involved compartment. The wound is left open and covered with sterile dressing until swelling decreases. Dressing changes, débridements, and partial wound closure are usually done in the operating room every 1 or 2 days until the skin can be closed. In some cases, skin grafts are necessary.

53. **How do you treat a simple clavicular fracture?**
These fractures are best managed with a **sling** and **activity restriction.** Union occurs in 2 to 4 weeks, but the sling may be removed once the child is comfortable. The residual bump (fracture callus) may take up to 2 years to smooth out (remodel). Traditionally, surgery has been considered necessary in few scenarios: open fractures, neurovascular injury, or skin compromise. However, there is a growing literature supporting surgical fixation of fractures with significant shortening of the bone (>2 to 3 cm) because these can cause problems with weakness and deformity in the affected shoulder.

54. **A teenager who punches a wall in anger typically incurs what fracture?**
Boxer fracture. This is a fracture of the distal fifth metacarpal, usually with apical dorsal angulation (Fig. 16-4). Up to 35 degrees of angulation can be accepted without compromise of function. Reduction often requires pin fixation.

55. **Children who fall on outstretched arms often suffer what type of fractures?**
Colles fractures. This is a group of complete fractures of the distal radius with varying displacement of the distal fragment. The fall, with the hand outstretched, wrist dorsiflexed, and forearm pronated, often results in a classic "dinner-fork" deformity of the wrist on examination.

56. **What does the presence of the posterior fat pad on an elbow radiograph suggest?**
Of the two fat pads that overlie the elbow joint, only the anterior one is visible on a lateral radiograph. If fluid accumulates in the joint space, as it does in cases involving bleeding, inflammation, or fracture, the fat pads are displaced upward and outward. The position of the anterior pad changes, and the posterior pad becomes visible. In the setting of acute trauma, the presence of a posterior fat pad is associated with a nearly 75% chance of occult fracture, and the elbow should be immobilized in a cast or splint with close follow-up scheduled. The most common injuries are a radial head fracture and a nondisplaced supracondylar humerus fracture.

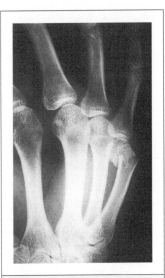

Figure 16-4. Boxer fracture with fracture of fifth (and fourth) metacarpal with volar displacement of the distal fragments after a punching injury. (From Katz DS, Math KR, Groskin SA [eds]: Radiology Secrets. Philadelphia, Hanley & Belfus, 1998, p 440.)

57. **In a teenager with wrist trauma, why is palpation of the anatomic "snuff box" a critical part of the physical examination?**
The anatomic snuff box (the in-pouching formed by the tendons of the abductor pollicis longus and extensor pollicis longus when the thumb is abducted [in hitchhiker fashion]) sits just above the scaphoid (carpal navicular) bone. The scaphoid is the carpal bone most commonly fractured, and it is at high risk for nonunion or avascular necrosis. Snuff-box tenderness, pain on supination with resistance, and pain on longitudinal compression of the thumb should increase suspicion for fracture of the scaphoid bone. Even when a radiograph is negative, if there is significant snuff-box tenderness, a fracture should be suspected and the wrist and thumb immobilized. A repeat radiograph in 2 to 3 weeks may better reveal a fracture. The use of CT or magnetic resonance imaging (MRI) can be used to more reliably identify a scaphoid fracture when the plain film is negative and the clinical suspicion is high.

Evenski AJ, Adamczyk MJ, Steiner RP, et al: Clinically suspected scaphoid fractures in children, *J Pediatr Orthop* 29:352–355, 2009.

58. **Name the eight carpal bones of the wrist.**
Disdaining some of the classic (mostly obscene) mnemonics, remember what will happen if a wrist fracture is missed:
Sinister **l**awyers **t**ake **p**hysicians **t**o **t**he **c**ourt **h**ouse; in order of proximal to distal, lateral to medial: **s**caphoid, **l**unate, **t**riquetrum, **p**isiform, **t**rapezium, **t**rapezoid, **c**apitate, and **h**amate.

59. **In pediatric fractures, what amount of angulation is acceptable before reduction is recommended?**
Acceptable angulation or displacement varies with a child's age. Younger children have remarkable healing potential to remodel with minimal to no residual deformity or limitation of rotation. As a rule, in children up to 8 years old, as much as 30 degrees of angulation *in the plane of motion* will heal satisfactorily without reduction. This means that a fracture that is flexed or extended in the wrist (in the direction the wrist typically moves) can be expected to model well. However, displacement with angulation toward the radius or ulna will not remodel so reliably, and rotational malalignment will not remodel at all. The degree of remodeling diminishes with age and growth remaining. In general, fractures closer to the growth plate will remodel more readily than midshaft fractures.

> Boutis K: Common pediatric fractures treated with minimal intervention, *Pediatr Emerg Care* 26:152–162, 2010.

60. **In which fractures will remodeling of bone *not* occur?**
The following fractures have a low chance of remodeling and may require closed or open reduction: intra-articular fractures (these must always be reduced anatomically to preserve joint function); plastic deformation (see previously), and fractures with excessive shortening or rotation. Angulation and translation deformities may remodel, but if the severity is too great, they may not remodel completely and leave residual deformity and dysfunction.

61. **How long should fractures be immobilized?**
Until they heal. But seriously, children's fractures generally heal more quickly than their counterparts in adults. The exact length of immobilization depends on several variables, including the child's age, the location of the fracture, and the type of treatment. As a rule of thumb, physeal, epiphyseal, and metaphyseal fractures heal more rapidly than diaphyseal fractures. On average, epiphyseal, physeal, and metaphyseal fractures heal in children within 3 to 5 weeks, whereas diaphyseal fractures may heal within 4 to 6 weeks.

> http://www.castroom.com.

62. **How long do fractured clavicles and femurs take to heal?**
- **Newborn:** Clavicle, 10 to 14 days; femur, 3 weeks
- **16-year-old child:** Clavicle, 6 weeks; femur, 6 to 10 weeks

63. **When is open reduction of a fracture indicated?**
An *open reduction* is an operative reduction of a fracture. Open reduction may be combined with internal fixation with pins, plates, or screws. Indications include the following:
- Failed closed reduction (often in older children with displaced fractures)
- Displaced intra-articular fractures
- Displaced Salter-Harris III and IV fractures (to prevent premature growth plate closure and realign the joint surface)
- Unstable fractures in patients with head trauma
- Open fractures (for irrigation and débridement)

HIP DISORDERS

64. **Why has DDH replaced CHD?**
The term *developmental dysplasia of the hip* (DDH) has replaced *congenital hip dislocation* (CHD) to reflect the evolutionary nature of hip problems in infants during the first months of life. About 2.5 to 6.5 infants per 1000 live births develop problems, and a significant percentage of these are not present on neonatal screening examinations. Clearly, the overt

pathologic process may not be present at birth, and periodic examination of the infant's hip is recommended at each routine well-baby examination until the age of 1 year.

DDH also refers to the entire spectrum of abnormalities involving the growing hip, ranging from dysplasia to subluxation to dislocation of the hip joint. Unlike CHD, DDH refers to alterations in hip growth and stability *in utero,* during the newborn period, and during the infant period. DDH also refers to hip disorders associated with neurologic disorders (e.g., myelomeningocele), connective tissue disorders (e.g., Ehlers-Danlos syndrome), myopathic disorders (e.g., arthrogryposis multiplex congenital), and syndromic conditions (e.g., Larsen syndrome).

Dezateux C, Rosendahl K: Developmental dysplasia of the hip, *Lancet* 369:1541–1552, 2007.

Bauchner H: Developmental dysplasia of the hip (DDH): an evolving science, *Arch Dis Child* 83:202, 2000.

65. **What are the Ortolani and Barlow maneuvers?**
The most reliable clinical methods of detection remain the Ortolani reduction and the Barlow provocative maneuvers. The infant should be lying quietly supine. Both examinations begin with the hips flexed to 90 degrees. To perform the *Ortolani maneuver,* the hip is abducted, and the examiner's index finger gently pushes up on the greater trochanter. This is a reduction maneuver that allows a dislocated femoral head to "clunk" back into the acetabulum (Fig. 16-5A). The *Barlow maneuver* is performed by adducting the flexed hip and gently pushing the thigh posteriorly in an effort to dislocate the femoral head (Fig. 16-5B). After 3 to 6 months of age, these tests are no longer useful because the hip becomes fixed in its dislocated position over time.

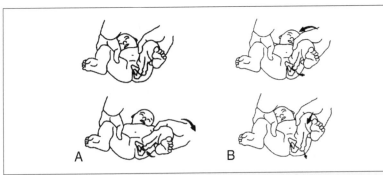

Figure 16-5. A, Ortolani maneuver. **B,** Barlow maneuver. (From Staheli LT [ed]: Pediatric Orthopedic Secrets. Philadelphia, Hanley & Belfus, 1998, p 166.)

KEY POINTS: THE FOUR "Fs" OF INCREASED RISK FOR DEVELOPMENTAL DISLOCATION OF THE HIP

1. First born

2. Female

3. Funny presentation (breech)

4. Family history (positive for developmental dysplasia of the hip)

66. **What is the Galeazzi sign?**

This test is performed by flexing both hips and knees together while evaluating the relative height of the knees. If one knee is significantly higher than the other, this can mean one of two things: the hip on the low side is dislocated, or the femur on the low side is short.

As opposed to the Ortolani and Barlow signs, the Galeazzi sign remains positive, and in fact usually becomes more obvious, as the child gets older.

67. **What is the significance of a "hip click" in a newborn?**

A *hip click* is the high-pitched sensation felt at the very end of abduction when testing for development dysplasia of the hip with the Barlow and Ortolani maneuvers; it occurs in 10% or less of newborns. Classically, it is differentiated from a hip "clunk," which is heard and felt as the hip goes in and out of joint. Although a debatable point, the hip click is thought to be benign. Its cause is unclear and may be the result of movement of the ligamentum teres between the femoral head and the acetabulum or the hip adductors as they slide over the cartilaginous greater trochanter. Worrisome features that might warrant evaluation (e.g., hip ultrasound, hip radiograph) include late onset of the click, associated orthopedic abnormalities, and other clinical features suggestive of developmental dysplasia (e.g., asymmetrical skin folds or creases, unequal leg length).

Witt C: Detecting developmental dysplasia of the hip, *Adv Neonatal Care* 3:65–75, 2003.

68. **What is the most reliable physical finding for a dislocated hip in the older child?**

Limited hip abduction. This is the result of shortening of the adductor muscles.

69. **What other diagnostic signs are suggestive of a dislocated hip?**

- **Asymmetry of the thigh and gluteal folds:** However, these may be present in many normal infants, and it is an unreliable sign if all other tests are normal.
- **Allis test:** With the hips flexed and the heels on the table, uneven knee level suggests hip dislocation.
- **Waddling gait, hyperlordosis of lumbar spine**: This is seen in older patients with bilateral dislocations.
- **Unilateral toe walking** is consistent with a significant leg length discrepancy as can be seen in a unilateral hip dislocation.

70. **What radiographic studies are most valuable for diagnosing DDH during the newborn period?**

In infants younger than 6 months, the acetabulum and the proximal femur are predominantly cartilaginous and thus not visible on plain radiograph. In this age group, these structures are best visualized with **ultrasound.** In addition to morphologic information, ultrasound provides dynamic information about the stability of the hip joint.

Weintroub S, Grill F: Ultrasonography in developmental dysplasia of the hip, *J Bone Joint Surg Am* 82:1004–1018, 2000.

71. **Should all infants be routinely screened by ultrasound for DDH?**

The answer is not clear. Because physical examination is not completely reliable and the incidence of late-diagnosed DDH has not declined, some investigators have recommended routine ultrasonographic screening. However, others argue that ultrasonography can lead to overdiagnosis and treatment. At present, the issue remains controversial.

Universal screening is more commonly done in Europe, whereas in the United States, selective screening on the basis of risk factors and physical examination findings is more the norm.

American Academy of Pediatrics: Clinical practice guideline: early detection of developmental dysplasia of the hip, *Pediatrics* 105:896–905, 2000.

72. **Who is at a higher risk for DDH?**

Dislocated, dislocatable, and subluxable hip problems occur in about 1% to 5% of infants. However, 70% of dislocated hips occur in **girls,** and 20% occur in infants born in **breech** position. Other risk associations include the following:
- Congenital torticollis
- Skull or facial abnormalities
- First pregnancy
- Positive family history of dislocation
- Metatarsus adductus
- Calcaneovalgus foot deformities in infants weighing <2500 g
- Amniotic fluid abnormalities (especially oligohydramnios)
- Prolonged rupture of membranes
- High birthweight

MacEwen GD: Congenital dislocation of the hip, *Pediatr Rev* 11:249–252, 1990.

73. **How is DDH treated?**

If the hip is dislocated, the first goal is to obtain a reduction and maintain that reduction to provide an optimal environment for femoral head and acetabular development. This is accomplished by keeping the legs abducted and the hips and knees flexed. The most commonly used devices are the Pavlik harness, the Frejka pillow, and the van Rosen splint. Double and triple diapers have *no role* in the treatment of DDH; they provide the parents with a false sense of security and do not provide reliable stabilization or positioning.

If the hip is merely shallow or loose and not frankly dislocated, the treatment is the same, but the harness or splint can come off once a day for an hour for bathing or play time.

Wenger DR, Bomar JD: Human hip dysplasia: evolution of current treatment concepts, *J Ortho Sci* 8:264–271, 2003.

74. **What is the significance of a positive Trendelenburg test?**

If a normal individual stands on one leg, the ipsilateral hip abductors (primarily the gluteus medius) prevent the pelvis from tilting, and balance is maintained (Fig. 16-6). Children older than 4 years can usually stand this way for at least 30 seconds. If the opposite side of the pelvis does tilt or the trunk lurches to maintain balance, this is a *positive Trendelenburg sign*. It may be an indicator of muscle weakness (as a result of muscular or neurologic pathology) or of hip instability (e.g., acetabular dysplasia).

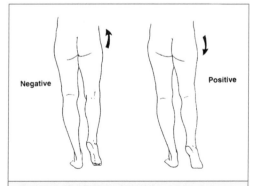

Figure 16-6. Trendelenburg sign. The pelvis tilts toward the normal hip when weight is borne on the affected side. (From Goldstein B, Chavez F: Applied anatomy of the lower extremities. Phys Med Rehabil State Art Rev 10:601-603, 1996.)

75. **What is a Trendelenburg gait?**

A *Trendelenburg gait* results from functionally weakened hip abductor muscles. It is commonly seen in children with a dislocated hip and Perthes disease. With a dislocated hip, the abductor muscles are at a mechanical disadvantage and are effectively weakened, which makes it difficult for them to support the child's body weight. As a result, the pelvis tilts away from the affected hip. In an effort to minimize this imbalance during the stance phase of gait, children lean over the affected hip.

76. **What is the most common cause of a painful hip in a child younger than 10 years?**

Acute transient synovitis is a self-limited inflammatory condition that occurs before adolescence, has no known cause, and generally has a benign clinical outcome. Some theorize that it is an immune response to a viral illness, and many patients give a history of having a recent viral illness—but then again, viral illnesses are very common in childhood. This disorder, although benign, can cause considerable anxiety among physicians and family members during its clinical course because it can mimic other, more sinister, conditions such septic arthritis, osteomyelitis, Legg-Calvé-Perthes (LCP) disorder, juvenile rheumatoid arthritis, SCFE, and tumor. It may occur anytime from the toddler age group to the late juvenile years, but the peak age of onset is between 3 and 6 years, and it is more common among boys. Acute transient synovitis remains a diagnosis of exclusion. Treatment consists of rest and calming of the synovitis with anti-inflammatory agents. Most patients experience complete resolution of their symptoms within 2 weeks of onset; the remainder may have symptoms of lesser severity for several weeks.

Caird MS, Flynn JM, Leung YL, et al: Factors distinguishing septic arthritis from transient synovitis of the hip in children, *J Bone Joint Surg Am* 88:1251–1257, 2006.

Do TT: Transient synovitis as a cause of painful limps in children, *Curr Opin Pediatr* 12:48–51, 2000.

77. **How can transient synovitis be differentiated from septic arthritis?**

See Table 16-3.

TABLE 16-3.	TRANSIENT SYNOVITIS VERSUS SEPTIC ARTHRITIS	
	Transient Synovitis	**Septic Arthritis**
History	Preceding upper respiratory infection ± low-grade fever	Fever
		Usually large joint involvement (hip, ankle, knee, shoulder, elbow)
	Hip or referred knee pain	
	Limp	
Physical	Refusal to bear weight	Exquisite pain, swelling, warmth
	Can delicately elicit range of motion in affected hip joint	Marked resistance to mobility
Laboratory	Erythrocyte sedimentation rate normal or mildly elevated	Erythrocyte sedimentation rate markedly elevated
	Mild peripheral leukocytosis	Leukocytosis with left shift
	Negative blood culture	Often positive blood culture
	Joint fluid cloudy	Joint fluid purulent
	Negative Gram stain	Often positive Gram stain

78. **What is LCP disease?**

    LCP disease (also called Perthes, Legg-Perthes or Legg-Calvé-Perthes after the three physicians who independently described it) is a disorder of the femoral head of unknown etiology that is characterized by ischemic necrosis, collapse, and subsequent repair (Fig. 16-7). Children typically present with a limp that is often painless. Over time, they often develop pain that localizes to the groin or is referred to the thigh or knee.

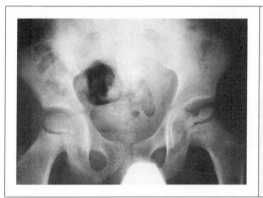

Figure 16-7. Anteroposterior view of the pelvis demonstrates fragmentation and irregularity of the left femoral head in a patient with Legg-Calvé-Perthes disease. The right hip is normal. (From Katz DS, Math KR, Groskin SA [eds]: Radiology Secrets. Philadelphia, Hanley & Belfus, 1998, p 405.)

79. **What are the pathologic stages of LCP disease?**

    LCP is a condition of aseptic necrosis of the femoral head involving children primarily between the ages of 4 and 10 years.

    ■ **Incipient or synovitis stage:** Lasting 1 to 3 weeks, this first stage is characterized by an increase in hip-joint fluid and a swollen synovium associated with reduced hip range of motion.

    ■ **Avascular necrosis:** Lasting 6 months to 1 year, the blood supply to part (or all) of the head of the femur is lost. The portion of the bone involved dies, but the contour of the femoral head remains unchanged.

    ■ **Fragmentation or regeneration and revascularization:** In the last and longest pathologic stage of LCP, which lasts 1 to 3 years, the blood supply returns and causes both the resorption of necrotic bone and the laying down of new immature bone. As the dead bone is removed, the integrity of the head is weakened and it collapses. Permanent hip deformity can occur during this last stage.

    It is important to note that plain radiographs may lag behind the progression of the disorder by as much as 3 to 6 months. Radionuclide bone scans and MRI are much better because ischemia and avascular necrosis can be detected much earlier.

80. **What is the prognosis for children with LCP disease?**

    The two main prognostic factors for LCP disease include the age of the child at diagnosis and the amount of epiphyseal involvement. Children younger than 6 years tend to have a more favorable prognosis, and those with less epiphyseal involvement also tend to have a better prognosis. Epiphyseal involvement has been classified by Salter into type A (with <50% epiphyseal involvement) and type B (with >50% head involvement).

81. **Which conditions are associated with coxa vara?**

    Coxa vara is a condition of a decreased femur shaft-neck angle. The three most common associations are **developmental coxa vara, avascular necrosis** of the femoral head, and **cleidocranial dysostosis**.

82. **What condition does the child in Figure 16-8 have?**
This is **femoral anteversion** (or medial femoral torsion), which is a common cause of in-toeing in younger children. The child is demonstrating the reverse tailor, or "W" position, which is a sign of the internally rotated hip.

Staheli LT: Torsional deformity, *Pediatr Clin North Am* 33:1382, 1986.

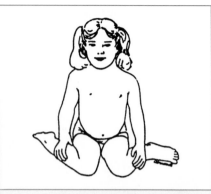

Figure 16-8. Reverse tailor position or "W" position.

83. **How is the extent of femoral anteversion measured?**
With the child lying prone and knees flexed at 90 degrees, the hip normally cannot be rotated internally (i.e., feet pushed outward) more than 60 degrees (angle A in Fig. 16-9). In addition, external rotation (angle B in Fig. 16-9) should exceed 20 degrees. A normal child averages about 35 degrees. Motion outside these ranges indicates that the cause of in-toeing is likely the result of physiologic femoral anteversion (or, less commonly, hip capsular contractions, as are seen in patients with cerebral palsy).

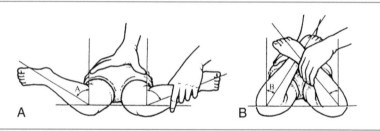

Figure 16-9. Measurement of femoral anteversion. (From Dormans JP: Orthopedic management of children with cerebral palsy. Pediatr Clin North Am 40:650, 1993.)

84. **Is sitting in the "W" position harmful?**
In a word, *no*. Although there is great confusion about this among many physicians and patients alike, there is absolutely no evidence that sitting in the "W" position has a harmful effect on the development of the hip and knee. Similarly, use of special orthopedic shoes or the infamous boots and bars that hold the feet turned in has no effect on the bony alignment of the proximal femur.

85. **Is there ever an indication to treat femoral anteversion?**
The neurologically normal child almost never requires treatment for anteversion. Although some children may walk with their feet turned in, especially early in life, this tends to improve as they age and improve in strength, coordination, and balance. An exception is the child with so-called *miserable malalignment syndrome,* who has severe femoral anteversion along with external tibial torsion. This child walks with the feet straight ahead (the tendency to in-toe is counterbalanced by the external rotation of the foot through the tibia), but the knees are pointed in; this places severe stress across the patellofemoral joint, and significant knee pain and disability follow. The treatment is quite significant, involving osteotomies of the femurs and tibias, but most patients have much improved knee mechanics and decreased pain.

86. **What symptoms do children with slipped capital femoral epiphysis (SCFE) have?**
SCFE involves progressive displacement with external rotation of the femur on the epiphyseal growth plate. The patient has intermittent or constant hip, thigh, or knee pain that has often been present for weeks or months. A limp, a lack of internal rotation, and an inability to flex the hip without also abducting may be noted. It is important to realize that any patient with knee pain may have underlying hip pathology.

87. **What systemic conditions are associated with SCFE?**
Children with SCFE tend to have delayed skeletal maturation and obesity and usually present between the ages of 8 and 14 years. It is more common in boys and in blacks. Systemic conditions associated with SCFE include hypothyroidism, panhypopituitarism, hypogonadism, rickets, and irradiation.

88. **What does FAI stand for?**
Femoral acetabular impingement syndrome. This is a relatively recently recognized entity thought to be a significant cause of hip pain and disability in adolescents and young adults. Similar to the way the rotator cuff of the shoulder can be damaged when impinged between the humeral head and acromion, the labrum of the hip (a structure analogous to the meniscus in the knee) can be torn when pinched between the acetabulum and femoral head or neck.

89. **What newer treatments are available for the treatment of hip pathology, including DDH, FAI, and SCFE?**
During the past decade, hip arthroscopy has become much more frequently used to diagnose and treat hip pain due to labral tears as well as to recontour the bony aspects of the hip joint when some types of dysplasia exist. Even more recently, some hip centers around the country have been describing their experience with repairing hip pathology through surgical dislocation of the hip. This technique has been eschewed in the past because of concerns about osteonecrosis of the femoral head as a complication. However, newer techniques have shown extremely low rates of this complication, and this procedure allows more direct and effective treatment of many hip problems, including unstable SCFE and FAI.

Khanduja V, Villar RN: Arthroscopic surgery of the hip: current concepts and recent advances, *J Bone Joint Surg Br* 12:1557–1566, 2006.

Rebello G, Spencer S, Mills M, et al: Surgical dislocation in the management of pediatric and adolescent hip deformity, *Clin Orthop* 467:724–731, 2009.

INFECTIOUS DISEASES

90. **Where does acute hematogenous osteomyelitis most commonly localize in children?**
- Lower extremity (femur, tibia, fibula): 70%
- Upper extremity (humerus, radius, ulna): 15%
- Foot: 4%
- Pelvis: 4%
- Vertebrae, skull, ribs, sternum, scapulae: 2%

Gold R: Diagnosis of osteomyelitis, *Pediatr Rev* 12:292–297, 1991.

91. **What is the most common cause of acute hematogenous osteomyelitis?**
Staphylococcus aureus (>90% of cases). Other less common bacterial causes can include *Salmonella* (especially in patients with sickle cell disease), *Pseudomonas aeruginosa* (following puncture wounds of the foot), *Kingella kingae*, *Streptococcus pneumoniae*, *Streptococcus pyogenes*, and in neonatal period *Streptococcus agalactiae* (group B strep) and gram-negative enteric bacteria.

92. **Diagnosis of osteomyelitis: CRP or ESR?**
    The trend is toward **C-reactive protein** (CRP). It responds more quickly than erythrocyte sedimentation rate (ESR) in the setting of acute inflammation and normalizes faster as the infection comes under control. A persistently abnormal CRP appears to be a better indicator of ineffective therapy, need for initial or repeated drainage, and likelihood of a worsening radiographic appearance.

93. **Diagnosis of osteomyelitis: MRI or bone scan?**
    The trend is toward **MRI**. MRI can precisely delineate area of infection, distinguish bone from soft tissue infection, and guide surgical intervention (Fig. 16-10). Its sensitivity can be as high as 97%. In infants, sedation will likely be needed. Technicium-99 m bone scans have a slightly lower sensitivity (80% to 90%). In the neonatal period, false-negative studies can be a result of decreased bone mineralization. Fractures can also cause increased uptake and sometimes can be confused with infection. No sedation is needed.

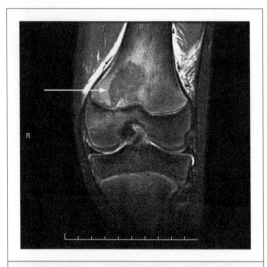

Figure 16-10. MRI or distal femur with metaphyseal lesion and overlying muscular edema consistent with osteomyelitis. (From Bergelson JM, Shah SS, Zaoutis TE [eds]: Pediatric Infectious Diseases: The Requisites in Pediatrics. Philadelphia, Mosby, 2008, p 239.)

Lim DJ, Eppes SC: Osteomyelitis. In Bergelson JM, Shah SS, Zaoutis TE, editors: *Pediatric Infectious Diseases: The Requisites in Pediatrics*, Philadelphia, 2008, Mosby Elsevier, p 238.

94. **What are the phases of a bone scan?**
    There are three phases in a bone scan defined by the time elapsed since injection of the radionuclide dye.
    - **Phase I**—*Angiographic phase:* During the first few seconds, the dye passes through the large blood vessels and provides early assessment of regional vascularity and perfusion.
    - **Phase II**—*Blood pool phase:* Usually obtained during the first minutes after an injection, this phase highlights the movement of the dye into the extracellular spaces of soft tissue and bone.
    - **Phase III**—*Delayed phase:* By 1.5 to 3 hours after injection, the dye localizes in the bone with minimal soft tissue imaging.
    The three-phase process is used to differentiate soft tissue from bony abnormalities.
    At times, a phase IV study may be done by rescanning for the same dye at 24 hours, which further minimizes soft tissue background activity.

95. **As osteomyelitis progresses, how soon do radiographic changes occur?**
    - **3 to 4 days:** Deep muscle plane shifted away from periosteal surface
    - **4 to 10 days:** Blurring of deep tissue muscle planes

- **10 to 21 days:** Changes in bone occur (e.g., osseous lucencies, punched-out lytic lesions, periosteal elevation)
- **>30 days:** bones sclerosis may be evident

96. **How often are blood cultures positive in patients with osteomyelitis?**
   50% of the time or less. Because this rate is relatively low, direct bone aspiration should be strongly considered, especially in the setting of an abscess. Aspiration raises the yield up to 70% and can facilitate antibiotic therapy. Empirical therapy is typically needed and usually is directed at probable methicillin-resistant *S. aureus* (MRSA) if the prevalence of MRSA in the community is higher than 10%.

   Afghani B, Kong V, Wu FL: What would pediatric infectious disease consultants recommend for management of culture-negative acute hematogenous osteomyelitis? *J Pediatr Orthop* 27:805–809, 2007.

KEY POINTS: OSTEOMYELITIS

1. The most common causative organism in healthy children is *Staphylococcus aureus*.

2. In children (unlike adults), spread of bacteria to bone is hematogenous rather than by local trauma.

3. In children with a puncture wound through a sneaker and osteomyelitis, think of *Pseudomonas aeruginosa*; however, the most common organism is still *S. aureus*.

4. Because of intravascular sludging and infarction, patients with sickle cell disease are at increased risk, especially for *Salmonella* infections.

5. Blood cultures are positive in less than 50% of cases; consider aspiration for greater likelihood of bacteriologic diagnosis.

6. Bone changes on radiograph may not occur for 10 to 15 days.

97. **What percentage of septic arthritis is culture negative?**
   Several studies have established that 30% to 60% of patients with clinically apparent septic arthritis have negative cultures of joint fluid. Reasons (both postulated and confirmed) for this observation include the fastidious nature of some less common etiologies of infectious arthritis (e.g., *K. kingae*), the loss of viability of some organisms on transport to the laboratory (e.g., *Neisseria* species), and perhaps a substance or cell population in the aspirate fluid that is bacteriostatic during *in vitro* culture conditions. Prompt processing of specimens and the use of several culture techniques (e.g., solid media plus liquid culture systems such as those used for blood cultures) can increase the yield of joint fluid cultures.

98. **How have the initial antibiotic choices for suspected bacterial bone and joint infections changed during the past decade?**
   The rapid growth of MRSA has required reassessment of initial choices. Previously, antistaphylococcal penicillins (e.g., oxacillin) or first-generation cephalosporins (e.g., cefazolin) were the first-line intravenous therapy. However, rates of MRSA are substantial in nearly all states. MRSA infections, especially those organisms with virulence factors, are associated with higher rates of local and systemic complications compared with methicillin-sensitive *S. aureus*. Many experts recommend the initial use of antibiotics directed against MRSA, such as vancomycin, linezolid, or clindamycin.

   Saphyakhajon P: Empiric antibiotic therapy for acute osteoarticular infections with suspected methicillin-sensitive *Staphylococcus aureus* or *Kingella*, *Pediatrics* 27:765–767, 2008.

99. **How long should antibiotics be continued in patients with osteomyelitis and septic arthritis?**
The precise answer is unclear, but infections caused by *S. aureus* or enteric gram-negative bacteria must be treated for longer periods than those caused by *Haemophilus influenzae*, *Neisseria meningitidis*, or *S. pneumoniae*. A minimum of 4 to 6 weeks is likely necessary for the former group, and 2 to 3 weeks are needed for the latter. If diagnosis has been delayed, if initial clinical response is poor, or if the CRP remains elevated, longer durations may be needed.

100. **Are oral antibiotics appropriate in the treatment of osteomyelitis?**
Traditional teaching has been to treat acute osteomyelitis for 4 to 6 weeks with intravenous antibiotics, usually through a central venous catheter. Evidence is increasing that the use of prolonged intravenous therapy and the use of early transition to oral therapy are equally effective. Factors that can contribute to the decision to opt for oral therapy include an identified organism, patient compliance, and the use of surgical débridement.

Zaoutis T, Localio AR, Leckerman K, et al: Prolonged intravenous therapy versus early transition to oral antimicrobial therapy for acute osteomyelitis in children, *Pediatrics* 123:636–642, 2009.

101. **When is open surgical drainage indicated in cases of osteomyelitis?**
    - Abscess formation in the bone, subperiosteum, or adjacent soft tissue
    - Bacteremia persisting >49 to 72 hours after the initiation of antibiotic treatment
    - Continued clinical symptoms (e.g., fever, pain, swelling) after 72 hours of therapy
    - Development of a sinus tract
    - Presence of a sequestrum (i.e., detached piece of necrotic bone)

Darville T, Jacobs RF: Management of acute hematogenous osteomyelitis in children, *Pediatr Infect Dis J* 23:255–257, 2004.

102. **Why are treatment failures more common in osteomyelitis than in septic arthritis?**
    - Antibiotic concentrations are much greater in joint fluid than in inflamed bone. Concentrations in joint fluid may actually exceed peak serum concentrations, whereas those in bone may be significantly less than serum concentrations.
    - Devitalized bone may serve as an ongoing nidus for infection and it has no blood flow to bring in antibiotics.
    - Diagnosis of osteomyelitis is more likely to be delayed than that of septic arthritis.

103. **How do the features of osteomyelitis in the neonate differ from those seen in the older child and adult?**
    - Multiple foci of infection are frequently seen.
    - Septic arthritis is a frequent association, probably reflecting the spread of infection through blood vessels penetrating the epiphyseal plates.
    - The pathogens causing neonatal osteomyelitis are the same as those responsible for sepsis neonatorum.

104. **How is the diagnosis of diskitis established?**
Diskitis, which is the infection and/or inflammation of the intervertebral disk, most commonly occurs in children between the ages of 4 and 10 years. The etiology is often unclear, but a bacterial cause (particularly *S. aureus*) is identified by blood cultures in about 50% of cases. The diagnosis can be difficult because the symptoms can be vague and vary greatly. Symptoms include generalized back pain with or without localized tenderness; limp; refusal to sit up, stand, or walk; back stiffness with loss of lumbar lordosis; abdominal pain; and unexplained low-grade fever. MRI can help distinguish between diskitis and vertebral osteomyelitis.

Early SD, Kay RM, Tolo VT: Childhood diskitis, *J Am Acad Orthop Surg* 11:413–420, 2003.

KNEE, TIBIA, AND ANKLE DISORDERS

105. What is the difference between valgus and varus deformities?
Some things appear to be destined to be learned, forgotten, and relearned many times as a rite of passage: the Krebs cycle is one; this is another. The terms refer to angular deformities of the musculoskeletal system. If the distal part of the deformity points toward the midline, the term is *varus*. If the distal part points away from the midline, it is *valgus*. For example, in patients with knock knees, the lower portion of the deformity points away, so the term is *genu valgum*.

Another method is to consider the body in the supine (anatomic) position. Draw a circle around the body. All angles conforming to the curve of the circle are varus; all angles going against the circle are valgus. Bowleggedness conforms to the circle around the body and is, therefore, *genu varum*.

106. Are children normally knock-kneed or bowlegged?
The answer is *yes*. Both can be normal depending on the age of the child. Most children at birth are bowlegged (genu varum) up to 20 degrees, but this tendency progressively diminishes until about 24 months, when the trend toward knock knees (genu valgum) begins. Knock knees are most noticeable at about 3 years of age (up to 15 degrees) and then begin to diminish. By 8 years of age, most children are—and will remain—in neutral alignment, meaning that with their knees extended, their knees and ankles both touch (Fig. 16-11).

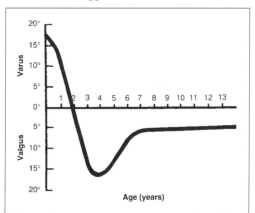

Figure 16-11. Development of the tibiofemoral angle during growth. (From Bruce RW Jr: Torsional and angular deformities. Pediatr Clin North Am 43:875, 1996.)

107. Which bowlegged infants or toddlers require evaluation?
Radiographs should be considered if bowleggedness demonstrates any of the following features:
- Present after 24 months (the time of normal progression to physiologic genu valgum)
- Worse after age 1 year as the infant begins to bear weight and walk
- Unilateral deformity
- Visually >20 degrees of varus angulation across the knee

It is important to remember that clinical or radiographic evaluation of alignment in the legs requires the knees to be pointed straight ahead. If the knees are pointed in or out, flexion at the knee can be easily mistaken for bowing of the legs.

108. What are the causes of pathologic genu varum (bowleggedness) or genu valgus (knock knees)?
Genu varum
- Physiologic bow legs
- Infantile tibia vara
- Hypophosphatemic rickets

- Metaphyseal chondrodysplasia
- Focal fibrocartilaginous dysplasia

Genu valgum
- Hypophosphatemic rickets
- Previous metaphyseal fracture of the proximal tibia (Cozen fracture)
- Multiple epiphyseal dysplasia
- Pseudoachondroplasia

Sass P, Hassan G: Lower extremity abnormalities in children, *Am Fam Physician* 68:461–468, 2003.

109. **Which children are more likely to develop Blount disease?**
Tibia vara, or Blount disease, is a medial angulation of the tibia in the proximal metaphyseal region as a result of a growth disturbance in the medial aspect of the proximal tibial epiphysis. In the infantile type, the child is usually an obese early walker, and he or she develops pronounced bowlegs during the first year of life. Black females are particularly at risk for severe deformity. In the adolescent variety, the onset occurs during late childhood or early adolescence, and the deformity is usually unilateral and milder. Although bracing can be effective in infantile cases diagnosed in the first 2 years of life, correction of severe deformity usually requires surgical intervention.

110. **How does tibial torsion change with age?**
Tibial torsion, the most common cause of in-toeing in children between the ages of 1 and 3 years, gradually rotates externally with age. For excessive internal rotation, bracing was used extensively in the past, but its efficacy is questionable because the natural history of the condition is self-resolution. Measurement is done by measuring the angle made by the long axis of the foot and the thigh when the knee is flexed 90 degrees.

111. **How effective is the Denis Browne splint for the treatment of tibial torsion?**
Not at all. The splint consists of a metal bar connected to shoes and holds the feet in varying degrees of external rotation. The splint was used frequently in the past for children with tibial torsion. However, there is absolutely no scientific evidence that this device alters the natural history of tibial torsion, and the use of this device for treatment of tibial torsion is rapidly fading.

112. **Why are ligamentous injuries less common in children?**
In children, ligaments tend to be stronger than the cartilaginous growth plates, and thus the growth plate will often fail (i.e., fracture) before the ligament tears.

113. **How are ankle sprains graded?**
Between 80% and 90% of ankle sprains are the result of excessive inversion and/or plantar-flexion causing injury to the lateral ligaments (anterior talofibular and calcaneofibular). A **grade 1 ankle sprain** is a mild, partial tear of the ankle ligament and results in no instability. A **grade 2 sprain** is a high-grade partial tear. Clinically differentiating between a grade 1 and 2 can be challenging. A **grade 3 sprain** is a complete tear of the ligament. This will result in some instability of the ankle, which can be detected with the ankle drawer test. This test is performed by immobilizing the lower tibia with one hand as the other hand grasps the heel and pulls the foot forward. There is always some motion (test the unaffected side to get an idea of what is normal for that patient), but with a complete tear, there is marked laxity with a poor end point.

114. **Which ankle sprains should be evaluated with a radiograph?**
More than 5,000,000 radiographs are estimated to be taken annually in children and adults for ankle injuries, yet there are no widely accepted guidelines. One set of guidelines (the Ottawa Ankle Rules) suggests obtaining a radiograph if there is malleolar pain and one or both of the following conditions is present: (1) the inability to bear weight for four steps

immediately after the injury and during office or emergency room evaluation; (2) bone tenderness at the posterior edge or tip of either malleolus. When these simple criteria were used in studies involving children and adults, no fractures were missed, and unnecessary radiographs were reduced by 25%.

Clark KD, Tanner S: Evaluation of the Ottawa Ankle Rules in children, *Pediatr Emerg Care* 19: 73–78, 2003.

115. **Should ankle sprains be cast?**
     No. If inversion ankle sprains are not complicated by a fracture or peroneal tendon dislocation, casting is not warranted. It has no benefit over early immobilization with a wrap, such as commercially available air stirrups. Additionally, complete immobilization may delay rehabilitation.

116. **What is the most significant mistake made during the evaluation of knee pain?**
     Failure to evaluate the hip as a source of the pain. Hip pathology frequently masquerades as knee or distal thigh pain (e.g., Perthes disease, SCFE). More than one knee has undergone a diagnostic arthroscopy for hip pathology.

117. **In acute injury, what are the main causes of blood in the knee joint?**
     Acute hemarthrosis is most commonly the result of the following:
     ■ Rupture of the anterior or posterior cruciate ligaments
     ■ Peripheral meniscal tears
     ■ Intratrabecular fracture
     ■ Major disruption or tear in the joint capsule

118. **Do meniscal tears occur in younger children?**
     Rarely do meniscal tears occur before the age of 12 years. A discoid meniscus is a congenitally abnormal meniscus that is shaped like a hockey puck instead of a "C." Because there is meniscus in the weight-bearing portion of the knee, and because the meniscus is not designed for this, these all eventually tear and become symptomatic. Meniscal tears in children not associated with a discoid meniscus are typically associated with a significant injury. They produce pain, swelling, and limping. Be sure to look for an associated injury to the anterior cruciate ligament.

119. **A 5-year-old boy with a painless swelling in the back of his knee has what likely condition?**
     Popliteal cysts. Also called *Baker cysts*, these occur more frequently in boys, are usually found on the medial side of the popliteal fossa, and are painless. In children, the cysts are rarely associated with intra-articular pathology. The mass should transilluminate on physical examination, confirming the fluid-filled nature of the lesion. The natural history is for the cyst to disappear spontaneously after 6 to 24 months. Surgery is not required except in extraordinary circumstances such as unremitting pain. Atypical findings (e.g., tenderness, firmness, history of rapid enlargement, pain) are justification for further diagnostic evaluation.

Seil R, Rupp S, Jochum P, et al: Prevalence of popliteal cysts in children: a sonographic study and review of the literature, *Arch Orthop Trauma Surg* 119:73–75, 1999.

120. **A teenager has chronic knee pain, swelling, and occasional "locking" of the knee joint, and his radiograph reveals increased density and fragmentation at the weight-bearing surface of the medial femoral condyle. What condition does he likely have?**
     Osteochondritis dissecans. In this disease, there is focal necrosis of a region of subchondral bone, typically in the lateral half of the medial femoral condyle. The cause is unknown, but antecedent trauma is common, and children (usually boys) with this condition are typically

very active. These cases present with activity-related pain; locking, buckling, and stiffness may be seen as well. A plain radiograph can reveal the diagnosis, but MRI is more sensitive when the clinical suspicion is high and radiographic findings are equivocal. Extended immobilization and activity restriction are the primary treatment in skeletally immature patients who have a favorable natural history—the lesions typically heal without surgery. For older adolescents and skeletally mature individuals, surgery is frequently required to stabilize the lesion and encourage healing. If the fragment does not heal, it may detach and become a loose body. This is a major problem because the lost articular cartilage cannot be replaced, and the risk for arthritis is high.

121. **What predisposes a child or teenager to recurrent dislocation of the patella?**
   - **Problems with alignment:** Genu valgum, laterally displaced tibial tubercle, patella alta
   - **Developmental problems:** Hypoplasia of the lateral femoral condyle, vastus medialis (VMO) insufficiency, abnormal attachment of the iliotibial tract
   - **Generalized ligamentous laxity:** Down syndrome, Ehlers-Danlos syndrome, Marfan syndrome, Turner syndrome

122. **How does patellofemoral stress syndrome occur?**
   This major cause of chronic knee pain in teenagers results from **malalignment of the extensor mechanism of the knee.** It is most commonly seen as an "overuse" entity in sports that involve running and full-knee flexion (e.g., track, soccer). It has been inappropriately called *chondromalacia patella*, which is a specific pathologic diagnosis of an abnormal articular surface that occurs in a minority of these patients. The patella serves as the fulcrum on which the quadriceps extend the knee. The multiple muscle bellies of the quadriceps may act asymmetrically, causing greater stress on the lateral aspect of the patella. This is particularly a problem for individuals with problems placing them at risk for patellar symptoms, including femoral anteversion, external tibial torsion, high (alta) patella, abnormally developed quadriceps, excessive flattening of the trochlear groove, or an increased Q angle. Treatment consists of ice, rest, nonsteroidal anti-inflammatory drugs, quadriceps strengthening, hamstring stretching, and possibly patellar-stabilizing braces.

123. **What is the Q angle?**
   This angle describes the lines of force acting on the patella. The angle is formed by the intersection of a line drawn from the anterior-superior iliac spine to the patella, and a line from the patella to the tibial tubercle. For teenage boys, the average Q angle is 14 degrees, and for girls it is 17 degrees. Angles of more than 20 degrees create a bowstringing effect that places a lateral stress on the patella and predispose individuals (particularly runners) to chronic knee pain.

SPINAL DISORDERS

124. **What are the different forms of scoliosis?**
   Scoliosis is a lateral curvature of the spine (i.e., coronal plane deformity) that has several general causes. The most common form is *idiopathic scoliosis*, which arises in otherwise normal children for reasons that are not fully understood, but there is an underlying genetic cause. Idiopathic scoliosis is subdivided according to age at which the disease is diagnosed: adolescent ($\geq$10 years), juvenile (3 to 10 years), and infantile (0 to 3 years). *Congenital scoliosis* occurs when there is a problem with the way the vertebrae form during embryogenesis. This form of scoliosis may be associated with anomalies of the cardiac and renal systems, which are developing at the same time. *Neurogenic scoliosis* is

associated with a variety of spastic and paralytic neuromuscular diseases such as cerebral palsy, muscular dystrophy, and myelomeningocele. Finally, there are *miscellaneous* causes of scoliosis that can be associated with connective tissue disorders like Marfan and Ehlers-Danlos syndromes. Scoliosis is also seen in increased rates in children who underwent major abdominal or thoracic surgery in infancy (such as open heart surgery or congenital diaphragmatic hernia repair).

National Scoliosis Foundation: http://www.scoliosis.org.

125. **How is screening for spinal deformity performed?**
The child should be undressed or dressed only in underwear with a gown open at the back. The child is asked to bend forward while standing, and the contour of the back is examined from behind and the side. This examination is then repeated with the child sitting. The following signs can suggest scoliosis:
- Shoulder or scapular asymmetry
- Asymmetry of paraspinal muscles or rib cage (the so-called rib hump) in the thoracic spine noted on forward bending (>0.5 cm in lumbar region and >1.0 cm in thoracic region; a scoliometer may be used for this determination)
- Sagittal plane deformity such as increased kyphosis when viewed from the side
- Waist-crease asymmetry that does not disappear when sitting (many waist-crease asymmetries are the result of leg-length discrepancies). This finding is very helpful in obese patients whose paraspinal prominence may be obscured by their subcutaneous adipose tissue.

Scoliosis Research Society: http://www.srs.org.

126. **What constitutes an abnormal scoliometric measurement?**
The *scoliometer* (also called an inclinometer) is a type of protractor used to measure the vertebral rotation and rib humping that is seen in scoliosis with the forward-bending test. An angle of 5 degrees or less is usually insignificant, whereas an angle of 7 degrees or more warrants orthopedic referral and consideration of standing posteroanterior and lateral radiographs for more precise assessment of curvature.

127. **Are males or females more likely to have scoliosis?**
It depends on the age and the cause of the scoliosis. For idiopathic scoliosis seen in infancy, males outnumber females by a 3:2 margin. As age increases, females catch up, and by adolescence, females are five to seven times more likely than males to have scoliosis.

128. **How valuable are school-based screening programs for scoliosis?**
This is controversial. Many states mandate school scoliosis screening. Experts in favor of these programs contend that reliable screening procedures exist and that early identification will lead to earlier nonoperative care and to the prevention of progression and of the need for surgical intervention. Opponents argue that the low incidence of children requiring treatment, the low positive-predictive value of screening programs, and high numbers of children unnecessarily referred do not justify the programs. Additionally, the effectiveness of nonoperative interventions has not been clearly defined. Organizations differ in their recommendations. The American Academy of Orthopaedic Surgeons and the American Academy of Pediatrics, while recognizing the limitations of screening, argue that girls should be screened twice (ages 10 and 12 years) and boys once (ages 13 or 14 years). The U.S. Preventive Services Task Force recommends against the routine screening of asymptomatic adolescents for idiopathic scoliosis.

Richards BS, Vitale MG: Screening for idiopathic scoliosis in adolescents, *J Bone Joint Surg Am* 90:195–198, 2008.

U.S. Preventive Services Task Force: Screening for idiopathic scoliosis in adolescents: recommendation statement, *Am Fam Physician* 71:1975–1976, 2005.

129. **How is scoliosis measured by the Cobb method?**
This is the standard technique used to quantify scoliosis in posteroanterior radiographs. One line is drawn along the vertebra tilted the most at the top of the curve, and another is drawn at the bottom of the curve. The curvature is represented by angle "a," which can be measured in two ways, as illustrated in Figure 16-12.

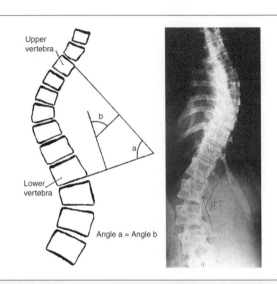

Figure 16-12. Measurement of the Cobb angle. (From Katz DS, Math KR, Groskin SA [eds]: Radiology Secrets. Philadelphia, Hanley & Belfus, 1998, p 321.)

KEY POINTS: SCOLIOSIS

1. Scoliosis of >10 degrees is relatively common (1% to 2%), but progression to ≥25 degrees and required treatment are rare.

2. Bracing does not permanently correct scoliosis, but it may prevent progression.

3. Establishing the maturity level of the skeleton is important because the risk for progression is increased with immaturity.

4. In adolescents, progressive curves are seven times more likely to appear in girls than in boys.

5. All scoliosis is not idiopathic: assess for limb-length discrepancy, congenital anomalies, and neurologic abnormalities, especially reflexes.

130. **What is the natural history of adolescent idiopathic scoliosis (AIS)?**
Untreated idiopathic scoliosis that is greater than 50 degrees at skeletal maturity is likely to continue to progress throughout life. The rate of progression tends to be slow, on the order of 1 degree per year, but over the expected lifetime of the patient, that could be 60 degrees or more of progression. However, even with this progression, AIS is not a fatal

disease, and there is little if any excess mortality seen in the few long-term natural history studies. Only when curves are greater than 90 to 100 degrees is there a clinically important effect on cardiopulmonary function. Some studies have shown psychosocial problems related to a patient's dissatisfaction with their appearance, but not all studies have reproduced this finding. Back pain may be increased in this population compared with age-matched norms, but there is no indication that surgery improves this.

Weinstein SL, Dolan LA, Cheng JCY: Adolescent idiopathic scoliosis, *Lancet* 371:1527–1537, 2008.

Weinstein SL, Dolan LA, Spratt KF, et al: Health and function of patients with untreated idiopathic scoliosis: a 50-year natural history study, *JAMA* 289:559–567, 2003.

131. **What is the recommended treatment of AIS?**
There are three approaches to the treatment of scoliosis: *observation*, *bracing*, and *surgery*. Therapy is dependent on the extent of curvature and the likelihood of progression (based on skeletal age, menarchal status, and chronologic age). In general, skeletally immature patients with curvatures of less than 25 degrees should be re-evaluated in 4 to 6 months, whereas those who are skeletally mature typically do not need re-evaluation. For skeletally immature patients with curvatures between 25 and 45 degrees, some bracing is usually used (particularly if increases in scoliosis are noted over a 3- to 6-month period), whereas ongoing re-evaluation is needed for the skeletally mature patients
in 6 to 12 months. Surgery is generally indicated for curvatures greater than 45 to 50 degrees.

Bracing does not reverse curvature but debatably may limit progression and the need for surgery.

Cruz I Jr, Smith BG: Scoliosis in children and adolescents: an update, *Contemp Pediatr* 27:42–53, 2010.

132. **What are the risk factors for progression of AIS?**
Idiopathic scoliosis is a growth phenomenon, and the rate of progression of the curve is proportional to the rate of growth. This is why many curves become clinically apparent in adolescence just after the growth spurt. Therefore, the risk for progression is greater in younger children (who have more growth remaining), and the larger the curve, the more likely it is to progress. Most other risk factors for progression are merely a surrogate for growth remaining, such as skeletal age and menarchal status.

133. **Have any genes related to AIS been identified?**
Yes! There is now a commercially available screening test that can ascertain the risk for progression of scoliosis based on a panel of genetic markers. Idiopathic scoliosis is likely not caused by one gene, but this panel of about 50 markers has been found to have an excellent negative predictive value (it accurately identifies patients at low risk for progression), although the positive-predictive value is less certain. As of now, this test is only available for white females 10 years of age or older. Over time, this type of test should become available for different populations with idiopathic scoliosis.

Oglivie J: Adolescent idiopathic scoliosis and genetic testing, *Curr Opin Pediatr* 22:67-70, 2010.

134. **Is it helpful to identify patients at high risk for progression at an early age?**
An emphatic *yes*. During the past few years, nonfusion techniques to definitively treat scoliosis have been promoted. In one such technique, staples are placed in the vertebral bodies across the growth plates on the concave side of the curve to stop growth on that side to allow the spine to grow into a corrected position over time. This technique is powerful, but is most effective when used to treat small curves in the 20- to 30-degree range. The problem arises in identifying the patients with small curves who are at risk for progression because most 20- to 30-degree curves will not reach surgical criteria. Genetic testing would be one way to identify such patients. Currently, this technique is reserved mostly for very young children who are at high risk for progression based on their growth remaining.

135. **What diagnosis should you consider in a teenage boy with very poor posture who is not flexible?**
    Scheuermann kyphosis. This is a wedge-shaped deformity of the vertebral bodies of unclear etiology that causes juvenile kyphosis (abnormally large dorsal thoracic or lumbar curves). Common in teenagers, it is distinguished from simple poor posture ("postural round-back deformity") by its sharp angulation and inability to correct by having the patient stand up straight or lie on top of a bolster. Radiographic studies reveal anterior vertebral body wedging and irregular erosions of the vertebral end plate. Treatment consists of exercise, bracing, and, rarely, surgical correction (for severe, painful deformities).

136. **What is the difference between spondylolysis and spondylolisthesis?**
    Spondylolysis is a condition in which there is a defect in the pars interarticularis (vertebral arch) of a vertebra that is most common at L5. This can be a congenital problem but is commonly seen as a stress fracture in athletes who do a lot of hyperextension of the lower back (classically gymnasts and football offensive linemen). **Spondylolisthesis** is a condition (often resulting from spondylolysis) that is characterized by forward slippage of one vertebra on the lower vertebrae. Pain is the most common presenting symptom for both conditions. The etiology is unclear, but various theories relate it to hereditary factors, congenital predisposition, trauma, posture, growth, and biomechanical factors. Treatment includes watchful waiting, limitation of activity, exercise therapy, bracing, casting, and surgery, depending on the patient's age, the magnitude of the slippage, the extent of pain, and the predicted likelihood of progression of the deformity.

    Klein G, Mehlman CT: Nonoperative treatment of spondylolysis and grade 1 spondylolisthesis in children and young adults, *J Pediatr Orthop* 29:146–156, 2009.

SPORTS MEDICINE

137. **Which sports injuries are the most common in school-aged children and adolescents?**
    Some 75% of injuries in school-aged children involve the lower extremities, and most injuries to the knee and ankle are reinjuries as a result of incomplete healing from a previous problem. Contusions and sprains are the most common types of injuries, with fractures and dislocations accounting for an additional 10% to 20%. Cranial injuries are the most common cause of sports fatality.

    Adolescent boys who participate in contact team sports, particularly football and wrestling, are at the highest risk for injuries. Among girls, softball and gymnastics have the highest injury rates.

    Only 10% of sports injuries are caused by an opponent; most injuries are caused by stumbling, falling, or misstepping. The latter finding suggests that improving intrinsic factors (e.g., raising the level of physical fitness, avoiding overuse, and strengthening joint stability) may be more important for the prevention of injuries than external factors (e.g., rule changes, equipment).

138. **What are overuse injuries?**
    Overuse injuries refer to chronic injuries caused by repetitive stress on the musculoskeletal system without sufficient recovery time. Contributing factors can include extremity malalignment (e.g., foot hyperpronation, excess femoral anteversion), scoliosis, and muscle weakness or imbalance. Improper equipment and hard training surfaces can also contribute to the problem.

    Soprano JV, Fuchs SM: Common overuse injuries in the pediatric and adolescent athlete, *Clin Pediatr Emerg Med* 8:7–14, 2007.

139. **Why have many Little Leagues banned the throwing of a curve ball?**
To minimize the cases of Little League elbow, or medial epicondylitis, another apophysitis that in this case results from overuse of the flexor-pronator muscles at the attachment to the medial epicondylar growth plate. The throwing of a curve ball stresses the ulnar collateral ligament on the medial elbow. Severe strain can result in partial separation of the apophysis, and occasionally bony avulsions can occur.

140. **What is the most likely diagnosis if a 12-year-old basketball player has painful swelling below both knees?**
Osgood-Schlatter disease. This is a traction apophysitis and results from repetitive stress (pull of the patellar tendon) on the tibial tubercle, which is connected to the tibial shaft through a cartilaginous plate. The cartilage is unable to handle the tensile forces created by the quadriceps muscle, and it hypertrophies and becomes inflamed. This process often occurs around the time of the adolescent growth spurt and is related to the level of physical activity. Physical examination reveals tenderness to palpation and a very prominent tibial tubercle. The pain is exacerbated with resisted knee extension.
Appropriate clinical management includes the judicious use of anti-inflammatory medications, restricted activities, quadriceps stretching and strengthening, and cross training. The condition is usually self-limited and resolves with skeletal maturity, although the bump remains. Immobilization, which may lead to disuse atrophy, is rarely necessary.

141. **A 12-year-old gymnast, one of the school's best tumblers, who develops chronic wrist pain has what likely condition?**
Epiphysiolysis of the distal radius. Also known as *gymnast's wrist*, this is the widening and resorption of the distal radial physis. The compression loads on the dorsiflexed wrist, often with rotational components, can result in significant radiographic changes. Treatment is rest of a duration depending on the extent of radiographic findings.

142. **What is the likely diagnosis in a fifth-grade football player with heel pain and a positive "squeeze test"?**
Sever disease, or apophysitis of the calcaneus. Caused by traction on the calcaneus at the insertion sites of the gastrocnemius-soleus muscles, microavulsions occur where bone meets cartilage. Pain is reproduced with compression of the medial and lateral aspects of the heel (the "squeeze test"). Treatment involves Achilles stretching, viscoelastic heel cups, and nonsteroidal anti-inflammatory drugs. Failure to improve suggests a possible calcaneal stress fracture, and immobilization may be required.

Soprano JV, Fuchs SM: Common overuse injuries in the pediatric and adolescent athlete, *Clin Pediatr Emerg Med* 8:9–11, 2007.

143. **If a ninth-grade soccer player with knee swelling "felt a pop" while scoring a goal, what are three possible diagnoses?**
A pop or snap sensation in the setting of acute knee injury is usually associated with the following:
■ Anterior cruciate ligament injury
■ Meniscal injury
■ Patellar subluxation

144. **What is the most accurate physical examination modality to assess anterior cruciate ligament (ACL) injury?**
Lachman test. With the patient lying in the supine position, the patient's lower thigh just above the knee is stabilized by one hand of the examiner, and the knee is flexed to 20 to 30 degrees. The examiner then attempts with the other hand to pull the tibia anteriorly in relation

to the stabilized femur. Increased displacement or absence of a solid stop (a "soft end point") compared with the uninjured knee suggests ACL injury (Fig. 16-13).

Spindler KP, Wright RW: Anterior cruciate ligament tear, *N Engl J Med* 359:2135–2142, 2008.

Scholten RJ, Opstelten W, DeVille WL, et al: Accuracy of physical diagnostic tests for assessing ruptures of the anterior cruciate ligament: a meta-analysis, *J Fam Pract* 52:689–694, 2003.

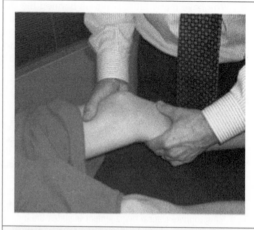

Figure 16-13. Lachman test for anterior cruciate ligament stability. (From Anderson SJ: Sports injuries. Curr Probl Pediatr Adolesc Health Care 35:137, 2005.)

145. **In what settings do ACL injuries occur in teenage athletes?**

These injuries tend to occur when landing from a jump, decelerating quickly, or changing direction suddenly. Up to 90% occur without contact with another athlete. Mechanisms include excessive femoral internal rotation, valgus stress (medially directed force) to the knee with the foot fixed, and hyperextension of the knee.

LaBella CR: Common acute sports-related lower extremity injuries in children and adolescents, *Clin Pediatr Emerg Med* 8:31–42, 2007.

146. **Why are girls more likely than boys to experience an ACL injury in high school sports?**

The disparity is striking, with girls two to eight times more likely to injure their ACL than boys. ACL injuries are uncommon in prepubertal athletes but increase through adolescence. The increased risk for females is incompletely understood but may be multifactorial, including differences in leg alignment, with more girls having a valgus deformity (knock knee); smaller notch width for the ACL in girls; hormonal (estrogen) effects on ACL laxity (risk increases during the preovulatory stage of menstrual cycle); and possible poorer neuromuscular control in girls compared with boys.

Spindler KP, Wright RW: Anterior cruciate ligament tear, *N Engl J Med* 359:2135–2142, 2008.

147. **How is a concussion defined?**

The American Academy of Neurology defines concussion as a "trauma-induced alteration in mental status that may or may not involve a loss of consciousness."

Practice parameter: the management of concussion in sports (summary statement). Report of the Quality Standards Subcommittee, *Neurology* 48:581–585, 1997.

148. **How should a player with a suspected on-field concussion be assessed?**

The basics—airway, breathing, circulation, and possibility of a cervical spine injury—need to be initially assessed to ensure no medical emergency is likely. Testing should involve a detailed neurologic examination as well as orientation to person, place, time, recent memory, performance of simple tasks (e.g., repeating numbers, spelling backward, serial subtractions) and postural stability. Players with loss of consciousness (LOC), with abnormal neurologic examination, or who worsen or fail to improve on ongoing mental status testing should be transported to an emergency department.

Meehan WP III, Bachur RG: Sport-related concussion, *Pediatrics* 1123:114–123, 2009.

Patel DR: Managing concussion in a young athlete, *Contemp Pediatr* 23:62–69, 2006.

149. **Is an athlete with a first concussion at increased risk for a second?**
Yes. LOC with a concussion is associated with a sixfold increased risk for future concussion compared with concussion and no LOC. After any concussion, risk for a second is increased in the ensuing 7 to 10 days. Recovery times are also longer after subsequent concussions compared with those without a previous history of concussion. An uncommon phenomenon, the "second-impact" syndrome, has been described, with death resulting from a second injury to the head in an athlete who had sustained an initial concussion from which the athlete had not fully recovered.

Meehan WP III, Bachur RG: Sport-related concussion, *Pediatrics* 1123:114–123, 2009.

150. **When should an athlete who has suffered a concussion be allowed to return to play?**
This is quite controversial, but a guiding rule is that no athlete should be allowed to return until all signs and symptoms have resolved. Such recovery typically includes neuropsychological testing because symptom reporting only by the athlete can be erroneous. Some schools use abbreviated "baseline" testing specifically for athletic purposes. When a player has been cleared to return, the return should be in stepwise fashion—light aerobic activity, noncontact drills, full-contact training—with symptom-free activity before medical clearance for game play.

Kirkwood MW, Yeates KO, Wilson PE: Pediatric sport-related concussion: a review of the clinical management of an oft-neglected population, *Pediatrics* 117:1359–1371, 2006.

ACKNOWLEDGMENT

The editors gratefully acknowledge contributions by Drs. Francis Y. Lee, John P. Dormans, Richard S. Davidson, Mark Magnusson, David P. Roye, and Joshua E. Hyman that were retained from previous editions of *Pediatric Secrets*.

CHAPTER 17

PULMONOLOGY

Robert W. Wilmott, MD, and Bradley A. Becker, MD

ALLERGIC RHINITIS

1. **How common is allergic rhinitis?**
   Very common. Between 10% and 30% of children experience rhinitis as the most common manifestation of allergic disease.

2. **In addition to chronic congestion, what features on physical examination suggest chronic allergic rhinitis?**
   - "Allergic facies": Open mouth, midface hypoplasia
   - "Allergic salute": Nasal crease on bridge of nose as a result of chronic upward rubbing with the palm of the hand
   - Diminished sense of taste and smell
   - Dental malocclusion
   - Allergic "shiners" (dark circles under the eyes)
   - Increased infraorbital folds
   - Cobblestoning of conjunctiva and posterior oropharynx
   - Violet discoloration of the nasal mucosa

3. **What are the major risk factors for allergic rhinitis?**
   - Positive family history
   - Heavy maternal cigarette smoking during the first year of life
   - Early introduction of solid foods (controversial)
   - Individuals born during pollen season
   - Higher serum immunoglobulin E (IgE) levels (>100 IU/mL before 6 years of age)
   - Atopic dermatitis
   - Ownership of pets

   Wang D-Y: Risk factors of allergic rhinitis: genetic or environmental? *Ther Clin Risk Manag* 1: 115–125, 2005.

4. **How does the time of year help identify the potential cause of allergic rhinitis?**
   Tree pollen is usually associated with the onset of the growing season. After local tree pollination, grass pollens appear; this may occur earlier in locales where there are short winters. Weed pollen is associated with the late-summer pollen peak, and ragweed is the primary weed pollen in eastern and central North America. Fungal aeroallergens span the growing season. Relative concentrations of household animal allergens, dust mites, and indoor fungi generally increase when doors and windows are closed. However, dust mites and molds proliferate in areas of high humidity and may cause perennial symptoms.

   Naclerio R, Solomon W: Rhinitis and inhalant allergens, *JAMA* 278:1842–1848, 1997.

5. **Which variables affect allergy skin testing in children?**
   - **Test site:** The forearm is less reactive than the back. The lower back is less reactive than the mid and upper back.
   - **Patient age:** Wheals on skin testing increase in size from infancy on and then often decline after 50 years of age. Infants react primarily with a small wheal and a large erythematous flare.
   - **Seasonality:** Allergen skin test sensitivity is increased after the pollen season and then declines until the next season.
   - **Medications:** These can inhibit allergen skin test response for various lengths of time: cetirizine (3 to 10 days), loratadine (3 to 10 days), diphenhydramine (1 to 3 days), chlorpheniramine (1 to 3 days), and hydroxyzine (1 to 10 days).
   - **Test technique:** Prick skin tests are more specific than intradermal skin tests.

   Demoly P, Michel FB, Bousquet J: In vivo methods for study of allergy skin tests, techniques, and interpretation. In Middleton E, Reed CE, Ellis EF, et al, editors: *Allergy: Principles and Practice*, St. Louis, 1998, Mosby, pp 430–439.

6. **What is an antigen-specific IgE ImmunoCAP?**
   An IgE ImmunoCAP (Phadia, Inc., Uppsala, Sweden) is an *in vitro* automated laboratory method used to quantify the amount of allergen-specific IgE in a patient's serum. The test allergen is bound to a solid phase matrix and then incubated with the serum. If it contains the allergen-specific IgE, the patient's IgE will bind to the ImmunoCAP antigen. Nonspecific IgE is removed by washing. Fluorescent-labeled anti-IgE is then added and binds to the IgE-antigen complex. Fluorescence is measured and compared to a standard curve.

   Sampson HA, Ho DG: Relationship between food-specific IgE concentrations and the risk of positive food challenges in children and adolescents, *J Allergy Clin Immunol* 100:444–451, 1997.

7. **Summarize the pros and cons of skin testing versus *in vitro* testing (e.g., IgE ImmunoCAP) for allergies.**
   ***In vitro* tests**
   - No risk for anaphylaxis
   - Results not influenced by medications (e.g., antihistamines), dermatographism, or extensive dermatologic disease
   - More costly
   - Better predictive value for some common food allergens

   Skin testing
   - Less costly
   - More sensitive than *in vitro* tests
   - Results immediately available

8. **What are the recommended treatments for children with chronic allergic rhinitis?**
   - Environmental control measures for allergen avoidance are the mainstay of treatment. Relevant sensitivities are based on positive skin or serum-specific IgE testing that correlates with symptoms on allergen exposure.
   - Pharmacotherapy (including nasal corticosteroid sprays), antihistamines (given orally or by nasal spray), or oral antileukotrienes
   - Immunotherapy is reserved for those with persistent symptoms despite the above treatment and for those who want control of symptoms with less medications.

   American Academy of Allergy, Asthma and Immunology: http://www.aaaai.org.

KEY POINTS: ALLERGIC RHINITIS

1. History (family, environmental, associated symptoms) is key to diagnosis.

2. With two atopic parents, the risk to the child is 50% to 70%.

3. IgE ImmunoCAP testing is indicated in patients with severe skin disorders or those unable to temporarily discontinue H_1-blocking antihistamines.

4. Sensitivity of testing: intradermal (may yield false-positive results) > skin prick > IgE ImmunoCAP

5. Allergic features: Shiners (dark circles under eyes), increased infraorbital folds, transverse nasal bridge crease, cobblestoning of conjunctiva and posterior oropharynx

6. Immunotherapy: Consider this when allergen avoidance and pharmacotherapy have produced suboptimal results.

9. **What are the major indoor allergens?**
   Dust mite, animal dander, cockroach, and **mold**.

10. **How can you rid the home of cat allergen?**
    - Remove upholstered furniture, carpet, and other sources harboring the allergen.
    - Obtain new bedding or impermeable bedding covers.
    - The cat's roaming areas should be limited, particularly the bedroom. The bedroom is the most important room to maintain as free of cat allergen as possible. Keeping the cat outside the home is an option for some.
    - Use high-efficiency particulate air filters or electrostatic air cleaners.
    - Consider a "felinectomy."

11. **How can house dust mite (HDM) concentrations be minimized?**
    Allergens from HDMs are among the most common triggers for allergic rhinitis and asthma. They are found throughout homes, but accumulate in bedding, soft furnishings, and carpet. HDM allergen reduction methods include the following:
    - Encasing pillows, mattresses, and box springs in allergen-proof, zippered fabric or plastic covers.
    - Bedding may be washed in hot (55°C [131°F]) water. Drying the bedding in high heat in a dryer is an alternative that may prevent scalding injuries in children from having the water heater temperature raised above 50°C (120°F).
    - Humidity should be reduced indoors using a dehumidifier or air conditioning with the windows closed.
    - Wall-to-wall carpeting should be removed as much as possible and replaced with throw rugs. These should be regularly washed or dry cleaned.

    Wood RA: Environmental control. In Leung DYM, Sampson HA, Geha RS, Szefler SJ, editors: *Pediatric Allergy: Principles and Practice*, St. Louis, 2003, Mosby, p 270.

12. **Which children should be considered for immunotherapy?**
    Immunotherapy is the treatment of choice for hymenoptera venom sensitivity—in carefully selected patients—to prevent life-threatening allergic reactions. Immunotherapy should be considered as treatment for IgE-mediated diseases (e.g., allergic rhinitis, allergic asthma) when allergen avoidance and adjunctive pharmacotherapy have produced suboptimal results. Although allergen immunotherapy may be helpful in patients whose asthma is difficult to

control, allergen immunotherapy is contraindicated in patients with unstable asthma and in those individuals whose FEV_1 levels are less than 70% of the predicted value.

Golden DBK: Insect allergy. In Adkinson NF, Yunginger JW, Basse WW, et al, editors: *Middleton's Allergy: Principles and Practice*, ed 6, St. Louis, 2003, Mosby, pp 1475–1486.

Matsui EC, Eggleston PA: Immunotherapy for allergic disease. In Leung DYM, Sampson HA, Geha RS, Szefler SJ, editors: *Pediatric Allergy: Principles and Practice*, St. Louis, 2003, Mosby, pp 277–285.

13. **How common is exercise-induced bronchospasm in children with allergic rhinitis?**
Up to 40% of patients with allergic rhinitis but no history of asthma have abnormal pulmonary function tests in response to exercise compared with 63% of asthmatic children and 7% of control children.

Bierman EW: Incidence of exercise-induced asthma in children, *Pediatrics* 56:847–850, 1975.

ASTHMA

14. **If both parents are asthmatic, what is the risk that their child will have asthma?**
60%. For a child with only one parent with asthma, the risk is estimated to be about 20%. If neither parent has asthma, the risk is 6% to 7%.

15. **When does asthma usually have its onset of symptoms?**
About 50% of childhood asthma develops before the age of 3 years, and nearly all has developed by the age of 7 years. The signs and symptoms of asthma, including chronic cough, may be evident much earlier than the actual diagnosis but may be erroneously attributed to recurrent pneumonia.

American Lung Association: http://www.lungusa.org.

16. **Which children with wheezing at an early age are likely to develop chronic asthma?**
Although about one third of children will have an episode of wheezing before they are 1 year old, most (80%) do not develop persistent wheezing after age 3 years. Risks factors for persistence include the following:
- Positive family history of asthma (especially maternal)
- Increased IgE levels
- Atopic dermatitis
- Rhinitis not associated with colds
- Secondhand smoke exposure

Taussig LM, Wright AL, Holberg CJ, et al: Tuscon Children's Respiratory Study: 1980 to present, *J Allergy Clin Immunol* 111:661–675, 2003.

17. **What historical points are suggestive of an allergic basis for asthma?**
- Seasonal nature with concurrent rhinitis (suggesting pollen)
- Symptoms worsen when visiting a family with pets (suggesting animal dander)
- Wheezing occurs when carpets are vacuumed or bed is made (suggesting mites)
- Symptoms develop in damp basements or barns (suggesting molds)

18. **What are other potential triggers for asthma?**
- Cold air
- Emotional extremes (stress, fear, crying, laughing)
- Environmental (pollutants, cigarette smoke)
- Exercise

- Foods, food additives
- Gastroesophageal reflux disease
- Hormonal (menstrual, premenstrual)
- Irritants (strong odors, paint fumes)
- Medications (nonsteroidal anti-inflammatory drugs, aspirin, β-blockers)
- Substance abuse
- Upper airway infections (rhinitis, sinusitis)
- Weather changes

19. **What distinguishes EIA from EIB?**
Exercise-induced asthma (EIA) is a common component of those who have been diagnosed with asthma. Significant symptoms (e.g., cough, chest tightness, wheezing, dyspnea) are noted after exercise in up to 90% of asthmatic children, although abnormal pulmonary function tests can be found in nearly 100% of these patients. *Exercise-induced bronchospasm (EIB)* now more commonly refers to those with airway narrowing in response to exercise who have not been diagnosed with asthma. Up to 12% of adolescent athletes and 40% of college varsity athletes may manifest EIB. Among atopic children, the incidence of EIB has been estimated to be as high as 40%.

Parsons JP, Kaeding C, Phillips G, et al: Prevalence of exercise-induced bronchospasm in a cohort of varsity college athletes, *Med Sci Sports Exerc* 39:1487, 2007.

20. **What is the time course of EIB?**
Symptoms, most commonly cough, peak 5 to 10 minutes after the conclusion of exercise and usually resolve within 30 to 60 minutes.

21. **How is EIB diagnosed?**
- **Exercise challenge:** EIB is likely if the peak flow rate or FEV_1 drops by 15% after 6 minutes of vigorous exercise, either in a laboratory or field setting. This exercise can include jogging on a motor-driven treadmill (15% grade at 3 to 4 mph), riding a stationary bicycle, or running up and down a hallway or around a track in field testing. The greatest reduction in EIB is usually seen 5 to 10 minutes after exercise. As further verification of the diagnosis, if the patient has developed a decreased peak flow (and possibly wheezing), two puffs of a β_2-agonist should be administered to attempt to reverse the bronchospasm.
- **Eucapnic voluntary hyperventilation (EVH):** Involves breathing a dry gas at an increased respiratory rate in an effort to induce bronchospasm and a decrease of FEV_1 of more than 10%.
- **Osmotic challenge:** Inhalation of hypertonic saline or dry powder mannitol to induce bronchospasm.
- **Pharmacologic challenge:** A direct measurement using agents that act on smooth muscle (e.g., histamine, methacholine). A decrease of FEV_1 of more than 20% is diagnostic for EIB.

Cuff S, Loud K: Exercise-induced bronchospasm, *Contemp Pediatr* 25:88–95, 2008.

22. **What mechanisms lead to airway obstruction during an acute asthma attack?**
The main causes of airflow obstruction in acute asthma are airway inflammation, including edema, bronchospasm, and increased mucus production. Chronic inflammation eventually results in airway remodeling, which may not be clinically apparent.

23. **All that wheezes is not asthma. What are other noninfectious causes?**
- **Aspiration pneumonitis:** Especially in a neurologically-impaired infant or an infant with gastroesophageal reflux, and especially if there is coughing, choking, or gagging with

feedings. If there is a clear association with feedings, consider the possibility of tracheoesophageal fistula.

- **Bronchiolitis obliterans:** Chronic wheezing often after adenoviral infection
- **Bronchopulmonary dysplasia:** Especially if there has been prolonged oxygen therapy or ventilatory requirement during the neonatal period
- **Ciliary dyskinesia:** Especially if recurrent otitis media, sinusitis, or situs inversus is present
- **Congenital malformations:** Including tracheobronchial anomalies, tracheomalacia, lung cysts, and mediastinal lesions
- **Cystic fibrosis:** If wheezing is recurrent, failure to thrive, chronic diarrhea, or recurrent respiratory infections
- **Congenital cardiac anomalies:** Especially lesions with large left-to-right shunts
- **Foreign-body aspiration:** If associated with an acute choking episode in an infant older than 6 months
- **Vascular rings, slings, or compression**

24. **How is the severity of an acute asthma attack estimated?**
    See Table 17-1.

TABLE 17-1. CRITERIA FOR ASSESSING THE SEVERITY OF AN ACUTE ASTHMA ATTACK

Sign or Symptom	Mild	Moderate	Severe
PEFR*	70%-90% predicted of personal best	50%-70% predicted of personal best	<50% predicted of personal best
Respiratory rate, resting or sleeping	Normal to 30% increase above the mean	30%-50% increase above the mean	Increase >50% above the mean
Alertness	Normal	Normal	May be decreased
Dyspnea†	Absent or mild; speaks in complete sentences	Moderate; speaks in phrases or partial sentences; infant's cry softer and shorter, infant has difficulty suckling and feeding	Severe; speaks only in single words or short phrases; infant's cry softer and shorter, infant stops suckling and feeding
Pulsus paradoxus‡	<10 mm Hg	10-20 mm Hg	20-40 mm Hg
Accessory muscle use	No intercostal retraction to mild retractions	Moderate intercostal retraction with tracheosternal retractions; use of sternocleidomastoid muscles; chest hyperinflation	Severe intercostal retractions, tracheosternal retractions with nasal flaring during inspiration; chest hyperinflation

(continued)

TABLE 17-1.   CRITERIA FOR ASSESSING THE SEVERITY OF AN ACUTE ASTHMA ATTACK *(continued)*

Sign or Symptom	Mild	Moderate	Severe
Color	Good	Pale	Possibly cyanotic
Auscultation	End-expiratory wheeze only	Wheeze during entire expiration and inspiration	Breath sounds becoming inaudible
Oxygen saturation	>95%	90%-95%	<90%
P_{CO_2}	<35	<40	>40

*Peak expiratory flow rate (PEFR) assessed for children 5 years of age or older.
†Parents' or physicians' impression of degree of child's breathlessness.
‡Pulsus paradoxus does not correlate with phase of respiration in small children.
Within each category, the presence of several parameters, but not necessarily all, indicates the general classification of the exacerbation.
Data from Gentile DA, Michaels MG, Skones DP: Allergy and immunology. In Zitelli BJ, Davis HW (eds): Atlas of Pediatric Physical Diagnosis, 4th ed. St. Louis, Mosby, 2002, p 98.

25. **Is a chest radiograph necessary for all children who wheeze for the first time?**
A chest radiograph should be considered for a first-time wheezing patient in the following situations:
- Findings on physical examination that may suggest other diagnoses
- Marked asymmetry of breath sounds (suggesting a foreign-body aspiration)
- Suspected pneumonia
- Suspected foreign-body aspiration
- Hypoxemia or marked respiratory distress
- Older child with no family history of asthma or atopy
- Suspected congestive heart failure
- History of trauma (e.g., burns, scalds, blunt or penetrating injury)

26. **What are the usual findings on arterial blood gas sampling during acute asthma attacks?**
The most common finding is hypocapnia (i.e., low CO_2) because of hyperventilation. Hypoxemia may also be present unless the child is being treated with oxygen. Therefore, hypercapnia is a serious sign that suggests that the child is tiring or becoming severely obstructed. This finding should prompt reevaluation and consideration of admission to a high-acuity unit.

27. **What are the indications for hospital admission in patients with asthma?**
After therapy in the emergency department, admission is advisable if a child has any of the following:
- Depressed level of consciousness
- Incomplete response with moderate retractions, wheezing, peak flow of less than 60% predicted, pulsus paradoxus of more than 15 mm Hg, Sao_2 of 90% or less, Pco_2 of 42 mm Hg or more
- Breath sounds significantly diminished
- Evidence of dehydration

- Pneumothorax
- Residual symptoms and history of severe attacks involving prolonged hospitalization (especially if intubation was required)
- Parental unreliability

An equally difficult (and very unpredictable) challenge relates to predicting which patients will relapse after responding to therapy and subsequently require hospitalization. This is a major problem because rates of relapse can approach 20% to 30%.

28. **Is a nebulizer more effective than a metered-dose inhaler (MDI) with a spacer for the treatment of asthma?**

For the treatment of exacerbations of asthma, nebulizers are primarily used in children younger than 2 years because of the ease of administration. Although an MDI with a spacer is used more commonly among older children, several studies in emergency rooms indicate that they are equally or more effective as nebulizers among young children, even those with moderate or severe acute asthma. Furthermore, the MDI with a spacer requires less treatment time and has fewer side effects, and it is often preferred by patients and parents.

Dolovich MB, Ahrens RC, Hess DR, et al: Device selection and outcomes of aerosol therapy: evidence based guidelines, *Chest* 127:335–371, 2005.

Castro-Rodriguez JA, Rodrigo GJ: Beta-agonists through metered-dose inhaler with valved holding chamber versus nebulizer for acute exacerbation of wheezing or asthma in children under 5 years of age: a systematic review with meta-analysis, *J Pediatr* 145:776–779, 2004.

29. **List the possible acute side effects of albuterol and other β-agonists.**
- **General:** Hypoxemia, tachyphylaxis
- **Renal:** Hypokalemia
- **Cardiovascular:** Tachycardia, palpitations, premature ventricular contractions, atrial fibrillation
- **Neurologic:** Headache, irritability, insomnia, tremor, weakness
- **Gastrointestinal:** Nausea, heartburn, vomiting

Fortunately these side effects are uncommon.

30. **What is the role of magnesium sulfate in acute asthma attacks?**

Magnesium sulfate is a known smooth muscle relaxant most commonly used in the treatment of preeclampsia. In asthmatic patients, when used in conjunction with standard bronchodilators and corticosteroids, magnesium sulfate can provide additional bronchodilation. Its use is less well studied in children compared with adults. Its role in acute asthma is unclear, but currently it is most commonly used when severely ill patients have failed to respond to conventional therapy.

Caroll W, Lenney W: Drug therapy in the management of acute asthma, *Arch Dis Child Educ Pract Ed* 92:3p82–ep86, 2007.

31. **How is chronic asthma severity classified among children 5-11 years of age?**

The National Heart, Lung, and Blood Institute and National Asthma Prevention Program (NAEPP) define severity in terms of impairment and risk. Four categories are listed: **intermittent, mild persistent, moderate persistent,** and **severe persistent.** Categorization which is also separately done for 0–4 years and ≥ 12 years, helps to guide therapy (Table 17-2).

National Asthma Education and Prevention Program Expert Panel Report 3: *Guidelines for the Diagnosis and Management of Asthma. Full Report 2007*, Bethesda, MD, August 2007, National Heart, Lung, and Blood Institute. NHLBI publication 08-4051. Available at: http://www.nhlbi.nih.gov/guidelines/asthma/asthgdln.htm. Accessed June 16, 2010.

TABLE 17-2. CATEGORIZATION OF ASTHMA SEVERITY

Intermittent	Mild Persistent	Moderate Persistent	Severe Persistent
Symptoms ≤2 times per week	Symptoms >2 times per week but not daily	Daily symptoms	Continual symptoms
Asymptomatic between exacerbations	Exacerbations may affect activity	Exacerbations affect activity	Limited physical activity
Nocturnal awakenings: ≤2 times per month	Nocturnal awakenings: 3-4 times per month	Nocturnal awakenings: >1 time per week but not nightly	Nocturnal awakenings: ≥7 times per week
β-Agonist use: ≤2 times per week	β-Agonist use: >2 times per week, but <1 time per day	β-Agonist use: daily	β-Agonist use: several times per day
FEV_1/FVC: >85%	FEV_1/FVC: >80%	FEV_1/FVC: 75-80%	FEV_1/FVC: <75%
Oral steroid need: 0-1 times per year	Oral steroid need: ≥2 times per year	Oral steroid need: ≥2 times per year	Oral steroid need: ≥2 times per year
No impairment with normal activity	Minor limitation of normal activity	Some limitation of normal activity	Extremely limited normal activity

32. **What is the treatment of choice for patients with *persistent* asthma?**
    Inhaled corticosteroids. Daily administration significantly improves symptoms, reduces exacerbations, and allows healing of the chronic inflammatory changes that have taken place in the airways over time. Dosing and the use of adjunctive medications (e.g., long-acting inhaled $β_2$-agonists, leukotriene-receptor antagonists) depend on the severity of the persistence.

     Rachelefsky G: Inhaled corticosteroids and asthma control in children: assessing impairment and risk, *Pediatrics* 123:353–366, 2009.

33. **Do inhaled steroids affect growth in children?**
    Results are conflicting but tend to indicate that mild growth suppression occurs among children receiving moderate to high doses, particularly in more severe asthmatic children and primarily during the first year of therapy (about 1 cm). These are generally not progressive. Asthma *per se* can also inhibit growth, and inhaled steroid therapy does not appear to affect eventual adult height. It is important that children who require the extended use of inhaled steroids are monitored for height and height velocity and cataracts.

     Guilbert TW, Morgan WJ, Zeiger RS, et al: Long-term inhaled corticosteroids in preschool children at high risk for asthma, *N Engl J Med* 354:1985–1997, 2006.

34. **What is anti-IgE treatment for asthma?**
    Omalizumab is a humanized monoclonal anti-IgE approved for adjunctive therapy of severe persistent asthma in patients aged 12 years and older with an elevated total IgE and sensitivity to perennial allergens. It prevents IgE binding to its high-affinity receptors on mast

cells and basophils. Omalizumab has been shown to reduce asthma exacerbations. Rarely, symptoms of anaphylaxis may develop up to 24 hours after administration, so the clinician administering the drug should be prepared to treat anaphylaxis, and the patient should carry self-injectable epinephrine for 1 day after administration.

Fanta CH: Asthma, *N Engl J Med* 360:1002–1014, 2009.

35. **Is there a role for complementary and alternative medicines in the treatment of asthma?**

There are no clear directions or guidelines for the use of complementary and alternative medicines for children with asthma, although these therapies are often independently used by families. Hypnosis, yoga, relaxation techniques, acupuncture, and massage have shown benefit in some studies, but a recent review of studies involving mind-body techniques, relaxation, manual therapies, and diet has found a tendency to little or no significant difference between sham (placebo) and active therapy.

Markham AW, Wilkinson JM: Complementary and alternative medicines (CAM) in the management of asthma: an examination of the evidence, *J Asthma* 41:131–139, 2004.

36. **How useful are pulmonary function tests when evaluating and following children with asthma?**

Spirometry is used for both the diagnosis and monitoring of asthma in children 5 years of age and older. The diagnosis of asthma requires airflow obstruction with at least a 12% improvement, or reversibility, in FEV_1 from baseline with the inhalation of a short-acting β-agonist. Patient history and physical examination do not adequately predict the degree of a patient's airflow obstruction. Spirometry is also used to monitor asthma after diagnosis and treatment. The goals of asthma therapy include normal or near-normal lung function with treatment. Spirometry should be performed on the patient after treatment has been initiated or changed, based on abnormal lung function, to assess improvement. It should also be performed during periods of prolonged loss of asthma control. Otherwise, in symptomatically controlled patients, it should be repeated at least yearly to monitor the patient long term. *Hand-held peak flow* measurements are useful for monitoring patients, but not for initial diagnosis.

National Asthma Education and Prevention Program Expert Panel Report 3: *Guidelines for the Diagnosis and Management of Asthma. Full Report 2007*, Bethesda, MD, August 2007, National Heart, Lung, and Blood Institute. NHLBI publication 08-4051. Available at: http://www.nhlbi.nih.gov/guidelines/asthma/asthgdln.htm. Accessed June 16, 2010.

KEY POINTS: ASTHMA

1. Characterized by recurrent reversible airway obstruction and inflammation, often with identifiable triggers

2. Typical abnormalities on spirometry include the following: decreased FEV_1 and FEV_1/FVC ratio; increase in FEV_1 (>12%) with bronchodilator or decrease in FEV_1 (>15%) with methacholine or histamine.

3. Classification is based on frequency of symptoms and exacerbations, nighttime awakenings, limitation of normal activities, use of oral steroids and lung function—intermittent, mild persistent, moderate persistent, and severe persistent.

4. $Paco_2$ measurements that are normal (40 mm Hg) or rising in an asthmatic patient with tachypnea or significant respiratory distress are worrisome for evolving respiratory failure.

5. Signs of impending respiratory failure include severe retractions, accessory muscle use (especially sternocleidomastoids), decreased muscle tone, and altered mental status.

37. **What proportion of asthmatic children "outgrow" their symptoms?**
Popular pediatric teaching has been that most children with asthma outgrow their symptoms. However, studies suggest that this is erroneous and that only 30% to 50% become free of symptoms, primarily those with milder disease. Many children who appear to outgrow symptoms have recurrences during adulthood. Studies also indicate that many infants who wheeze with viral infections, and are asymptomatic between illnesses, tend to outgrow their asthma. Children whose initial wheezing occurs later in life, with allergen sensitization as a major factor, tend to have more persistence of recurrent bronchospasm. Although the overall trend is for asthma to become milder, a large percentage of adults have persistent obstructive disease, both recognized and unrecognized.

Sears MR, Greene JM, Willan AR, et al: A longitudinal, population-based, cohort study of childhood asthma followed to adulthood, *N Engl J Med* 349:1414–1422, 2003.

BRONCHIOLITIS

38. **What is the most important cause of lower respiratory tract disease among infants and young children?**
Respiratory syncytial virus (RSV). Up to 100,000 children are hospitalized annually in the United States as a result of this pneumovirus, which is different from—but closely related to—the paramyxoviruses. Disease most commonly occurs during outbreaks in winter or spring in the United States and during the winter months of July and August in the southern hemisphere. In the first 2 years of life, 90% of children will become infected with RSV and up to 40% will develop some lower respiratory disease.

Hall CB, Weinberg GA, Iwane MK, et al: The burden of respiratory syncytial virus infection in young children, *N Engl J Med* 360:588–598, 2009.

39. **What other agents cause bronchiolitis?**
RSV is estimated to cause 50% to 80% of cases. Other agents responsible for bronchiolitis include human metapneumovirus (second most common cause), parainfluenza virus, influenza virus types A and B, and adenovirus. Of these, adenovirus is most likely to result in rare serious sequelae, such as obliterative bronchiolitis.

Bush A, Thomson AH: Acute bronchiolitis, *BMJ* 335:1037–1041, 2007.

40. **What are the best predictors of the severity of bronchiolitis?**
The single best predictor at an initial assessment appears to be **oxygen saturation,** which can be determined by pulse oximetry. An Sao_2 of less than 95% correlates with more severe disease; a low Sao_2 is often not clinically apparent, and objective measurements are necessary. An arterial blood gas with a Pao_2 of 65 or less or a $Paco_2$ of more than 40 mm Hg is particularly worrisome. Other predictors of increased severity include the following:
- An ill or "toxic" appearance
- History of prematurity (gestational age, <34 weeks)
- Atelectasis on chest radiograph
- Respiratory rate of more than 60 breaths/minute
- Infant less than 3 months old

41. **What are the typical findings on a chest radiograph in a child with bronchiolitis?**
The picture is varied. Most commonly, there is hyperinflation of the lungs. About 25% of hospitalized infants have atelectasis or infiltrates. Bilateral interstitial abnormalities with peribronchial thickening are common, or patients may have lobar, segmental, or subsegmental consolidation that can mimic bacterial pneumonia. Bacteremia or secondary bacterial pneumonia, however, is unusual in patients with bronchiolitis. With the possible exception of atelectasis, the chest radiograph findings do not correlate well with the severity of the disease.

42. **Which patients with bronchiolitis are at risk for apnea?**
Apnea in patients hospitalized with bronchiolitis has ranged from 3% to 20% in studies. Concerns of apnea are often used as rationale for hospitalization. Higher-risk patients are those born at term and younger than 1 month, preterm infants (<37 weeks' gestation) and younger than 48 weeks' postconception, and those with an observed apneic episode before evaluation. If none of these clinical criteria are present, the risk of apnea is less than 1%.

Willwerth BM, Harper MB, Greenes DS: Identifying hospitalized infants who have bronchiolitis and are at high risk for apnea, *Ann Emerg Med* 48:4441–4447, 2006.

43. **Is the use of steroids justified for bronchiolitis?**
Although corticosteroids have been used by clinicians for many years for the treatment of bronchiolitis, the preponderance of multiple controlled studies has shown no immediate or long-term advantage with their use, either by the systemic or inhaled route.

Yanney M, Vyas H: The treatment of bronchiolitis, *Arch Dis Child* 93:793–798, 2008.

44. **Are bronchodilators effective as a therapy for bronchiolitis?**
The use of bronchodilator therapy for bronchiolitis is controversial. Infants with a strong family history of asthma are those most likely to respond. Nebulized epinephrine (with both α- and β-adrenergic action) may be more effective than β_2-agonists such as albuterol. In infants with significant wheezing, a trial of a bronchodilator therapy may be considered. Continuation of bronchodilators should be based on a positive clinical response using an objective means of evaluation.

Zorc JJ, Hall CB: Bronchiolitis: recent evidence in diagnosis and management, *Pediatrics* 125:342–349, 2010.

Subcommittee on Diagnosis and Management of Bronchiolitis: Diagnosis and management of bronchiolitis, *Pediatrics* 118:1774–1793, 2006.

45. **Is there a vaccine to prevent RSV infection?**
No, there is not yet a safe and effective vaccine against RSV, although vaccines are in development.
Palivizumab (Synagis), a monoclonal antibody directed against RSV, is effective for prophylaxis of RSV infection in infants. It is given intramuscularly and must be given once per month during the RSV season. This drug is not indicated for the treatment of RSV infection.

KEY POINTS: BRONCHIOLITIS

1. The most common causes are respiratory syncytial virus and metapneumoviruses.

2. The illness severity is greatest between 2 and 6 months of age.

3. Atelectatic changes on chest radiograph are common.

4. In most cases, supportive care is all that is needed.

5. In more severe cases, the value of bronchodilators and corticosteroids is controversial.

46. **Does infection with RSV confer lifelong protection?**
No. In fact, reinfection is very common. In day care centers, up to 70% of infants who acquire RSV infections during the first year of life are reinfected during the subsequent 2 years. Primary infections tend to be the most severe episodes, with subsequent illnesses being more muted. In older children and adults, RSV infections present with the same symptoms as "colds," and reinfection is also common.

47. **If a 5-month-old child is hospitalized as a result of RSV bronchiolitis, what should the parents be told about the likelihood of future episodes of wheezing?**
In follow-up studies, 40% to 50% of these infants have subsequent recurrent episodes of wheezing, usually during the first year after illness. Subclinical pulmonary abnormalities may also persist. The question of whether the pulmonary sequelae are the result of the bronchiolitis or of a genetic predisposition to asthma remains unclear. Factors such as pulmonary abnormalities before the illness, passive cigarette smoke exposure, atopic diathesis, and immunologic responses of virus-specific IgE determine the risk for recurrence.

CLINICAL ISSUES

48. **How is hemoptysis differentiated from hematemesis?**
See Table 17-3.

TABLE 17-3. HEMOPTYSIS VERSUS HEMATEMESIS		
	Hemoptysis	Hematemesis
Color	Bright red and frothy	Dark red or brown
pH	Alkaline	Acid
Consistency	May be mixed with sputum	May contain food particles
Symptoms	Preceded by gurgling	Preceded by nausea
	Accompanied by coughing	Accompanied by retching

Rosenstein BJ: Hemoptysis. In Hilman BC, editor: *Pediatric Respiratory Disease*, Philadelphia, 1993, WB Saunders, p 533.

49. **What are the indications for surgical repair of pectus excavatum?**
This is still an area of considerable controversy. Nearly 1 in 400 children have this congenital chest wall anomaly. Children with pectus excavatum (Fig. 17-1) tend to have reduced total lung capacity, reduced vital capacity, increased residual volume, and reduced stroke volume during maximal exercise.
However, most patients are still in the normal range for these values. The most common complaints relate to poor self-image and decreased exercise tolerance. Counseling is often sufficient for the cosmetic aspects, but many older patients report an improvement in exercise tolerance following repair, despite what appear to be minor changes in cardiac

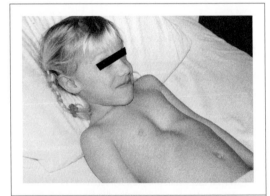

Figure 17-1. Pectus excavatum. (From James EC, Corry RJ, Perry JF: Principles of Basic Surgical Practice. Philadelphia, Hanley & Belfus, 1987, p 173.)

function. Whether the reason is cosmetic or to improve maximal exercise, operative repair should be delayed until the child is older than 16 years to decrease the risk for recurrence during the pubertal growth spurt.

Kelly RE Jr: Pectus excavatum: historical background, clinical picture, preoperative evaluation and criteria for operation, *Semin Pediatr Surg* 17:181–193, 2008.

50. **What are the most common causes of chronic cough?**
Postnasal drip (also known as upper airway cough syndrome) and **asthma** and asthma-like symptoms. The differential diagnosis of chronic cough is very long and includes congenital anomalies, infectious or postinfectious cough, gastroesophageal reflux, aspiration, physical and chemical irritation, and psychogenic cough. After a thorough history and physical examination, evaluation with a chest radiograph and spirometry can also help to establish the diagnosis.

Asilsoy S, Bayram E, Agin H, et al: Evaluation of chronic cough in children, *Chest* 134: 1122–1128, 2008.

Goldsobel AB, Chipps BE: Cough in the pediatric population, *J Pediatr* 156:352–356.e1, 2010.

51. **When should the diagnosis of psychogenic cough be considered?**
A psychogenic cough should be considered in children with a persistent dry, honking, explosive daytime cough that disappears with sleep or at the weekend. It often starts after an upper respiratory infection. The patient complains of a tickle or "something in the throat." Physical examination and laboratory work are normal, and conventional therapies are ineffective. Behavior management is the preferred treatment, although, in some cases, psychological intervention is required. Speech therapy and hypnosis have also been employed successfully.

52. **What medications are most effective for cold symptoms in children?**
Multiple studies have failed to show benefit over placebo of any particular medication, including dextromethorphan, diphenhydramine, codeine, and echinacea. In addition, because the use of over-the-counter cold and cough products with antihistamines and decongestants have been implicated with many adverse events, a U.S. Food and Drug Administration advisory committee has recommended against their use in children younger than 6 years. Many manufacturers have voluntarily removed such products intended for children younger than 2 years. Supportive care with patience and self-resolution of symptoms (tincture of time) remain the mainstay of treatment.

Lokker N, Sanders L, Perrin EM, et al: Parental misinterpretations of over-the-counter pediatric cough and cold medication labels, *Pediatrics* 123:1464–1471, 2009.

Pediatric fatalities associated with over the counter (non-prescription) cough and cold medications, *Ann Emerg Med* 53:411–417, 2009.

53. **What constitutes passive cigarette smoke?**
Passive cigarette smoke consists of both the smoker's exhalation (mainstream smoke, about 15% of total) and the more noxious sidestream (the unfiltered burning end of the cigarette, about 85% of total).

54. **What are the possible risks of passive cigarette smoke exposure?**
- Decreased fetal growth and persistent adverse effects on lung function across childhood from smoking in pregnancy
- Increased incidence of sudden infant death syndrome
- Increased incidence of acute and chronic middle ear effusions
- Increased frequency of upper and lower respiratory tract infections
- Appearance of wheeze illness at an earlier age with more frequent exacerbations
- Impaired lung function during childhood from second-hand smoke after birth

Longer-term issues of increased cancer rates and cardiovascular disease remain under study. In addition, if a parent smokes, a child is twice as likely to become a smoker.

The Health Consequences of Involuntary Exposure to Tobacco Smoke: A Report of the Surgeon General, 2007, Available at: http://www.surgeongeneral.gov/library/secondhandsmoke.pdf. Accessed on June 16, 2010.

55. How is clubbing diagnosed?

Digital clubbing is the presence of increased amounts of connective tissue under the base of the fingernail. This may be determined by the following:

- **Rock the nail** on its bed between the examiner's finger and thumb. In patients with clubbing, the nail seems to be floating.
- **Visual inspection** reveals that the distal phalangeal depth (DPD), which is the distance from the top of the base of the nail to the finger pad, exceeds the interphalangeal depth (IPD), which is the distance from the top of the distal phalangeal joint to the underside of the joint. Normally, the DPD/IPD ratio is less than 1, but in patients with clubbing, it is more than 1.
- **The diamond (or Schamroth) sign:** Normally, if the nails of both index fingers or any other two identical fingers are opposed, there is a diamond-shaped window present between the nail bases (Fig. 17-2); this window disappears in patients with clubbing.

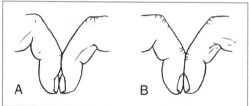

Figure 17-2. A, Normal child with a diamond-shaped window between the nail bases when the fingers are opposed. **B,** In digital clubbing, the diamond-shaped window is obliterated by the increased amount of soft tissue under the base of the nail.

56. What are the causes of digital clubbing?

- **Pulmonary:** Bronchiectasis (as in cystic fibrosis, bronchiolitis obliterans, ciliary dyskinesia), pulmonary abscess, empyema, interstitial fibrosis, malignancy, pulmonary atrioventricular fistula
- **Cardiac:** Cyanotic congenital heart disease, chronic congestive heart failure, subacute bacterial endocarditis
- **Hepatic:** Biliary cirrhosis, biliary atresia, α_1-antitrypsin deficiency
- **Gastrointestinal:** Crohn disease, ulcerative colitis, chronic amebic and bacillary diarrhea, polyposis coli, small bowel lymphoma
- **Endocrine:** Thyrotoxicosis, thyroid deficiency
- **Hematologic:** Thalassemia, congenital methemoglobinemia (rare)
- **Idiopathic:** May be a variation of normal and not indicative of underlying disease
- **Hereditary:** May be a variation of normal and not indicative of underlying disease

Modified from Hilman BC: Clinical assessment of pulmonary disease in infants and children. In Hilman BC, editor: *Pediatric Respiratory Disease*, Philadelphia, 1993, WB Saunders, p 61.

57. What is the pathophysiology of clubbing?

The answer is unclear. The increased connective tissue under the nail beds that causes digital clubbing may be caused by the presence of vasoactive substances that are increased because of hypoxia; increased production in chronic inflammatory disease; or decreased lung clearance. Possible mediators include platelet-derived growth factor and prostaglandin E_2.

58. **Nasal polyps are associated with which conditions?**
    - ■ **Children:** Nasal polyps are rare in children except as a manifestation of cystic fibrosis (Fig. 17-3). About 3% of children with cystic fibrosis have nasal polyps, which are often a recurrent problem.
    - ■ **Adolescents:** There is a wider range of possible diagnoses, including cystic fibrosis, allergic rhinitis, chronic sinusitis, malignancy, "triad asthma" (asthma, nasal polyps, aspirin sensitivity), and ciliary dyskinesia syndrome (e.g., Kartagener syndrome).

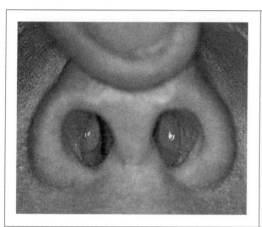

Figure 17-3. Nasal polyps in a patient with cystic fibrosis. (From Zitelli BJ, Davis HW: Atlas of Pediatric Physical Diagnosis, 4th ed. St. Louis, Mosby, 2002, p 550.)

59. **A patient with chronic sinusitis and recurrent pulmonary infections has a chest radiograph that demonstrates a right-sided cardiac silhouette. What diagnostic test should be considered next?**

    Bronchial or nasal turbinate mucosal biopsy for electron microscopic evaluation of cilia. **Kartagener syndrome** is one of the ciliary dyskinesia (or immotile cilia) syndromes. The presenting symptoms are a constellation of recurrent pulmonary infections, chronic sinusitis, recurrent otitis media, situs inversus, and infertility (in males). Structural ciliary abnormalities (most common are absent dynein arms) result in abnormal ciliary beat frequency and decreased clearance of respiratory secretions, thereby predisposing the patient to infection. In addition, because spermatozoa have tails with the same ultrastructural abnormalities as respiratory cilia, they move less well, causing infertility. The cause of the situs inversus (Fig. 17-4) is not fully understood, but it occurs in about 50% of individuals with primary ciliary dyskinesia. It has been

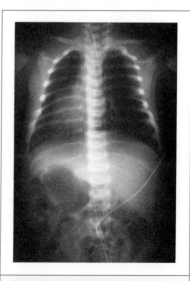

Figure 17-4. Dextrocardia with situs inversus. (From Clark DA: Atlas of Neonatology. Philadelphia, WB Saunders, 2000, p 115.)

suggested that cilia are important for proper organ orientation during embryonic development and that dysfunctional cilia make organ orientation a random event, leading to situs inversus 50% of the time.

60. **What percentage of children snore?**
Between 5% and 10% of preadolescent children are reported by their parents to snore at night.

61. **In which children who snore should obstructive sleep apnea (OSA) be suspected?**
At night, the child with OSA may have persistent snoring interrupted by periods of silence during which respiratory efforts are made, but there is no air movement. Increased work of breathing, with retractions; prominent mouth breathing; unusual sleep postures; frequent nighttime awakenings; enuresis; and night sweats are symptoms of OSA. During the day, there may be excessive daytime sleepiness, learning problems, morning headaches, or personality changes.

62. **What evaluations should be performed on a child with suspected OSA?**
    - **Physical examination:** Mouth breathing while awake, dysphagia, midface or mandibular hypoplasia, tonsillar hypertrophy, cleft palate, palatal deformity caused by adenoidal hypertrophy, failure to thrive (FTT), or obesity
    - **Lateral airway radiograph:** One of the easiest and most direct means of assessing upper airway calibre. Less commonly required are videofluoroscopy of the upper airway, computed tomography, or magnetic resonance imaging.
    - **Flexible nasopharyngoscopy:** Useful for dynamic assessment of the nasal cavities, upper airway, and larynx
    - **Detailed nocturnal polysomnography** (overnight sleep study or polysomnogram [PSG]): Until consistent clinical correlates can be found, the gold standard for the definitive diagnosis of OSA
    - **Cardiologic assessment** (chest radiograph, electrocardiogram, and echocardiography): Used for children with documented OSA and severe or sustained oxygen desaturation

    Wetmore RF: Sleep-disordered breathing. In Wetmore RF, editor: *Pediatric Otolaryngology: The Requisites*, Philadelphia, 2007, Mosby Elsevier, pp 190–201.

63. **What are the potential long-term consequences of OSA?**
The most severe complications of OSA in children are right ventricular hypertrophy, hypertension, polycythemia, compensatory metabolic alkalosis, life-threatening cor pulmonale, and respiratory failure. Later in life, OSA is associated with an increased risk for cardiovascular morbidity and mortality. It is strongly implicated in the development of hypertension, ischemic heart disease, arrhythmias, and sudden death (in individuals with coexisting ischemic heart disease); it also contributes to the risk for stroke.

    Chan J, Edman JC, Koltai PJ: Obstructive sleep apnea in children, *Am Fam Physician* 69:1147–1154, 2004.

64. **What is the most common cause of infantile stridor?**
Congenital laryngomalacia occurs as a result of prolapse of the poorly supported supraglottic structures: the arytenoids, the aryepiglottic folds, and the epiglottis. Stridor is loudest after crying or exertion, but it typically does not interfere with feeding, sleep, or growth. Symptoms usually resolve by the time the infant is 18 months old.

65. **How can you clinically distinguish bilateral from unilateral vocal cord paralysis in an infant?**
Normally, the vocal cords are tonically abducted, with voluntary adduction resulting in speech. With unilateral paralysis, one cord is ineffective for speech, and hoarseness results.

The infant's cry may be weak or absent. Stridor is usually minimal but may be positional (e.g., sleeping on the side with the paralyzed cord up may allow it to fall to midline and produce obstructive sounds). With bilateral paralysis, hoarseness is less apparent, and the cry remains weak, but stridor (both inspiratory and expiratory) is usually quite prominent; in addition, the infant is more likely to have frank symptoms of pulmonary aspiration.

66. **What is the most common cause of chronic hoarseness in children?**
Screamer's nodes. These are vocal cord nodules caused by vocal abuse, such as repetitive screaming, yelling, and coughing. They are the cause of a hoarse voice in more than 50% of children when hoarseness persists for more than 2 weeks.

67. **Which clinical features are suggestive of foreign-body aspiration?**
Symptoms and history
- Child less than 4 years old
- Boys twice as common as girls
- Coughing
- Hemoptysis
- Respiratory infection not resolving with treatment
- History of choking
- Difficulty breathing

Signs
- Fixed, localized wheeze
- Wheezing in a child who has no history of asthma
- Reduced breath sounds over one lung, one lobe, or one segment
- Mediastinal shift
- One nipple higher than the other as a result of unilateral hyperinflation
- Stridor

68. **Are chest radiographs useful for evaluating a foreign-body aspiration?**
Unfortunately, only about 10% to 15% of aspirated foreign bodies are radiopaque. Thus, inspiratory films are often normal. Features suggesting a foreign-body aspiration are as follows:
- Expiratory chest radiograph showing asymmetry in lung aeration as a result of obstructive emphysema (the foreign body often acts as a ball-valve mechanism, allowing air in but not out)
- Right and left lateral decubitus films that show the same asymmetry (these views are often used in uncooperative children who cannot or will not exhale on command)
- Obstructive atelectasis

69. **What are the possible mechanisms for the development of lung abscesses in children?**
- **After pneumonia:** Particularly *Staphylococcus aureus, Haemophilus influenzae, Streptococcus pneumoniae*, and *Klebsiella pneumoniae*
- **Hematogenous spread:** Especially if an indwelling central catheter or right-sided endocarditis is present
- **Penetrating trauma**
- **Aspiration:** Especially in neurologically compromised patients
- **Secondary to infection of an underlying pulmonary anomaly:** Such as a bronchogenic cyst

Campbell PW: Lung abscess. In Hilman BC, editor: *Pediatric Respiratory Disease*, Philadelphia, 1993, WB Saunders, pp 257–262.

70. **What are the typical clinical findings in patients with bronchiectasis?**
Bronchiectasis is the progressive dilation of bronchi, most likely from acute and/or recurrent obstruction and infection. It may result from a variety of infections (e.g., adenoviral, rubeola,

pertussis, tuberculosis), and it is often associated with underlying pulmonary susceptibility (e.g., cystic fibrosis, ciliary dyskinesia syndromes, immunodeficiencies). Clinical findings can be variable but usually include persistent cough, chronic production of purulent sputum, recurrent fevers, and digital clubbing. Inspiratory crackles are often heard over the affected area. Hemoptysis and wheezing can occur but are uncommon.

71. **A novice teenage mountain-climber develops headache, marked cough, and orthopnea at the end of a rapid 2-day climb. What is the likely diagnosis?**
    Acute mountain sickness with high-altitude pulmonary edema. This condition results from insufficient time to adapt to altitude changes above 2500 to 3000 meters, with alveolar and tissue hypoxia as a result of pulmonary hypertension and pulmonary edema. In severe cases, cerebral edema can result. Treatment consists of returning the patient to a lower altitude and administering oxygen. If descent and supplemental oxygen are not available, portable hyperbaric chambers and nifedipine should be used until descent is possible.

    Gallagher SA, Hackett PH: High-altitude illness, *Emerg Med Clin North Am* 22:329–355, 2004.

    Bartsch P, Mairbaurl H, Swenson ER, Maggiorini M: High altitude pulmonary edema, *Swiss Med Wkly* 133:377–384, 2003.

72. **What is the likely diagnosis of a child with diffuse lung disease, microcytic anemia, and sputum that contains hemosiderin-laden macrophages?**
    Pulmonary hemosiderosis. This condition, the presenting symptoms of which can include chronic respiratory problems or acute hemoptysis, is characterized by alveolar hemorrhage and microcytic hypochromic anemia with a low serum iron level. Hemosiderin ingested by alveolar macrophages can often be detected in sputum or gastric aspirates after staining with Prussian blue. Most commonly, the condition is idiopathic and isolated, but it can be associated with cow milk hypersensitivity (Heiner syndrome), glomerulonephritis with anti–basement membrane antibodies (Goodpasture syndrome), and collagen vascular disease.

73. **How should a child with a spontaneous pneumothorax be managed?**
    If the pneumothorax is small and the child is asymptomatic, observation alone is appropriate. Administration of 100% oxygen may speed resorption of the free air, but this technique is less effective in children in older age groups. If the pneumothorax is larger than 20% (as measured by the [diameter of pneumothorax]^3/[diameter of hemithorax]^3) and/or the patient has evolving respiratory symptoms, insertion of a thoracostomy tube and application of negative pressure should be considered. Signs of tension pneumothorax (e.g., marked dyspnea, tachypnea and tachycardia, unilateral thoracic hyperresonance with reduced breath sounds, tracheal shift) necessitate emergent aspiration and tube placement. Adolescents with spontaneous pneumothoraces have a high recurrence rate because of the common association with subpleural blebs. As a follow-up measure, many authorities recommend chest computed tomography with contrast because significant blebs can be treated by surgical pleurodesis.

74. **Describe the clinical and radiographic features of a tension pneumothorax.**
    - **Clinical:** Increasing respiratory distress, hypoxemia, hypercarbia, hypotension
    - **Radiographic:** Hyperlucency of the hemithorax, shifting of the mediastinum, flattening of the diaphragm, widening of the intercostal spaces (Fig. 17-5)

75. **What physical examination features suggest a pleural effusion?**
    - Dullness to percussion
    - Diminished or absent breath sounds on the side of the effusion
    - Diminution in tactile fremitus

- Presence of a friction rub on auscultation
- Egophony ("e" to "a" changes)

76. **In children with pleural effusions, how are exudates distinguished from transudates?**
Exudative pleural effusions meet at least one of the following criteria:
- Pleural fluid protein–to–serum protein ratio of greater than 0.5
- Pleural fluid lactate dehydrogenase (LDH)–to–serum LDH ratio of greater than 0.6
- Pleural fluid LDH more than 0.6 of the serum value
If none of these criteria are met, the patient has a transudative pleural effusion.

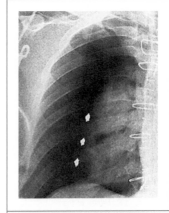

Figure 17-5. Tension pneumothorax. (From Katz DS, Math KR, Groskin SA [eds]: Radiology Secrets. Philadelphia, Hanley & Belfus, 1998, p 61.)

77. **What pediatric diseases are associated with exudative and transudative pleural effusions?**
Exudates result from conditions of increased capillary permeability, whereas transudates occur with increased capillary hydrostatic pressure.
Exudative
- Pneumonia
- Tuberculosis
- Malignancy
- Chylothorax

Transudative
- Congestive heart failure
- Cirrhosis
- Nephrotic syndrome
- Upper airway obstruction
In children, the most common cause for a pleural effusion is pneumonia ("parapneumonic"), whereas, in adults, the most common etiology is congestive heart failure.

Beers SL, Abramo TJ: Pleural effusions, *Pediatr Emerg Care* 23:330–334, 2007.

78. **What are possible treatments for infected parapneumonic effusions?**
Although uncomplicated pleural effusions can usually be managed conservatively without the need for surgery, about 5% of patients with pleural effusions progress to empyema (Fig. 17-6). The precise approach to therapy is controversial and often varies by institution, but options include medical management alone or in combination with thoracentesis, chest tube drainage, video-assisted thoracoscopic surgery (VATS) with chest tube drainage, intrapleural fibrinolytic therapy, and thoracotomy. In general, a simple diagnostic and therapeutic thoracentesis is done with insertion of a chest tube in the early exudative phase of an empyema when fluid is accumulating. VATS therapy is more commonly the treatment of choice in early organizing empyemas (a fibrinopurulent phase), whereas thoracotomy, often combined with pleural stripping, is used in later, more advance empyemas when scar formation can result in lung entrapment.

St. Peter S, Tsao K, Harrison C, et al: Fibrinolysis vs. thoracoscopic surgery for pediatric empyema, *J Pediatr Surg* 44:106–111, 2009.

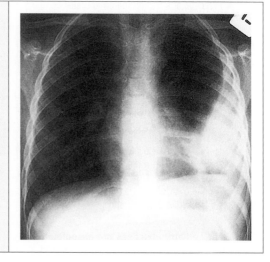

Figure 17-6. Large left empyema with passive atelectasis of the adjacent lung. (From Chernick V, Boat TF, Wilmott RW, Bush A [eds]: Kendig's Disorders of the Respiratory Tract in Children, 7th ed. Philadelphia, Saunders, 2006, p 374.)

79. **What is the value of chest physiotherapy in patients with pediatric pulmonary disease?**

    The main function of chest physiotherapy is to assist with the removal of tracheobronchial secretions to lessen obstruction, reduce airway resistance, enhance gas exchange, and reduce the work of breathing. Its use has been advocated in patients with chronic sputum production (e.g., cystic fibrosis), primary pneumonia, and atelectasis; for intubated neonates; and for postextubation and postoperative patients. Clinical benefits in each category—with the exception of diseases of chronic sputum production—remain highly anecdotal and understudied. Limited evidence does not support a role in bronchiolitis and asthma.

    American Association for Respiratory Care: http://www.aarc.org.

    Lannefors L, Button BM, McIlwaine M: Physiotherapy in infants and young children with cystic fibrosis: current practice and future developments, *J R Soc Med* 97(Suppl 44):S8–S25, 2004.

80. **Who was Ondine, and what was her curse?**

    Ondine was a legendary water nymph who fell in love with Hans, a mortal. She put a curse on him with the stipulation that, should he ever betray her, he would suffocate by not breathing when he fell asleep. Unfortunately, Hans fell for the charms of Bertha, and he eventually succumbed to the curse while dozing. The term *Ondine curse* has been used to describe the syndrome of sleep apnea as a result of reduced respiratory drive, although the term *central hypoventilation syndrome* (CHS) is used more correctly. This rare condition is often associated with other abnormalities of brainstem function. CHS can be idiopathic, or it can be a complication of an earlier insult to the developing brain. In some families, it is genetic. Children with CHS are initially treated by tracheostomy and mechanical ventilation during sleep. Results with phrenic nerve pacing have been good in older infants and children. Familial recurrence of CHS has suggested a genetic etiology and mutations in the *PHOX2B* gene have been reported in studies from France and the United States.

    Weese-Mayer DE, Berry-Kravis EM: Genetics of congenital central hypoventilation syndrome: lessons from a seemingly orphan disease, *Am J Respir Crit Care Med* 170:16–21, 2004.

CYSTIC FIBROSIS

81. **What is the basic defect in patients with cystic fibrosis (CF)?**
A defect in the **CF transmembrane conductance regulator (CFTR) protein.** This is a key ion channel that regulates chloride and sodium transfer across the apical membrane of epithelial cells and other cells. In patients with CF, chloride is poorly secreted into the airway lumen, and there is increased absorption of sodium from the luminal surface of the airway or duct, thereby resulting in respiratory and pancreatic secretions that are relatively dehydrated and viscid. These hyperviscous secretions obstruct pancreatic ducts, resulting in steatorrhea from exocrine pancreatic insufficiency, and they interfere with pulmonary mucociliary clearance, thereby causing chronic respiratory disease. In the sweat gland, CFTR is involved in the reabsorption of chloride, and abnormal CFTR function in patients with CF leads to the production of sweat with increased sodium and chloride concentrations. More than 1500 mutations of the gene that codes for this protein have been identified.

O'Sullivan BP, Freedman SD: Cystic fibrosis, *Lancet* 373:1891–1904, 2009.

82. **What is the incidence of CF in various ethnic groups?**
   - Whites: 1 in 3300 live births
   - Hispanics: 1 in 8000 to 9500 live births
   - Native Americans (in the United States): 1 in 11,200 live births
   - Blacks: 1 in 15,300 live births
   - Asians: 1 in 32,100 live births

Cystic Fibrosis Foundation: http://www.cff.org.

83. **What are the presenting signs and symptoms of CF?**
These can be remembered with the acronym **CF PANCREAS**:
   - **C**hronic cough and wheezing
   - **F**ailure to thrive
   - **P**ancreatic insufficiency (signs of malabsorption, including bulky, foul stools)
   - **A**lkalosis and hyponatremic dehydration
   - **N**eonatal intestinal obstruction (meconium ileus) and nasal polyps
   - **C**lubbing of the fingers and chest radiographs with changes
   - **R**ectal prolapse
   - **E**lectrolyte elevation in sweat (salty skin)
   - **A**bsence or congenital atresia of the vas deferens
   - **S**putum with *Staphylococcus* or *Pseudomonas* (mucoid)

Schidlow DV: Cystic fibrosis. In Schidlow DV, Smith DS, editors: *A Practical Guide to Pediatric Respiratory Diseases*, Philadelphia, 1994, Hanley & Belfus, p 76.

84. **How is the diagnosis of CF made?**
It is made on the basis of the following:
   - Result of a sweat test
   - Mutational analysis in the presence of clinical characteristics of CF (this is performed if the sweat test is equivocal)

85. **What constitutes an abnormal sweat test?**
Sweat gland secretions should be obtained by pilocarpine iontophoresis. A level of sweat chloride of more than 60 mEq/L is abnormal; 40 to 60 mEq/L is borderline; and less than 40 mEq/L is normal.

86. **How are newborns screened for CF?**
Newborns with CF have elevated levels of immunoreactive cationic trypsinogen, which is a precursor of trypsin. If the initial screen for this compound is elevated, mutational analysis of DNA and sweat testing follow in an attempt to confirm the diagnosis. Most states offer CF screening, but there is some debate about whether the clinical benefits of early identification outweigh the clinical and psychosocial risks of screening.

Ross LF: Newborn screening for cystic fibrosis: a lesson in public health disparities, *J Pediatr* 153: 308–313, 2008.

Balfour-Lynn IM: Newborn screening for cystic fibrosis: evidence for benefit, *Arch Dis Child* 93:7–9, 2008.

87. **What are the mainstays of pulmonary therapy for children with CF?**
   - Airway clearance techniques (e.g., chest physiotherapy, mechanical vests, flutter valve)
   - Mucolytic agents (e.g., recombinant human DNAse, acetylcysteine)
   - Anti-inflammatory agents (e.g., ibuprofen, inhaled corticosteroids)
   - Bronchodilators (e.g., β_2-agonists)
   - Antibiotics (oral, inhaled, and intravenous)

O'Sullivan BP, Freedman SD: Cystic fibrosis, *Lancet* 373:1891–1904, 2009.

KEY POINTS: CYSTIC FIBROSIS

1. This is the most common lethal inherited disease in whites.

2. Cystic fibrosis gene: There are more than 1500 known mutations; ΔF508 is the most common in North America (75%).

3. Key to diagnosis: Sweat test (sweat chloride >60 mEq/L is abnormal)

4. A chronic obstructive pulmonary disease

5. Gastrointestinal manifestations can include pancreatic insufficiency, bowel obstruction, rectal prolapse, intussusception, gastroesophageal reflux, and cholelithiasis.

6. Pulmonary colonization with *Pseudomonas aeruginosa* or *Burkholderia cepacia* is a poor prognostic sign.

88. **Which features of CF have prognostic significance?**
   - **Gender:** Males have better survival rates than females, although the gap is narrowing.
   - **Colonization with virulent bacteria:** *Pseudomonas aeruginosa*, methicillin-resistant *S. aureus* (MRSA), and *Burkholderia cepacia* are more serious pathogens, which are often resistant to multiple drugs and difficult to clear after the patient becomes persistently infected. *Stenotrophomonas maltophilia* is an emerging problem; patients who are chronically colonized with these organisms have significantly poorer survival rates than other patients with CF.
   - **Diabetes mellitus** is a negative prognostic factor that is associated with increased rates of decline in pulmonary function.
   - **Malnutrition** is also associated with increased rates of decline in pulmonary function.
   - **Cor pulmonale** is one of the late complications of CF because progressive obstructive airway disease leads to the development of pulmonary hypertension and respiratory failure. The patient's prognosis is poor after the development of cor pulmonale.

- **Pneumothorax** is associated with moderate to advanced lung disease in patients with CF. Therefore, air leak has traditionally been regarded as a poor prognostic sign. The prognosis has been improving now that pneumothoraces are being managed aggressively.
- **Worsening pulmonary function tests:** Patients with an FEV_1 level that is less than 30% of predicted have an increased 2-year mortality rate.

Montgomery GS, Howenstine M: Cystic fibrosis, *Pediatr Rev* 30:302–309, 2009.

Kulich M, Rosenfeld M, Goss CH, Wilmott R: Improved survival among young patients with cystic fibrosis, *J Pediatr* 142:631–636, 2003.

PNEUMONIA

89. **What agents cause pneumonia in children?**
See Table 17-4.

TABLE 17-4. AGENTS THAT CAUSE PNEUMONIA

Age	Viral	Bacterial	Atypical

Birth to 3 wk	Cytomegalovirus
	Herpes simplex virus
		Group B
		  streptococcus
		Gram-negative enteric
		  bacilli (e.g.,
		  Escherichia coli)
		*Listeria
		  monocytogenes*
			*Ureaplasma
			  urealyticum*

3 wk to 3 mo	Respiratory syncytial virus
	Parainfluenza viruses
	Human metapneumovirus
	Influenza A and B
	Adenovirus
	Bocavirus
	Rhinovirus
		*Streptococcus
		  pneumoniae*
		Bordetella pertussis
		*Staphylococcus
		  aureus*
			*Chlamydia
			  trachomatis*

3 mo-5 yr	Respiratory syncytial virus
	Parainfluenza viruses
	Influenza A and B
	Human metapneumovirus
	Adenovirus
	Bocavirus
	Rhinovirus
		*Streptococcus
		  pneumoniae*
		*Haemophilus
		  influenzae*
		  (nontypeable)
		*Staphylococcus
		  aureus*
			*Mycoplasma
			  pneumoniae*
			*Chlamydophila
			  pneumoniae*

**5 yr to
  adolescence**
	Influenza A and B	*Streptococcus
		  pneumoniae*
		*Staphylococcus
		  aureus*
			*Mycoplasma
			  pneumoniae*
			*Chlamydophila
			  pneumoniae*

90. **What are important trends in the etiology of pneumonia in the United States?**
    - **Bacterial:** The introduction of the heptavalent pneumococcal vaccine has substantially reduced hospitalizations for pneumonia.
    - **Viral:** More common in younger age groups, and most frequently RSV. Human metapneumovirus, described initially in 2001, can mimic the clinical picture of RSV. The pandemic of influenza H1N1 places it in the differential diagnosis of community-acquired pneumonia in all age groups.
    - **Atypical pneumonia:** Caused by *Mycoplasma pneumoniae* and *Chlamydophila* (formerly *Chlamydia*) *pneumoniae*, these infections were previously thought to be uncommon in preschool-aged children. In this age group, the incidence is thought to be increasing. Both organisms become more prevalent in school-aged children and are the most common etiology for pneumonia in older children.

    Grijalva CG, Griffin MR, Nuorti JP, et al: Pneumonia hospitalizations among children before and after introduction of the pneumococcal conjugate vaccine—United States, 1997–2006. *MMWR Morb Mortal Wkly Rep* 58:1, 2009.

91. **Are throat or nasopharyngeal cultures helpful for the diagnosis of pneumonia?**
    As a rule, the correlation between throat and nasopharyngeal bacterial cultures and lower respiratory tract pathogens is poor and of limited value. Healthy children may be colonized with a wide variety of potentially pathologic bacteria (e.g., *S. aureus*, nontypeable *Haemophilus influenzae*), which can be considered part of the normal flora; *Bordetella* pertussis is an exception. Polymerase chain reaction studies to identify respiratory viruses, *C. pneumoniae or M. pneumoniae*, is more useful because these organisms are much less commonly carried asymptomatically.

92. **How often are blood cultures positive in children with suspected bacterial pneumonia?**
    10% of the time or less in hospitalized patients. In outpatients with community-acquired pneumonia, the likelihood is lower (<3%). Thus, the sicker the patient, the greater the potential yield. The incidence of bacteremia is unclear because the true denominator in the equation (the number of true bacterial pneumonias) is difficult to ascertain due to imprecision with making a definitive diagnosis. The low rate of positive blood cultures does suggest that most bacterial pneumonias are not acquired by hematogenous spread.

93. **How often are pleural fluid cultures positive in children with suspected bacterial pneumonia?**
    Between 60% and 85% are positive if antibiotics have not already been initiated. This high yield emphasizes the importance of recognizing a pleural effusion in patients with pneumonia and the value of early thoracentesis before starting antibiotic therapy.

94. **How common is an occult pneumonia in a febrile child with leukocytosis?**
    In a search for a focus of infection, the chest is always a suspect. Before the introduction of the pneumococcal conjugate vaccine, children younger than 5 years without clinical evidence of pneumonia but with a temperature of 39°C or higher and a total white blood cell count of 20,000 or more had a positive chest radiograph for pneumonia in 19% of cases. Since the introduction of the vaccine, the likelihood of occult pneumonia has fallen but is still significant at 9%.

    Rutman MS, Bachur R, Harper MB: Radiographic pneumonia in young, highly febrile children with leukocytosis before and after universal conjugate pneumococcal vaccination, *Pediatr Emerg Care* 25:1–7, 2009.

    Bachur R, Perry H, Harper MB: Occult pneumonias: empiric chest radiographs in febrile children with leukocytosis, *Ann Emerg Med* 33:166–173, 1999.

95. **Can a chest radiograph reliably distinguish between viral and bacterial pneumonia?**
No. Viral infections more commonly have interstitial, perihilar, or peribronchial infiltrates; hyperinflation; segmental atelectasis; and hilar adenopathy. Effusions are uncommon. However, there can be considerable overlap in features with bacterial (and chlamydophilal and mycoplasmal) pneumonia. Bacterial pneumonia more commonly results in lobar and alveolar infiltrates, but the sensitivity and specificity of this finding are not very high.

Kronman MP, Shah SS: Pediatric community-acquired pneumonia, *Contemp Pediatr* 26:44–50, 2009.

96. **What are indications for hospital admission in children with pneumonia?**
■ All who appear toxic, dyspneic, or hypoxic
■ Suspected staphylococcal pneumonia (e.g., pneumatocele on chest radiograph)
■ Significant pleural effusion
■ Suspected aspiration pneumonia (because of the higher likelihood of progression)
■ Children who cannot tolerate oral medications or who are at significant risk for dehydration
■ Suspected bacterial pneumonia in very young infants, especially with multilobar involvement
■ Poor response to outpatient therapy after 48 hours
■ Those whose family situation and chances for reliable follow-up are suboptimal

97. **What clinical clues suggest atypical pneumonia?**
Atypical pneumonia refers to one caused by certain bacteria, including *Mycoplasma pneumoniae, Chlamydophila pneumoniae* and *Legionella pneumophila*. These infections tend to start gradually, have minimal or a nonproductive cough, and have frequent constitutional signs (e.g., headache, rash, pharyngitis). Chest radiographs tend to show patchy, peribronchial infiltrates with only occasional lobar consolidation.

98. **What are the causes of "afebrile infant pneumonia" syndrome?**
The syndrome is usually the result of *Chlamydia trachomatis*, cytomegalovirus, *Ureaplasma urealyticum*, or *Mycoplasma hominis*. Affected infants develop progressive respiratory distress over several days to a few weeks, along with poor weight gain. A maternal history of a sexually transmitted infection is common. Chest radiographs reveal bilateral diffuse infiltrates with hyperinflation. There may be eosinophilia and elevated quantitative immunoglobulins (IgG, IgA, IgM). The etiologic causes overlap in clinical picture, although a history of conjunctivitis suggests chlamydia.

99. **What are the clinical characteristics of chlamydial pneumonia in infants?**
■ Illness occurs between 2 and 19 weeks after birth. Most infants show symptoms by 8 weeks of age.
■ Onset is gradual, with upper respiratory prodromal symptoms lasting longer than 1 week.
■ Nearly 100% of patients are afebrile.
■ Less than half have inclusion conjunctivitis.
■ Respiratory signs and symptoms include the following: staccato cough, tachypnea, diffuse crackles, and occasional wheezing.
■ Chest radiograph reveals bilateral hyperexpansion and symmetrical interstitial infiltrates.
■ Seventy percent have an elevated absolute eosinophil count ($>400/mm^3$).
■ More than 90% have increased quantitative immunoglobulins (IgG, IgM).

100. **How helpful are cold agglutinins in the diagnosis of *M. pneumoniae* infections?**
Cold agglutinins are IgM autoantibodies that are directed against the I antigen of erythrocytes, which agglutinate red blood cells at $4°C$. Up to 75% of patients with mycoplasma infections will develop them, usually toward the end of the first week of illness, with a peak at 4 weeks. A titer of 1:64 supports the diagnosis. Other infectious agents, including adenovirus, cytomegalovirus,

Epstein-Barr virus, influenza, rubella, *Chlamydia*, and *Listeria*, can also give a positive result. A single cold agglutinin titer of 1:64 is therefore suggestive but not conclusive evidence of infection with *M. pneumoniae*. Culture and serologic studies are time-consuming, so rapid diagnosis using a specific polymerase chain reaction test for *M. pneumoniae* has been developed.

Waites KB: New concepts of *Mycoplasma pneumoniae* infections in children, *Pediatr Pulmonol* 36: 267–278, 2003.

101. **When do the radiologic findings of pneumonia resolve?**
Although there is a wide range, as a rule, most infiltrates that result from *S. pneumoniae* resolve in 6 to 8 weeks, and those that are caused by RSV resolve in 2 to 3 weeks. However, with some viral infections (e.g., adenovirus), it may take up to 1 year for radiographs to normalize. If significant radiologic abnormalities persist for more than 6 weeks, there should be a high index of suspicion for a possible underlying problem (e.g., unusual infection, anatomic abnormality, immunologic deficiency).

Regelmann WE: Diagnosing the cause of recurrent and persistent pneumonia in children, *Pediatr Ann* 22:561–568, 1993.

102. **Do children with pneumonia need follow-up radiographs to verify resolution?**
Generally, no. Exceptions would include children with pleural effusions, those with persistent or recurrent signs and symptoms, and those with significant comorbid conditions (e.g., immunodeficiency).

Mahmood D, Vartzelis G, McQueen P, Perkin MR: Radiological follow-up of pediatric pneumonia: principle and practice, *Clin Pediatr* 46:160–162, 2007.

103. **What are the causes of recurrent pneumonia?**
- **Aspiration susceptibility:** Oropharyngeal incoordination, vocal cord paralysis, gastroesophageal reflux
- **Immunodeficiency:** Congenital, acquired
- **Congenital cardiac defects:** Atrial septal defect, ventricular septal defect, patent ductus arteriosus
- **Abnormal secretions or reduced clearance of secretions:** Asthma, cystic fibrosis, ciliary dyskinesia
- **Pulmonary anomalies:** Sequestration, cystic adenomatoid malformation, tracheoesophageal fistula
- **Airway compression or obstruction:** Foreign body, vascular ring, enlarged lymph node, malignancy
- **Miscellaneous:** For example, sickle cell disease, sarcoidosis

Kaplan KA, Beierle EA, Faro A, et al: Recurrent pneumonia in children: a case report and approach to diagnosis, *Clin Pediatr* 45:15–22, 2006.

KEY POINTS: PNEUMONIA

1. Effusion or pneumatocele suggests a bacterial cause.

2. Radiographic findings in patients with mycoplasmal infections are highly variable.

3. In half of patients with chlamydial pneumonia, conjunctivitis precedes pneumonia.

4. Hilar adenopathy suggests tuberculosis.

5. In a febrile infant with a white blood cell count higher than 20,000/mm^3, consider a chest radiograph to look for occult pneumonia.

104. **How does the pH of a substance affect the severity of disease in aspiration pneumonia?**
A low pH is more harmful than a slightly alkaline or neutral pH, and it is more likely to be associated with bronchospasm and pneumonia. The most severe form of pneumonia is seen when gastric contents are aspirated; symptoms may develop in a matter of seconds. If the volume of aspirate is sufficiently large and the pH is less than 2.5, the mortality rate may exceed 70%. The radiographic picture may be that of an infiltrate or pulmonary edema. Unilateral pulmonary edema may occur if the child is lying on one side.

105. **How should children with aspiration pneumonia be managed?**
Acute aspiration can often be treated supportively without antibiotics because the initial process is a chemical pneumonitis. If secondary signs of infection occur, antibiotics should be started after appropriate cultures; either penicillin or clindamycin is a reasonable choice to cover the oropharyngeal anaerobes that predominate. If the aspiration is nosocomial, antibiotic coverage should be extended to include gram-negative organisms.

PULMONARY PRINCIPLES

106. **In addition to underlying immunologic immaturity, why are infants more susceptible to an increased severity of respiratory disease?**
   - Very compliant chest wall (allows passage through birth canal but limits inspiratory effort as it distorts with increased respiratory loading)
   - Respiratory muscles more easily fatigued as a result of decreased muscle mass and fewer type I muscle fibers (slow twitch, high oxidative fibers)
   - Chest wall elastic recoil is low in infancy (airway closure occurs at a higher relative lung volume)
   - High airway compliance facilitates airway collapse and air trapping
   - Collateral ventilation poorly developed, thus increasing likelihood of atelectasis during illness
   - Higher airway mucous gland concentration in infants than in adults

107. **At what age do alveoli stop increasing in number?**
Although extra-acinar airway development is complete by 16 weeks of gestation, alveolar multiplication continues after birth. Early studies suggested that postnatal alveolar multiplication ends at 8 years of age. However, more recent studies have shown that it is terminated by 2 years of age and possibly between 1 and 2 years of age. After the end of alveolar multiplication, the alveoli continue to increase in size until thoracic growth is completed.

108. **What is the normal respiratory rate in otherwise healthy children?**
Rates in children who are awake can be widely variable, depending on the psychological state and activity. Rates while sleeping are much more reliable and are a good indicator of pulmonary health. As a general rule in an afebrile, otherwise healthy and calm, resting infant or child, the expected maximal respiratory rate declines with increasing age. In the absence of other signs and symptoms, term newborns breathe up to a mean of 50 breaths/minute, decreasing to 40 breaths per minute by 6 months and to 30 breaths per minute at 1 year. Beyond 1 year of age, the rate declines gradually, reaching the typical adult rate of 14 to 20 breaths/minute by the middle teenage years. Counting respiratory rates over 1 minute gives a more accurate measurement than extrapolating rates over shorter periods to 1 minute.

109. **What is the significance of grunting respirations?**
Grunting respirations are moaning, crying-like noises heard during expiration and thought to be a physiologic attempt to maintain alveolar patency. In patients seen in hospital settings,

grunting is associated with a higher likelihood of serious infections, including pneumonia, pyelonephritis, and peritonitis.

Bilavsky E, Shouval DS, Yarden-Bilavsky H, et al: Are grunting respirations a sign of serious bacterial infection in children? *Acta Paediatr* 97:1086–1089, 2008.

110. **What is normal oxygen saturation in healthy infants who are younger than 6 months?**
In a longitudinal study using pulse oximetry, baseline saturation was higher than 95% (normal was 98%, with the lower 10th percentile at 95%). However, acute desaturations are common; almost all are associated with brief episodes of apnea while sleeping.

Hunt CE, Corwin MJ, Lister G, et al: Longitudinal assessment of hemoglobin saturation in healthy infants during the first six months of life, *J Pediatr* 134:580–586, 1999.

111. **What is the difference between Kussmaul, Cheyne-Stokes, and Biot types of breathing patterns?**
    - **Kussmaul:** Deep, slow, regular respirations with prolonged exhalation; seen in diabetic ketoacidosis and salicylate ingestion
    - **Cheyne-Stokes:** Crescendo-decrescendo respirations alternating with periods of apnea (no breathing); causes include heart failure, uremia, central nervous system trauma, increased intracranial pressure, and coma
    - **Biot** (also known as ataxic breathing): Characterized by unpredictable irregularity; breaths may be shallow or deep and stop for short periods; causes include respiratory depression, meningitis, encephalitis, and central nervous system lesions involving the respiratory centers

112. **Why a sigh?**
A sigh is just a sigh in Casablanca, but it is also a very effective antiatelectatic maneuver. By definition, it is a breath that is more than three times the normal tidal volume.

113. **Is there a respiratory basis for yawning?**
Although a respiratory function for yawning is frequently suggested, scientific support for this belief is minimal. Increasing the concentration of CO_2 in inspired air increases the respiratory rate but does not change the rate of yawning. Relief of hypoxia and opening areas of microatelectasis are other theories that are not supported by scientific studies. Some studies hypothesize that yawning may be an arousal reflex.

114. **What are "coarse" breath sounds?**
In a patient with coarse breath sounds, the loudness of expiration equals the loudness of inspiration on auscultation. In large airways, expiratory breath sounds are louder than inspiratory breath sounds as a result of turbulence. Coarse breath sounds can be physiologic (as when listening just below the center of the clavicle to primarily bronchial sounds) or pathologic (if interposed fluid allows for the transmission of large airway sounds or if airways are widened [e.g., bronchiectasis]).

115. **At what concentration is inspired oxygen toxic?**
In addition to atelectasis, high oxygen concentration can cause alveolar injury with edema, inflammation, fibrin deposition, and hyalinization. The precise level of hyperoxia that results in injury is unclear and varies by age and underlying lung pathology, but a reasonable rule is to assume that a concentration of more than 80% for longer than 36 hours is likely to result in significant ongoing damage; 60% to 80% is likely to be associated with more slowly progressive injury. An inspired oxygen concentration of 50%, even when administered for extended periods of time, is unlikely to cause pulmonary toxicity.

Jenkinson SG: Oxygen toxicity, *J Intensive Care Med* 3:137–152, 1988.

116. **Why is a child who is receiving 100% oxygen more likely to develop atelectasis than one who is breathing room air?**

Nitrogen is more slowly absorbed than oxygen by alveoli. In room air (with its 78% nitrogen), alveolar collapse is minimized by the continued presence and pressure of nitrogen gas (the "nitrogen stint"). With 100% oxygen breathing, however, the high solubility of oxygen in blood can lead to absorption atelectasis in areas of poor ventilation and intrapulmonary shunting.

117. **At what Pao_2 does cyanosis develop?**

Cyanosis develops when the concentration of desaturated (i.e., reduced) hemoglobin is at least 3 gm/dL centrally or 4 to 6 g/dL peripherally. However, multiple factors affect the likelihood that a given Pao_2 will result in clinically apparent cyanosis: anemia (less likely), polycythemia (more likely), reduced systemic perfusion or cardiac output (more likely), and hypothermia (more likely). Cyanosis is generally a sign of significant hypoxia. In a patient with adequate perfusion and a normal hemoglobin, central cyanosis is commonly noted when the Pao_2 is about 50 mm Hg.

118. **What are the causes of a reduced Pao_2 associated with an increased A-aDo_2 (alveolar-arterial oxygen tension difference)?**

- **Right-to-left shunting:** Intracardiac, abnormal arteriovenous connections; intrapulmonary shunts that result from perfusion of airless alveoli (e.g., pneumonia, atelectasis), often referred to as ventilation-perfusion mismatching
- **Maldistribution of ventilation:** Asthma, bronchiolitis, atelectasis, and so forth
- **Impaired diffusion:** An uncommon mechanism because many of the conditions previously thought to have a "diffusion block" (e.g., respiratory distress syndrome) also have a major component of shunting; may be seen when interstitial edema affects the septal walls (e.g., in early pulmonary edema and interstitial pneumonia)
- **Decreased central venous oxygen content:** As a result of a sluggish circulation (e.g., shock) or increased tissue oxygen demands (e.g., sepsis)

119. **How does the pulse oximeter work?**

The key principle behind pulse oximetry is that oxygenated hemoglobin allows for more transmission of red light than does reduced hemoglobin. By contrast, transmission of infrared light is unaffected by the amount of oxyhemoglobin present. A light source of red and infrared wavelengths is applied to an area of the body thin enough that the light can traverse a pulsating capillary bed and be detected by a light detector on the other side. Each pulsation increases the distance the light has to travel, which increases the amount of light absorption. A microprocessor derives the arterial oxygen saturation by comparing absorbencies at baseline and during the peak of a transmitted pulse.

120. **What are the disadvantages or limitations of pulse oximetry?**

- Patient movement disturbs measurements.
- Poor perfusion states affect accuracy.
- Fluorescent or high-intensity light can interfere with results.
- It is unreliable if abnormal hemoglobin is present (e.g., methemoglobin).
- It is unable to detect hypoxia until the Pao_2 decreases below 80 mm Hg.
- Accuracy diminishes with arterial saturations below 70% to 80%.

121. **In infants with unilateral lung disease, should the good lung be up or down?**

The good lung should be **up.** This is another example of why children are not simply small adults. It is well established that adults with unilateral lung disease treated in a decubitus position will have an increase in oxygen saturation when the good lung is placed down; this occurs because of an increase in ventilation to the dependent lung. Studies have shown that the opposite occurs in infants and children because ventilation is preferentially distributed toward the uppermost lung. This positional redistribution of ventilation appears to change to an adult pattern during the late teenage years.

Davies H, Helms P, Gordon I: Effect of posture on regional ventilation in children, *Pediatr Pulmonol* 12:227–232, 1992.

ACKNOWLEDGMENT

The editors gratefully acknowledge contributions by Drs. Ellen R. Kaplan, Carlos R. Perez, William D. Hardie, Barbara A. Chini, and Cori L. Daines that were retained from the first three editions of *Pediatric Secrets*.

CHAPTER 18

RHEUMATOLOGY

Carlos D. Rosé, MD, CIP, Balu H. Athreya, MD,
Elizabeth Candell Chalom, MD, and Andrew H. Eichenfield, MD

CLINICAL ISSUES

1. **What is an ANA?**
   Antinuclear antibody (ANA) is made up of circulating γ-globulins directed against several known and unknown nuclear proteins. Unfortunately, the classic immunofluorescence technique is being replaced by a still nonvalidated enzyme-linked immunosorbent assay (ELISA) technique in order to save costs. When it is measured by an immunofluorescent technique, it is also called *fluorescent antinuclear antibody* (FANA). It is expressed as a titer, usually with a cutoff of 1:40. It is positive in 97% of patients with systemic lupus erythematosus (SLE), usually at a titer at or above 1:320, and in 60% to 80% of patients with juvenile rheumatoid arthritis (JRA), usually at a lower titer. It is also positive in 10% to 30% of normal children and because of that should not be used as a screening test when the child does not present objective physical findings of arthritis.

2. **What is an ANA profile?**
   Out of the many nuclear antigens that can make the FANA test positive, there are some with clinical value in pediatrics. They are grouped under the so-called ANA profile. These are individual antibodies measured by ELISA (commercial laboratories) or Western blot (specialized laboratories).

3. **Should I order a profile instead of an ANA because it has more specificity?**
   No. This test has value only in the right clinical context (see later) and when there is a documented positive ANA by immunofluorescence.

4. **What is the significance of the various antibodies included in the ANA profile?**
   - *Anti–double-stranded DNA:* Associated with systemic lupus erythematosus. This test has to be ordered separately; it is not usually part of the profile.
   - *Antihistone:* Associated with drug-induced lupus
   - *Anti-Ro* (also called anti-SS A): Associated with Sjögren syndrome and neonatal lupus
   - *Anti-La* (also called anti-SS B): Associated with Sjögren syndrome and neonatal lupus

5. **A 6-year-old girl with a 2-month history of joint pain (onset after a viral illness) has a normal physical examination, complete blood cell count, and erythrocyte sedimentation rate (ESR), but a positive ANA titer of 1:160. What are some of the possible explanations for this positive ANA?**
   - Laboratory variation
   - Nonspecific response to viral illness
   - Preclinical state of SLE (least likely)
   - Normal population frequency (about 8% at that titer)
   - Other autoimmune or paraneoplastic conditions

   Tan EM, Feltkamp TE, Smolen JS, et al: Range of antinuclear antibodies in "healthy" individuals, *Arthritis Rheum* 40:1601–1611, 1997.

6. **Is Raynaud phenomenon a disease?**
   In 1874, Maurice Raynaud, while still a medical student, described a triad of episodic pallor, cyanosis, and erythema after exposure to cold stress; the term *Raynaud phenomenon* describes this clinical triad. When this phenomenon is associated with a disease such as scleroderma or lupus, it is called *Raynaud syndrome*; when the phenomenon is seen as an isolated condition without any other rheumatic disorder, it is called *Raynaud disease*, although some patients on long-term follow-up may develop an associated disease (e.g., CREST syndrome [a limited form of systemic sclerosis]). Rheumatologists are commonly consulted for adolescents with blue dusky hands and feet. If there is no pallor, it is probably benign acrocyanosis (Crocq disease), a benign variant of no clinical relevance. It may occur in association with weight loss in athletes or children treated with amphetamine derivatives for attention-deficit/hyperactivity disorder.

   Nigrovic PA, Fuhlbrigge RC, Sundel RP: Raynaud's phenomenon in children: a retrospective review of 123 patients, *Pediatrics* 111:715–721, 2003.

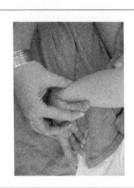

Figure 18-1. Abnormal contact between the thumb and forearm in a young girl with benign hypermobility joint syndrome.

7. **When is a child considered to have hypermobile joints?**
   The presence of three of the following features suggests true hypermobility:
   - Apposition of the thumb to the flexor aspect of the forearm (Fig. 18-1)
   - Hyperextension of the fingers so that they lie parallel to the dorsum of the forearm
   - Hyperextension at the elbow of greater than 10 degrees
   - Knee hyperextension of greater than 10 degrees
   - Ability to touch the floor with the heel and also with the palms of the hands from a standing position without flexing the knee

8. **Which children can demonstrate a Gorlin sign?**
   Gorlin sign is the ability to touch the tip of the nose with the tongue. It is seen in conditions associated with hypermobility syndromes, such as Ehlers-Danlos syndrome.

9. **In what settings can reactive arthritis occur?**
   Reactive arthritis in its broadest sense refers to a pattern of arthritis associated with a nonarticular (remote) infection. By definition, it is an inflammatory arthritis, but a live organism cannot be isolated by culture of synovial fluid or synovial biopsy. A restricted definition of the syndrome includes arthritis after enteric (e.g., *Salmonella*, *Shigella*, *Yersinia*, *Campylobacter*, *Giardia*) or genitourinary infections (e.g., *Chlamydia*).

   Flores D, Marquez J, Garza M, Espinoza LR: Reactive arthritis: newer developments, *Rheum Dis Clin North Am* 29:37–59, 2003.

10. **What conditions are associated with gastroenteritis and arthritis?**
    Noninfectious
    - Ulcerative colitis
    - Crohn disease
    - Behçet disease
    - Henoch-Schönlein purpura
    - Celiac disease

Infectious
- *Salmonella*
- *Shigella*
- *Yersinia*
- *Campylobacter*
- Tuberculosis
- Whipple disease
- Giardiasis

11. **One week after mild trauma, an 8-year-old girl has pain and tenderness in the right foot and leg, both of which are cold, exquisitely tender to the touch, with mottled discoloration. What is the likely diagnosis?**

    Complex regional pain syndrome, type 1. More commonly called *reflex sympathetic dystrophy*, this poorly understood entity is often confused with arthritis because of localized severe pain in one of the extremities. However, there are several features that separate it from arthritis. The pain is not confined to a single joint; it is regional in nature, involving portions of an extremity; and it often follows minor trauma. The pain is very severe, and even light touch causes pain (i.e., hyperesthesia). Several dysautonomic changes (e.g., mottling, color changes, sweating) may occur. Laboratory findings are normal. Autonomic dysfunction can be confirmed by technetium scan or magnetic resonance imaging (MRI), which demonstrates reduced blood flow. Regional osteopenia as a result of disuse may develop.

    Because the role of the sympathetic nervous system is unclear and dystrophy may not occur in all cases, the terminology change has been advised by the International Association for the Study of Pain. In type 1, all of the features of the complex are present without definable nerve injury. In type 2, a definable nerve injury is present.

    Gauntlett-Gilbert J, Meadows C, Connell H, Ramanan AV: When painkillers don't kill pain, *Arch Dis Child Educ Pract Ed* 93:9–13, 2008.

    Sherry DD, Malleson PN: The idiopathic musculoskeletal pain syndromes in childhood, *Rheum Dis Clin North Am* 28:669–685, 2002.

12. **How is complex regional pain syndrome managed?**

    Although many children are cast because of suspected hairline fractures, immobilization is contraindicated. Treatment is aimed at providing pain relief using analgesics and other nonmedical modalities. A good explanation of the mechanism of pain and assurance that this condition is controllable are essential when managing these children and their families. A physical therapy program should be started immediately, with emphasis on passive and active range of motion exercises and the maintenance of function. Aquatherapy is particularly useful in these children to initiate therapy. Desensitization of the painful area using one of several modalities (e.g., biofeedback, transcutaneous electrical nerve stimulation, visualization, acupuncture) should be part of the program. A positive attitude on the part of physicians and therapists is essential. In extreme situations, sympathetic blockade may be needed. Newer therapies also include electrical stimulation of the spinal cord and the use of intrathecal baclofen (a γ-aminobutyric acid receptor agonist that inhibits sensory input to the neurons of the spinal cord).

    Lee BH, Scharff L, Sethna NF, et al: Physical therapy and cognitive-behavioral treatment for complex regional pain syndromes, *J Pediatr* 141:135–140, 2002.

    van Hilten BJ, van de Beek WJ, Hoff JI, et al: Intrathecal baclofen for the treatment of dystonia in patients with reflex sympathetic dystrophy, *N Engl J Med* 343:625–630, 2000.

13. **Do children develop fibromyalgia?**

    Children as young as 9 years old have been described as having this syndrome. *Fibromyalgia* is a condition that is characterized by musculoskeletal aches and pains, fatigue, disturbed sleep patterns, and tenderness over various parts of the body. These tender points are specific for the diagnosis (Fig. 18-2). There should be tenderness over at least 4 of these 11 points for proper classification of individuals. In addition, there should be no tenderness over nonspecific sites such as the forehead or the pretibial region.

Aches and pains are extremely common in children and may be the result of serious medical diseases (e.g., leukemia), mental illness (e.g., depression), and psychosocial stress. Differentiation of chronic musculoskeletal pain of nonorganic origin may be difficult in children and adolescents.

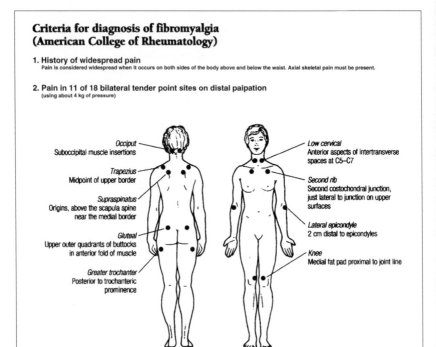

Criteria for diagnosis of fibromyalgia (American College of Rheumatology)

1. History of widespread pain
Pain is considered widespread when it occurs on both sides of the body above and below the waist. Axial skeletal pain must be present.

2. Pain in 11 of 18 bilateral tender point sites on distal palpation
(using about 4 kg of pressure)

Occiput
Suboccipital muscle insertions

Trapezius
Midpoint of upper border

Supraspinatus
Origins, above the scapula spine near the medial border

Gluteal
Upper outer quadrants of buttocks in anterior fold of muscle

Greater trochanter
Posterior to trochanteric prominence

Low cervical
Anterior aspects of intertransverse spaces at C5–C7

Second rib
Second costochondral junction, just lateral to junction on upper surfaces

Lateral epicondyle
2 cm distal to epicondyles

Knee
Medial fat pad proximal to joint line

Figure 18-2. American College of Rheumatology criteria for the diagnosis of fibromyalgia. (From Ballinger S, Bowyer S: Fibromyalgia: the latest "great" imitator. Contemp Pediatr 14:147, 1997.)

DERMATOMYOSITIS AND POLYMYOSITIS

14. **What are the criteria used for the diagnosis of juvenile dermatomyositis and polymyositis?**
   - Symmetrical proximal muscle weakness (e.g., Gower sign)
   - Elevated serum enzymes in muscle (creatine kinase [CK], lactic dehydrogenase [LDH], aspartate transaminase [AST], and/or aldolase)
   - Abnormal electromyogram (increased insertional activity, myopathic pattern, polymorphic potentials)
   - Inflammation and/or necrosis on muscle biopsy
   - Characteristic skin eruption

   The presence of rash distinguishes dermatomyositis from polymyositis. Three out of four criteria plus a pathognomonic rash establish the diagnosis of dermatomyositis, and a confirmatory biopsy is not necessary. If fewer criteria are met, a biopsy may be needed for diagnosis.

Compeyrot-Lacassagne S, Feldman BM: Inflammatory myopathies in children, *Pediatr Clin North Am* 52:493–520, 2005.

Ramanan AV, Feldman BM: Clinical features and outcomes of juvenile dermatomyositis and other childhood-onset myositis syndromes, *Rheum Dis Clin North Am* 28:833–857, 2002.

15. **What skin changes are pathognomonic for dermatomyositis?**
Gottron patches
(Fig. 18-3). These begin as inflammatory papules over the dorsal aspect of interphalangeal joints and the extensor aspect of the elbows and knee joints. The papules become violaceous and flat topped and may coalesce to become patches. Eventually, the lesions show atrophic changes and become hypopigmented.

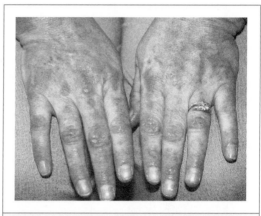

Figure 18-3. Gottron papules. (From Fitzpatrick JE, Aeling JL: Dermatology Secrets, 2nd ed. Philadelphia, Hanley & Belfus, 2001, p 257.)

16. **What are the other classic cutaneous findings of dermatomyositis among children?**
- Periorbital edema and erythema with violaceous color of the upper eyelid (heliotrope rash)
- Rash over the upper chest in the shawl distribution
- Photosensitivity
- Cutaneous vasculitis with ulceration
- Nail-fold capillary abnormalities

17. **Which infectious agents are known to cause myositis?**
- **Viral:** Notably Coxsackie (named after Coxsackie, NY) and influenza A and B
- **Bacterial:** *Staphylococcus* and *Yersinia* (causing pyomyositis)
- **Protozoal:** *Toxoplasma* and trichinosis
- **Spirochetal:** *Borrelia*
  The most common cause of acute muscle disease associated with pain, difficulty walking, and a high level of creatine kinase is viral myositis.

JUVENILE IDIOPATHIC ARTHRITIS

18. **Why is JRA becoming juvenile idiopathic arthritis (JIA)?**
The Europeans and Canadians have never liked the term "rheumatoid" embedded in JRA, which has been used in the United States since 1977, because it suggests homology with the adult disease (rheumatoid arthritis). In the same year of 1977 in the city of Basel, European investigators coined the term JCA, which included pretty much all forms of primary childhood arthritis. The International League of Associations of Rheumatology (ILAR) ended the transatlantic dispute and has come up with the new name—JIA (juvenile **idiopathic** arthritis).

At least there is some consistency because the "J" and the "A" remain unchanged. "J" stands for *juvenile* (before the 17th birthday for disease onset), and "A" for *arthritis*, meaning joint inflammation. The new classification went through multiple revisions and is still work in progress. The potential advantages are (1) the end of the confusion and (2) the hopeful beginning of the solution by recognizing at least that we do not know what causes the disease (it may pay to be humble). The fact that the term JRA continues to be used in the United States and Latin America ensures the terminology turmoil will persist for a while.

19. **What is synovitis, and at what point is it considered chronic?**
Synovial inflammation (synovitis) is the primary pathologic lesion in JIA. It is chronic at 6 weeks in the United States and at 3 months in Europe.

20. **What is the most common chronic arthritis seen in children?**
JIA, with a point prevalence of about 1:1000.

21. **What are the diagnostic criteria for the classification of JIA?**
JIA is a diagnosis of exclusion. Features include the following:
- Onset at ≤16 years of age
- Clinical arthritis with joint swelling or effusion, increased heat, and limitation of range of motion with tenderness
- Duration of disease of ≥6 weeks

22. **What are the characteristics of the seven main subsets of JIA?**
The seven major subgroups are distinguished by the number of joints, presence of rheumatoid factor, and different combination of extra-articular manifestations (Table 18-1).

23. **Describe the pattern of fever and rash of the systemic-onset subset of JIA.**
Systemic-onset JRA (Still disease) accounts for about 15% of cases of children with JIA. Affected individuals typically have fever of unknown origin with once- or twice-daily (i.e., quotidian) temperature spikes, often higher than 40°C. Shaking chills often precede the fever. The temperature characteristically returns to 37°C or lower; continuous fever should suggest other diagnoses.

A blotchy, light pink, evanescent rash that blanches on compression and that may show perimacular pallor accompanies the fever in more than 90% of cases (Fig. 18-4). The rash of systemic JIA is diagnostic only after the diagnosis is made (by exclusion). Arthritis may not be present during the first several weeks of illness. Serositis, hepatosplenomegaly, and lymphadenopathy are other significant findings in patients with this form of the disease.

Ravelli A, Martini A: Juvenile idiopathic arthritis, *Lancet* 369:767–778, 2007.

24. **Why is it sometimes difficult to distinguish systemic JIA from leukemia?**
Up to 20% of patients with leukemia have some degree of musculoskeletal symptoms, including joint pain and occasional swelling. In both diseases, there is anemia, fever, and weight loss. Both can appear with hepatosplenomegaly and lymphadenopathy. In leukemia, however, the fever is not usually spiking, and platelets tend to be low to low normal. A good examination of a peripheral smear is crucial. A high lactic dehydrogenase level is very suggestive of leukemia, and the technetium-99 bone scan shows a different pattern of uptake. More than one bone marrow biopsy may be necessary.

Ostrov BE, Goldsmith DP, Athreya BH: Differentiation of systemic juvenile rheumatoid arthritis from acute leukemia near the onset of disease, *J Pediatr* 122:595–598, 1993.

Tuten HR, Gabos PG, Kumar SJ, Harter GD: The limping child: a manifestation of acute leukemia, *J Pediatr Orthop* 18:625–629, 1998.

TABLE 18-1. SUBSETS OF JUVENILE IDIOPATHIC ARTHRITIS

Subset	No. of Joints	Age	Uveitis	RF	ANA	HLA-B27	Remission	Other Symptoms
Systemic	Any	0-16 mo	–	–	–	–	50%	Fever, visceromegaly, serositis, rash
Oligopersistent	1-4	2 yr	++++	–	++++	–	60%	None
Oligoextended*	>5	2 yr	++++	–	++++	–	20%	None
Polyarticular RF(–)	>5	3 yr	+++	–	+++	–	15%	Subcutaneous nodules (small)
Polyarticular RF(+)	>5	12-17 yr	None	+	++	–	0%	Subcutaneous nodules (large)
Enthesitis-related arthritis	Any number	8-16	Acute	–	–	+	Unknown	Tendinous involvement Enthesitis[†]
Psoriatic arthritis	Any number	Any	+	–	+/–		Low	Dactylitis, psoriasis of nails and skin, tendinous involvement
Other arthritis[‡]	N/A	N/A	N/A	N/A	N/A	N/A	N/A	N/A

*After a typical oligoarticular onset with an oligoarticular course for 6 months, the new joints become recruited.
[†]Inflammation at the insertion point of tendons, capsule, and ligaments.
[‡]Any form of chronic arthritis that fails to meet criteria for any of the other subsets.

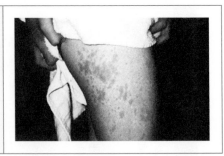

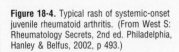

Figure 18-4. Typical rash of systemic-onset juvenile rheumatoid arthritis. (From West S: Rheumatology Secrets, 2nd ed. Philadelphia, Hanley & Belfus, 2002, p 493.)

25. **In a patient with suspected rheumatic disease, what clinical features are more suggestive of malignancy?**
Particularly concerning are nonarticular bone pain, back pain as the principal symptomatic feature, bone tenderness, and severe constitutional symptoms. Children with rheumatic joint problems are typically stiff, and they may complain about pain. The pain of malignancy is out of proportion to the amount of swelling around the joint, and it tends to be worse at night. It is vital to think about the possibility of malignancy in children with rheumatic complaints.

 Cabral DA, Tucker LB: Malignancies in children who initially present with rheumatic complaints, *J Pediatr* 134:53–57, 1999.

26. **What is the value of measuring ANA and rheumatoid factor (RF) in patients with JIA?**
After JIA has been diagnosed on clinical grounds, results of these tests help assign the patient to the appropriate category (e.g., Oligociarticular or RF-positive polyarticular). Because ANA can be present in 10% to 30% of normal children, this test should not be used as a screening test to diagnose JIA in children who experience noninflammatory pain. These tests are also useful as prognostic indicators. The presence of ANA increases the risk for uveitis, thereby making ophthalmologic surveillance more important. RF is valuable as a marker of poor prognosis in adolescents with polyarticular arthritis.

27. **Are radiographs helpful for diagnosing JIA?**
No. There are no characteristic radiographic changes at onset. The value of radiology is to rule out other skeletal conditions and to provide a documented baseline status.

28. **A patient with JIA who becomes ill with thrombocytopenia, profound anemia, and markedly elevated transaminases probably has what complication?**
Macrophage activation syndrome (MAS). This is new conceptualization of an old problem seen in children with systemic-onset JIA both at onset (even at presentation) and late during the course of disease. It is characterized by a massive upregulation of T-cell and macrophagic function, with vast release of proinflammatory cytokines leading to hemophagocytosis (the hallmark). It is believed that, in most cases, MAS is triggered by a viral infection. MAS is the single most important contributor of mortality (which lately has improved), together with gastrointestinal bleeding and infection among patients with systemic JIA. The name and nosologic classification of this entity are currently being debated by experts in the field.

29. **What are the main features of the macrophage activation syndrome?**
 ■ Worsening of fever and rash
 ■ Profound anemia (due in part to hemophagocytosis), leukopenia, and thrombocytopenia

- Disseminated intravascular coagulation with hypofibrinogenemia and pseudonormalization of ESR
- Liver dysfunction
- Hypertriglyceridemia
- Hyponatremia (pseudo)
- Massive increase in ferritin levels
- Occasional central nervous system involvement
- Generalized musculoskeletal pain

Ramanan AV, Schneider R: Macrophage activation syndrome—what's in a name! *J Rheum* 30:2513–2516, 2003.

KEY POINTS: JUVENILE IDIOPATHIC ARTHRITIS

1. Sine qua non: Persistence for ≥ 6 weeks

2. Seven subtypes differentiated by number of involved joints, presence of rheumatoid factor, and extra-articular involvement

3. Characteristic finding: Morning stiffness or soreness that improves during the day

4. No diagnostic laboratory tests are diagnostic

5. Patients <7 years old with antinuclear antibody–positive oligoarticular juvenile idiopathic arthritis at highest risk for uveitis

30. **What has been the traditional first-line approach to JIA medical management?**
The so-called first-line therapy consists of **nonsteroidal anti-inflammatory drugs (NSAIDs).** Given at the correct dose, they exert pain relief and suppress inflammation (decrease in morning stiffness), with a peak action at 4 to 6 weeks. The classic representatives of this group are aspirin, ibuprofen, naproxen, tolmetin, and indomethacin. Choice among them is made on the basis of availability in liquid form, half-life, side-effect profile, individual doctor preferences, and results of an individual trial. Most of their action is through inhibition of cyclooxygenase. About one third of patients have their symptoms controlled through the use of NSAIDs; two thirds require more aggressive drug therapy. For patients with oligoarticular disease, intra-articular injection of corticosteroids is also considered first-line therapy.

31. **What second-line agents have been used in the treatment of JIA?**
    - Gold salts
    - Penicillamine
    - Hydroxychloroquine
    - Sulfasalazine
    - Methotrexate

    Of these, only methotrexate has been proved beneficial in a randomized, double-blind, placebo-controlled trial.

    Giannini EH, Brewer EJ, Kuzmina N, et al.: Methotrexate in resistant juvenile rheumatoid arthritis: results of the USA-USSR double blind placebo controlled trial, *N Engl J Med* 326:1043–10499, 1992.

32. **When are corticosteroids indicated for children with JIA?**
    - Life-threatening disease (e.g., carditis, myocarditis)
    - Unremitting fever unresponsive to NSAIDs

- Unrelenting polyarthritis with severe limitations requiring intensive physical therapy to achieve ambulatory status
- Topical therapy for uveitis (rarely, systemic steroids are needed for children with aggressive uveitis unresponsive to topical therapy)

33. **What are the most common side effects of prolonged corticosteroid therapy?**
Effects can be minimized by alternate-day therapy, but sometimes the treatment is worse than the disease. Commonly encountered problems associated with high-dose corticosteroid use in children can be remembered using the mnemonic **CUSHINGOID MAP**:
- **C**ataracts
- **U**lcers
- **S**triae
- **H**ypertension
- **I**nfectious complications
- **N**ecrosis of bone (avascular)
- **G**rowth retardation
- **O**steoporosis
- **I**ncreased intracranial pressure (pseudotumor cerebri)
- **D**iabetes mellitus
- **M**yopathy
- **A**dipose tissue hypertrophy (obesity, "buffalo hump")
- **P**ancreatitis

34. **What are biologic agents?**
These are genetically engineered products that act by blocking specific immune pathways, such as cytokine signaling, to lessen inflammation. Etanercept, the first biologic agent used in the treatment of JIA, blocks the actions of tumor necrosis factor-α, a proinflammatory cytokine. A growing variety of other agents are used, including adalimumab, another antibody to tumor necrosis factor, and abatacept, which is a costimulation blocker that acts by blocking receptors on antigen-presenting cells. Others act as interleukin receptor antagonists. Biologic agents have become important therapeutic options for patients with JIA resistant to or intolerant of conventional treatments.

   Lovell DJ, Reiff A, Jones OY, et al: Long-term safety and efficacy of etanercept in children with polyarticular-course juvenile rheumatoid arthritis, *Arthritis Rheum* 54:1987–1994, 2006.

35. **Which children with JIA require the most frequent monitoring for uveitis?**
Uveitis (also called *iridocyclitis*) is inflammation of the iris and the ciliary body. It occurs on average in 20% of patients with pauciarticular JRA and in 5% of patients with polyarticular disease. Table 18-2 summarizes the American Academy of Pediatrics guidelines for frequency of slit-lamp examination developed by the sections of ophthalmology and rheumatology. Patients at high risk require quarterly examinations; those at moderate risk need biannual examinations; and those at low risk can be examined annually.

   Nguyen QD, Foster CS: Saving the vision of children with juvenile rheumatoid arthritis-associated uveitis, *JAMA* 280:1133–1134, 1998.

36. **What is the earliest sign of uveitis among patients with JIA?**
When the anterior chamber of the eye is examined with a slit lamp, a "**flare**" is the earliest sign. This is a hazy appearance as a result of an increased concentration of protein and inflammatory cells. Later signs can include a speckled appearance of the posterior cornea (as a result of keratic precipitates), an irregular or poorly reactive pupil (as a result of synechiae between the iris and lens), band keratopathy, and cataracts.

   Foster CS: Diagnosis and treatment of juvenile idiopathic arthritis-associated uveitis, *Curr Opin Ophthalmol* 14:395–398, 2003.

TABLE 18-2. FREQUENCY OF OPHTHALMOLOGIC EXAMINATION IN PATIENTS WITH JIA

Type	Antinuclear Antibodies	Age at Onset	Duration of Disease (Years)	Risk Category	Eye Examination Frequency (Months)
Oligo- or polyarthritis	+	≤6	≤4	High	3
	+	≤6	>4	Moderate	6
	+	≤6	>7	Low	12
	+	>6	≤4	Moderate	6
	+	>6	>4	Low	12
	−	≤6	≤4	Moderate	6
	−	≤6	>4	Low	12
	−	>6	N/A	Low	12
Systemic disease (fever, rash)	N/A	N/A	N/A	Low	12

Data from Cassidy J, Kivlin J, Lindsley C, Nocton J: Ophthalmologic examinations in children with juvenile rheumatoid arthritis. *Pediatrics* 117:1843-1845, 2006.

37. **What are the juvenile spondyloarthropathies under the revised classification system?**
The spondyloarthropathies are now considered one of the subsets of JIA and are recognized under the heading enthesitis-related arthritis.

38. **What are the characteristic clinical features of the juvenile spondyloarthropathies?**
 - Affect males older than 8 years of age
 - Enthesitis (inflammation of tendon, capsule, and ligament insertion sites) characteristic
 - Prodromal oligoarthritis involving large joints of the lower extremities including the hip
 - Involvement of the sacroiliac joints and of the back, which is manifested as pain, stiffness, and reduced range of motion
 - Associated with HLA-B27 (≤90% in children with ankylosing spondylitis and 60% of those with other spondyloarthropathies)
 - Seronegativity: ANA and rheumatoid factors typically negative

39. **How is enthesitis diagnosed clinically?**
The *enthesis* is the site of attachment of ligaments, tendons, capsule, and fascia to bone. Enthesopathy is unique to the spondyloarthropathies and appears as painful localized tenderness at the tibial tubercle (which may be mistaken for Osgood-Schlatter disease), the peripheral patella, and the calcaneal insertion of the Achilles tendon and plantar fascia (which may be mistaken for Sever disease). Thickening of the Achilles tendon and tenderness of the metatarsophalangeal joints are associated findings. MRI can be extremely helpful. The T2-weighted image may show bone marrow edema adjacent to the enthesis.

40. **Why is the diagnosis of ankylosing spondylitis difficult to make in children?**
A child may have undifferentiated spondyloarthritis (an enthesitis-related arthritis) that is characterized by enthesitis and recurrent episodes of lower-extremity oligoarthritis for several

years before he or she develops back symptoms. To fulfill the criteria for ankylosing spondylitis, clinical features of lumbar spine pain, limitation of lumbar motion, and radiographic signs of sacroiliitis must be present. The average time from onset of symptoms to diagnosis in an adult with ankylosing spondylitis is 5 years; many adolescents are adults before they fulfill the criteria (Fig. 18-5). MRI is very helpful to document early sacroiliitis.

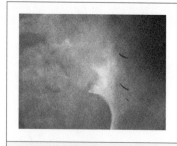

Figure 18-5. Periarticular sclerosis in a boy with chronic sacroiliitis and a diagnosis of spondyloarthropathy.

41. Where are the dimples of Venus?
The dimples of Venus are prominent paravertebral indentations in the lower back of some individuals. A line drawn between the dimples marks the lumbosacral junction; this is the midpoint for the Schober test, which is a measure of anterior flexion of the lumbosacral spine.

LYME DISEASE

42. What criteria are used to diagnose Lyme disease?
Classification criteria (i.e., case definition) as determined by the Centers for Disease Control and Prevention include the following:
- Erythema migrans: enlarging circular erythematous lesion (minimum size, 5 cm), *or*
- At least one clinical manifestation (arthritis, cranial neuropathy, atrioventricular block, aseptic meningitis, radiculoneuritis) and isolation or serologic evidence of *Borrelia burgdorferi* infection

43. How is Lyme disease confirmed in the laboratory?
Although attempts to demonstrate borrelial DNA in infected tissues by polymerase chain reaction has met with some success and cultures occasionally render positive results, the main diagnostic tool continues to be serology. Immunoglobulin M (IgM) peaks about 4 weeks after infection, and IgG does so at 6 weeks. This is the main reason why antibodies may not be detected during the early dermatologic and neurologic stages.

There are two detection techniques: ELISA and Western blot. Both are available for IgG and IgM. ELISA measures whole components of *Borrelia*. It is a very sensitive test, but with many false-positive results. A negative ELISA requires no further investigation at a given time. All positive ELISAs—particularly those with borderline positivity—should be confirmed by Western blot. This is the so-called two-tier system.

A newer test—the C6 peptide ELISA—measures IgG to a relatively invariant lipoprotein on the spirochete and as a single test has been shown to be as sensitive and almost as specific as the two-tier system.

Steere AC, McHugh G, Damle N, et al: Prospective study of serologic tests for Lyme disease, *Clin Infect Dis* 47:188–195, 2008.

44. Describe the classic rash of Lyme disease.
Erythema migrans (previously known as *erythema chronicum migrans*) is the distinctive cutaneous lesion of Lyme disease. The lesion begins as a small red macule or papule and enlarges in an annular centrifugal fashion to about 10 to 15 cm or more in diameter. The lesions may have varying intensities of redness within the plaque, partial central clearing, or a

ring-within-a-ring configuration. Occasionally, the central area may become indurated, vesicular, or crusted. Erythema migrans lesions usually appear within 11 days of the bite of an infected *Ixodes* tick (range, 2 to 30 days). Multiple lesions are present in only about 20% of cases.

45. **If infection ensues after a tick bite, how does Lyme disease progress?**
   - **Early localized disease:** 2 to 30 days. Sixty to 80% of children will develop erythema migrans. Some may have a flu-like illness with fever, myalgia, headache, fatigue, arthralgia and malaise.
   - **Early disseminated disease:** 3 to 12 weeks. Clinical manifestations reflect hematogenous spread to other sites; these include secondary erythema migrans, cranial nerve palsies (primarily facial nerve), and aseptic meningitis. Much more rarely seen in children (compared with adults) are radiculoneuritis and carditis (with varying degrees of heart block).
   - **Late disease:** 2-12 months. In children, the most common manifestation is arthritis. Rarely, encephalomyelitis can develop. There is controversy regarding chronic Lyme disease.

   Kest HE, Pineda C: Lyme disease, *Contemp Pediatr* 25:56–64, 2008.

   Feder HM Jr, Johnson BJB, O'Connell S, et al: A critical appraisal of "chronic Lyme disease." *N Engl J Med* 357:1422–1430, 2007.

KEY POINTS: LYME DISEASE

1. Spirochete *Borrelia burgdorferi* is the culprit.

2. Only one third of patients recall the tick bite.

3. The erythema migrans rash is virtually diagnostic.

4. Enzyme-linked immunosorbent assay testing has a high false-positive rate; confirm with Western blot analysis.

5. Potential complications include arthritis, aseptic meningitis and cranial nerve palsies, and atrioventricular block.

6. Lyme meningitis (compared with viral meningitis): Cranial neuropathy and papilledema are more common, with longer duration of symptoms before diagnosis.

46. **How is the diagnosis of Lyme meningitis established?**
   The diagnosis is often inexact and is commonly made on the basis of the finding of cerebrospinal fluid pleocytosis and the presence of erythema migrans and/or positive serology. Both ELISA and Western blot testing may be negative or indeterminate early during the course of infection, when dissemination to the central nervous system has occurred. Specific testing of the cerebrospinal fluid for intrathecal production of specific antibody and demonstration of *B. burgdorferi* DNA by polymerase chain reaction testing are not readily available, and the latter is relatively insensitive.

47. **How are Lyme disease and viral meningitis clinically differentiated?**
   Both are predominantly summertime illnesses, but the distinction is critical because Lyme meningitis requires weeks of intravenous antibiotics. In addition to the possible presence of erythema migrans, other areas of clinical distinction in patients with signs and symptoms of meningitis include the following:
   - Cranial neuropathy, especially peripheral seventh-nerve palsy, is strongly suggestive of Lyme meningitis.

- Papilledema is more commonly seen in patients with Lyme meningitis.
- Longer duration (7 to 12 days versus 1 to 2 days) of symptoms, including headache before lumbar puncture, is more typical of Lyme meningitis.
- Rash of erythema migrans
- Cerebrospinal fluid pleocytosis should not have more than 10% neutrophils in Lyme meningitis

  Either the rash of erythema migrans, papilledema, or a cranial nerve palsy is seen in more than 90% of patients with Lyme meningitis but in almost none with viral meningitis.

Avery RA, Frank G, Glutting, Eppes SC: Prediction of Lyme meningitis in children from a Lyme disease-endemic region: a logistic-regression model using history, physical, and laboratory findings, *Pediatrics* 117:e1–e7, 2006.

Shah SS, Zaoutis TE, Turnquist JL, et al: Early differentiation of Lyme from enteroviral meningitis, *Pediatr Infect Dis J* 24:542–545, 2005.

48. **Should lumbar punctures be done for patients with facial palsy and suspected Lyme disease?**
    This remains debated because studies in the late 1990s revealed "occult meningitis" (i.e., cerebrospinal fluid [CSF] pleocytosis) in patients without meningeal signs but with Lyme facial palsy. However, the clinical significance of an abnormal CSF is unclear, and there has been no apparent increase in late-stage Lyme disease in those treated with oral antibiotics alone. Consequently, most experts advise no lumbar puncture for suspected or confirmed Lyme facial palsy, unless there is severe or prolonged headache, nuchal rigidity, or other meningeal signs.

49. **How is Lyme arthritis differentiated from septic arthritis?**
    The inflammation generated by Lyme arthritis is significantly less intense than septic arthritis. With Lyme arthritis, which typically involves a single large joint (knee $\geq$90%), range of motion is less limited, and weight bearing is sometimes possible. On joint aspiration, septic arthritis more typically shows more than 100,000 cells/mL^3.

50. **What is the prognosis for children diagnosed with Lyme arthritis?**
    Multiple studies have shown that the long-term prognosis for treated patients is excellent, with little morbidity. Clinicians should be aware that persistent synovitis after the completion of a single course of 4 weeks of antibiotics is not rare and not the result of antibiotic failure. In fact, up to two thirds of patients with Lyme arthritis require 3 months to achieve resolution, and 15% have symptoms of their arthritis for more than 12 months.

Gerber MA, Zemel LS, Shapiro ED: Lyme arthritis in children: clinical epidemiology and long-term outcome, *Pediatrics* 102:905–908, 1998.

Wang TJ, Sangha O, Phillips CB, et al: Outcomes of children treated for Lyme disease, *J Rheumatol* 25:2249–2253, 1998.

51. **What should be suspected if a patient with Lyme disease develops fever and chills after starting antibiotic treatment?**
    The **Jarisch-Herxheimer reaction.** This reaction consists of fever, chills, arthralgia, myalgia, and vasodilation, and it follows the initiation of antibiotic therapy in certain illnesses (most typically syphilis). It is thought to be mediated by endotoxin release as the organism is destroyed. A similar reaction occurs in 40% or less of patients treated for Lyme disease, and it may be mistaken for an allergic reaction to the antibiotic.

52. **Should we follow Lyme disease course and response to therapy with titers?**
    No! As a result of the continued secretion of antibodies by memory cells, serology (particularly with ultrasensitive commercial kits) may remain positive for up to 10 years after

microbial eradication. The misinterpretation of positive serology as a proxy for active infection is behind many unnecessary antibiotic courses in endemic areas.

Kalish RA, McHugh G, Granquist J, et al: Persistence of immunoglobulin M or immunoglobulin G antibody responses after active Lyme disease, *Clin Infect Dis* 33:780–785, 2001.

53. **Is antibiotic prophylaxis indicated for all tick bites?**
No. In most regions, the rate of tick infestation is low, and thus the likelihood of transmission is also low. Even in endemic areas, the risk for Lyme disease to a placebo group after tick bites was only 1.2%. The tick has to be attached for at least 24 to 48 hours before the transmission of infection occurs. Treating all tick bites with antibiotics is impractical (some children would be on oral antibiotics throughout the summer). One study did show that a single 200-mg dose was effective for preventing Lyme disease if it was given within 72 hours of the tick bite. Consequently, antibiotic prophylaxis is not routinely recommended, but, in unique circumstances (e.g., endemic areas, prolonged attachment, pregnancy), prophylaxis could be considered.

Nadelman RB, Nowakowski J, Fish D, et al, Tick Bite Study Group: Prophylaxis with single-dose doxycycline for the prevention of Lyme disease after an *Ixodes scapularis* tick bite, *N Engl J Med* 345:79–84, 2001.

Shapiro ED, Gerber MA, Holabird NB, et al: A controlled trial of antimicrobial prophylaxis for Lyme disease after deer-tick bites, *N Engl J Med* 327:1769–1773, 1992.

54. **What are other means of preventing Lyme disease?**
■ Avoidance of tick-infested areas
■ Use of light-colored, long-sleeved clothing, with pants tucked into sneakers
■ Insect repellents (N,N-diethylmetatoluamide [DEET]; permethrin)
■ "Tick checks" after potential exposures
■ Proper tick removal: Pulling straight out, with tweezers close to skin

Hayes EB, Piesman J: How can we prevent Lyme disease? *N Engl J Med* 348:2424–2430, 2003.

RHEUMATIC FEVER

55. **What is acute rheumatic fever?**
A postinfectious, immune-mediated, inflammatory reaction that affects the connective tissue of multiple organ systems (heart, joints, central nervous system, blood vessels, subcutaneous tissue) and that follows infection with certain strains of group A β-hemolytic streptococci (GABHS). The major manifestations are carditis, polyarthritis, chorea, erythema marginatum, and subcutaneous nodules. In the developing world, acute rheumatic fever and rheumatic heart diseases are the leading causes of cardiovascular death during the first five decades of life.

56. **What are the major Jones criteria for rheumatic fever?**
The mnemonic **J♥NES** may be useful:
■ **J**oints: Migratory arthritis
■ **♥**: Heart disease
■ **N**odules: Subcutaneous nodules
■ **E**rythema: Erythema marginatum
■ **S**ydenham: Sydenham chorea

57. **What is acceptable proof of antecedent streptococcal pharyngitis when diagnosing acute rheumatic fever?**
■ **Throat culture:** This is the gold standard for diagnosis of GABHS. Positive cultures, however, do not distinguish GABHS pharyngitis from a carrier state.
■ **Streptococcal antigen tests:** Rapid diagnostic tests for the detection of GABHS antigens in pharyngeal secretions are acceptable evidence of infection because they are highly specific. Again, positive tests do not distinguish true infection from a carrier state.

- **Antistreptococcal antibodies:** At the time of clinical presentation with rheumatic fever, throat cultures are usually negative. It is reasonable to assess the levels of antistreptococcal antibodies in all cases of suspected rheumatic fever because the antibodies should be elevated at the time of presentation.

Gerber MA, Baltimore RS, Eaton CB, et al: Prevention of rheumatic fever and diagnosis of acute streptococcal pharyngitis, *Circulation* 119:1541–1551, 2009.

58. **Which antistreptococcal antibodies are most commonly measured?**
The most commonly employed test measures antibodies to antistreptolysin O. The cutoff for a positive test in a school-aged child is 320 Todd units (240 in an adult); levels peak 3 to 6 weeks after infection. If the test is negative—as may be the case in 20% or less of patients with acute rheumatic fever (ARF) and in 40% of those with isolated chorea—other antistreptococcal antibodies may be detected. The most practically available of these identifies antibodies to deoxyribonuclease B (positive cutoff, 240 units in children, 120 in adults). Alternatively, subsequent convalescent samples run simultaneously with the acute sample may detect rising titers of either antistreptolysin O or antideoxyribonuclease B.

59. **What are the common manifestations of carditis in patients with ARF?**
In his *Etudes Médicales du Rhumatisme*, Lasègue remarked that "rheumatic fever licks the joints . . . and bites the heart," meaning that the severity of the two manifestations tends to be inversely related. In more recent outbreaks of ARF, 80% or less of patients have had evidence of carditis. ARF causes a pancarditis, which potentially affects all layers (from the pericardium through the endocardium) and may include the following:
- **Valvulitis:** This is heralded by a new or changing murmur. The most common manifestation is isolated mitral regurgitation, and this is followed in frequency by a mid-diastolic rumble of unclear pathophysiology (Carey-Coombs murmur), and then by aortic insufficiency in the presence of mitral regurgitation. Isolated aortic insufficiency is uncommon, and so are stenotic lesions.
- **Dysrhythmias:** Electrocardiogram abnormalities typically involve some degree of heart block.
- **Myocarditis:** When mild, this may manifest as resting tachycardia out of proportion to fever. However, when it is clinically more severe and in combination with valvular damage, myocarditis may lead to congestive heart failure.
- **Pericarditis:** Patients may have chest pain or friction rub. Pericarditis and myocarditis virtually never occur in isolation.

Messeloff CR: Historical aspects of rheumatism, *Med Life* 37:3–56, 1930.

60. **How quickly can valvular lesions occur in children with ARF?**
New murmurs appear within the first 2 weeks in 80% of patients, and they rarely occur after the second month of illness. Hence, during an episode, one normal echocardiogram in the first 2 weeks should be sufficient to eliminate carditis.

61. **What are the typical characteristics of arthritis in patients with ARF?**
Migratory polyarthritis is usually the earliest symptom of the disease, and it typically affects the large joints, the knees, the ankles, the elbows, and the wrists (hips are not commonly involved). The joints are extraordinarily painful; weight bearing may not be possible. Physical examination discloses warmth, erythema, and exquisite tenderness such that the weight of even bedclothes and sheets may not be tolerable. This tenderness is typically out of proportion with the degree of swelling.

62. **What is the effect of aspirin therapy on the arthritis of rheumatic fever?**
This type of arthritis is exquisitely sensitive to even modest doses of salicylates, which effectively arrest the process within 12 to 24 hours. If aspirin or other NSAIDs are employed

early during the course of the condition, the arthritis will not migrate, and a delay in diagnosis may result. Such medications should be withheld until the clinical course of the illness has become clear. Conversely, if there is not a dramatic response to aspirin, a diagnosis other than rheumatic fever should be considered.

63. **How long does the arthritis associated with ARF usually persist?**
In untreated cases of ARF, arthritis affects a number of joints sequentially for less than a week each; the entire process rarely lasts more than a month. Treatment with aspirin or NSAIDs will shorten the clinical course.

64. **What is the rash of rheumatic fever?**
Erythema marginatum. This rash occurs in less than 5% of cases of ARF. If you see it and call a colleague to the bedside to confirm it, it is likely to have disappeared in the meantime. It is an evanescent, pink to slightly red, nonpruritic eruption with pale centers and serpiginous borders; it may be induced by the application of heat, and it always blanches when palpated. The outer edges of the lesion are sharp, whereas the inner borders are diffuse (Fig. 18-6). It is most often found on the trunk and proximal extremities (but not the face). Erythema marginatum is seen almost solely in patients with carditis.

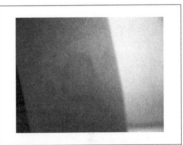

Figure 18-6. Classic rash of erythema marginatum on the arm of a child with acute rheumatic fever.

65. **What is Sydenham chorea?**
Purposeless, involuntary, irregular movements of the extremities that are associated with muscle weakness and labile emotional behavior. These symptoms are believed to result from inflammation of the cerebellum and of the basal ganglia.

66. **Who was Saint Vitus?**
Saint Vitus was a Sicilian youth who was martyred in the year 303. In the Middle Ages, individuals with chorea would worship at shrines dedicated to this saint. Accordingly, Sydenham chorea is also known as "Saint Vitus dance." Saint Vitus is the patron saint of dancers and comedians.

67. **Are corticosteroids of benefit for the treatment of ARF?**
Controlled studies in the 1950s failed to show any definite benefit of corticosteroids for the treatment of rheumatic carditis. Nonetheless, it is generally recommended that patients with severe carditis (e.g., congestive heart failure, cardiomegaly, third-degree heart block) receive prednisone (2 mg/kg per day) in addition to conventional therapy for their heart failure. The unusual patient with well-documented rheumatic arthritis that does not respond to salicylates or NSAIDs will benefit symptomatically from prednisone.

68. **Can antibiotic prophylaxis for rheumatic fever ever be discontinued?**
The optimal duration of antistreptococcal prophylaxis after documented ARF is the subject of some debate. It is clear that the risk for recurrence decreases after 5 years have elapsed from the most recent attack. Most clinicians therefore recommend discontinuing prophylaxis in patients who have not had carditis after 5 years or on the 21st birthday (whichever comes later). Those at high risk for contracting streptococcal pharyngitis (e.g., school teachers, health care professionals, military recruits, others living in crowded conditions) and anyone

with a history of carditis should receive antibiotic prophylaxis for longer periods. Recommendations vary, ranging from 10 years to the 40th birthday (whichever is longer) to lifelong prophylaxis, depending on the extent of residual heart disease.

69. **Where do PANDAS live in the world of pediatric rheumatology?**
In 1989, Swedo and colleagues characterized the psychiatric abnormalities found in children with Sydenham chorea, noting a high prevalence of obsessive-compulsive disorder (OCD) behaviors. They also described a syndrome, which they dubbed **PANDAS** (**p**ediatric **a**utoimmune **n**europsychiatric **d**isorders **a**ssociated with **s**treptococcal infection), in which OCD and Tourette syndrome in some children appeared to be triggered or exacerbated by streptococcal infections in the absence of classic chorea or other manifestations of rheumatic fever.

The existence of PANDAS remains controversial. There has been no prospective study of group A streptococcal infection to confirm the association of streptococcal pharyngitis with these behavioral abnormalities. The symptoms of tic disorders and OCD tend to fluctuate spontaneously and may be nonspecifically exacerbated by illness. In some cases, the only link to streptococcal infection has been a single throat culture or serologic test, thereby bringing the specificity of the condition into question. PANDAS currently remains a yet-unproven hypothesis.

Kurlan R, Johnson D, Kaplan EL: Streptococcal infection and exacerbations of childhood tics and obsessive-compulsive symptoms: a prospective blinded cohort study, *Pediatrics* 121:1188–1197, 2008.

Kurlan R, Kaplan EL: The pediatric autoimmune neuropsychiatric disorders associated with streptococcal infections (PANDAS) etiology for tics and obsessive-compulsive symptoms: hypothesis or entity? Practical considerations for the clinician, *Pediatrics* 113:883–886, 2004.

Swedo SE, Rapaport JL, Cheslow DL, et al: High prevalence of obsessive-compulsive symptoms in patients with Sydenham chorea, *Am J Psychiatry* 146:246–249, 1989.

SYSTEMIC LUPUS ERYTHEMATOSUS

70. **What is systemic lupus erythematosus (SLE)?**
A multisystem autoimmune disorder that is characterized by the production of autoantibodies and a wide variety of clinical and laboratory manifestations.

Lupus Foundation of America: http://www.lupus.org.

71. **What laboratory tests should be ordered in a child who is suspected of having SLE?**
A useful screening test for SLE is the FANA test. Up to 97% of patients with SLE have positive ANAs at some point during their illness (although not necessarily at the time of diagnosis). In a patient with characteristic signs and symptoms, a positive ANA may help confirm suspicions of SLE. Unfortunately, however, up to 10% of the normal childhood population may also have a positive ANA. Therefore, a positive ANA in the absence of any objective findings of SLE means very little. Other autoantibodies are much more specific, but they are less sensitive for SLE. These include antibodies to double-stranded DNA and the extractable nuclear antigen Sm. Complement levels are often depressed in patients with active SLE, and sedimentation rates are often elevated. The combination of a positive anti–double-stranded DNA antibody level and a low C_3 level is nearly 100% specific for SLE. Anemia, leukopenia, lymphopenia, and/or thrombocytopenia may also be seen.

Gill JM, Quisel AM, Rocca PV, Walters DT: Diagnosis of systemic lupus erythematosus, *Am Fam Physician* 68:2179–2186, 2003.

Gottlieb BS, Ilowite NT: Systemic lupus erythematosus in children and adolescents, *Pediatr Rev* 27:323–330, 2006.

KEY POINTS: SYSTEMIC LUPUS ERYTHEMATOSUS

1. The hallmark of systemic lupus erythematosus (SLE) is the presence of autoantibodies at intermediate to high titers.

2. About 15% to 20% of SLE patients have the onset of disease during childhood.

3. Clinical presentations vary, but the most common presenting symptoms are arthritis, rash, and renal disease.

4. Neonatal SLE is caused by maternal autoantibodies; this leads to complete congenital heart block.

5. The presence of antiphospholipid antibodies predisposes the patient to venous thrombosis.

72. **What are the most common manifestations of SLE in children?**
    - Arthritis: 80% to 90%
    - Rash or fever: 70%
    - Renal disease, such as proteinuria or casts (every patient with SLE is likely to have some abnormality demonstrated on renal biopsy): 70%
    - Serositis: 50%
    - Hypertension: 50%
    - Central nervous system disease (psychosis/seizures): 20% to 40%
    - Anemia, leukopenia, thrombocytopenia: 30% each

    Iqbal S, Sher MR, Good RA, Cawkwell GD: Diversity in presenting manifestations of systemic lupus erythematosus in children, *J Pediatr* 135:500–505, 1999.

73. **Describe the neurologic manifestations of SLE.**
    Lupus cerebritis is a term that implies an inflammatory etiology of central nervous system disease. Microscopically, however, widely scattered areas of microinfarction and noninflammatory vasculopathy are seen in brain tissue; actual central nervous system vasculitis is rarely observed. A lumbar puncture may reveal cerebrospinal fluid pleocytosis or an increased protein concentration, but it can be normal as well. Neuropsychiatric manifestations (psychoses, behavioral changes, depression, emotional lability) or seizures are most commonly observed. An organic brain syndrome with progressive disorientation and intellectual deterioration can be seen. Cranial or peripheral motor or sensory neuropathies, chorea, transverse myelitis, and cerebellar ataxia are less common manifestations of central nervous system lupus. Severe headaches and cerebral ischemic events have also been seen.

    Steinlein MI, Blaser SI, Gilday DI, et al: Neurological manifestations of pediatric systemic lupus erythematosus, *Pediatr Neurol* 13:191–197, 1995.

74. **Which diseases should be considered in the differential diagnosis of children with a butterfly rash?**
    A malar rash is present in 50% of children with SLE. The typical butterfly rash involves the malar areas and crosses the nasal bridge, but it spares the nasolabial folds; occasionally, it is difficult to distinguish from the rash of dermatomyositis. (Accompanying erythematous papules on the extensor surfaces of the metacarpophalangeal and proximal interphalangeal joints are common in dermatomyositis, but these are not generally seen in patients with SLE.) Seborrheic dermatitis or a contact dermatitis may be similar to the rash of SLE. Vesiculation should suggest another disease, such as pemphigus erythematosus. A malar flush is clinically distinct and may be seen in children with mitral stenosis or hypothyroidism.

75. **Should children with SLE undergo a renal biopsy?**

This is an area of controversy because nearly all children with SLE will have some evidence of renal involvement. Usually, clinical disease (e.g., abnormal urine sediment, proteinuria, renal function changes) correlates with the severity of renal disease on biopsy, but this is not always the case. Extensive glomerular abnormalities can be found on biopsy with minimal concurrent clinical manifestations. For this reason, many authorities are aggressive with early biopsy. Three circumstances in particular warrant biopsy:

- A child with SLE and nephrotic syndrome—to distinguish membranous glomerulonephritis from diffuse proliferative glomerulonephritis (which would warrant more aggressive therapy)
- Failure of high-dose corticosteroids to reverse deteriorating renal function—to determine the likelihood of benefit from cytotoxic therapy
- A prerequisite to entry into clinical therapeutic trials

Petty RE, Laxer RM: Systemic lupus erythematosus. In Cassidy JT, Petty RE (eds): *Textook of Pediatric Rheumatology*, ed 5, Philadelphia, WB Saunders, 2005, pp 342-391.

76. **How can the result of renal biopsy affect treatment of SLE?**

Biopsy can reveal a spectrum of renal pathology, ranging from a normal kidney (rare) to mesangial nephritis or glomerulonephritis (focal or diffuse, proliferative or membranous). Histologic transformation from one group to another over time is not unusual. Treatment of lupus nephritis is based on the severity of the lesion. Mesangial disease may require little or no intervention. Patients with membranous nephropathy commonly have nephrotic syndrome and usually respond to prednisone. Focal proliferative glomerulonephritis is often controlled with corticosteroids alone, but diffuse proliferative glomerulonephritis often requires corticosteroids, intravenous pulse cyclophosphamide, and possibly other immunosuppressives.

77. **When should high-dose corticosteroid therapy be considered for SLE management?**

High-dose corticosteroids usually consist of either intravenous pulse methylprednisolone (30 mg/kg per dose with a maximal dose of 1 g given daily or on alternate days given as an intravenous bolus for up to three doses) or oral prednisone (1 to 2 mg/kg per day). Often, intravenous pulses are then followed by high-dose oral steroids. The main indications for high-dose steroids in cases of SLE are as follows:

- Lupus crisis (widespread acute multisystem vasculitic involvement)
- Worsening central nervous system disease (as long as steroid psychosis in not thought to be the etiology)
- Severe lupus nephritis
- Acute hemolytic anemia
- Acute pleuropulmonary disease

78. **What is the association of antiphospholipid antibodies and lupus?**

Antiphospholipid antibodies can cause recurrent arterial and/or venous thromboses (e.g., stroke, phlebitis, renal vein thrombosis, placental thrombosis leading to fetal demise). Antiphospholipid antibodies are usually detected as anticardiolipin antibodies or lupus anticoagulant. These antibodies are often seen in patients with SLE, but their prevalence among patients with pediatric lupus varies widely (30% to 87% for anticardiolipin antibodies and 6% to 65% for lupus anticoagulant), depending on the study cited. The pathogenesis of thrombosis in patients with antiphospholipid antibodies remains unclear.

Von Scheven E, Athreya BH, Rosé CD, et al: Clinical characteristics of antiphospholipid antibody syndrome in children, *J Pediatr* 129:339–345, 1996.

79. **Which laboratory tests are useful for monitoring the effectiveness of therapy in patients with SLE?**

Serologic studies can provide useful information about the activity of SLE. The ANA titer does not correlate with disease activity. However, anti–double-stranded DNA titers (if present) often drop, and complement levels may increase and return to normal with effective therapy. Sedimentation rates usually decrease, and complete blood cell counts may return to normal (or at least improve) with effective therapy and decreased disease activity.

80. **What are the most common manifestations of neonatal lupus erythematosus (NLE)?**

The syndrome of neonatal lupus erythematosus (NLE) was first described in babies born to mothers with SLE or Sjögren syndrome; however, it has now been found that 70% to 80% of mothers with these conditions are asymptomatic. NLE is most likely caused by the transmission of maternal IgG autoantibodies. The main manifestations are as follows:

■ **Cutaneous:** Skin lesions are found in about 50% of babies with NLE. Although the rash may be present at birth, it usually develops within the first 2 to 3 months of life. The lesions include macules, papules, and annular plaques, and they may be precipitated by exposure to sunlight. The lesions are usually transient and nonscarring.

■ **Cardiac:** Complete congenital heart block (CCHB) is the classic cardiac lesion of NLE; 90% of all CCHB is due to neonatal lupus. Most cases of CCHB appear after the neonatal period, and 40% to 100% of these patients eventually require a pacemaker, usually before they are 18 years old. The average mortality rate associated with CCHB during the neonatal period is 15%.

■ **Hepatic:** Hepatic involvement is seen in at least 15% of babies with NLE. Hepatomegaly with or without splenomegaly is usually seen. Hepatic transaminases are either mild or moderately elevated, or they may be normal. Clinically and histologically, the appearance is often one of idiopathic neonatal giant cell hepatitis.

■ **Hematologic:** Thrombocytopenia, hemolytic anemia, and/or neutropenia may be seen.

Silverman ED, Laxer RM: Neonatal lupus erythematosus, *Rheum Dis Clin North Am* 23:599–618, 1997.

81. **What is the pathophysiology of the CCHB of NLE?**

CCHB is caused by maternal autoantibodies that cross the placenta and deposit themselves in the conducting system—usually the atrioventricular node—of the fetal heart. This leads to a localized inflammatory lesion, which may then be followed by scarring with fibrosis and calcification. The autoantibodies found are usually anti-Ro antibodies, but anti-La antibodies can also be the etiologic agents.

Silverman ED, Laxer RM: Neonatal lupus erythematosus, *Rheum Dis Clin North Am* 23:599–618, 1997.

82. **What are the common features of drug-induced lupus?**

Fever, arthralgias and arthritis, and serositis can be seen in patients with drug-induced lupus. ANA and antihistone antibodies are often positive, but antibodies to double-stranded DNA are usually negative, and complements remain normal. Renal involvement, central nervous system disease, malar rash, alopecia, and oral ulcers are not usually seen in patients with drug-induced lupus, and their presence should raise suspicion for SLE.

83. **What are the most common causes of drug-induced lupus in children?**

Antiepileptic medications (especially ethosuximide, phenytoin, and primidone) are the most common causes, and at least 20% children taking antiepileptic drugs will develop a positive ANA. Minocycline, hydralazine, isoniazid, α-methyldopa, and chlorpromazine are also associated with drug-induced lupus, as are a variety of antithyroid medications and β-blockers. Actually, all the tetracyclines have been associated with a peculiar lupus-like syndrome that includes the following:

■ Acute symmetrical polyarthritis
■ Positive ANA
■ Mild liver dysfunction

This rather common syndrome is associated with the chronic use of tetracyclines in association with the treatment of acne. It usually resolves within 2 weeks of discontinuation of the medication, but it may last longer.

VASCULITIS

84. **What clinical features suggest a vasculitic syndrome?**
A multisystem disease with **fever, weight loss,** and **rash** is often the presenting picture in a vasculitic disorder. Many different types of rashes may be seen, the more common of which are palpable purpura, urticarial vasculitis, and dermal necrosis. Central nervous system involvement, arthritis, myositis, and/or serositis may be seen.

Blanco R, Martinez-Taboada VM, Rodriguez-Valverde V, Garcia-Fuentes M: Cutaneous vasculitis in children and adults: associated diseases and etiologic factors in 303 patients, *Medicine* 77:403–418, 1998.

85. **How are the primary systemic vasculitides classified?**
One scheme proposed by an international consensus classifies vasculitides on the basis of the size of the vessels that are predominantly affected. In the list below, conditions *in italics* are common pediatric diseases. Conditions marked with an asterisk (*) are not uncommon in pediatric rheumatology centers.
Large vessel vasculitis
■ Takayasu arteritis*
Medium-sized vessel vasculitis
■ *Kawasaki disease*
■ Polyarteritis nodosa and its limb-limited variant*
Small vessel vasculitis
■ Microscopic polyangiitis*
■ Wegener granulomatosis*
■ Churg-Strauss syndrome*
■ Immune complex mediated: *Henoch-Schönlein purpura, lupus vasculitis, serum-sickness vasculitis, drug-induced immune-complex vasculitis, infection-induced immune-complex vasculitis,* Sjögren syndrome vasculitis,* hypocomplementemic urticarial vasculitis,* Behçet disease*
■ Paraneoplastic small vessel vasculitis (mostly with acute myelocytic leukemia, acute lymphoblastic leukemia, or asparaginase treatment)*
■ Inflammatory bowel disease vasculitis, particularly ulcerative colitis–associated stroke and Polyarteritis nodosa-like syndrome associated with Crohn disease*

Jennette JC, Falk RJ, Andrassy K, et al: Nomenclature of systemic vasculitides: proposal of an international consensus conference, *Arthritis Rheum* 37:187–192, 1994.

86. **Which infectious agents are associated with vasculitis?**
■ **Viral:** Human immunodeficiency virus, hepatitis B and C viruses, cytomegalovirus, Epstein-Barr virus, varicella virus, rubella virus, and parvovirus B19
■ **Rickettsial:** Rocky Mountain spotted fever, typhus, rickettsialpox
■ **Bacterial:** Meningococcus, disseminated sepsis as a result of any organism, subacute bacterial endocarditis
■ **Spirochete:** Syphilis
■ **Mycobacterial:** Tuberculosis

87. **What are the conditions that are grouped under the term *pulmonary-renal syndromes?***
■ Wegener granulomatosis
■ Goodpasture syndrome
■ Churg-Strauss syndrome
■ SLE

88. **What is the clinical triad of Behçet disease?**
Aphthous stomatitis, genital ulcerations, and **uveitis.** Behçet disease is a vasculitis of unclear etiology. In two thirds of cases in children, polyarthritis and inflammatory gastrointestinal lesions occur, which can confuse the diagnosis with inflammatory bowel disease, particularly if the patient is younger than 5 years. Aseptic meningitis, sinus vein thrombosis, and other forms of deep vein thrombosis are characteristic of this disease.

89. **Should it be "Henoch-Schönlein purpura" or "Schönlein-Henoch purpura"?**
In 1837, Johann Schönlein described the association of purpura and arthralgia. Edward Henoch later added the additional clinical features of gastrointestinal symptoms in 1874 and renal involvement in 1899. Thus, purists would say that, more properly, the term should be "Schönlein-Henoch purpura." However, in 1801, William Heberdeen described a 5-year-old boy with joint and abdominal pains, petechiae, hematochezia, and gross hematuria in his *Commentaries on the History and Cure of Disease*, so the true purists might say that, most properly, the condition should be "Heberdeen syndrome."

90. **What are the characteristic laboratory findings of patients with Henoch-Schönlein purpura (HSP)?**
Acute-phase reactants, including the ESR and C-reactive protein, are commonly elevated, and there is frequently a mild leukocytosis. Thrombocytopenia is never seen. Microscopic hematuria and proteinuria are indicators of renal involvement. HSP purpura appears to be an IgA-mediated illness; elevated serum IgA has been noted and has been demonstrated by immunofluorescence in skin and renal biopsies. (The renal histology is indistinguishable from Berger disease.) Circulating immune complexes and cryoglobulins containing IgA are also commonly seen.

91. **What kinds of skin lesions are noted in patients with HSP?**
HSP is one of the hypersensitivity vasculitides and, as such, is characterized by leukocytoclastic inflammation of arterioles, capillaries, and venules. Initially, urticarial lesions predominate, and they may itch or burn; these develop into pink maculopapules (Fig. 18-7). With damage to the vessel walls, there is bleeding into the skin, which results in nonthrombocytopenic petechiae and palpable purpura. A migrating soft tissue edema is also commonly seen in younger children.

92. **In addition to the skin, what other organ systems are typically involved in HSP?**
Classically, HSP involves the musculoskeletal system, the gastrointestinal tract, and/or the kidneys.
■ The most common abdominal finding is gastrointestinal colic (70%). This is frequently associated with nausea, vomiting, and gastrointestinal bleeding. These findings may precede the skin rash in 30% of cases or less. Intussusception occurs in 5% cases or less.

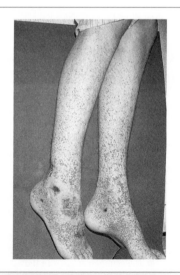

Figure 18-7. Numerous purpuric macules and papules on the legs and feet of a child with Henoch-Schönlein purpura. (From Gawkrodger DJ: Dermatology: An Illustrated Colour Text, 3rd ed. Edinburgh, Churchill Livingstone, 2002, p 78.)

- Renal involvement occurs in about 50% of reported cases, and it is usually apparent early during the course of the illness. It ranges in severity from microscopic hematuria to nephrotic syndrome.
- Joint involvement is very common (80%) and can be quite painful. Periarticular swelling of the knees, ankles, wrists, and elbows—rather than a true arthritis—is usually seen.
- Up to 15% of males can have scrotal involvement with epididymitis, orchitis, testicular torsion, and scrotal bleeding.
- Pulmonary hemorrhage is a rare complication of HSP that is mainly seen among adolescents and adults. It is associated with significant mortality.

Tizard EJ, Hamilton-Ayres MJJ: Henoch-Schönlein purpura, *Arch Dis Child Educ Pract Ed* 93:1–8, 2008.

93. **How often does chronic renal disease develop in children with HSP?**
The long-term prognosis of patients with HSP depends mainly on the initial renal involvement. Overall, less than 5% of patients with HSP develop end-stage renal disease. However, up to two thirds of children who have severe crescentic glomerulonephritis documented on biopsy will develop terminal renal failure within 1 year. Of those with nephritis or nephrotic syndrome at the onset of illness, almost half may have long-term problems with hypertension or impaired renal function as adults. Microscopic hematuria as the sole manifestation of HSP is common and is associated with a good long-term outcome.

Coppo R, Andrulli S, Amore A, et al: Predictors of outcome in Henoch-Schönlein purpura in children and adults, *Am J Kidney Dis* 47:993–1003, 2006.

Kawasaki Y, Suzuki J, Sakai N, et al: Clinical and pathological features of children with Henoch-Schönlein purpura nephritis: risk factors associated with poor prognosis, *Clin Nephrol* 60:153–160, 2003.

KEY POINTS: IN HENOCH-SCHÖNLEIN PURPURA

1. A small vessel vasculitis.

2. The classic clinical triad is as follows: purpura, arthritis, and abdominal pain.

3. Half of patients have abnormal urinalyses (hematuria, proteinuria; usually mild).

4. Steroid therapy is debated, but it should be considered for painful arthritis, abdominal pain, nephritis, edema, and scrotal swelling.

5. A few patients have long-term renal complications.

94. **Why is the diagnosis of intussusception often difficult in patients with HSP?**
- Intussusception can occur suddenly, without preceding abdominal symptoms.
- Nearly half of cases of HSP intussusception are ileoileal (compared with non-HSP intussusceptions, of which 75% are ileocolic). This increases the likelihood of a false-negative barium enema.
- The variety of possible gastrointestinal complications in patients with HSP (e.g., pancreatitis, cholecystitis, gastritis) can confuse the clinical picture.
- The common occurrence (50% to 75%) of melena, guaiac-positive stools, and abdominal pain in HSP without intussusception may lead to a lowered index of suspicion.

95. **When are corticosteroids indicated for the treatment of HSP?**
The precise indication for corticosteroids in patients with HSP remains controversial. Prednisone, 1 to 2 mg/kg per day (maximum: 80 mg/kg per day) for 5 to 7 days, is often used for severe intestinal symptoms and may decrease the likelihood of intussusception.

Corticosteroids may be helpful in the settings of significant pulmonary, scrotal, or central nervous system manifestations to minimize vasculitic inflammation; they are sometimes used if severe joint pain is present and NSAIDs are contraindicated. Steroids do not prevent the recurrence of symptoms, and symptoms may flare when steroids are discontinued. There is a great deal of controversy surrounding whether the early use of corticosteroids (oral or intravenous pulses) in patients with renal disease improves long-term outcome, but no benefit has yet been demonstrated in randomized controlled trials.

Chartapisak W, Opastiraku S, Willis NS, et al: Prevention and treatment of renal disease in Henoch-Schönlein purpura: a systematic review, *Arch Dis Child* 94:132–137, 2009.

Weiss PF, Feinstein JA, Luan X, et al: Effects of corticosteroid on Henoch-Schönlein purpura: a systematic review, *Pediatrics* 120:1079–1087, 2007.

96. **What is acute hemorrhagic edema of infancy (AHEI)?**
A simplistic answer is that AHEI is an infantile version of HSP, appearing during the first year of life. Erythematous, palpable, large purpuric lesions develop and when confluent are quite dramatic in appearance. Skin lesions are seen in the upper and lower extremities, and on the face, particularly in the ears, IgA deposition is common around the vasculitic lesions. Renal and gastrointestinal involvements are rare, and recovery is the rule in 2 to 3 weeks. It is also known as Finkelstein syndrome.

McDougall CM, Ismail SK, Ormerod A: Acute haemorrhagic oedema of infancy, *Arch Dis Child* 90:316, 2005.

97. **In which rheumatic diseases can "cauliflower ears" be seen?**
In babies with AHEI and in older children with relapsing polychondritis—a potentially serious disease primarily affecting cartilage of the ears, airways, sclera, and aortic valve ring.

INDEX

Note: Page numbers followed by *b* indicate boxes, *f* indicate figures and *t* indicate tables.